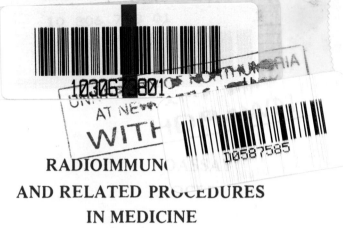

RADIOIMMUNOASSAY AND RELATED PROCEDURES IN MEDICINE 1977

VOL.II

PROCEEDINGS SERIES

RADIOIMMUNOASSAY AND RELATED PROCEDURES IN MEDICINE 1977

PROCEEDINGS OF AN INTERNATIONAL SYMPOSIUM ON
RADIOIMMUNOASSAY AND RELATED PROCEDURES IN MEDICINE
HELD BY THE
INTERNATIONAL ATOMIC ENERGY AGENCY
IN CO-OPERATION WITH THE
WORLD HEALTH ORGANIZATION
IN BERLIN (WEST), 31 OCTOBER – 4 NOVEMBER 1977

In two volumes

VOL.II

INTERNATIONAL ATOMIC ENERGY AGENCY
VIENNA, 1978

RADIOIMMUNOASSAY AND RELATED PROCEDURES IN MEDICINE 1977
IAEA, VIENNA, 1978
STI/PUB/469
ISBN 92–0–010178–X
Printed by the IAEA in Austria
June 1977

FOREWORD

The International Symposium on Radioimmunoassay and Related Procedures in Medicine held by the International Atomic Energy Agency in co-operation with the World Health Organization in Berlin (West) from 31 October to 4 November 1977 was the third in its subject field to have been organized by the Agency, its predecessors having been the Symposium on In Vitro Procedures with Radioisotopes in Clinical Medicine and Research held in co-operation with the World Health Organization in Vienna in 1969 and the Symposium on Radioimmunoassay and Related Procedures in Clinical Medicine and Research held in Istanbul in 1973. The proceedings of both these earlier meetings were published by the Agency.

Radioimmunoassay and related procedures for the measurement of hormones, vitamins, drugs and other classes of substances in the body fluids and tissues, above all in the blood, are now in the forefront of medical applications of radioactive materials. During the four years from 1973 to 1977, growth in the commercial availability of reagents and kits for established assays has brought many of these into routine use. This in turn has led to an increasing awareness of the need for assay standardization and quality control and to an increasing attention to techniques of assay data analysis. The rapidly expanding demands on assay services has stimulated interest in the possibilities for automation of assay procedures. Promising new assay methods have been further refined, notably solid-phase radioassay and radioreceptor assay. At the same time there has been a resurgence of interest in alternative assay methods not based on the use of radioactive materials, making a critical reappraisal of the entire subject field desirable. The importance of radioimmunoassay itself was underlined by the award in 1977 of a Nobel Prize in medicine to Rosalyn Yalow of the United States of America for her pioneer work on the method over the last two decades, particularly in relation to the measurement of protein hormones.

The latest symposium, which was attended by 314 participants from 33 countries and at which 68 papers, including seven invited review papers, were presented, provided opportunities for an exchange of information on all these topics. The introductory lecture by W.D. Odell of the United States of America, entitled "We don't look at hormones the way we used to", drew attention to the very great conceptual changes that have arisen in relation to hormones in recent years, largely as a result of the applications of radioimmunoassay and related procedures in endocrinology. The subject of assay standardization and quality control was considered at length in two round-table discussion sessions, one on assay design, standardization and within-laboratory quality control and one on external quality control, arranged in co-operation with the World Health Organization Special Programme of Research in Human Reproduction.

The proceedings, comprising two volumes, contain the full texts of all the papers presented at the symposium, together with an edited record of the discussions. Volume I covers those parts of the meeting dealing with methodology; an annex to this volume gives data on commercially available well scintillation counting systems and liquid scintillation counting systems. Volume II covers those parts dealing with applications and includes an edited record of the two round-table discussion sessions mentioned.

EDITORIAL NOTE

The papers and discussions have been edited by the editorial staff of the International Atomic Energy Agency to the extent considered necessary for the reader's assistance. The views expressed and the general style adopted remain, however, the responsibility of the named authors or participants. In addition, the views are not necessarily those of the governments of the nominating Member States or of the nominating organizations.

Where papers have been incorporated into these Proceedings without resetting by the Agency, this has been done with the knowledge of the authors and their government authorities, and their cooperation is gratefully acknowledged. The Proceedings have been printed by composition typing and photo-offset lithography. Within the limitations imposed by this method, every effort has been made to maintain a high editorial standard, in particular to achieve, wherever practicable, consistency of units and symbols and conformity to the standards recommended by competent international bodies.

The use in these Proceedings of particular designations of countries or territories does not imply any judgement by the publisher, the IAEA, as to the legal status of such countries or territories, of their authorities and institutions or of the delimitation of their boundaries.

The mention of specific companies or of their products or brand names does not imply any endorsement or recommendation on the part of the IAEA.

Authors are themselves responsible for obtaining the necessary permission to reproduce copyright material from other sources.

CONTENTS OF VOLUME II

II. STANDARDIZATION AND QUALITY CONTROL (Session V and Session VI, Part 1)

Round-table discussion on assay design, standardization and within-laboratory quality control, including the following papers: 3

Basic concepts in quality control
R.P. Ekins
Quality control for RIA: recommendations for a minimal program
D. Rodbard
Quality control and assay design
R.P. Ekins
The use of quality control within a laboratory
S.L. Jeffcoate

External quality-control surveys of peptide hormone radioimmunoassays in the Federal Republic of Germany: the present status (IAEA-SM-220/17) 81
H. Breuer, D. Jungbluth, I. Marschner, G. Röhle, P.C. Scriba, W.G. Wood
Discussion 90
Mise en place et premiers résultats d'un programme de contrôle de qualité national français en radioimmunologie (IAEA-SM-220/81) 91
Ch.-A. Bizollon, R. Cohen, D. Froget
Discussion 102
An elementary components of variance analysis for multi-centre quality control (IAEA-SM-220/59) 105
P.J. Munson, D. Rodbard
Discussion 124
The need for standardization of methodology and components in commercial radioimmunoassay kits (IAEA-SM-220/19) 127
W.G. Wood, I. Marschner, P.C. Scriba
Discussion 137
Performance of radioimmunoassays for digoxin as evaluated by a group experiment (IAEA-SM-220/7) 141
A. Dwenger, R. Friedel, I. Trautschold
Discussion 148

Quality control in RIA: a preliminary report on the results of the World Health Organization's programme for external quality control (IAEA-SM-220/115) 149
M.A. Cresswell, P.E. Hall, B.A.L. Hurn
Discussion 158
Round-table discussion on external quality control 159

III. APPLICATIONS

III.1. Assays for vitamins (Session VI, Part 2)

A novel radioassay for the determination of folate in serum and red cells and new observations on the stability of serum folate (IAEA-SM-220/32) 171
E.P.J. Lynch, K.C. Tovey, H. Guilford
Discussion 176
Studies on folate binding and a radioassay for serum and whole-blood folate using goat milk as binding agent (IAEA-SM-220/45) 177
R.D. Piyasena, D.A. Weerasekera, N. Hettiaratchi, T.W. Wikramanayake
Discussion 192
Estimation of folate binding capacity (unsaturated and total) in normal human serum and in β-thalassaemia (IAEA-SM-220/52) 193
S. Moulopoulos, J. Mantzos, E. Gyftaki, M. Kesse-Elias, V. Alevizou-Terzaki, E. Souli-Tsimili
Discussion 197
Assay of 25-OH vitamin D_3 (IAEA-SM-220/56) 199
Ph. De Nayer, M. Thalasso, C. Beckers
Discussion 208

III.2. Assays for steroids and other small molecules (Session VII)

Invited review paper

Recent advances in steroid radioimmunoassay (IAEA-SM-220/205) 213
S.L. Jeffcoate
Discussion 222
Radioimmunoassay of steroids in homogenates and subcellular fractions of testicular tissue (IAEA-SM-220/39) 225
S. Campo, G. Nicolau, E. Pellizari, M.A. Rivarola
Discussion 235

Sencillo método de dosificación de proteína transportadora de hormonas sexuales (PTHS) – sus valores en hombres, en mujeres y en el embarazo (IAEA-SM-220/100) 237
C.A. Tafurt, R. de Estrada
Discussion 243

A model for evaluating steroids acting at the hypothalamus-pituitary axis using radioimmunoassay and related procedures (IAEA-SM-220/41) 245
J. Spona, Ch. Bieglmayer, R. Schroeder, E. Pöckl
Discussion 256

Determination of estradiol, estrone and progesterone in serum and human endometrium in correlation with the content of steroid receptors and 17β-hydroxysteroid dehydrogenase activity during the menstrual cycle (IAEA-SM-220/85) 257
M. Schmidt-Gollwitzer, J. Eiletz, J. Pachaly, K. Pollow
Discussion 271

Specific bile acid radioimmunoassays for separate determinations of unconjugated cholic acid, conjugated cholic acid and conjugated deoxycholic acid in serum and their clinical application (IAEA-SM-220/4) 273
S. Matern, W. Gerok
Discussion 283

Radioimmunoassay of primary and secondary bile acids in serum with specific antisera and ^{125}I-labelled ligands (IAEA-SM-220/87) 285
O.A. Jänne, O.K. Mäentausta
Discussion 293

The radioimmunoassay of clomipramine (Anafranil-Geigy): a tricyclic antidepressant (IAEA-SM-220/37) 295
G.F. Read, D. Riad-Fahmy
Discussion 298

The specific radioimmunoassay in pharmacokinetics: its potency, requirements and development for routine use as illustrated by an assay for Pirenzepin (IAEA-SM-220/63) 299
G. Bozler
Discussion 308

The radioimmunoassay of biologically active compounds in parotid fluid and plasma (IAEA-SM-220/35) 309
R.F. Walker, G.F. Read, D. Riad-Fahmy
Discussion 315

III.3. Assays for thyroid-related hormones (Session VIII, Part 1)

Invited review paper

Pathophysiological aspects of recent advances in current thyroid function testing (IAEA-SM-220/206) 319
R.-D. Hesch
Discussion 339

Thyroxine and thyrotrophin radioimmunoassays using dried blood samples on filter paper for screening of neonatal hypothyroidism (IAEA-SM-220/55) 341
C. Beckers, C. Cornette, B. François, A. Bouckaert, M. Lechat

Le dosage radioimmunologique de la thyréostimuline hypophysaire à partir d'un échantillon de sang capillaire recueilli sur papier filtre: intérêt dans le dépistage de l'hypothyroïdie néonatale (IAEA-SM-220/71) 349
J. Ingrand, M.A. Dugue, A.M. Mamarbachi, P. Bourdoux, F. Delange
Discussion 360

Control of treatment of differentiated thyroid carcinoma by measurement of thyroglobulin in serum (IAEA-SM-220/23) 363
J. Hagemann, C. Schneider
Discussion 368

New concepts for the assay of unbound thyroxine (FT_4) and thyroxine binding globulin (TBG) (IAEA-SM-220/92) 369
G. Odstrchel, W. Hertl, F.B. Ward, K. Travis, R.E. Lindner, R.D. Mason
Discussion 376

Development of a two-site radioimmunoassay for antithyroglobulin antibodies using ^{125}I-thyroglobulin (IAEA-SM-220/54) 379
J.P. Léonard, F. Taymans, C. Beckers
Discussion 387

III.4. Assays for peptides (Session VIII, Part 2 and Session IX)

A radioimmunoassay of plasma corticotrophin (IAEA-SM-220/38) 391
L. Hummer
Discussion 402

Dosage radioimmunologique du fragment biologiquement actif de l'hormone parathyroïdienne humaine (IAEA-SM-220/74) 405
C. Desplan, A. Jullienne, D. Raulais, P. Rivaille, J.P. Barlet, M.S. Moukhtar, G. Milhaud
Discussion 416

Calcitonin radioimmunoassay: clinical application (IAEA-SM-220/103) ... 419
F. Raue, H. Minne, W. Streibl, R. Ziegler
Discussion ... 426
Etude de la spécificité du dosage radioimmunologique du procollagène de type I et de type III (IAEA-SM-220/25) ... 427
G. Heynen, M. Broux, B. Nusgens, C.M. Lapière, J.A. Kanis, S. Gaspar, P. Franchimont
Discussion ... 434

Invited review paper

Tumour-associated antigens (IAEA-SM-220/207) ... 435
K.D. Bagshawe
Discussion ... 466
A different approach to the radioimmunoassay of thyrotrophin-releasing hormone (IAEA-SM-220/90) ... 469
T.J. Visser, W. Klootwijk, R. Docter, G. Hennemann
Discussion ... 476
New immunogenic form for vasopressin: production of high-affinity antiserum and development of an RIA for plasma arginine-vasopressin (IAEA-SM-220/82) ... 479
G. Rougon-Rappuzi, B. Conte-Devolx, Y. Millet, M.A. Delaage
Discussion ... 486
Radioimmunoassay of arginine-vasopressin and clinical application (IAEA-SM-220/99) ... 489
H. Wagner, V. Maier, M. Häberle, H.E. Franz
Discussion ... 493
Dosage radioimmunologique des enképhalines (IAEA-SM-220/67) ... 495
P. Pradelles, C. Gros, C. Rougeot, O. Bepoldin, F. Dray, C. Llorens-Cortes, H. Pollard, J.C. Schwartz, M.C. Fournie-Zaluski, G. Cracel, B.P. Roques
Discussion ... 503
Dosage radioimmunologique du facteur thymique sérique (FTS) (IAEA-SM-220/68) ... 505
J.M. Pleau, D. Pasques, J.F. Bach, C. Gros, F. Dray
Discussion ... 510

Chairmen of Sessions ... 511
Secretariat of the Symposium ... 511
List of Participants ... 513
Author Index ... 537
Corrigenda to Vol.I ... 541

Session V and Session VI, Part 1

STANDARDIZATION AND QUALITY CONTROL

Chairmen

P.E. HALL
World Health Organization

R.P. EKINS
United Kingdom

ROUND-TABLE DISCUSSION ON ASSAY DESIGN, STANDARDIZATION AND WITHIN-LABORATORY QUALITY CONTROL

Chairman

P.E. Hall	(World Health Organization)

Panel Members

R.P. Ekins	(United Kingdom)
S.L. Jeffcoate	(United Kingdom)
D. Rodbard	(United States of America)

P.E. Hall *(Chairman)*: I should like to give a brief account of the background to this session, and the involvement of the World Health Organization's Special Programme of Research, Development and Research Training in Human Reproduction. The objectives of this Programme are to: (a) evaluate the safety and effectiveness of existing methods of fertility regulation; (b) improve existing methods; (c) develop new methods; (d) study psychosocial factors affecting family planning; and (e) investigate the delivery of family planning services.

Since many studies within the Programme involve the use of hormone assays and are being undertaken on a collaborative basis, we have been concerned about how we can obtain comparable assay results between centres participating in the Programme, as well as how centres can monitor their assay performance on a day-to-day basis.

Over the past two years we have developed a strategy which encompasses both the distribution of assay reagents to participating centres and also a quality-control programme for monitoring their assay performance. We have had the privilege of being able to work with many eminent scientists throughout the world and in particular we have had the pleasure of having the collaboration of Prof. Ekins, Dr. Jeffcoate and Dr. Rodbard in the area of assay quality control. In what follows, we shall present some concepts developed in their laboratories over the last few years and we shall indicate how these concepts can be utilized for quality-control purposes. We shall consider particularly what is quality control, why is it necessary, how is it done, and for what is it used.

Quality control has a dual purpose. In the short term it allows a critical analysis of assay results, indicating to the investigator the necessity of rejecting individual results within an assay or even the results of complete assays. In the longer term it is an integral part of the improvement of assay quality, since quality control allows the investigator to identify and eliminate factors which contribute to poor assay performance in his currently used method. There is thus a short loop in that one uses quality control for the day-to-day monitoring of assay performance and a longer loop in that one uses it over an extended period to optimize assay design and achieve improved assay performance (Fig.A).

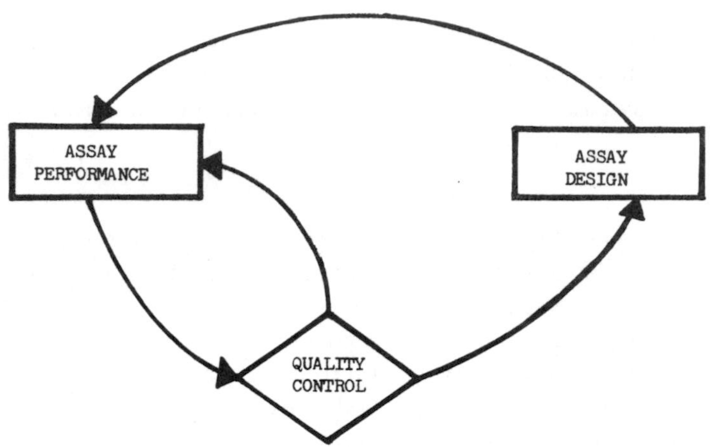

FIG.A. Purposes of quality control.

A further important aspect of quality control is that it must be purposeful and educational. All too often, quality-control measures are a very haphazard and casual part of laboratory practice. Some workers occasionally include a so-called quality-control specimen in their assays, but quality control should be an essential part of any assay system. Furthermore, there is a hierarchy in quality control. We are concerned firstly with what happens within an assay and secondly with what happens within a laboratory between assays. These aspects comprise internal quality control. We are concerned thirdly with what happens between laboratories using the same methodology and finally between laboratories using different methodologies. These aspects comprise external quality control (Fig.B).

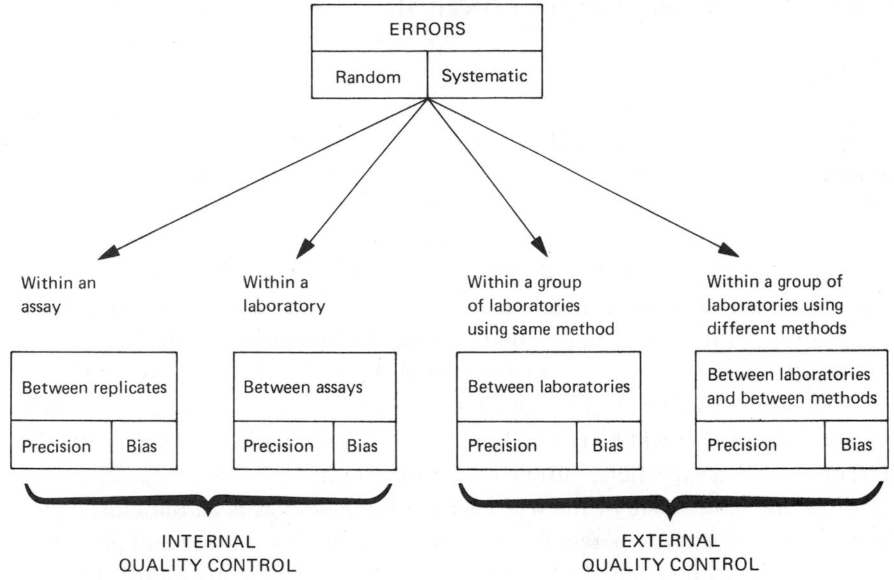

FIG.B. Nature of internal and external quality control.

At all levels of this hierarchy we utilize quality-control measures to allow us to assess errors, both random and systematic, which we may evaluate in terms of precision and bias.

Finally, let me reiterate that quality control is used both for the immediate analysis of assay results and for the eventual improvement of assay quality. I should now like to ask Prof. Ekins to set the scene and indicate what we are attempting to achieve in quality control. After Prof. Ekins' contribution I shall call on Dr. Rodbard to review actual methods available for assessing assay quality.

BASIC CONCEPTS IN QUALITY CONTROL

R.P. EKINS

The Middlesex Hospital Medical School,
London, United Kingdom

The concepts and techniques which we are presenting, in encapsulated form, today are those presented in a series of WHO Courses on Standardization and Quality Control of Radioimmunoassay of Hormones for Clinical Trials of Fertility-Regulating Agents in which Drs Hall, Jeffcoate, Rodbard and myself have recently participated. Each of these courses has been of a week's duration, and I am sure that it will be generally realized that we are limited today to presenting only a superficial outline of their content.

A particular feature of the WHO series of courses has been our endeavour not to restrict ourselves merely to a discussion of the standard techniques of quality control as practiced by clinical chemists for many years. These have traditionally centred on the inclusion of quality-control samples in each assay batch, and the assessment of the variation in results within and between batches, and between collaborating laboratories. Such procedures, which are clearly as relevant to radioimmunoassay techniques as to any other type of assay procedure, are obviously of fundamental importance in monitoring assay performance within the individual laboratory, in distinguishing 'outlier' samples and assay batches and in identifying differences in performance between laboratories. Of equal importance in our view, however, has been discussion of the reasons which lead to assays being occasionally of poor quality (i.e. yielding unacceptable variations within or between assay batches) or to the observation of widely divergent results between laboratories leading, in turn, to problems of standardization and interpretation.

In addition to examining the reasons for varying or divergent assay results, we have also attempted to delineate the particular factors which lead to improvements in assay reliability, and the measures which may be employed to reduce the differences in results between one laboratory and another. It is in relation to these aspects of the subject (i.e. those concerned with an understanding of the sources of assay variation, and of the measures relating to its elimination) that any consideration of quality control of radioimmunoassay techniques per se must inevitably differ from a more general discussion of quality control as applied to other assay methods.

The particular aspects of this subject with which I wish to deal in this opening presentation are primarily philosophical and conceptual in nature, and are intended to ensure that we all fully understand what we are talking about. A discussion of basic concepts and the clarification of terminology never seems to excite particular enthusiasm. Nevertheless, it has always been surprising to me, as something of an intruder into the field of assay methodology, that so many of its fundamental concepts, and the terminology upon which it relies, should be so imprecisely, or indeed illogically, defined. There is no doubt in my mind that the resulting confusion has had far-reaching practical effects and, in some cases, has entirely distorted the development of assay methodology. In particular, I have long argued that a misunderstanding of the concepts of 'sensitivity' and 'precision' has profoundly affected the way in which radioimmuno- and other 'saturation' assays are conventionally designed, and indeed has led to a long-standing neglect of technical factors which profoundly affect their performance.

VALID AND INVALID ASSAYS

Before discussing the exact concepts underlying such terms, however, I would like to examine briefly the meanings of the words 'measurement', 'assay' and 'amount' in the context of our present concern with the reproducibility and standardization of radioimmunoassay procedures.

Elsewhere in these Proceedings, I have attempted to distinguish between assays whose primary objective is the comparison of the effects produced in a selected biological environment of substances which may be chemically different, or heterogeneous, and assays in which the objective is the measurement of the 'amount' of a defined substance. Of these two forms of assay, the first are inevitably regarded as 'bioassays'; the second may be carried out using a 'biological' assay system, but are usually more conveniently performed using what may be generally termed 'chemical' reagents, albeit these may themselves (as, for example, in the case of antibodies) have been prepared by biological means. Aside from the difference in objective underlying these two forms of assay, they are primarily characterized by different criteria of 'validity' by which they should be assessed. Assays of the first kind are 'analytically valid' provided the effects produced in the biological system are essentially identical, i.e. the 'analytical validity' of an assay falling into this category depends upon the demonstration of 'functional' identity of the substances compared within the system. Such assays are clearly primarily concerned with evaluating the effect of, for example, different drugs or of their metabolites, the relative potencies of different hormone forms etc. Conversely, assays of the second type are 'analytically valid' only if the substance representing the subject of the measurement is molecularly homogeneous and identical in molecular structure to the 'standard' material employed to calibrate the assay system used.

This broad distinction has tended to become obscured by the fact that many conventional 'bioassay' systems, relying on the observation of the relative effects produced, typically, by the 'unknown' sample on one hand and the 'standard' or 'reference preparation' on the other, have nevertheless been fundamentally concerned with measurements of the amount of the substance in the 'unknown' sample. Implicit in the reasoning underlying such measurements has been the idea that the relative effects produced by 'unknown' and 'standard' reflected the 'amounts' of the substance in each implying in turn that the substance producing the effect was the same in both 'unknown' and 'standard' and comprised a molecular species of a single unique structure. Thus, if one sample elicited twice the response elicited by another, it has been conventional to deduce (assuming a linear response, and 'validity' of the assay) that the first sample contained twice the 'amount' of the substance contained by the second.

Recognition that many of the substances with which we are concerned in biological and medical science are molecularly heterogeneous totally invalidates these simple concepts, and must make us re-examine what we mean by the 'amount' of a substance if it is suspected not to comprise a single species of molecule, and what we mean by the 'assay' or 'measurement' of such a substance. Without dwelling on this question overlong, and in too great detail, suffice it to say that at the present time, the term 'amount' is sometimes implicitly applied to the effects produced by the substances under test, and sometimes to the mass or number of molecules of the substance on the assumption that it is molecularly homogeneous. In short, two different concepts shelter under the same term. As illustration of this distinction, one may contrast the concepts underlying the phrases 'amount (or concentration) of thyroxine' and 'amount (or concentration) of thyroid stimulating immunoglobulins (TSI)'; likewise, differing concepts essentially underlie statements relating to the 'amount of growth hormone' in a blood sample and the 'amount of growth hormone' in an ampoule intended for therapeutic administration.

In drawing attention to these questions, my particular intention is both to emphasize the lack of conceptual clarity underlying some of the terms we take for granted in the field of biological measurement and to try to identify some of the implications with respect to standardization and quality control of the differing concepts of measurement that I have discussed. In particular, there are two points which are of importance in this context.

(1) Radioimmunoassays are primarily intended to estimate the molecular concentration (or mass) of a substance characterized by a single molecular structure, and they are 'analytically invalid' if the assumptions relating to molecular homogeneity of the target substance (i.e. the 'analyte') are not fulfilled.
(2) The results obtained with any assay system (whether it is intended to compare biological effects (i.e. is 'functionally specific') or to estimate the molecular amount of a particular structurally unique substance (i.e. is 'structurally specific')) in which the substances present in 'unknown' or 'standard' are different, or heterogeneous in molecular structure, are particularly liable to variation as a

result of any change in the assay procedure. This, in turn, implies that such an assay system cannot be 'standardized' in the normal sense in which this term is used (i.e. by the use of a calibration or 'reference' preparation) – indeed it has been argued that there is virtually no justification for using 'standards' in such assay systems for this reason [1].

Having advanced these basic propositions, we should examine the particular characteristics of radioimmunoassay systems more closely. Such systems typically rely on antisera which comprise a heterogeneous population of antibodies displaying varying structural specificity; they also frequently depend on the use of 'standard' or 'reference' preparations which themselves comprise heterogeneous mixtures of substances of differing, albeit related, molecular structure. Finally, 'unknown' samples also typically contain a variety of molecules possessing sufficient structural resemblance to interact, to varying degrees, in the assay system. The upshot of this combination of circumstances is that many – perhaps, indeed, all – radioimmunoassays are, in some measure, 'analytically invalid'. Thus in no sense can the results of such assays be regarded as representing the number (or mass) of molecules of a single unique structure or the 'amount' (in this sense) of the substance of interest in the 'unknown' sample.

Although the measurements may be clinically useful, the penalties attaching to the use of 'analytically invalid' assay systems in terms of their standardization and day-to-day reproducibility may be severe. In particular, even if we confine our discussion in the first instance to the problem of replication of assay results within an individual laboratory, we are likely to find differences in results from batch to batch, since any environmental or procedural change between batches is likely to affect assay results. In short, as originally emphasized by Gaddum [2] and others, because an assay is 'analytically invalid' the assay results may only be reproduced by exact replication of the assay procedure – a general requirement which is almost incapable of fulfilment. In particular, of the factors most likely to change from assay batch to batch, the composition of the radioisotopically labelled antigen is most likely to vary. If this material is molecularly heterogeneous, the spectrum of molecules within it is likely to change with time (even with repeated purification) with consequent changes in assay results.

A further dimension, over and above within-laboratory assay variation, is added when consideration is extended to the variation of assay results resulting from the use in different laboratories of different assay reagents and/or protocols. As we have seen, 'invalidity' of assay systems – and the consequent variation in assay results between one assay and another – can arise from a variety of causes. One source of variation is the use by different laboratories of different 'standards' or 'reference preparations' and the extent of between-laboratory variation will almost certainly be reduced, though not necessarily eliminated, by the use of a common 'standard'. Likewise, adoption of common packages of primary reagents, including standards, antisera and labelled antigen removes further major sources of between-laboratory variation, but the results between laboratories may nevertheless still not coincide unless every detail of the assay protocol, and every general reagent (including buffers and adsorbents) are exactly replicated in every laboratory.

The magnitude of these effects clearly varies depending on the nature of the analyte: the measurement of a chemically defined substance, such as thyroxine, represents less of an analytical challenge than that of thyroid stimulating hormone (TSH) or luteinizing hormone (LH), 'standard' preparations of both of which are known to be heterogeneous. In short, the 'analytical invalidity' of the majority of radioimmunoassays is not an 'all-or-none' phenomenon, but varies in degree. The greater the extent of 'analytical invalidity', the greater the degree of variation between assay batches, and the more divergent the results that are likely to be encountered between different laboratories.

The particular conclusions that I would like to emphasize in summary of this discussion are:

(1) That as a fundamental prerequisite to a high degree of reproducibility of assay results, both between and within laboratories, all components of an assay system must be carefully selected to yield an assay system conforming as closely as possible to the criteria defining 'analytical validity'.

(2) That in the case of significant 'invalidity' of an assay system the only short-term strategy likely to yield convergence of results is exact replication of assay reagents and protocol both between assay batches, and between laboratories. 'Standardization' of such systems by distribution of common 'standards' at best leads to some convergence of assay results; at worst it may be misleading by suggesting that different laboratories are employing a 'common currency' in the expression of their assay results.

These conclusions have obvious implications vis-à-vis any hopes we may entertain to standardize radioimmunoassay procedures in the face of the widespread distribution of different assay kits, and lie at the root of the reagent distribution programmes now being undertaken both by the WHO and the United Kingdom.

ACCURACY, BIAS, PRECISION AND SENSITIVITY

I now want to turn to consideration of statistical terms (or concepts) of more immediate practical concern to this discussion. In particular, I want to discuss and clarify the meanings of the terms 'accuracy', 'bias', 'precision' and 'sensitivity'. A clear understanding of the meaning of these words is of fundamental importance, since they represent parameters which essentially define assay 'quality' (aside, perhaps, from the time required to perform an assay, which defines the 'turn-round time' of the system). Moreover, unless we clearly understand the concepts underlying these terms, and are able to perform the calculations required to express the concepts in the form of numerical indices, we are neither able to monitor assay performance nor to assess the practical usefulness of any experimental manœuvre we may perform in the laboratory to improve that performance. In practice, as we shall see, although it might be considered that such fundamental concepts are well understood, they have frequently **not** formed the basis of the technical development of radioimmunoassay procedures in the past.

First, let us consider the concept of 'accuracy'. This is a controversial term which signifies different things to different people, and for this reason it might be preferable if its use were abandoned in scientific literature. Nevertheless it represents a useful general concept which relates to the closeness of an assay result to the 'true' or 'correct' value. Both in the case of 'analytically invalid' assays, and in those situations in which we do not know what constitutes the 'true' result, we are forced to adopt the notion of the 'correct' value, which represents an agreed value for the result of the procedure. In common every-day parlance, we would regard a marksman as 'accurate' if the shots he fired were likely to strike their intended target.

Divergence of an assay result from the 'true' or 'correct' value arises as a result of error. Such error may be of a consistent or inconsistent (i.e. random) nature. Thus, in pipetting unknown serum samples into radioimmunoassay incubation tubes, we may use an incorrectly calibrated pipette, so that all 'unknown' sample volumes are, for example, 10% too low. This would clearly lead to results being constantly 10% in error (assuming that assay standards were pipetted with a correctly calibrated pipette). Conversely, we may use a correctly calibrated pipette for dispensing 'unknown' samples, but either as a result of technical inexpertise or because of some malfunction of the instrument used, repeated pipettings may vary to an extent of, for example, ± 5%. In this situation, although the mean of a large number of repeat determinations might centre on the true or correct value, individual measurements might fall too high or too low by an amount of the order of 5%.

These examples illustrate the two fundamental ways in which errors of measurement can be categorized; however, both forms of error can clearly lead to divergence of an individual measurement from the 'true' or 'correct' value. Likewise (returning to our previous analogy), the shots that the marksman fires may miss the target either because of misalignment of the sighting mechanism on his rifle, or because of his inability to hold the rifle steadily. In the latter case, although the general direction of his shots might centre on the target, the individual shots might be so widely scattered that the probability of an individual shot striking the target would be exceedingly small.

The terms conventionally employed to represent these two forms of error are 'bias' and 'imprecision'. The term 'bias' represents the consistent or systematic component of error leading to divergence of measurements from the 'true' or 'correct' value and may be estimated by carrying out a large number of repeat determinations on an individual 'unknown' sample, and assessing the divergence of the mean result from the 'true' value. Conversely, the term 'imprecision' refers to inconsistent or random errors, and is usually represented by the standard deviation (or coefficient of variation) of replicate measurements about the mean of the measurements. As in the case of the estimation of bias, assessment of 'imprecision' necessarily depends upon the performance of a large number of replicate measurements to yield a good estimate of their standard deviation.

Any individual assay measurement may yield a value which departs from the true value as a result either of 'bias' or 'imprecision', just as the individual shot fired by the marksman may miss the target because of misalignment of the rifle sighting mechanism or of his unsteady grip. Of course, in practice, both sources of error will inevitably contribute to divergence of the experimental result from the 'true' or 'correct' value and the assayist, on the basis of a single measurement, will normally be unable to assess the extent to which the result is 'incorrect' as a result either of 'bias' or 'imprecision'. Only as a result of repeated measurements, and appropriate statistical analysis, is the assayist able to estimate the contribution of errors of each category to the total error of the measurements. The statistical tools used in this assessment will be considered later in this discussion.

In discussing these concepts, you will note that I have temporarily abandoned the use of the word 'accuracy'. The reason for this is that there are two schools of thought regarding the definition of this term. On the one hand, the International Federation of Clinical Chemistry [3] (and clinical chemists in general) regard 'accuracy' as synonymous with lack of 'bias'; thus a measurement is 'inaccurate' in so far as the mean of a large number of replicate measurements departs from the 'correct' or 'true' value. Conversely, a method may be deemed as 'accurate' whatever its 'imprecision', and however widely individual measurements may scatter about the 'correct' or 'true' value.

In opposition to this view, many scientists (including statisticians, such as Prof. Finney, who have contributed greatly to the statistical analysis of bioassay and radioimmunoassay) regard the term 'accuracy' as embracing both 'bias' and 'precision'. Thus, a method may be regarded as 'inaccurate' because the measurement is 'incorrect'; moreover it is 'incorrect' because errors either of a consistent or random nature have deflected the measurement from the 'correct' or 'true' value. In so far as it is possible to assign a numerical value to this concept of 'accuracy', it may be represented by the equation:

$$\text{Accuracy} = \sqrt{\text{Bias}^2 + \text{Precision}^2}$$

I must here confess that my own personal preference is for a definition of 'accuracy' along these lines. Thus, it seems to me to be totally absurd – to revert

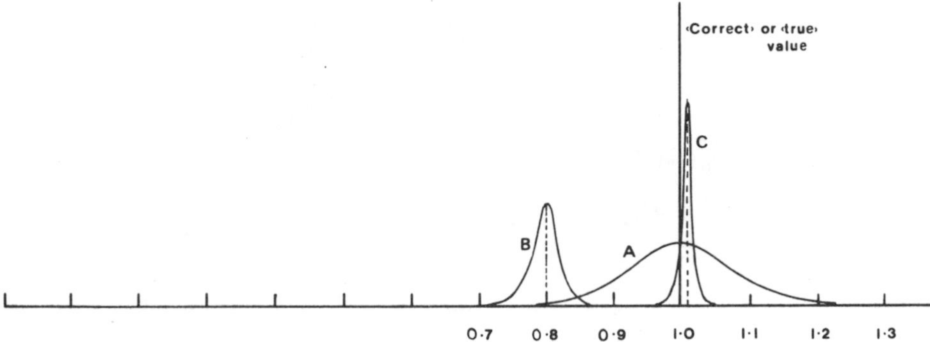

FIG.1. Distribution of assay results observed with three (hypothetical) assay systems. The 'true' or 'correct' assay result is represented by unity on the abscissa. Of the three assay systems, B is strongly biased towards a lower value, C is slightly positively biased, but is extremely precise, A is unbiased but yields widely dispersed values. Typical results yielded by pairs of duplicates are shown. Although the results yielded by assay C are (generally) closer to the 'true' value than those yielded by the other two assay systems, the identification of 'bias' and 'accuracy' requires that assay system A is deemed to be the most 'accurate'.

to our original analogy – to suggest (in line with the IFCC definition) that of two marksmen, the more 'accurate' is the one who, however wild his aim, discharges shots of which it can only be said that their average direction is in line with the target, whilst the marksman whose firearm is consistently misaligned by even the smallest amount is deemed to be less 'accurate'. In practice, the latter might well fire shots repeatedly falling closer to the target, whilst only occasionally might the first marksman do better. Likewise, in the case of assay procedures, the identification of 'bias' with 'accuracy' might well lead to the curious terminological and conceptual illogicality of an assayist selecting the less 'accurate' of two assay procedures on the grounds that it generally yielded individual assay results closer to the true value (Fig.1).

I recognize that in discussing these ideas it may be said that one is obsessively concerned with terminology, and I would generally agree that it matters little what word we use in any situation as long as we are clear as to the concept which it represents. The fundamental problem arises when terms are used loosely to represent different, and even conflicting concepts, as in the case of the word 'accuracy'. As I said earlier, it might be preferable to abandon the use of the word 'accuracy' altogether, although it would seem to me to be useful to have in our possession a term which reflects the overall liability of an assay procedure (or of the marksman) to error, regardless of the category into which the error falls. (We should also bear in mind that the designation of an error or variation as consistent or random depends upon the point of view from which it is seen: replicate samples may, for example, consistently differ, albeit the

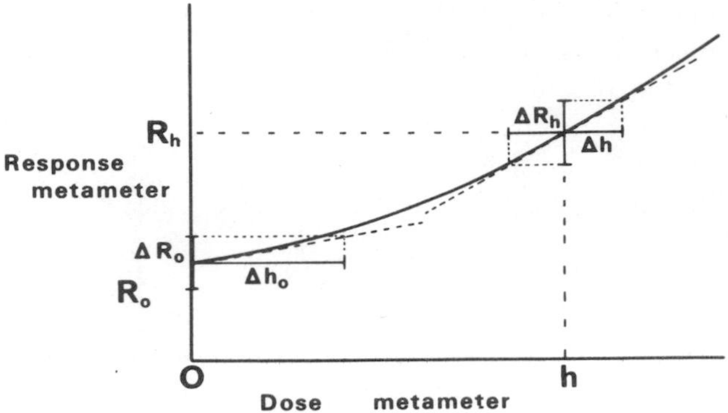

FIG.2. Relation between errors in response and dose metameters. The error (Δh) in the measurement of h is given by the error (ΔR_h) in the measurement of the assay response and the slope of the dose-response curve at the corresponding point on the dose-response curve. (Δh may be represented by the standard deviation σ_h, or any desired multiple of σ_h.) The error (Δh_0) in the measurement of h_0 defines the detection limit, or 'sensitivity', of the assay.

variation between individual replicates may nevertheless be expressed in terms of a standard deviation.) Moreover the concept of 'accuracy' embracing both 'bias' and 'precision' represents the meaning which is implied in the everyday usage of this word, and it would seem to me to be confusing to adopt a scientific definition which conflicts with its everyday connotation. The dangers associated with the use of a word to cover two disparate concepts are even more dramatically revealed in a consideration of the terms 'sensitivity' and 'precision'. I have frequently been involved in arguments regarding the meaning of these terms, and it would seem inappropriate to discuss them yet again were it not that already at this Symposium I have heard the word 'sensitivity' used in several different ways; moreover, in practice, extremely few assayists logically proceed from what I think are now generally accepted definitions of these terms to the practical design of assay systems.

Let us, therefore, first consider the concepts of precision. The 'precision' (or, more correctly, 'imprecision') of a measurement is commonly represented by the standard deviation or coefficient of variation of replicate measurements. (For the sake of simplicity we may assume that measurements are normally distributed about a mean as is usually the case in radioimmunoassays.) The 'precision' of a 'dose' measurement on an individual sample may be estimated by replicating the measurement several times within an assay batch, and calculating the standard deviation (or some multiple of this representing the possible error at a chosen confidence level) in the usual way. Alternatively, one may calculate the standard deviation σ_{R_h} or error ΔR_h of the response metameter R_h (e.g. counts bound) and divide this quantity by the slope of the dose-response curve at the relevant point (Fig.2). The results of these two calculations will normally be identical, assuming that the dose-response curve is essentially linear within the limits defined by the standard deviation of the response; otherwise there may be a slight, albeit usually insignificant, discrepancy between the two results. In short, by either routine, we may obtain an estimate of the standard deviation, σ_h, in the measurement of the analyte concentration, h, in any unknown sample.

What is the essential significance of such an estimate? Fundamentally, it tells us what is the smallest difference from what we may provisionally designate the basal value h that can be regarded as statistically significant. Clearly if we measure a second sample which yields a value h′, then the confidence with which we may say that the difference in the estimates (h′ – h) is 'real' depends upon the magnitude of the ratio $(h'-h)/\sigma_h$ (assuming that the standard deviation of measurements of h′ is roughly the same as that of h).

The situation in practice is slightly more complex than appears from this brief description; for example, in our measurements of both h and h′, we may rely on replicate determinations of each of the two samples, so that our question will take the form: is the difference between the two means, h and h′, statistically significant? In such circumstances, the relevant parameter is the standard error of the mean estimate in each case, and this clearly requires appropriate numerical adjustment to the corresponding standard deviations depending on the number of replicates taken for each of the two determinations.

Nevertheless, in spite of these numerical adjustments arising from the number of replicates included in the assay, the essential point at issue is that the standard deviation σ_h of measurements of h represents a fundamental indicator of the power of the system to distinguish samples containing higher or lower amounts of the analyte.

The next point to be emphasized is that σ_h will usually vary with the magnitude of h. This effect arises either because the standard deviation in the measurement of the response metameter, σ_R, is not constant (i.e. there is non-uniformity of variance), or because the slope of the response curve is not constant (i.e. the response curve is not linear). Inconstancy of either or both of these parameters implies that σ_h (i.e. (σ_R/slope)) will usually change with h. A useful way of portraying this variation is by means of what I have elsewhere termed the 'precision profile' of the assay [4]. This, quite simply, is a graphical representation of the way in which σ_h varies with h, taking the form, for example, of a simple plot of σ_h against h, or as the coefficient of variation, σ_h/h, against h. Alternatively, logarithmic scales can be used to represent the variables (Fig.3).

This is a very important concept in the context of quality control and assay design, albeit, frankly, there is nothing especially novel about it. The 'precision profile' corresponds conceptually very closely to Gaddum's 'index of precision',

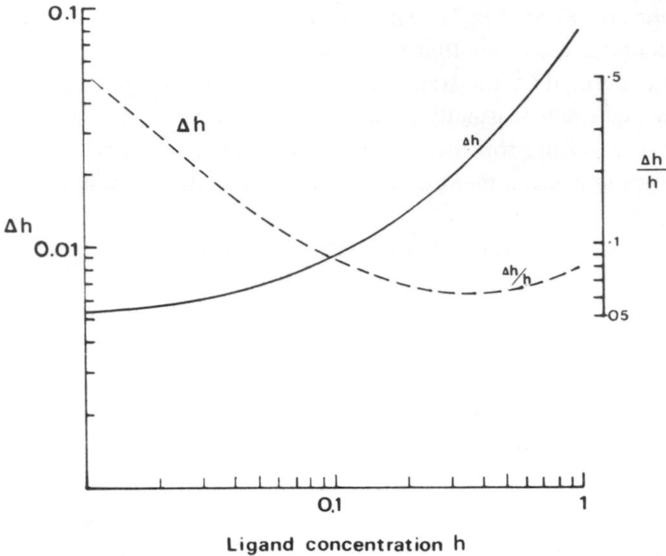

FIG.3. The assay 'precision profile' showing Δh (or σ_h) plotted as a function of analyte (ligand) concentration h. Both Δh and the relative error Δh/h are shown on logarithmic scales; likewise the analyte concentration h.

λ, which has been used for many years as a numerical indicator of performance of bioassay systems [5]. However, Gaddum's derivation of λ (also calculated as σ_R/slope) relied on the assumptions both of uniformity of variance along the (log) dose-response curve and of linearity (constancy of slope) of the curve. The value of λ (which, it may readily be shown, essentially represents the coefficient of variation in the measurement of any analyte concentration h) was thus conventionally regarded as approximately constant. This is clearly an approximation (as was acknowledged from the outset by Gaddum) since in no practical assay system can the coefficient of variation of measurement of the analyte remain constant, irrespective of the latter's magnitude. In many bioassay systems, and even in many radioimmunoassays, the approximations implied in the derivation of the index of precision are acceptable over a fairly wide range of analyte concentrations, and make λ a useful indicator of assay performance. Nevertheless, the more precisely defined 'precision profile' is a more exact portrayal of the performance of the system, and is particularly important in defining the optimal assay design of radioimmunoassay systems as will be discussed later.

A point of particular importance on the 'precision profile' is the intercept of the curve of σ_h against h with the vertical axis, corresponding to the standard deviation of 'zero dose' (or 'zero analyte') measurement. This value essentially defines the 'minimal detectable amount' of analyte (or 'lower limit of detection' of the assay) just as, in the more general case, the standard deviation of measurement of any defined analyte concentration defines the minimum detectable difference from that value. The 'minimal detectable amount' is, in practice, subject to the same numerical adjustments arising from the number of replicates used in the assay procedure (and the degree of confidence demanded) as discussed earlier. Thus, it is, in principle, possible to reduce its magnitude ad infinitum merely by increasing the number of replicates employed for the determination of each sample (standards and unknowns) in the assay system. Nevertheless, the standard deviation of 'zero dose' measurement (representing the standard error of 'singlicate' samples) constitutes a fundamental index of performance of the assay system which is independent of the number of replicates the assayist may happen to use in a particular assay run. The 'minimal detectable amount' is frequently equated with the 'sensitivity' of the assay, an assay being regarded as more 'sensitive' if the detection limit is smaller and vice versa.

'Sensitivity' represents a particularly abused term whose elimination from scientific literature has also often been proposed (e.g. [6]); nevertheless, accepting for the moment the use of the word discussed above, it is clearly imperative, in comparing the 'sensitivity' of various assay procedures, that a universal convention be applied to its calculation, implying agreement on the number of replicates and the confidence level involved in the derivation. Otherwise we encounter the absurd situation of assay systems being claimed as more 'sensitive' merely on the (concealed) grounds that a greater number of replicates have been used or a lower confidence level adopted in defining the detection limit. In practice, any survey of the current literature reveals both considerable ignorance of the correct way in which the detection limit should be calculated, and the absence of any clear convention regarding numbers of replicates and confidence level. This makes almost impossible any valid assessment of the relative performance of different assay techniques (see, for example, [7]) with regard to their 'sensitivity'.

Such problems pale into insignificance, however, compared with the identification of the term 'sensitivity' with the slope of the dose-response curve, which represents the conventional definition originally adopted by many workers in the field of radioimmunoassay and by official bodies [8, 9].

Although the logical absurdity of this definition has often been discussed and it has become more general, in recent years, to equate 'sensitivity' with the 'minimal detectable amount' rather than with the slope of the dose-response curve, the entire field of radioimmunoassay continues to be dominated by the latter definition and much of the mythology that currently attaches to this form of measurement is rooted in this fallacious concept. As illustrations of these mythologies, one may draw attention to the spurious belief that assays are most

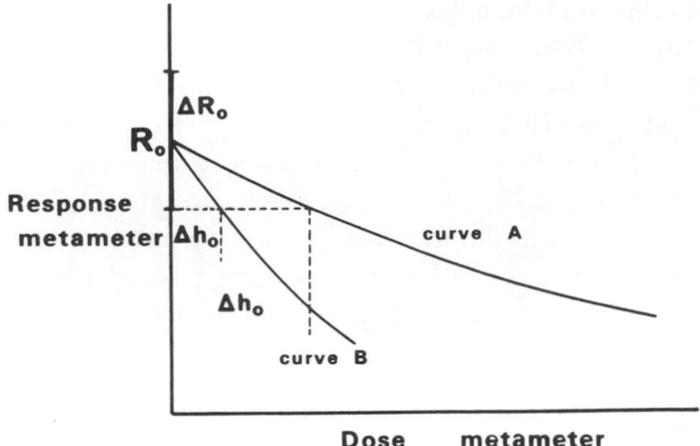

FIG.4. Illustration of a situation in which an increase *in the slope of the response curve may result in a reduction of the detection limit (Δh_0). Note that the 'absolute' error (e.g. the standard deviation) in R_0 is assumed to remain unchanged.*

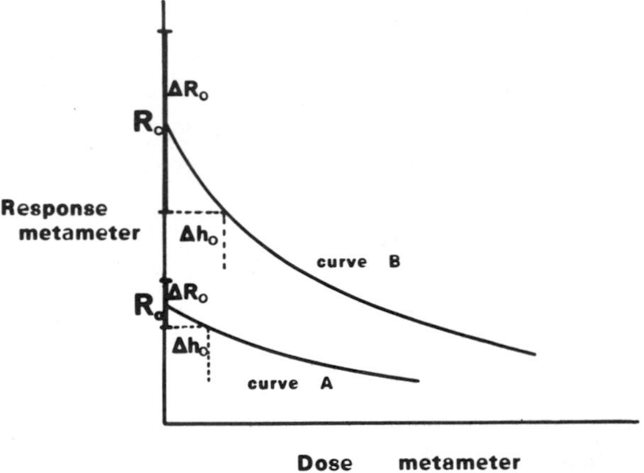

FIG.5. Illustration of a situation in which a decrease *in the slope of the response curve accompanied by decrease in the 'absolute' error in R_0 may result in a reduction of the detection limit (Δh_0). Note that although the 'absolute error' (e.g. the standard deviation) in R_0 is assumed to have been reduced in curve A, the relative error (e.g. coefficient of variation) in the measurement of the response may be closely similar for both curve A and curve B.*

'sensitive' when set up in such a way that 30–50% of the labelled analyte is bound at zero dose, and that degradation of the label necessarily affects assay performance. (Degradation of label, resulting in reduced antibody binding and 'flattening' of the dose-response curve, is typically regarded as implying a loss in assay 'sensitivity'. In certain situations, this may not be true, and assay performance may be minimally affected, even when the label is 60–80% impure and non-reactive.)

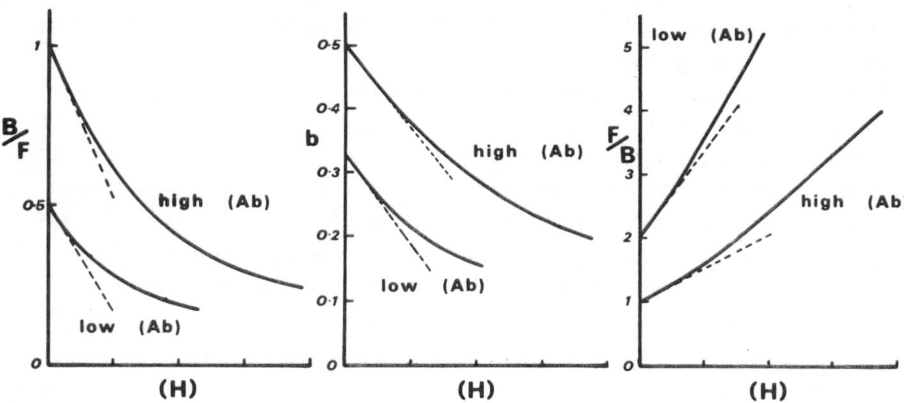

FIG.6. Identical radioimmunoassay data shown plotted in terms of (a) B/F, (b) fraction bound, b, (c) F/B. The change in slope of the response curve consequent upon a change of antibody concentration by a factor of 2 is shown in each case.

The implications of these two differing concepts of 'sensitivity', with respect to assay design, and indeed to the whole question of assessing assay performance, will be discussed later. At this point, it is sufficient to emphasize the distinction between the two definitions and illustrate one of the many absurdities that springs from regarding the slope of the dose-response curve per se as an indicator of 'sensitivity' (or 'precision'). Figure 4 illustrates circumstances in which increase in the slope of the dose-response curve correlates with decrease in the detection limit; Fig.5, in contrast, illustrates a situation in which, because of changes in the error of measurement of the response metameter, the curve with lower slope corresponds to the system yielding the smaller detection limit. The essence of these two illustrations is that the slope of the dose-response curve alone is not indicative of the magnitude of the detection limit, but only when taken in conjunction with errors in the measurement of the response as illustrated in Fig.2. As illustration of the nonsense that can arise as a result of disregarding the statistical analysis of assay data in assessing changes in assay performance, Fig.6 shows the changes in the slope of the dose-response curve resulting from a change in antibody concentration. The curves are here shown plotted in three conventional coordinate systems, with B/F, fraction bound, and F/B represented as functions of analyte concentration. It is evident from these figures that three assayists, plotting assay results respectively in the three coordinate frames shown, might be misled into believing that a reduction in antibody concentration would: (a) decrease, (b) not influence, (c) increase the 'sensitivity' of their assay systems. In reality, on the basis of the evidence shown, it is impossible to assess what the effect resulting from a change in antibody concentration on an assay performance would be. Absurd as this example reveals the identification of response curve slope with sensitivity to be, it is on such a basis that much current radioimmunoassay methodology implicitly rests.

These ideas will be explored further in my later presentation on quality control and assay design. Suffice it at this stage to delineate the basic concepts which must underlie any scientific assessment of assay performance. However, as a final addition to this brief introduction, it is important to emphasize that, just as we may represent within-assay performance by a 'within-assay precision profile', the same concept is applicable to between-assay batch performance, and between-laboratory performance. This implies a hierarchy of precision profiles containing at least three 'tiers'; others may be added by considering, for example, the 'between-laboratory/between-assay system precision profile', and so on. The statistical methods in calculating these 'profiles' will, of course, be discussed later. It may be appropriate to emphasize here that the particular 'profile' relevant to the assayist depends upon the precise context in which the assay is performed; for example, a clinician submitting a sample for measurement in any one of a number of laboratories contributing to a national assay service – as is currently in existence in the United Kingdom – will be primarily influenced by the 'between-laboratory/between-assay system profile' in assessing the errors in the assay results. Conversely, a sensible assayist interested in examining a change in hormone level arising from some physiological stimulus will be careful to measure samples in a single assay run, in which case the 'within-assay profile' will determine the significance of the observations.

Finally, for the sake of completeness (although it is a concept more open to criticism) it is possible to envisage 'bias profiles' totally analogous to 'precision profiles' on the assumption that the 'bias' of an assay vis-à-vis another is a consistent function of dose level, albeit not constant.

REFERENCES

[1] CORNFIELD, J., Statistics in Endocrinology (McARTHUR, J.W., COLTON, T., Eds), M.I.T. Press, Cambridge, Mass. (1970) 145.

[2] GADDUM, J.H., Pharm. Rev. 5 (1953) 87.

[3] BÜTTNER, J., BORTH, R., BOUTWELL, J.H., BROUGHTON, P.M.G., Clin. Chim. Acta 63 (1975) F25.

[4] EKINS, R.P., Hormone Assays and their Clinical Application (LORAINE, J.A., BELL, E.T., Eds), Churchill Livingstone, Edinburgh (1976) 1.

[5] GADDUM, J.H., Spec. Rep. Ser. Med. Res. Comm., London, No.183 (1933).

[6] JONES, R.C., Proc. Inst. Radio Eng. 47 (1959) 1495.

[7] KAISER, H., SPECKER, H., Z. Anal. Chem. 149 (1956) 46.

[8] YALOW, R.S., BERSON, S.A., Radioisotopes in Medicine: In Vitro Studies (Proc. Symp. Oak Ridge Associated Universities, 1967) (HAYES, R.L., GOSWITZ, F.A., MURPHY, B.E.P., Eds), USAEC Division of Technical Information (1968) 7.

[9] MACURDY, L.B., ALBER, H.K., BENEDETTI-PICHLER, A.A., CARMICHAEL, H., CORWIN, A.H., FOWLER, R.M., HUFFMAN, E.W.D., KIRK, P.L., LASHOF, T.W., Anal. Chem. 26 (1954) 1190.

QUALITY CONTROL FOR RIA

Recommendations for a minimal program

D. RODBARD
National Institute of Child Health and Human Development,
National Institutes of Health,
Bethesda, Maryland,
United States of America

INTRODUCTION

Quality control (QC) of radioimmunoassay is an indispensible part of the laboratory procedure. The basic principles of RIA quality control have been described in detail [1–9]. The QC of RIA is similar in many respects to QC in the general clinical chemistry laboratory: one seeks to monitor the validity, accuracy and precision (reproducibility, repeatability) of the assay system. The observed variability can be attributed to components arising within assays, between assays, and between laboratories, reagents and methods. QC relies on extensive statistical theory, practice and computational methods. The basic statistical principles have been described [10–14]. Each radioimmunoassay laboratory should have at least one person, preferably the laboratory director, who has completed a basic course in biostatistics (e.g. Ref. [15]). Further, it would be desirable that each laboratory have access to the services of a consulting statistician to assist in the design and implementation of a QC system custom tailored to its own requirements. The statistician can also assist in setting up appropriate computer programs for routine data processing.

In view of the extensive treatment in the literature, the present report is intended to review the essential features of a minimal 'prototype', with emphasis on the development of statistically valid, objective rules for rejection of an individual tube, a set of replicates, or the entire standard curve and assay.

STABILITY CONTROL AND CONFIRMATION OF VALIDITY

A major purpose of the QC program is to detect any deterioration (or improvement) of assay performance. Thus, QC should be an integral part of routine laboratory procedure and a part of every assay – not an idle exercise when publishing papers or as an annual affair to maintain accreditation. After each assay, one should ask: Is this a 'satisfactory' assay, i.e. is it 'in line' with previous assays, or is any one of a dozen or more aspects of the assay 'out of control'? An easy way to gain some assurance that the quality of the assay is satisfactory, is to ensure that the assay resembles previous ones as closely as possible in all readily measurable respects (assuming that previous assays were satisfactory and valid!). Thus, we construct control charts to examine several assay 'parameters', e.g. $\%(B/T)_0$ (per cent binding for zero dose), slope, intercept or ED_{50} (dose when $\%B/B_0 = 50\%$), ED_{80} (dose when $\%B/B_0 = 80\%$), minimal detectable dose [16], and 'residual variance' (or any other simple measure of the overall magnitude of the scatter of the points around the calibration curve). In addition, the affinity constant (K) and binding capacity ($[AB^{\circ}]$) from a Scatchard plot are important indices which reflect any deterioration of labelled antigen or antibody, failure to reach equilibrium and/or problems in separation of bound and free ligand. These analyses can be performed automatically by the same computer programs used for calculation of results for unknowns [17, 18]. However, it is essential to have an intelligent, critical and objective person available to scrutinize the results.

Construction of such 'control charts' does not evaluate the 'quality' of the assay; only its stability. Of course, if the assay had been thoroughly validated initially, then 'stability' presumably implies continued satisfactory quality. In assays where particular cross-reactivity problems frequently arise (e.g. dihydrotestosterone versus testosterone, 17α-hydroxyprogesterone versus progesterone, FSH versus LH versus TSH versus hCG, insulin versus proinsulin, etc.), it is desirable to test 'cross-reactivity' in every assay (or at least periodically) and display the results (e.g. per cent cross-reactivity) on a control chart. In assays where 'non-parallelism' of patient sera and standard materials is a recurrent problem, one should analyse a few QC samples (or unknowns) at two or three dilutions, calculate the slope and include a measure of 'parallelism' on the stability-control chart. One might use the slope of a logit-log plot [6], or simply the slope (derivative) of y versus log(X) at any specified response level for this purpose. It is often convenient to 'normalize' this slope, by subtracting (or dividing by) the corresponding slope of the standard curve at the same response level. Similarly, one can monitor the median slope for all unknown samples which have been analysed at two or more dose levels.

Every laboratory should be innovative in evaluating which 6 or 10 criteria give the most information on the stability of various assay systems. For example, in some assays, non-specific counts may be a serious problem; in others, the 'maximum bindability' of tracer may be a sensitive indicator of damaged tracer. In effect, we seek to verify the continued applicability of the several criteria used for the initial validation of the assay system (e.g. specificity, 'parallelism', recovery, comparison with independent assay methods, and significance of experimental manipulations or physiological results). By proper experimental design, one can re-confirm and update the measures of validity of the assay system with minimal expenditure of effort.

TABLE I. DEPENDENCE OF NUMBER OF DOSE LEVELS FOR STANDARD CURVE AND NUMBER OF QUALITY-CONTROL SAMPLES ON ASSAY SIZE

Number of unknown samples	Number of QC samples	Number of dose levels on standard curve
1– 10	3	6
10– 50	5	10
50– 200	7	12
200– 500	10	15
500–1500	12	15 for each 500

ASSAY QUALITY: WITHIN-ASSAY VARIABILITY

To evaluate the 'quality' of the assay, we first seek to estimate the within-assay precision. In general, this will vary systematically with dose level. There are two major approaches to evaluate this which may be termed (A) direct and (B) indirect.

(A) The 'direct' method using QC samples

The direct approach is to analyse a few samples in duplicate or triplicate in each of several assays. In general, the larger the assay, the greater the number of QC samples which should be included. Table I shows an arbitrary but representative guideline for number of dose levels for the standard curve and number of QC samples, as a function of assay size. The larger the assay, the smaller the percentage cost attributable to the standard curve and to the QC samples (which may be regarded as secondary standards). Also, the larger the assay, the greater the cost of either rejecting an assay when it should have been accepted, or accepting an assay when it should have been rejected (Type I or Type II errors, respectively). Hence, the added cost of additional QC samples is well justified. As a general rule, the number of standards and QC samples should increase (roughly) in proportion to the square root of the number of unknown samples in the assay. It is desirable that the number of replicates and dilutions used for each QC sample be the same as for the unknown samples.

For each QC specimen we calculate the sample mean ($\bar{X}$), variance (s^2), standard deviation (s) and per cent coefficient of variation ($\%CV = 100\ s/\bar{X}$). Unfortunately, the sample standard deviation based on duplicates or triplicates is very unreliable: it is subject to large 'random sampling error'. However, by combining results over several assays (to obtain a 'cumulative' average within-assay variability), and/or combining the results from several different samples

TABLE II. VALUES OF $R(=\sqrt{F} = s_1/s_2)$ CORRESPONDING TO UPPER 99.5th PERCENTILE OF F FOR VARIOUS DEGREES OF FREEDOM df_1 AND df_2

df_2 \ df_1	1	2	3	4	9
10	3.58	3.07	2.84	2.70	2.44
20	3.15	2.64	2.41	2.27	1.99
60	2.91	2.41	2.17	2.03	1.73
120	2.86	2.35	2.12	1.98	1.68
∞	2.81	2.30	2.07	1.93	1.62

(which is possible if they have about the same variance, or if their variances can be equalized by use of a square root, log or other transformation), one can obtain very reliable information with minimal expenditure of time or effort in terms of extra 'tubes' or computation. While the necessary calculations can be done easily by manual methods, ideally one should utilize automated, computerized methods [9, 17–19] to avoid numerical computational errors, assure consistency of computing format and avoid the need for approximations. Further, the computer program can alert the user when the variability of 'today's assay' is statistically significantly larger than that on the previous 10 or 20 assays. This avoids the tedium of having to refer to statistical tables to interpret the results.

If a sample has been analysed in replicate and s^2 has been calculated, one can calculate the F ratio

$$F = \frac{s_1^2}{s_2^2} \tag{1A}$$

where s_1^2 is the variance (square of the standard deviation) of today's results, based on df_1 degrees of freedom, and s_2^2 is the previous cumulative within-assay variance, based on df_2 degrees of freedom. This F ratio may be compared with the percentiles of the F distribution for df_1, df_2 degrees of freedom. It is desirable to use the 99, 99.5 or even 99.9th percentile to be conservative. If the F ratio calculated by Eq. (1A) were greater than the 99.5th percentile of the F distribution (available in most statistical texts or tables, e.g. [20]), then one is alerted that a '1 in 200' event has occurred. If one were to have three independent QC samples, and were to make three separate tests, then the chance of obtaining such a warning would be approximately 3 in 200. When using more than three QC samples, one may wish to use a higher percentile (e.g. 99.9th percentile) of the F distribution. Rather than using the 'F ratio' which is the ratio of two variances, it may be more convenient to use the ratio of the standard deviation for the current assay, divided by the previous cumulative standard deviation. This ratio may be designated as $R = \sqrt{F}$:

$$R = \sqrt{F} = \frac{s_1}{s_2} \qquad (1B)$$

Table II shows a few selected critical values of R. (When df_1 is 1, corresponding to duplicate measurements, this ratio is identical with Student's t distribution for df_2 degrees of freedom.) Thus, if the standard deviation for duplicates on the present assay were more than 3.58 times a previous estimate of the within-assay standard deviation (based on 10 assays, 10 df), then one would reject the (null) hypothesis that the two estimates were drawn from the same population at the $P = 0.005$ level and infer that there has been a 'significant' deterioration of assay precision.

This test is not very sensitive: even if one were to have three independent QC samples, each in duplicate, in each of 20 previous assays and with optimal pooling of information, we would have the critical values for R corresponding to $df_1 = 3$, $df_2 = 60$ in Table II. Hence, one would receive a 'warning' that the precision of the assay was deteriorating only if the overall standard deviation (and corresponding %CV) were to increase by a factor of 2.17.

(B) Indirect measurement of within-assay precision, based on the relationships σ_y^2 versus y and y versus X

In view of the conservative nature of the direct approach (based on a very limited amount of information), one should also utilize a more efficient, indirect approach which uses information from all of the samples in the assay which have been analysed in replicate.

In this approach one exploits the fact that the standard deviation of the potency estimate at dose level X (s_x) can be estimated if one knows the standard deviation of the response (s_y) and the slope of the dose-response curve (dy/dX) evaluated at this point:

$$\sigma_x = \frac{\sigma_y}{dy/dX} = \frac{\sigma_y}{\text{slope}} \qquad (2)$$

Thus, the task of finding σ_x for any given point on the dose-response curve reduces the two steps:

Step 1. Find the relationship between σ_y^2 or σ_y and y;

Step 2. Describe the shape of the dose-response curve in quantitative terms so that one can calculate the slope (derivative) for any dose level.

Step 1. Suppose both standards and unknowns have been analysed in

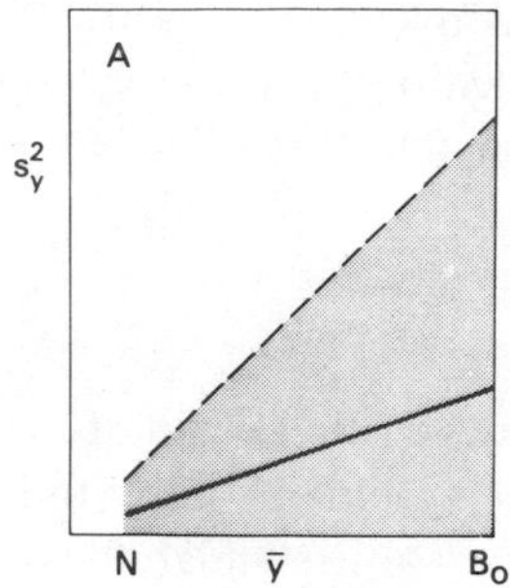

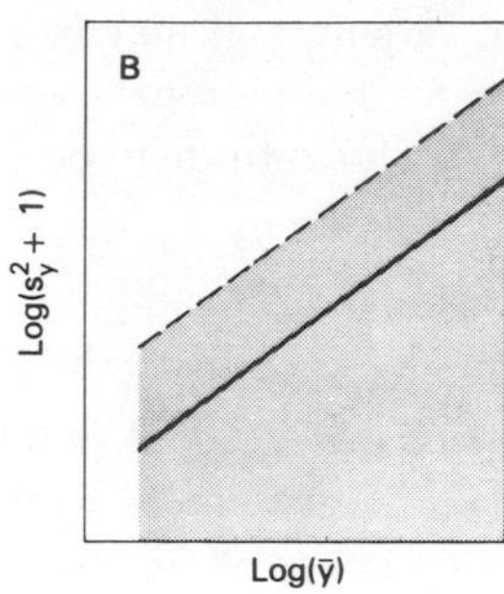

FIG.1. Relationship between σ_y^2 and y, shown on linear (panel A) and log-log coordinates (panel B). For each set of replicates, one calculates s_y^2 and $\bar{y}$, where y is the original response variable ('raw counts'). Although s^2 is subject to large sampling error, an underlying relationship is usually found (solid line), based on pooled information from standards and unknowns over several assays. The 99.5% upper limit of acceptability for a standard or unknown is shown by the dashed line; replicates falling above this line should be rejected.

duplicate. For each pair of tubes, we calculate the mean response, $\bar{y}$, the sample standard deviation of response, s_y, and the sample variance, s_y^2. (Here y denotes observed counts, unless otherwise indicated.) Then we plot s_y^2 versus $\bar{y}$ (Fig. 1A), using different symbols for standards and unknowns. Alternatively, one may plot $(\sigma_y^2 + 1)$ versus $\bar{y}$ on log-log paper (Fig. 1B). The log-log plot has several advantages:

(1) it readily covers a wide range of σ_y^2;

(2) one can show both σ_y^2 and σ_y on the vertical scale, using a four-cycle semi-log paper on the left ordinate, and a two-cycle semi-log paper on the right ordinate, since $\log(\sigma^2) = 2 \log(\sigma)$;

(3) a power-function relationship between σ_y^2 and y [21] corresponds to a linear relationship between $\log(\sigma_y^2)$ and $\log(\bar{y})$;

(4) the upper 99.5% confidence limits for σ will appear as a straight line, parallel to the predicted value of σ^2;

(5) $\log(\sigma_y^2)$ shows better uniformity of variance than σ_y^2.

These plots (Fig. 1) will usually appear to be a random scattergram, due to the enormous variability of s^2 based on only one or two df. (For 1 df, the 95% confidence limits for s^2 would be 5.02 times larger or 1018 times smaller than the true σ^2; the 99% confidence limits for s^2 would be 7.88 times larger or 25465 times smaller than the true value, based on the χ^2 distribution.) However, one may divide the scattergram into 5 or 10 regions or bins (either containing equal numbers of points or equally spaced in terms of $\bar{y}$), and find the **median** variance in each region. Then, one 'fits' the relationship between σ_y^2 and $\bar{y}$, either by a straight line, a parabola, or a power function [2, 4, 8, 21], i.e.

$$\sigma_y^2 = a_0 y^J \quad \text{(3A)}$$

The latter is easily 'fit' by use of linear regression

$$\log(\sigma_y^2 + 1) = \log(a_0) + J \log(\bar{y}) \tag{3B}$$

The power function is preferable if the 'y' values represent the 'raw' data, e.g. counts bound, but this model may fail if y represents B/T, B/F, %B/B_0, or B_0/B.[1] One should superimpose the 'fitted function' on the scattergram. Usually, the variance of y increases nearly in direct proportion to y (i.e. J = 1, so $\sigma_y^2 = a_0 y$). This is a general rule, observed in a large number of assays [8, 21, 22].

The relationship between σ_y^2 and y should first be estimated for the standard curve. This is usually based on a very small number of 'points' and, hence, degrees of freedom. A similar analysis for the unknowns will often provide a wealth of information. If one has 200 unknown samples analysed in duplicate, then he will be able to estimate σ_y^2 with (approximately) 200 degrees of freedom. One should then test whether the same relationship between σ_y^2 and y can be used for both the standards and unknowns for the present assay. If so, one should pool the information; if not, one should investigate the assay procedure to identify the source of this discrepancy.

Next, one should test whether the values for a_0 and J on today's assay are 'compatible' with the distribution of a_0 and J on previous assays. First, it might be desirable to fix J at its best estimate for several assays and then re-estimate a_0 for each assay. If today's value for a_0 were above the estimated 99.5th percentile of the distribution of a_0 for previous assays, then one may infer that the variability is statistically significantly higher than on the previous assays. This may be due to 'bad luck', or more likely, a malfunctioning pipetting machine or an unskilled or careless operator. In any event, it calls for appropriate action. If the present value for a_0 were more than 4 times the previous cumulative mean (i.e. σ is increased by a factor of 2 across the board), this might call for rejection of the assay, and a major overhaul of operations. This comparison with previous assays should be done separately for standards and unknowns, and the results compared. This provides a more sensitive test of homogeneity of results. It is possible that a small difference between standards and unknowns would be undetectable on any one assay, but would become evident when results are pooled or averaged over several assays.

One may then proceed to use the relationship between σ_y^2 and y as a basis for rejection of outliers. For any given response level, y, one has a very reliable

---

[1] By virtue of subtraction of the non-specific counts to calculate B/T or B/B_0, one violates the condition that $\sigma^2(0) = 0$. If y represents a response other than 'raw' counts, then in lieu of $\log(s_y^2 + 1)$, one should use $\log(s_y^2 + \epsilon)$, where ϵ represents a small constant, in Eq. (3B). A reasonable value for ϵ might be 10 times smaller than the smallest non-zero value of s_y^2. (ϵ is needed to prevent the appearance of log(0).)

estimate of the true or expected variance, σ_y^2. This is 'known' with a reliability corresponding (approximately) to the total number of degrees of freedom for the individual estimates of σ^2. Hence, one may calculate the upper acceptance limits (UL) for the sample variance s^2 for an unknown as

$$UL = F \sigma_y^2 \tag{4}$$

where df_1 is the number of degrees of freedom for the estimate of variance for replicates for an unknown (or standard), df_2 is the number of degrees of freedom for the estimate of σ^2, P is the rejection probability level and F is the tabulated value of the F distribution for df_1, df_2, at the $100(1 - P)$ percentile. This approach provides an objective criterion for rejection of replicates which have poor precision. When s^2 is greater than UL, the set of values should be rejected.[2] The probability of falsely rejecting a set of replicates can be set at any arbitrarily selected nominal value, e.g. $P = 0.01$, 0.005 or 0.001. For example, if one uses the upper 99.5 percentile of the F distribution (so that he would expect to reject only 1 of 200 samples which were actually in control, i.e. $P = 0.005$), and if the relationship between σ_y^2 and $\bar{y}$ were based on about 120 df, then the critical F ratio of observed to expected variance, s^2/σ^2, would be 8.18 when using duplicates ($df_1 = 1$), 5.54 for triplicates ($df_1 = 2$) or 4.50 for quadruplicates ($df_1 = 3$). (The corresponding ratios in terms of $R = s/\sigma$, given in Table II, are 2.86, 2.35 and 2.12, respectively.) Hence, our ability to reject samples on the basis of poor reproducibility increases as we increase the number of replicates.[3] The experimentalist must balance this increase in information against the increased cost of the assay, and the fact that overall assay precision often deteriorates as the size of the assay increases as a result of fatigue, changes in time or temperature of reactions, need for different batches of reagents or different runs in a centrifuge, etc.

Step 2. How does one evaluate the precision (%CV) for an unknown, given the value of σ_y^2? To do so, one must evaluate the slope of the calibration curve at each dose level. This is easily calculated, irrespective of the method used for construction of the dose-response curve. We shall give explicit instructions for four cases: (I) point-to-point linear interpolation; (II) polynomial or spline fit; (III) logit-log [1–4, 6] and (IV) the four-parameter logistic method [6, 16, 21].

---

[2] Alternatively, one can set an upper limit on s as $R \times \sigma$, where R is the square root of F. Then, one should reject a set of replicates if $s/\sigma > R$.

[3] For every unknown specimen in the assay analysed in replicate, we obtain an estimate of the observed standard deviation of the response (s_y), and the expected standard deviation (σ_y). The ratio of these, $R = s_y/\sigma_y$, may be printed out next to each potency estimate. If it exceeds the value calculated from the percentiles of the F distribution, one is warned that this potency estimate is unreliable. The 'gap' test [12] (or similar) may be used to identify 'outliers' if triplicates or quadruplicates have been used.

I. (A) Point-to-point linear interpolation in terms of y (counts) versus arithmetic dose:

1. Plot the curve;
2. Calculate $\bar{y}$ for each dose;
3. Calculate the slope between two dose levels, $\Delta y/\Delta X$;
4. Plot slope = $\Delta y/\Delta X$ versus X; this results in a step function; consider the slope between two points to apply to a 'dose' halfway between them.
5. 'Smooth' this relationship (by eye), and use the 'smoothed' slope for any given dose level.

I. (B) If using y = counts versus $X' = \log_{10}(X)$, follow steps 1–5 above and then use the relationship

$$(\text{slope versus X}) = \frac{\Delta y}{\Delta X} \cong \frac{[\text{slope versus } \log_{10}(X)]}{(2.303)X} \tag{5}$$

II. Polynomial or spline fit with $X' = \log_{10}(X)$, follow steps 1–5 above and Here the dose-response curve is described either segmentally or globally by

$$y = a_0 + a_1X' + a_2(X')^2 + a_3(X')^3 + a_4(X')^4 \tag{6}$$

Then the slope dy/dX is given by

$$\frac{dy}{dX} = \frac{a_1 + 2a_2X' + 3a_3(X')^2 + 4a_4(X')^3}{(2.303)X} \tag{7}$$

III. Logit-log method: if using a linear relationship

$$Y' = \text{logit}(Y) = \alpha + \beta X' \tag{8}$$

where X' is $\log_{10}(X)$ and $Y = B/B_0$, then

$$dY'/dX' = \beta \tag{9A}$$

$$dY/dX' = \beta(1 - Y)(Y) \tag{9B}$$

$$dY/dX = \frac{\beta(1 - Y)(Y)}{(2.303)X} \tag{9C}$$

$$dy/dX = \frac{(\bar{B}_0 - \bar{N})\beta(1 - Y)(Y)}{(2.303)X} \tag{9D}$$

Note: If $X' = \log_e(X)$, then omit the factor 2.303 in Eqs (7), (9C) and (9D).

IV. Four-parameter logistic:
Here, the dose-response curve is described by

$$y = \frac{a - d}{1 + (X/c)^b} + d \tag{10}$$

and

$$\text{slope} = dy/dX = \frac{-(a-d)\,b(X/c)^b}{X[1 + (X/c)^b]^2} = \frac{-b(a-y)(y-d)}{X(a-d)} \tag{11}$$

This corresponds to the expression for the logit-log method, making the substitutions: $a = B_0$, $d = N$, $c = \text{antilog}(-\alpha/\beta)$, and $b = -\beta/(2.303)$. Hence, Eqs (9D) and (11) can be used interchangeably, noting that $Y = (y - d)/(a - d)$.

Methods II–IV have the advantage that the dose-response curve is defined mathematically, and hence one can calculate the slope (derivative) everywhere by means of a simple formula (e.g. Eqs (9D) or (11)). Likewise, the use of the mass-action law equations (e.g. in Ref. [16]) permits the slope to be expressed analytically. Method I, which has abrupt discontinuities in slope at each dose level, requires some means to estimate a 'smoothed' slope. Similar analyses to estimate the slope may be used for **any** method of dose interpolation.

Having completed **Step 2**, to obtain the slope, the predicted σ_x for any point on the standard curve is given by

$$\sigma_x = \frac{\sigma_y}{\text{slope}} = \frac{(a_0 y^J)^{1/2}}{\text{slope}} \tag{2A}$$

or

$$\%CV_x = \frac{\sigma_x}{X} \cong 100\,\frac{(a_0 y^J)^{1/2}}{\text{slope } X} \tag{2B}$$

Automated computerized display of σ_x or $\%CV_x$ versus X or y has been implemented in terms of the logistic family of methods using high-speed digital computers (e.g. [2, 4, 6, 17]). However, these analyses can readily be performed on the smallest hand-held calculators or microprocessors. The 'precision profile', i.e. a plot of σ_x or $\%CV_x$ versus X (or Y) can be generated by the eight-line program in BASIC shown in Fig. 2. This program will generate a table of X, y, B/B_0, the predicted standard deviation of X (σ_x) and the per cent error in

BASIC program to calculate predicted precision at any point on the dose-response curve

```
1    INPUT A, B, C, D, SO, AO, J
2    PRINT "DOSE"; "COUNTS"; "B/BO"; "STD.DEV. X"; "%CV"
3    FOR Y1= 0.95 TO 0.05 STEP – 0.05
4    Y= D + (A – D)* Y1
5    X= C * ((A – Y)/(Y – D)) ↑ (1/B)
6    S= SQR(SO * AO * Y↑J) * X * (A – D)/B/(A – Y)/(Y – D)
7    PRINT X; Y; Y1; S; 100*S/X
8    NEXT Y1
```

FIG.2. A short program in BASIC to calculate the standard deviation of the potency estimate and the corresponding $\%CV_x$ for dose, as $\%B/B_0$ ranges from 95% to 5%. This assumes a power-function relationship between σ_y^2 and y, and the four-parameter logistic (or logit-log) relationship to describe the dose-response curve. Here A, B, C, D, X and Y correspond to a, b, c, d, X and y of Eq.(10), A0 and J are the parameters of Eq.(3) and S0 is the residual variance of the weighted least-squares curve-fitting procedure, Y1 is B/B_0, and S is the predicted σ_x. If A0 is not statistically significantly different from unity, one may omit this term.

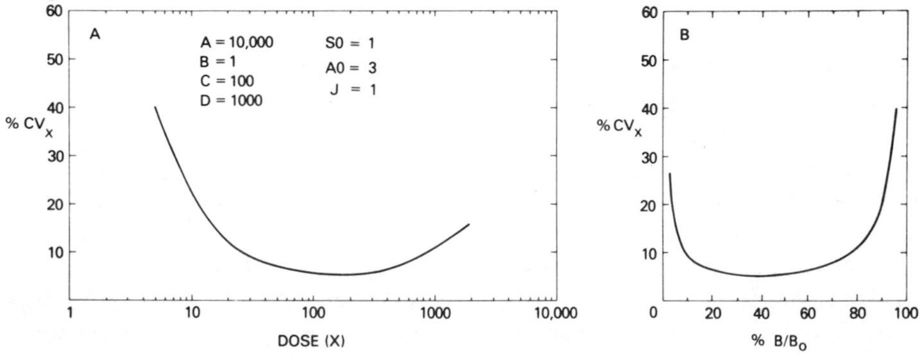

FIG.3. Relationship between $\%CV_x$ and log(X) (panel A), or between $\%CV_x$ and $Y = \%B/B_0$ (panel B). This permits one to compare the precision of the quality-control samples, both within-assays and between-assays, with the predicted within-assay precision estimated by the 'indirect' approach, based on the relationships of σ_y^2 versus y and of y versus X.

X ($\%CV = 100\,\sigma_x/X$) for various dose levels as B/B_0 varies from 0.05 to 0.95 in increments of 0.05. One may then plot σ_x or $\%CV_x$ versus X, y or B/B_0. Graphs of $\%CV_x$ versus B/B_0 or versus log(X) (i.e. X on a semilog paper) are usually preferable (Fig. 3).

One can then compare the observed, empirical $\%CV_x$ for the few QC samples analysed using the 'direct' method (above) with that predicted by the 'indirect' method [9]. Ideally, they should agree within the limits of random sampling variation (as given by the F distribution). One should not be surprised if the QC samples behave somewhat better, on the average, than that predicted by the indirect method. If the QC samples were not handled in a 'blind' fashion, they will usually receive extra special tender loving care, which leads to a biased estimate of assay precision. Hence, if there is a discrepancy, then the most trustworthy values are likely to be the ones based on the 'indirect' analysis which uses all available information on all standards and unknowns.

The analyses just described provide a measure of precision for tubes which have been analysed in immediate juxtaposition. Hence, these analyses represent a form of 'ideal conditions' variability, and do not provide any information about, nor protection against, the possibility of systematic drift throughout an assay. In the event of significant 'drift' in the assay, both the direct and indirect approaches just described will severely underestimate the error between samples dispersed throughout the assay. The only protection against this is to use 'drift control samples' (thus adding another component of variance to the ANOVA), and/or randomization of all tubes in the assay.

DISCUSSION

We have focused on the problem of estimation of within-assay variance, either directly or indirectly. This is the first measure of precision, and often the one of greatest importance: this is the best attainable precision. If this deteriorates, it is likely that all other levels of precision will also deteriorate. Also, in view of the well-known observation that within-assay precision is two- to threefold better than between-assay precision, the experimentalist should always design his studies (be they clinical or for basic research) such that all relevant comparisons can be made within an assay – and, if possible, within a small region of a given assay. Likewise, in multi-centre studies, the experimental design should permit all important comparisons to be made within laboratories and, if possible, within assays. Thus, the statistician should be consulted to assist in optimal allocation of samples to assays and laboratories.

In addition to the measurements of within-assay precision, one must also estimate the component of between-assay variance [6, 7, 9]. One should consider the local 'contrast' between today's result and the result on recent assays (local between-assay variance), and compare this with the previous cumulative between-assay variance [6, 9]. Further, the analyses described in Ref. [9] allow one to evaluate whether to reject an assay or whether it is permissible to invoke a 'correction factor'.

The same kind of analyses can be used to evaluate variability between laboratories, or between groups of laboratories employing different reagents or methods [19]. The ANOVA approach may even be used to evaluate pipetting machines and technicians [7]. Thus, the ANOVA methods provide us with an objective, easily calculated, numerical measure of the components of variability introduced from different sources, and permits us to evaluate the 'confidence limits' for these estimates of variance.

The role of intuition: Many experimentalists have argued that formal QC procedures are inadequate or even unnecessary. Simply by 'looking' at the assay, they claim to be able to detect if anything is wrong. There may be some merit to this: by scanning the results, the eye can search for dozens, perhaps hundreds of patterns. For example, (a) are all of the results too high or too low? (b) Are the results expressed in the correct units? (c) What percentage of clinical samples are in the normal (or hyper- or hypo-active) range? Is this in accord with results on the last 10 or 20 assays? If not, is this due to a change in the patient population or in the assay method?

The above questions can be attacked, quantitatively, by simply constructing frequency distributions for today's results and for those from previous assays. The Kolmogorov-Smirnov test may be used to test for a significant change in the overall distribution, while a simple **t** test for proportions should indicate whether the per cent normal (or hyper- or hypo-active) is in accord with long-term expectations.

In addition, most RIAs provide considerable information which may be regarded as internal validity checks. For example, the assay may contain successive eluates from a chromatographic column. Accordingly, one can expect a smooth concentration profile, with a contour which may be predictable on the basis of previous experiments. Further, many of the samples are likely to contain none of the substance of interest, and thus their response should be nearly at B_0. Thus, instead of having only 3 or 4 'tubes' for B_0, we may have 30 or 40, spaced throughout the assay. These provide a sensitive measure of assay drift. Similarly, in clinical applications, we have 'experiments' which serve to confirm the reliability of the assay: a 'certain percentage' of pregnancy tests should be positive in a stable obstetrical clinic; a 'certain percentage' of patients with galactorrhea will have hyperprolactinemia. We can define 'typical' patterns of response during provocative tests (glucose, insulin, arginine tolerance tests; responses to stimulation by TRH, LHRH, TSH, ACTH, etc.), and expect these in a 'certain percentage' of patients. In patients with choriocarcinoma, the results of the current assay for hCG should be 'in line' with the extrapolated results based on previous assays. If there is an abrupt discontinuity for several such subjects, we are 'warned' that the results of the current assay are 'out of line'. (In such an application, several previously assayed samples should be included in the present assay, and thus serve as additional QC samples which provide additional information on between-assay variability.) Hence, an assay containing several hundred samples provides a wealth of information – which may exceed that provided by the few formal QC samples. However, rather than analysing these data subjectively by 'intuition', one should specify many of these criteria in a formal manner, and then evaluate each of them using objective, statistical methods. The use of easily calculated non-parametric statistics [15] seems ideally suited to this purpose, and may correspond well to the logic used in the intuitive approach. Ideally, in this manner, one could utilize information from virtually all of the samples in the assay, to evaluate assay performance in terms of our expectations of the results of the clinical or basic 'experiments' embedded in the assay. Thus, in the final analysis, we must ask 'Do the results make sense?'

ACKNOWLEDGEMENTS

P.J. Munson and D.W. Wilson provided many stimulating discussions and helpful suggestions. T. Broderick provided excellent secretarial assistance.

NOMENCLATURE

α, β	coefficients of logit-log equation
a, b, c, d	coefficients, e.g. for four-parameter logistic equation
$[Ab^\circ]$	total concentration of antibody combining sites
a_0, J	coefficients of power function relationship between σ_y^2 and y.
ANOVA	Analysis of variance
$\%(B/T)_0$	%B/T (bound-to-total ratio corrected for non-specific counts) when X = 0
B/B_0	$\%B/T/\%(B/T)_0$; response variable expressed in normalized scale from 0 to 1 (specifically bound counts relative to counts bound for zero dose).
%CV	Coefficient of variation (standard deviation expressed as per cent of mean)
df	degrees of freedom
F	ratio of two independent estimates of variance
K	equilibrium constant of association (L/M)
QC	Quality control
R	$\sqrt{F}$; ratio of two standard deviations
s	sample standard deviation
s^2	sample variance

s_0^2	residual variance
σ	expected standard deviation
σ^2	expected (predicted) variance
X	dose
$\bar{X}$	mean X
X'	transformed dose variable, usually $\log_{10}(X)$
y	response variable: untransformed ("raw") counts
Y	transformed response variable, usually B/B_0
Y'	$\text{logit}(B/B_0) = \log_e \{Y/(1-Y)\}$, where $Y = B/B_0$

REFERENCES

[1] RODBARD, D., RAYFORD, P.L., COOPER, J., ROSS, G.T., J. Clin. Endocrinol. Metab. 28 (1968) 1412.

[2] RODBARD, D., COOPER, J.A., In Vitro Procedures with Radioisotopes in Medicine (Proc. Symp. Vienna, 1969), IAEA, Vienna (1970) 659.

[3] RODBARD, D., RAYFORD, P.L., ROSS, G.T., "Statistical quality control of radioimmunoassays", Statistics in Endocrinology (McARTHUR, J.W., COLTON, T., Eds), MIT Press, Cambridge, Mass. (1970) 411.

[4] RODBARD, D., "Statistical Aspects of Radioimmunoassays", Competitive Protein Binding Assays (ODELL, W.D., DAUGHADAY, W.H., Eds.), J.B. Lippincott Co., Philadelphia, Pa., (1971) 204.

[5] Standarization of Radioimmunoassay Procedures, Report of an International Atomic Energy Agency Panel, Int. J. Appl. Radiat. Isot. **25** (1974) 145.

[6] RODBARD, D., Clin. Chem. **20** (1974) 1255.

[7] RUSSELL, C.D., DE BLANC, H.J., WAGNER, H.N., Johns Hopkins Med. Bull. **135** (1974) 344.

[8] RODBARD, D., LENOX, R.H., WRAY, H.L., RAMSETH, D., Clin. Chem. **22** (1976) 350.

[9] McDONAGH, B.F., MUNSON, P.J., RODBARD, D., Comput. Programs Biomed. 7 (1977) 179.

[10] HARRIS, E.K., DEMETS, D.L., Clin. Chem. **18** (1972) 244.

[11] HARRIS, E.K., KANOFSKY, P., SHAKARJI, G., COTLOVE, E., Clin. Chem. **16** (1970) 1022.

[12] YOUDEN, W.J., STEINER, E.H., Statistical Manual of the Assoc. of Official Analytical Chemists (Association of Official Analytical Chemists) Washington, D.C. (1975) 88 pp.

[13] FINNEY, D.J., Statistical Method in Biological Assay, Griffin, London (1964).

[14] DUNCAN, A.J., Quality Control and Industrial Statistics, 4th edn, Richard D. Irwin, Homewood, Ill. (1974).

[15] COLQUHOUN, D., Lectures on Biostatistics, Clarendon Press, Oxford (1971) (see esp. Chapter 13, pp. 279–343).

[16] RODBARD, D., MUNSON, P.J., DE LEAN, A., These Proceedings, Vol. 1, p. 469.

[17] RODBARD, D., FADEN, V.B., Radioimmunoassay Data Processing, 3rd edn, National Technical Information Service, Springfield, Va. 22141 (1975) (PB 246222 for magnetic tape and PB 246223-4 for printed listings).
[18] DUDDLESON, W.G., MIDGLEY, A.R., NISWENDER, G.D., Comput. Biomed. Res. 5 (1972) 205.
[19] MUNSON, P.J., RODBARD, D., "An elementary components of variance analysis for multi-centre quality control", These Proceedings, Vol. 2.
[20] ABRAMOWITZ, M., STEGUN, I.A. (Eds), Handbook of Mathematical Functions, (Ninth Printing), US Govt. Printing Office, Washington, DC (1970).
[21] FINNEY, D.J., Biometrics 32 (1976) 721.
[22] MIDGLEY, A.R., Jr., NISWENDER, G.D., REBAR, R.W., "Principles for the assessment of the reliability of radioimmunoassay methods (precision, accuracy, specificity, sensitivity", Immunoassay of Gonadotrophins, Transactions of the First Karolinska Symposium on Research Methods in Reproductive Immunology, Stockholm 1969 (DICZFALUSY, E., Ed.), Reproductive Endocrinology Research Unit, Karolinska Sjukhuset, Stockholm (1969) 163 : Acta Endocrinol. Suppl. 142 (1969) 163.

P.E. HALL *(Chairman):* Thank you, Prof. Ekins and Dr. Rodbard. I now invite questions.

P.G. MALAN: With regard to Dr. Rodbard's review, I can confirm that the response-error relationship does in fact provide a very reasonable basis for looking at errors in assays. For the past two years we have been processing our data on this basis. The variation between one assay and the next is not very great if one uses the techniques of binning and pooling the results that he has described and in fact it can be used as one parameter of quality control.

May I turn to your extremely useful normalization technique for comparing and combining assays. We have found the non-parametric analytical technique described by Steiner an extremely powerful one for detecting bias and rejecting individual results or the results of complete assays before pooling the variances in order to perform analyses such as you have described.

D. RODBARD: I would agree with you that non-parametric or ametric statistical methods, particularly those based on ranks, percentiles and such concepts, are extremely useful, particularly because they give uniformity of variance and so allow the application of classical analysis of variance and related techniques with greater validity. Their drawback is that they involve the loss of some of the information in the original measurement scale. I think that if it is possible to retain the original measurement scale, we all prefer to do so, the more so since radioimmunoassay data are really very metric. Even so, the non-parametric methods are just about as informative and I would encourage their use.

D. FULD: For the past two years, we have also studied the relationship of the variance of y versus mean y (σ_y^2 versus $\bar{y}$). By examining the median variance for each small region of y, one can find the overall relationship as described by

Dr. Rodbard. Further, we have examined the frequency distribution for the ratio of the variance of y to the mean y value. In effect, we are looking at the frequency distribution for the slope of a line from the origin to the set of values $(\bar{y}, \sigma_y^2)$. It appears that these slopes are distributed in a manner similar to a Gaussian distribution. These results are compatible with your discussion of the minimal detectable dose, wherein you assume that the response variable y is subject to chi-square distribution. Thus, when we seek to combine the information from all of the replicated samples in an assay, an alternative approach is to look at the mean or the median of the ratio, variance of y divided by $\bar{y}$, or $\sigma_y^2/\bar{y}$.

Regarding your use of the 'Studentizing' transformation to achieve or attempt to achieve uniformity of variance for empirical quality-control data, I would like to express serious reservations. As a general rule, many elementary statistics books indicate a minimum of 30 values is needed to obtain a reliable mean, and at least 50 values are needed to have a reliable estimate of the standard deviation. Hence, I am concerned that use of a mean and standard deviation based on as few as 10 degrees of freedom will introduce serious instability into the calculations. For this reason, we have adopted an alternative approach. In a preliminary analysis, we found that as a general rule the standard deviation of the potency estimate is very nearly proportional to the potency estimate. In other words σ_x is proportional to x, and the coefficient of variation of the potency estimate nearly constant over a wide working range for each assay. Accordingly, rather than using an empirical Studentizing transformation, it may be preferable simply to take each of the values for the three (or more) quality-control samples, and simply divide each of these original measurements by the mean value for the respective quality-control pool measured in several assays. We are attempting to equalize the variance, but rather than utilizing the observed standard deviation (which is subject to enormous random sampling errors), we are 'correcting' or 'normalizing' the data by using the basic rule that σ_x is proportional to x, and taking advantage of the fact that the mean can be much more reliably estimated than the standard deviation, when dealing with small numbers of observations.

D. RODBARD: Thank you very much for your comments, Dr. Fuld. I am pleased to see that you also find that the variance of y is almost directly proportional to y in literally dozens of assay systems. Your data may be the most extensive yet available in the world. I might comment that the general linear relationship between variance of y and y does not hold for all assay systems. Occasionally, we find some degree of curvature, and in such cases it is useful to utilize a power function as suggested by Finney. Nevertheless, a linear relationship is usually a satisfactory approximation. I am also pleased to see that your results indicate that the original response variables (in terms of counts bound) are subject to a Gaussian distribution.

I agree that, ideally, one should have at least 10 to 20 degrees of freedom in order to obtain a 'reliable' mean and even more than this in order to obtain a reliable estimate of the sample standard deviation (s). Obviously, the more degrees of freedom, the better. Unfortunately, we rapidly encounter the problem of diminishing returns, since the precision of σ increases with increasing numbers of observations, but only approximately in proportion to the square root of n. I would agree that the use of the Studentizing transformation to achieve uniformity of variance, to combine results from different quality-control samples, should be based on a very reliable estimate of the standard deviation, preferably with 30 degrees of freedom or more. Failure to obtain reliable estimates of the mean and/or standard deviation effectively results in the introduction of random errors and decreases the efficiency of the analysis. Certainly, one should not attempt to utilize the Studentizing transformation with less than 10 degrees of freedom. In the case of limited data, it may be useful to utilize non-parametric statistical methods as suggested by Dr. Malan, to avoid the problems of non-uniformity of variance. Alternatively, when the coefficient of variation is constant, and σ_x is proportional to x over the range of interest, then a logarithmic transformation is a simple method to obtain uniformity of variance. Alternatively, one can divide by the overall mean for respective samples, so that all values are essentially expressed as percentages of the overall mean. In effect, we are saying that the percentage changes or percentage errors are (more or less) constant over the range of interest. One may utilize the transformation $x' = 100\,x/\bar{x}$, where all results are expressed as a percentage of the overall mean. Alternatively, for each result for each quality-control sample we may first subtract the mean, and then divide by the mean, utilizing the formula $x' = (x-\bar{x})/\bar{x}$. Here we are transforming all of the observations to examine the percentage change from the overall mean.

Your approach, Dr. Fuld, should be more reliable than the Studentizing transformation when basing analyses on a small number of observations. However, the Studentizing transformation is extremely general, and allows one to handle other cases where the standard deviation of x is any arbitrary function of x. Moreover, your approach is relatively insensitive to outliers. When utilizing a Studentizing transformation, it is desirable to have some rules built in to reject outliers, which may otherwise severely bias the results. In practice, we have found the Studentizing transformation to be an extremely useful approach to combine results from different quality-control samples, and still retain uniformity of variance, to permit calculation of an analysis of variance, and thus provide optimal pooling of information.

P.E. HALL *(Chairman)*: Thank you. I now call on Prof. Ekins to discuss assay quality control in relation to assay design.

QUALITY CONTROL AND ASSAY DESIGN

R.P. EKINS
The Middlesex Hospital Medical School,
London, United Kingdom

I want in this presentation to return to the question of the interaction of the parameters relating to assay performance with assay design, and again, as in my earlier presentation, I think it preferable to emphasize general concepts rather than embark on a detailed discussion of the statistical techniques involved. This is not to imply that the latter are unimportant – nevertheless my general feeling is that many assayists are confused at a conceptual level regarding assay design, rather than that the statistical techniques involved (which are mostly both standard and simple, albeit a little time-consuming) represent much of a problem.

The fundamental starting point of my presentation is that the overriding objective of radioimmunoassay design is the selection of individual reagents, and a method of combination of those reagents, such that the 'accuracy' of measurement of the analyte at the concentration at which it occurs in a biological fluid of interest is maximized. This implies that we must minimize errors giving rise to bias and imprecision (both within and between batch) in our system. Clearly there is very little point in developing highly sophisticated statistical procedures for monitoring assay performance unless we use them to improve the assay method and generally ensure that the system that we are keeping under surveillance is 'optimized', both with respect to bias and precision, within the constraints imposed by time and money.

There is neither particular need, nor opportunity, to present in detail here the measures that the assayist should take to minimize assay bias. Clearly there are two complementary ways of achieving this objective, on the one hand by choosing specific reagents (for example, antibody) of the highest possible structural specificity; on the other hand, by ensuring that all samples in the assay system (including both unknowns and standards) are as alike as one another as possible, both in terms of general composition, and of the physical environment to which they are exposed. This implies, in turn, that assay standards should, when relevant, be made up in 'analyte'-free serum (unless doing otherwise is proved not to affect assay results); it likewise implies that the kinetic characteristics of the system must be carefully investigated, since it is generally impossible to process all samples simultaneously, and the biasing effects of differences in timing in any of the steps involved in the assay procedure must be carefully investigated. Examination of these and other aspects of an assay protocol are a fundamental prerequisite to the establishment of any reliable assay procedure.

USE OF THE PRECISION PROFILE AND THE RESPONSE-ERROR RELATIONSHIP IN ASSAY DESIGN

In this particular presentation, the principal issue with which I wish to deal is the fundamental importance of the precision profile as (aside from the assessment of bias) constituting the chief guideline in the setting up of assays. This concept has lain at the root of a controversy regarding radioimmunoassay design in which I was involved with Drs Berson and Yalow over many years (e.g. Refs [1, 2]), and which I think has confused the field ever since. Central to my own thinking on this issue has been that, in the setting up of an assay, the essential objective in the selection of reagent concentrations is maximization of the precision of measurement of the analyte concentration ('dose'). In the particular case of the selection of reagents to maximize assay sensitivity, this objective may be rephrased as 'minimization of the lower limit of detection' or (tautologically) as 'maximization of the precision of measurement at zero dose'. Each of these concepts implies appropriate statistical analysis; this is in sharp contrast to Berson and Yalow's philosophy, and indeed to the approach formally adopted by most workers in the field.

As we have seen earlier, the precision profile can readily be computed (even using simple, paper-and-pencil methods, though these are time-consuming) by estimation of the relationship between the error (i.e. standard deviation) in the response metameter, and the magnitude of the response. This we may call the 'response-error relationship' (RER) (Fig. 1a, b). The combination of the error in the response at any point of the response curve with the slope of the curve at the same point yields the precision of the corresponding dose measurement as discussed earlier. In practice, the RER may be established either by taking a large number of replicates at various points along the response curve, or by setting up a large number of duplicates of samples falling randomly along the curve. The essential objective in either case is the generation of sufficient data to ensure statistically reliable estimates of the standard deviation of the response over the entire span of response values. (We have used both methods in my own laboratory for many years, each being particularly appropriate at different stages during the work-up of a particular assay technique (e.g. Ref.[4].)

The RER is of importance in a variety of different contexts. Clearly it is vital to the calculation of the precision of dose measurements per se; it is also of importance in 'weighting' data when fitting dose-response curves using computer techniques (and even, implicitly, when curve fitting 'by eye'). These aspects have been the particular concern of Dr. Rodbard, and in many of his publications he and his colleagues have discussed the calculations involved in the characterization of the RER or (as he prefers) the relationship between 'σ_y and y'. (My personal preference is to endow the relationship with a name, since σ_y and y are non-specific terms relating to any y coordinate.) Moreover, earlier

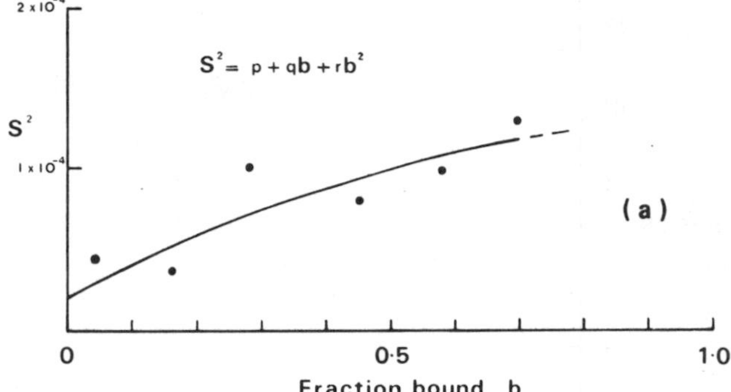

FIG.1a. Typical response-error relationship (RER) that might be observed in assay in which 'bound' fraction alone is counted and constitutes response metameter. (A suggested equation, roughly commensurate with the observed data, is shown.) The exact form of the curve will depend, in practice, on the nature of the experimental system, and on the fraction(s) counted.

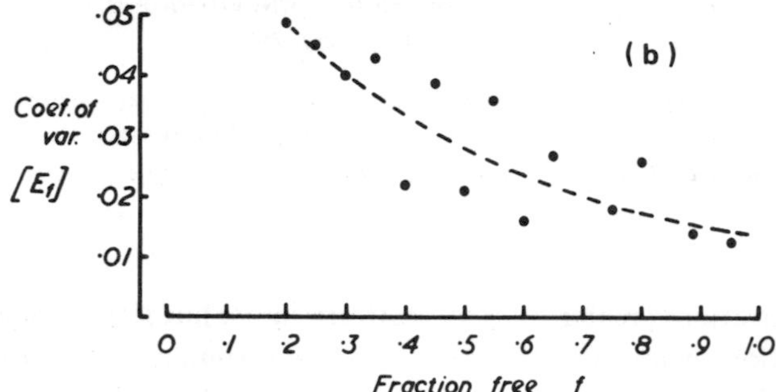

FIG.1b. Response-error relationship (RER) observed in an actual assay for aldosterone in which the free fraction alone is counted and comprises the response metameter.

in this symposium, I also showed how, with the advent of microprocessor-controlled counters, the RER can be employed to define useful sample counting times. Within the present context, the essential importance of the RER is that it constitutes a prerequisite to the determination of the precision profile. The significance of the precision profile, in turn, is that, unless it is experimentally determined, it is impossible to establish formally which of two assay systems is 'better' (in terms of their within-assay reproducibility), nor to evaluate the usefulness of any change in assay reagents or procedure. This point is illustrated in Fig.2 which shows the precision profiles yielded by three different (hypothetical) assay systems. These curves tell us that assay system 1 is the most precise for

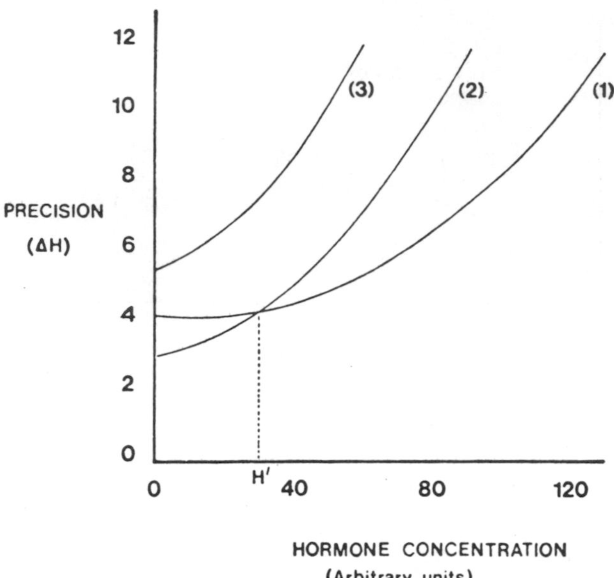

FIG.2. Comparison of three assay systems. Assay system 2 is the most sensitive, but system 1 is the most precise for concentrations greater than 35 units. Assay system 3 is inferior in performance to 1 and 2; nevertheless it approaches system 1 in sensitivity.

analyte concentrations greater than 35 arbitrary units, but is less precise than 2 at concentrations below 35. The most sensitive system is 2, since the precision of measurement of zero analyte (or zero dose), is maximal using this system.

Figure 2 is somewhat over-simplified since, in practice, the RER upon which the precision profile is based is itself subject to error. This arises from the limited amount of data which can, in practice, be utilized in establishing the exact shape and position of the curve defining the RER. I will not discuss this question in detail here, nor will I discuss the variety of mathematical expressions which can be proposed as representing the RER in different assay systems. The particular point which I wish to emphasize is that, in consequence of the statistical uncertainty attaching to the experimental determination of the RER, the corresponding precision profile is perhaps better represented as a shaded band rather than a line, and that a corresponding uncertainty attaches to the question: which of two assays is more precise at any particular analyte concentration.

To emphasize the significance both of the RER and of the precision profile in this context, the following group of figures illustrates the steps involved in assessing the performance of two assays: Fig.3 shows the response curves yielded by the two systems, Figs 4a and 4b show plots of the differences between duplicates observed in sets of samples (both standards and unknowns) included

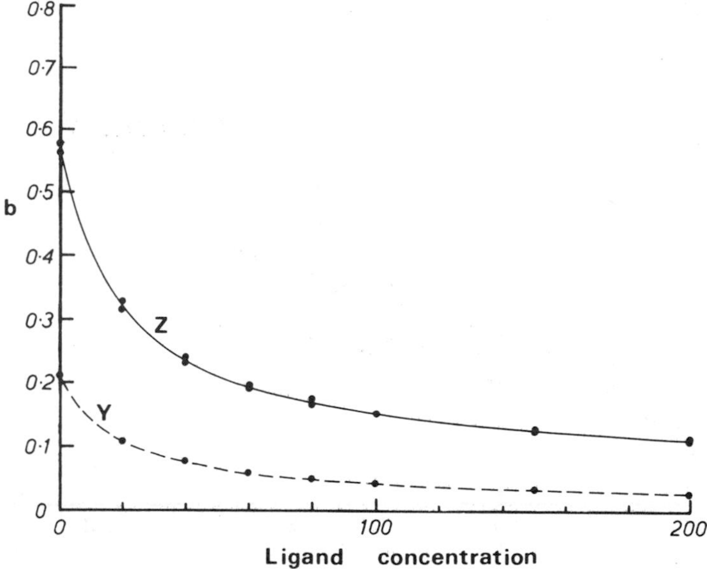

FIG.3. Response curves (plotted as fraction of label 'bound', b, versus ligand concentration) in two assay systems Y and Z.

in each system. The difference between duplicates can be used to yield an estimate, albeit a poor one, of the standard deviation of the corresponding replicate population, since

$$\sigma = \frac{\text{difference between duplicates}}{\sqrt{2}}$$

The RER corresponding to each set of duplicates is shown on the (somewhat simplistic) assumption that σ_R is linearly related to R (in this case, fraction bound). Finally, by dividing the estimate of standard deviation taken from the smoothed RER by the corresponding slope of the response curve, we can calculate the precision of the dose measurement for selected values of the dose, and plot the precision profile as shown in Fig.5. The upshot of these calculations is that we can rationally decide which of the two systems, X or Y, is the more precise, and over which analyte range.

Now in illustrating the approach, I am more concerned with the concept than with the statistical detail, which has been or will be presented in greater depth elsewhere in this discussion. The essential message that I wish to convey is that in evaluating the effect on assay performance of any change in assay procedure, such as an increase or decrease in concentration of the antibody or

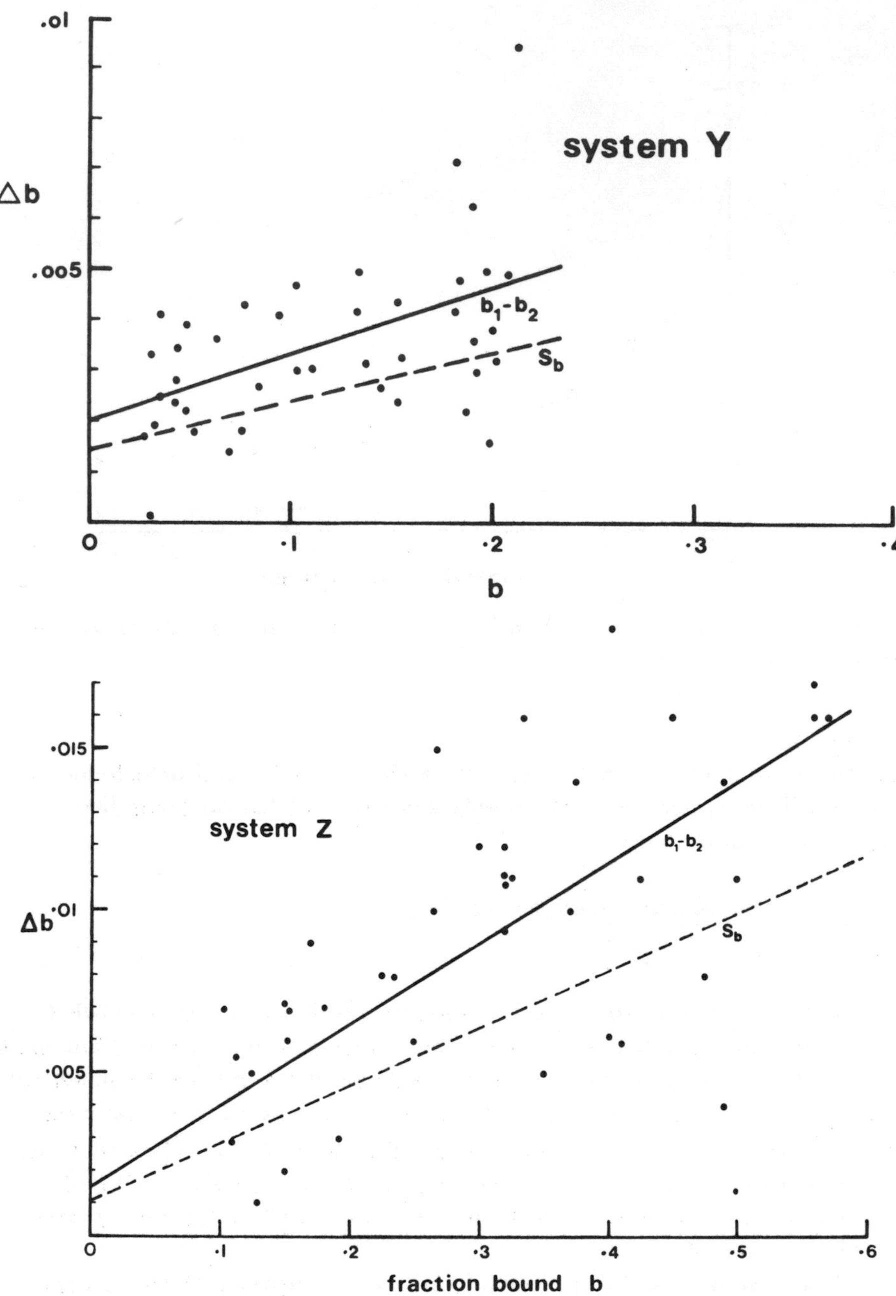

FIG.4. Observed differences between duplicate measurements, Δb (= $\overline{b_1 - b_2}$), plotted as function of fraction bound, b, in assay systems Y and Z. Also plotted is the standard deviation in b, S_b (= $\Delta b/\sqrt{2}$). Linear relationships are portrayed for the sake of simplicity.

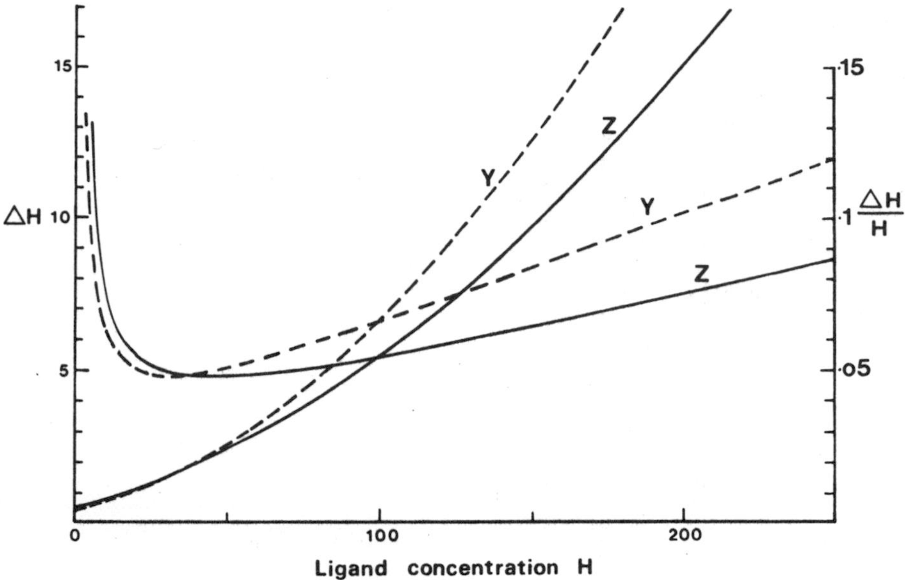

FIG.5. Precision profiles plotted from the data shown in Figs 3 and 4. Note that assay system Y is marginally more sensitive; assay system Z is more precise for values of H greater than 40 (approx.).

amount or specific activity of the labelled antigen employed, or such as would result from progressive degradation of the latter, it is almost totally irrelevant to base conclusions on the effect in the dose-response curve per se. The fundamental question must be what is the effect of the change on the precision profile?

OPTIMIZATION OF ASSAY PERFORMANCE

Simple as is the idea that it is the effect on assay precision which should guide the assayist in evaluating changes in assay procedure, and which should properly underlie the theory of saturation assay (including radioimmunoassay) methodology, it is one which is consistently ignored. To illustrate this point, the following discussion is addressed to the perennial question: what concentration of antibody, and what level of tracer binding, is necessary to obtain maximal assay sensitivity? In illustrating the correct and incorrect approaches to answering this question, I shall rely on two model assay systems (A and B) differing only in the extent of 'non-specific' binding occurring in each system, this being assumed to be zero (no 'misclassification error') in system A, and 2% in system B. In each model system I shall also assume that the 'bound' radioactivity is counted.

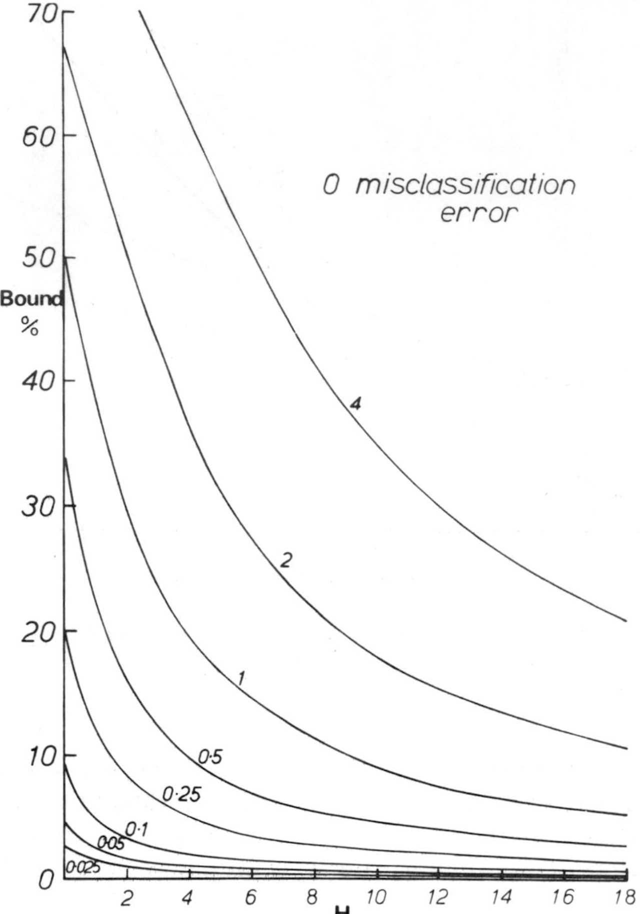

FIG.6. Family of dose-response curves theoretically anticipated in a saturation assay system without misclassification error as binding protein (antibody) concentration is increased. Concentrations of both binding protein and ligand are expressed in units of 1/K, where K = equilibrium constant.

Figures 6 and 7 show the respective families of dose-response curves that would be anticipated on the basis of the law of mass action as the concentration of antibody is progressively reduced in the two systems. As is evident, the only significant difference between the two sets of curves is that as antibody concentration approaches zero, or antigen concentration approaches infinity, the percentage of label bound approaches zero in system A and 2% (the 'non-specific' level) in system B. It is also evident that maximal slope at zero dose occurs in each case at an antibody concentration of 0.5 units, under which conditions 33% of the label is bound in system A and 35% in system B.

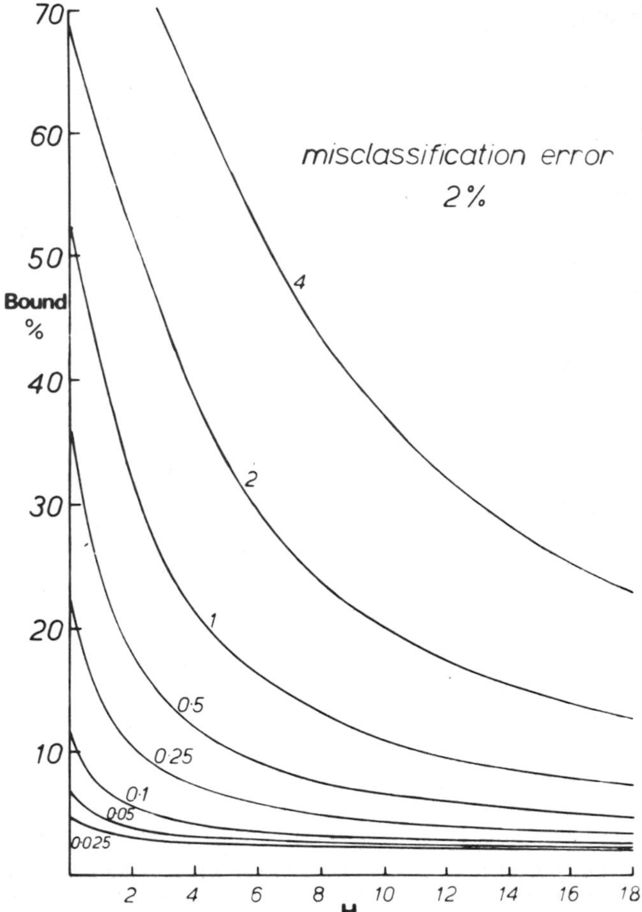

FIG. 7. Identical family of response curves to that shown in Fig. 6 anticipated in a system with a 2% 'misclassification' error.

It was the observation that maximal slope of the dose-response curve occurs using an antibody concentration binding one third of the labelled antigen that persuaded Yalow and Berson originally to maintain that maximal assay sensitivity is attained under these conditions (e.g. Ref.[5]), and this propostion has very largely subsequently dominated the radioimmunoassay field for many years. In subsequently defending this contention, Yalow and Berson have discussed the effect of increase in the slope of the dose-response curve assuming, for example a 10% statistical error in the measurement of the response [1, 6]. Moreover, by counting all samples to 1% precision, the error of the response variable could implicitly be held constant. They concluded that "assuming the experimental error is unchanged, increasing the sharpness of the dose-response curve results in a reduction

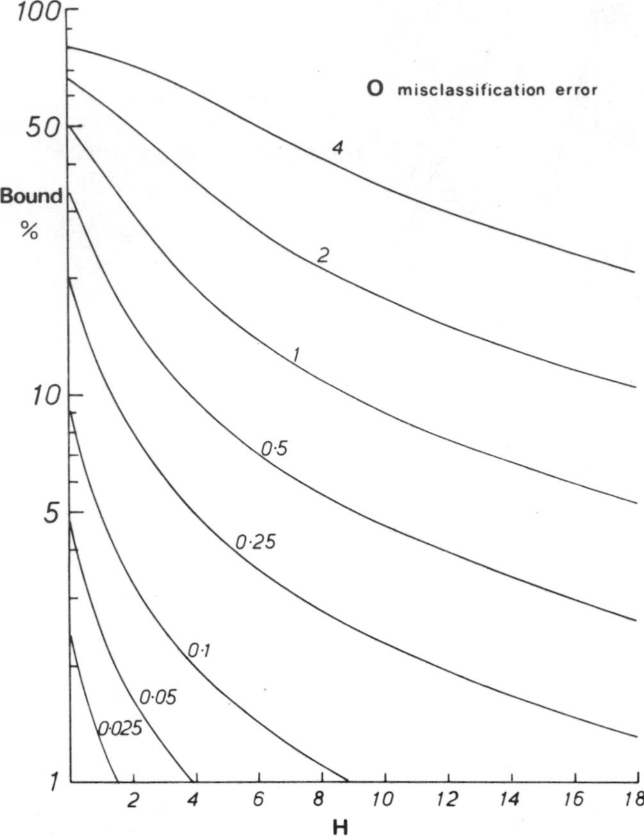

FIG.8. Family of curves corresponding to that shown in Fig.6, plotted in terms of log (percentage bound). In this coordinate system, a constant relative error in the measurement of percentage bound may be portrayed by a line of constant length on the logarithmic scale. The curve with a maximal slope at zero dose thus corresponds to the conditions of maximal sensitivity (assuming constant relative error in the response).

in minimal detectable quantity. Accordingly, we have defined sensitivity in terms of the slope of the dose-response curve".

Such a proposition is, of course, entirely valid assuming constancy of the experimental error, and provided that the dose-response curve is plotted in a co-ordinate frame in which the experimental error is portrayed as constant. Thus, assuming a constant coefficient of variation (e.g. 10%) in the response metameter, the appropriate method representing the response (fraction bound) is as the logarithm of the response, since in a plot of log of (fraction bound) against dose, a constant relative error may be represented as a line of constant length. In these

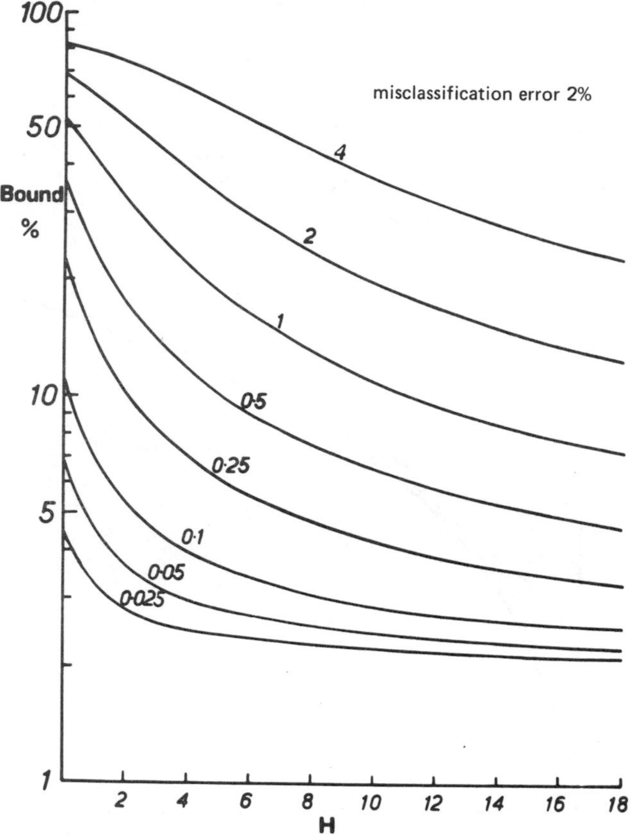

FIG. 9. Family of curves corresponding to that shown in Fig. 7, plotted in terms of log (percentage bound).

circumstances (and in these circumstances only), the slope of the response curve at any point may legitimately be taken as directly indicative of the corrresponding error in the dose measurement.

The effect of thus transforming the curves shown in Figs 6 and 7 is shown in Figs 8 and 9 in the percentages of label bound presented on logarithmic scales. The striking conclusion that may be drawn from these two sets of curves is that in system A, with no 'non-specific' binding, maximal slope at zero dose (implying a minimal detection limit) occurs as both the antibody concentration and the percentage of the label bound approach zero, whereas in system B, with a 'non-specific' binding of 2%, it occurs at an antibody concentration such that the percentage bound is in the region of 10–15%.

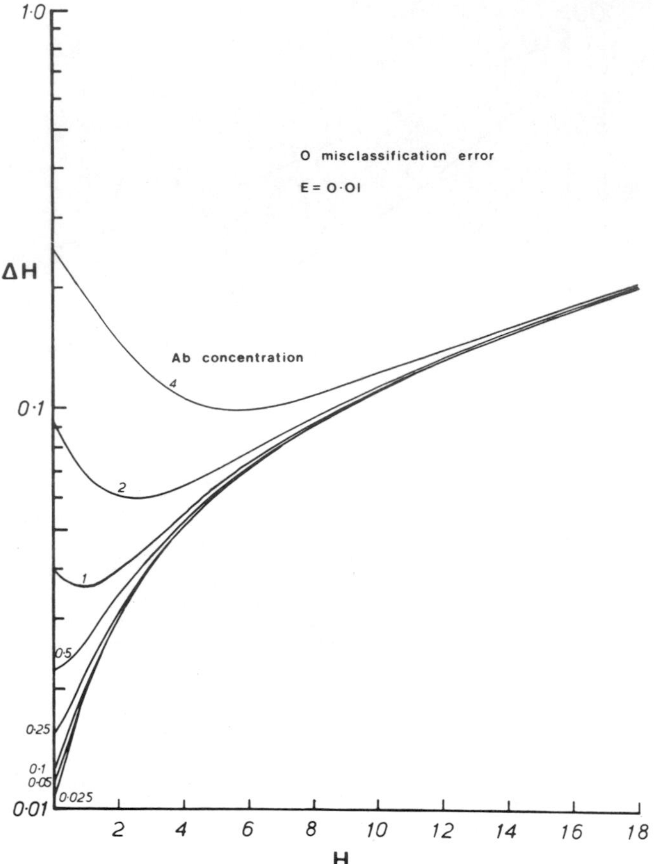

FIG.10. Precision profiles corresponding to family of curves shown in Fig.6, assuming constant relative error of 1% in measurement of 'bound' activity. Note that maximal precision at all dose levels is obtained with binding protein (antibody) concentration of zero.

However, the alternative and generally more satisfactory method of displaying the same conclusion is by calculating and plotting the corresponding precision profiles as shown in Figs 10 and 11. In deriving these particular sets of curves the assumption has been made throughout that the response (fraction or percentage bound) is estimated with a coefficient of variation of 1%. Again, we reach the conclusion that maximal precision at zero dose (i.e. maximal sensitivity) is attained by using an antibody concentration approaching zero in the absence of a'non-specifically bound' moiety.

These two sets of curves also point to a second striking conclusion; by eliminating 'non-specific' binding, maximal precision at all other analyte concentrations is obtained under conditions approaching zero binding of antigen. In contrast, in the presence of a 2% non-specific binding factor, there exists, at any predefined dose level, an optimal concentration of antibody which maximizes

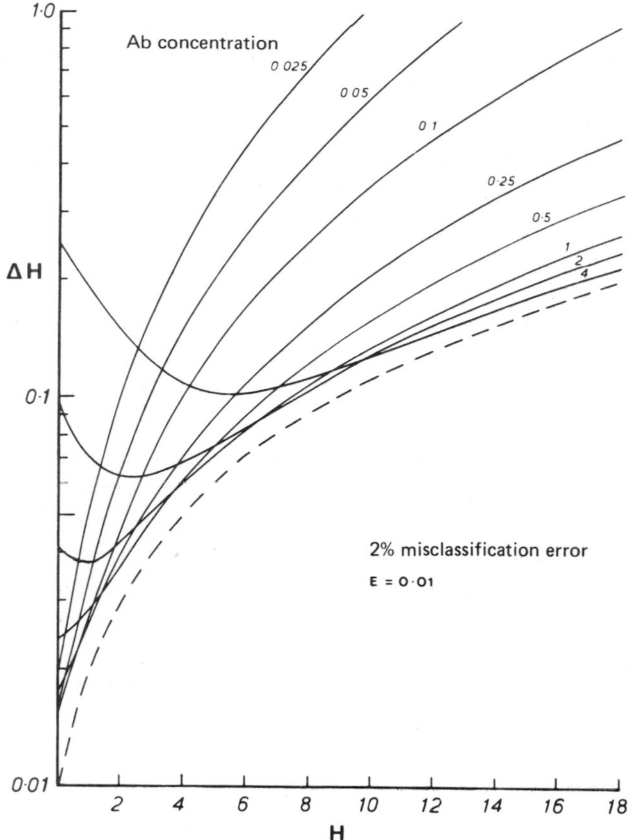

FIG.11. Precision profiles corresponding to family of curves shown in Fig. 7, under same assumptions as for Fig.10. Note that maximal precision at zero dose (maximal sensitivity) is obtained with binding protein (antibody) concentration of 0.1 units (approx. 11% binding) and that maximal precision at concentrations greater than zero is obtained using binding protein concentrations which depend on analyte concentration in question.

the precision of the dose measurement. However, in the latter situation, the dose range over which acceptable precision is attained is considerably restricted.

In presenting these figures, I recognize that they represent an over-simplification of the true situation arising in a radioimmunoassay. In particular, I have not taken into account the measurement of the labelled antigen per se. In short, it is clearly impossible to work with a 'bound fraction' equal to zero when one is relying on counting the activity in this moiety, and the conclusions discussed above are, in consequence, clearly erroneous. Moreover, for a variety of reasons (including the inevitable increase in the error of measurement of labelled antigen as the bound antigen falls) the assumption on which these curves has been based (that of a constant coefficient of variation in the measurement of the response) can never be fully maintained at all levels of the response. Nevertheless, my fundamental purpose here is both to demonstrate the correct approach to the question of the choice of assay reagents and assay design, and to expose, in a simple, non-mathematical way, one of the logical fallacies upon which radioimmunoassay practice currently rests.

Although Figs 10 and 11 are, for the reasons given above, somewhat simplistic and unreal, they point to conclusions which are broadly verifiable both by more exact algebraic [7] or computer analysis based on theoretical models of 'saturation assay' systems, and by careful experiment. In particular, certain types of radioimmunoassay do yield, in practice, a response-error relationship approximating to a constant relative error (i.e. σ_R proportional to R), and very low levels of 'non-specific' binding. Thus, the solid-phase assay systems developed by Dr. Wide display characteristics broadly in line with the above propositions; indeed, Dr. Wide takes particular care to ensure, by repeated washing of the solid-phased antibody, that 'non-specific' binding values generally fall to below 0.1% (personal communication). Under these conditions, maximal sensitivity – in accordance with valid theoretical prediction – is achieved with levels of bound antigen at zero dose falling to as low as 2%.

The almost universal belief that radioimmunoassay and other saturation assays must be set up in such a way that 30–50% of the labelled antigen is bound at zero dose is, in fact, a pure fantasy without fundamental scientific basis. In so far as the belief possesses theoretical justification, this rests on the existence in many assays of relatively high values for 'non-specific' binding which in turn have the effect, as demonstrated in Fig.11, of increasing the optimal concentration of antibody (and of zero-dose binding) required to yield maximal assay sensitivity. Nevertheless, although the effects of a high 'non-specific' binding value can be mitigated by an increase of antibody concentration (and implicitly of 'specific' binding) this is achieved at the expense of a loss in assay working range, and of a prolongation in assay incubation times.

There is a further highly important consequence of the toleration of a high level of 'non-specific' binding, that is, the vulnerability of such an assay system to impurity of the labelled material used. If all activity other than 'specifically bound' labelled antigen is removed from, for example, the solid-phased antibody employed in Dr. Wide's systems, then the existence of even very high levels of 'non-immunoreactive' impurities in the labelled preparation are entirely inconsequential. The practical implication of this is that the labelled reagent may be usable for very long periods, without significant loss in assay performance even when non-immunoreactive impurities reach levels of the order of 75% or more.

Of course, as the immunoreactive content of the labelled material falls, so will the fraction of the label which appears in the 'specifically bound' moiety. Correspondingly, the commonly employed 'percentage bound versus dose' response curve will flatten, giving rise to the erroneous belief that the performance of the assay will necessarily have deteriorated. In many assay systems, this will indeed be the case; in others, however, particularly those characterized by very low 'non-specific' binding, the performance may remain unaffected. This will be revealed, not by examination of the dose-response curve in isolation, but by comparison of the precision profiles yielded by pure and degraded label. This proposition was dramatically verified in a recent WHO Course held in Costa Rica, where the precision profiles yielded by two comparable assays, in one of which the labelled material had been deliberately degraded by 50%, were essentially identical. Such observations are of particular importance, of course, to kit manufacturers, and indeed to organizations such as the WHO, concerned in distributing reagents on a national or world-wide scale, and faced with the problem of maintaining assay performance in the face of distributed radioactive labels of uncertain purity.

In presenting the effects of antibody concentration on the precision profile as shown in Figs 10 and 11, I must emphasize that the RER observed in many assays may not take a simple form such as is implied in constancy of relative or percentage error, and that no simple transformation of the response variable, such as its transformation as log (fraction bound), yields a coordinate system in which the slope of the response curve thus correlates with precision of the dose measurement. In such cases, the formal calculation of the precision profile is obligatory in assessing the effect of any change in assay parameters.

There is much that I have necessarily omitted in this general presentation of quality control in relation to assay design. I have nevertheless felt it appropriate to address myself to the fundamental concepts which should govern an approach to these questions, and in particular to the proposition that the fundamental goals are the maximization of assay precision, and the minimization of assay bias at the dose level or over the dose range of interest. Although I imagine that no one would dissent from this view, I have attempted to demonstrate that, in practice, as a result of a basic misunderstanding of the concepts of sensitivity and precision, the radioimmunoassay field has acquired a set of mythologies which has little theoretical basis, and which has deflected attention from some of the factors which profoundly affect assay performance. In particular, I have attempted to reveal the fallacy of relying on the shape, slope and appearance of the assay dose-response curve as a guide to assay performance, and to emphasize the importance of the precision profile as the sole legitimate parameter whereby any change in assay design may be evaluated. This necessarily implies assessment of the statistical characteristics of the assay system, and in particular the evaluation, following any methodological changes (e.g. changes in antibody concentration, separation procedure, labelled antigen preparation, etc.) of the response-error relationship in addition to the corresponding dose-response curve. It is because this is not customarily done that we are forced to live with so much mythology, so much bad assay design and so much inferior assay performance. Underlying the whole of this presentation is the view that the monitoring of assays for bias and precision by conventional quality-control methods is futile if the assays have not initially been designed on the basis of their performance with regard to each of these parameters.

REFERENCES

[1] DISCUSSION, Statistics in Endocrinology (McARTHUR J.W., COLTON, T., Eds), M.I.T. Press, Cambridge, Mass. (1970) 379.

[2] DISCUSSION, Protein and Polypeptide Hormones, Part 3 (MARGOULIES, M., Ed.), Excerpta Medica Foundation, Amsterdam, New York, London (1969) 672.

[3] EKINS, R.P., NEWMAN, G.B., PIYASENA, R., BANKS, P., SLATER, J.D.H., J. Steroid Biochem. **3** (1972) 289.

[4] ALBANO, J.D.M., EKINS, R.P., MARITZ, G., TURNER, R.C., Acta Endocrinol. **70** (1972) 487.

[5] YALOW, R.S., BERSON, S.A., Radioisotopes in Medicine: In Vitro Studies (Proc. Symp. Oak Ridge Associated Universities, 1967) (HAYES, R.L., GOSWITZ, F.A., MURPHY, B.E.P., Eds), USAEC Division of Technical Information (1968) 7.

[6] BERSON, Solomon A., YALOW, Rosalyn S., Methods in Investigation and Diagnostic Endocrinology (BERSON, Solomon A., YALOW, Rosalyn S., Eds), North-Holland Publishing Co., Amsterdam (1973) 84.

[7] EKINS, R.P., NEWMAN, G.B., "Theoretical aspects of saturation analysis", Steroid Assay by Protein Binding, Transactions of the Second Karolinska Symposium on Research Methods in Reproductive Immunology, Stockholm, 1970 (DICZFALUSY, E., Ed.), Reproductive Endocrinology Research Unit, Karolinska Sjukhuset, Stockholm (1970) 11 : Acta Endocrinol. **64** Suppl. (1970) 11.

P.E. HALL *(Chairman):* Thank you again, Prof. Ekins. I invite questions on this paper.

D. FULD: Whilst I have found your paper very interesting, I have doubts as to the value of the methods that you have described in the routine daily quality control of assays, especially with kits.

P.E. HALL *(Chairman):* May I interpose a comment. We have seen, both from Prof. Ekins' and Dr. Rodbard's papers, that we can use both the response-error relationship and the dose-error relationship, or the precision profile, as quality-control parameters on a day-to-day basis; we can also use these same concepts for assay design. This has been quite clearly brought out and I anticipate that Dr. Jeffcoate will take it a stage further in his presentation.

R.P. EKINS: May I respond to Dr. Fuld's point very briefly. I have concentrated entirely in this presentation upon the importance of the response-error relationship and implicitly the precision profile in relation to assay design. Nevertheless, the same concepts are clearly applicable to the comparison of any two or more assay systems, including the comparison of assay kits. Before embarking on a quality-control programme to monitor the day-to-day performance of one's kit, it is clearly of importance to decide which of the available kits to buy.

It is at this point of decision, ideally, that the kit user should either establish for himself, or be presented with, the precision profile of the assay system, not only **within** batch, but also **between** batches. He should also have some indication of the bias of the system or, where the true result of the determination is not known, as with the majority of the protein hormones, be provided with data correlating the assay results with relevant physiological or clinical findings. Reproducibility of results is nevertheless very important, and data relating to this aspect of performance are essential.

V. KRUSE: I understand the significance of the misclassification error. How important is it to make this error low and what price must one pay to achieve this?

R.P. EKINS: Misclassification of free and bound activity is of enormous importance in radioimmunoassay. The effect of a high 'non-specific bound' moiety in the bound fraction is to constrain very greatly the operating or working range of the assay system. If one can reduce the non-specific contribution to zero, the result is a more sensitive assay, achieved with a reduction in incubation time and an increase in the working range. Such an assay is also far less vulnerable to degradation of the label, i.e. it is more 'rugged'. Many people tolerate misclassification errors of the order of 10% or more. Most assayists feel very comfortable with 'non-specific' counts of the order of 2%. In contrast, we see in Dr. Wide, for example, a meticulous and experienced assayist who takes great care to reduce non-specific counts to less than 0.1%. The very good reasons he has for doing this emerge when one examines the fundamental theory of radioimmunoassay, as I have endeavoured to do, albeit somewhat simplistically, in the illustrations I showed. As for your second question, I can do no more than assert that the benefits in terms of assay quality, speed of turn-round and overall efficiency which result from adopting assay designs in line with the concepts I have attempted to convey are very great. The work of Dr. Wide's laboratory is an excellent example of this.

R.M. LEQUIN: How do you overcome the problem that lower binding implies lower counts. Do you add more tracer and, if so, does that not impair the sensitivity?

R.P. EKINS: In my presentation I have deliberately over-simplified some of the details in order to convey fundamental concepts which are unfamiliar, or even resisted, by many people. It is true, of course, that as one reduces the amount of binding, one inevitably reduces the number of bound counts and usually increases, in consequence, the statistical errors of counting. This in turn results in an increase in the overall relative error of measurement of the assay response. On the other hand, one may, concomitantly, be increasing the slope of the dose-response curve. The net result may be an increase in precision. There is, in short, an optimum situation which may, in well-designed assays in which non-specific binding is eliminated, lie in a region of antibody concentration where only 2–10% of the label is bound. In certain simple situations, it is possible to establish the optimum concentrations of reagents algebraically (see, for example, Ekins and Newman, 1970[1]); however, in those circumstances in which the RER is represented by a complex algebraic equation, the algebraic approach to assay design becomes too difficult, and one must (as both we in our laboratory and, subsequently, Dr. Rodbard have done) build computer models to optimize assay design. In this presentation, I have been primarily concerned to establish the basic approach to the assessment of assay performance, and to show the direction in which such assessment leads us. So antipathetic are many practising assayists to the notion that a good assay can operate with less than 50% binding at zero dose that many kit manufacturers dare not sell kits that do not conform to this particular mythology.

J. GRENIER: May I suggest to Dr. Ekins that use of the precision profiles may not be the only way to look at the quality of a kit. A very important way, I think, is to compare values obtained with the kit and those obtained by a reference method of established accuracy. There is no merit in having a high sensitivity and elaborate data analysis if the values are wrong by a factor of two or more.

R.P. EKINS: You are absolutely right of course. In a presentation of such restricted duration, I have perhaps neglected to emphasize that the chosen method must be unbiased. Nevertheless, from your comments it appears that you have been primarily concerned with the measurement of substances such as the steroid hormones, for which reference methods yielding the 'true' value for the measurement exist. Naturally if the assessment of bias is possible, then it becomes mandatory to make this assessment in evaluating assay performance. On the other hand, when we enter the protein field, we are in an entirely different situation in which we are not even certain that a quantity such as 'the concentration of TSH in blood' has any absolute meaning, quite aside from there being no reference methods to measure it. Under these circumstances, assay reproducibility, as determined from within- and between-assay and between-laboratory precision profiles, is the only quality-control parameter left. Of course, a substitute for 'bias' in such assays is 'clinical usefulness', but as far as I am aware no one has yet attempted a formal quality-control programme based upon some form of numerical index of clinical utility, albeit this forms a semi-intuitive aspect of every experienced assayist's assessment of assay performance.

P.E. HALL *(Chairman)*: Thank you. I now call on on Dr. Jeffcoate to pursue some of the concepts already brought up by Prof. Ekins and Dr. Rodbard, and their practical applications in quality-control procedures.

---

[1] EKINS, R.P., NEWMAN, G.B., "Theoretical aspects of saturation analysis", Steroid Assay by Protein Binding, Transactions of the Second Karolinska Symposium on Research Methods in Reproductive Immunology, Stockholm, 1970 (DICZFALUSY, E., Ed.), Reproductive Endocrinology Research Unit, Karolinska Sjukhuset, Stockholm (1970) 11: Acta Endocrinol. **64** Suppl. 147 (1970) 11.

THE USE OF QUALITY CONTROL WITHIN A LABORATORY

S.L. JEFFCOATE
Chelsea Hospital for Women,
London, United Kingdom

1. INTRODUCTION

Most of the ideas and concepts that are discussed in this paper were generated in the minds and laboratories of Prof. Ekins and Dr. Rodbard, and they have crystallized over the past 12 months as a result of the efforts of Dr. Hall of WHO's Special Programme of Research in Human Reproduction in attempts to assess and improve the quality of the assays being done by laboratories world-wide, collaborating with WHO. I take a simple-minded approach to RIA and the results that I shall present are all experimental results obtained with no greater computing facilities than a piece of paper, a pencil and the human brain. Sophisticated computing facilities are not needed to perform quality-control procedures in RIA.

2. PRECISION, BIAS AND ACCURACY

An assay result can be in error either because of a random error, the index of which we call precision, or it can be wrong as the result of systematic error, associated with the particular method or laboratory; this is what we prefer to call bias. Thus any particular estimate can be wrong as a result of either poor precision or poor bias or both. These can be included together under the term accuracy (though others use this as a synonym for bias). 'Precision' is illustrated in Fig. 1; two methods, A and B, yield the same mean result, but A is much more precise than B. 'Bias', a systematic displacement of all observation in a sample from the true or accepted value, is illustrated in Fig.2. Here, methods A and C are equally precise but method C yields on average a mean result which is biased from that of A (giving the 'correct' result) by an amount 'b'. What is meant by the correct' value will depend on the situation. In some instances it is known but in others (most) it is not. As shown in Fig.3, we can look at a method and combine the elements of imprecision and bias together to get an estimate of the 'accuracy' of a method by taking the sum of the squares of the precision (the standard deviation) and the bias and taking the square root. This is illustrated schematically in Fig.4 which might represent the results from a number of different laboratories, for instance in an interlaboratory quality-control scheme. The precision of the laboratories (or methods) is plotted along the horizontal axis so that labs X and C are highly precise whereas labs B and E are least precise. Bias is shown plotted at right angles in the vertical axis, positive bias away from the correct value being

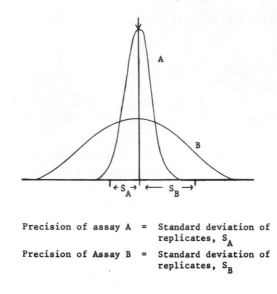

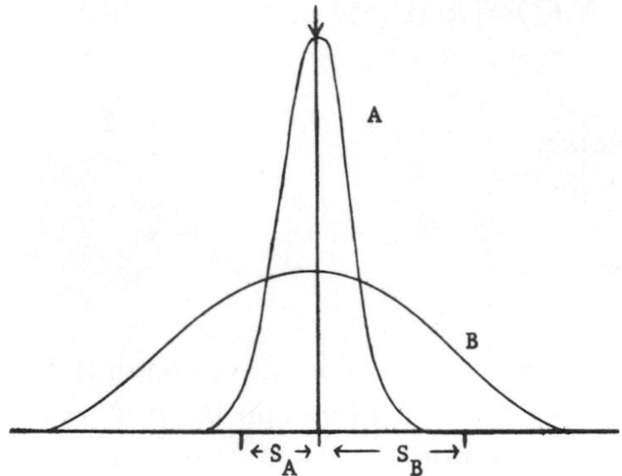

Precision of assay A = Standard deviation of replicates, S_A

Precision of Assay B = Standard deviation of replicates, S_B

FIG.1. Precision of an assay. Both assays are unbiased compared with the 'correct' value indicated by the arrow.

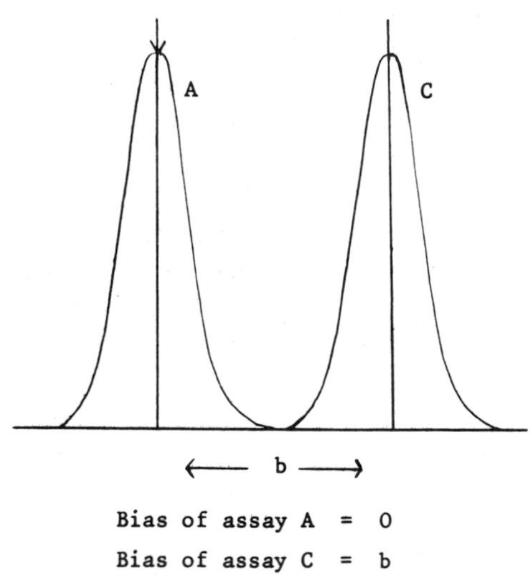

FIG.2. Bias of an assay. Assay C, though equally precise, is biased compared with assay A.

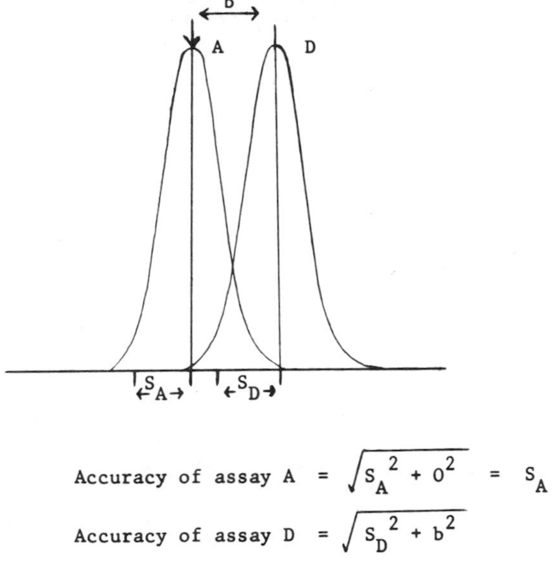

$$\text{Accuracy of assay A} = \sqrt{s_A^2 + 0^2} = s_A$$

$$\text{Accuracy of assay D} = \sqrt{s_D^2 + b^2}$$

FIG.3. Accuracy of an assay, combining the elements of bias and imprecision.

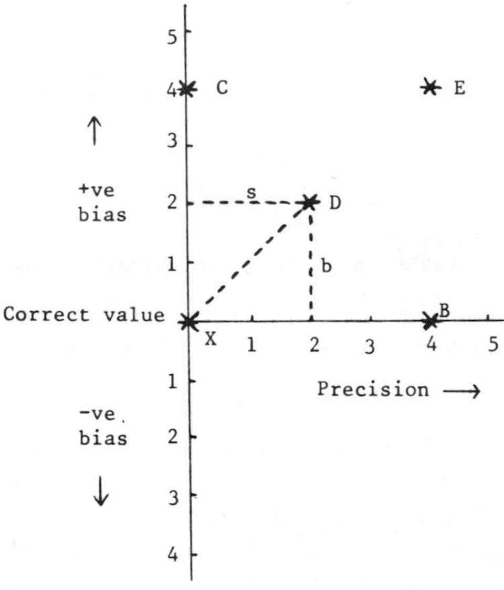

FIG.4. Precision/bias plot. The 'accuracy' (as defined in Fig.3 and text) is given by the direct distance away from the correct value at zero imprecision.

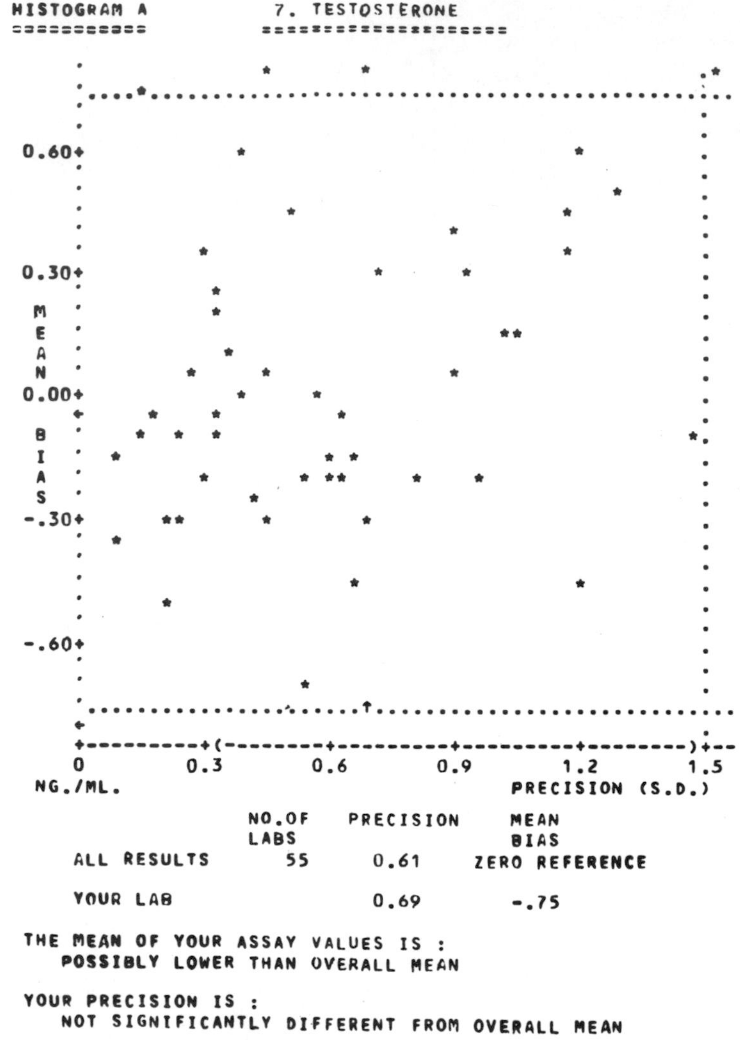

FIG.5. Precision/bias plot from WHO External Quality-Control Programme, 1976. End of period report for the testosterone assay. Each symbol represents one laboratory.

shown upwards and negative bias downwards. So the further the laboratory is up or down from the correct value, the more biased it is. Thus labs X and B are unbiased whereas C and E show marked positive bias. We can combine these two parameters by measuring the direct distance of the result from the correct value which by pythagorean geometry is the hypotenuse of a right-angled triangle. Thus it is the square root of the sum of the squares of the two sides and the same as the formula shown in Fig.3. Figure 5 shows the end of period report (for testosterone) from the World Health Organization External Quality Control Scheme for 1976 in which over 100 laboratories contributed. The individual laboratories' results are scattered about a precision-bias plot, the most imprecise laboratories being on the right of the figure, the most biased laboratories at the top and the bottom, and the most accurate laboratories are those which show the least distance measured directly to the centre point (half-way up on the left).

3. LOOKING AT THE PRECISION OF A SINGLE ASSAY

Let us look at an assay to show how some of the concepts described earlier can be used to assess its quality. A typical assay is shown in Fig.6. A number of standards and unknowns are set up usually in replicate and often, as in the case shown, in duplicate. Also included are a number of quality-control samples, preferably containing high, middle and low values spanning the range of physiological or pathological values expected in the samples. The overall precision of such an assay can be calculated in several ways. First, we can plot (or calculate without actually plotting) the response-error relationship (RER). The variation in the replicates is plotted against the mean of the replicates as shown in Fig.7. The variation can be the standard deviation or the variance, or (for duplicates) the differences. The regression line fitted to these points has a slope which is a measure of the overall precision of the assay. This can be measured and recorded. We also look at the precision of the quality-control samples. Each sample appears six times in the assay, twice each at the beginning, in the middle and at the end, and thus a good estimate of the overall within-assay precision of those samples can be obtained. This will form a relatively simple precision profile. Figure 8 shows a full precision profile plotted using data from the WHO Matched Reagent Programme for progesterone: the two laboratories are about 3000 miles apart, and were using exactly the same materials and methods. It is also possible to use the precision profile to choose between reagents, and in the example shown in Fig.9 we were trying to choose between two cortisol antisera for use in the WHO programme. There were three different laboratories (1, 2 and 8) testing two antisera (J and K). In an international reagent programme, it is necessary to see that the method is going to travel, so at the outset the testing is done internationally. The three laboratories 1, 2 and 8 were in different continents and although there are some differences between the three laboratories, they all show that antiserum K had a precision greater than that of antiserum J at low levels. This was a situation where the difference was marked; in situations where the differences are not marked it becomes more important to use the precision profiles concept.

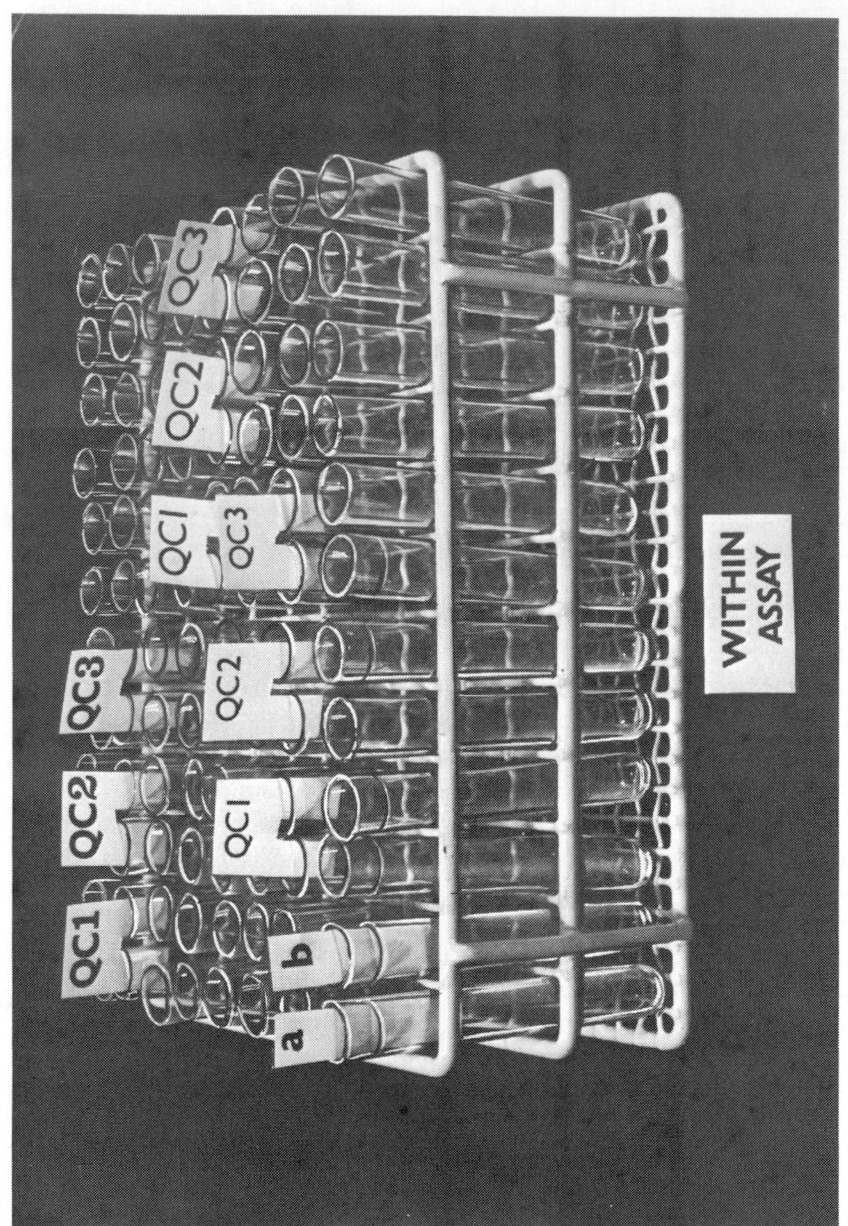

FIG. 6. Typical assay composed of duplicates, a and b, standards and unknown samples (not indicated) and samples of quality-control pools (QC_1, QC_2 and QC_3) at three different concentrations placed at three different positions in the assay.

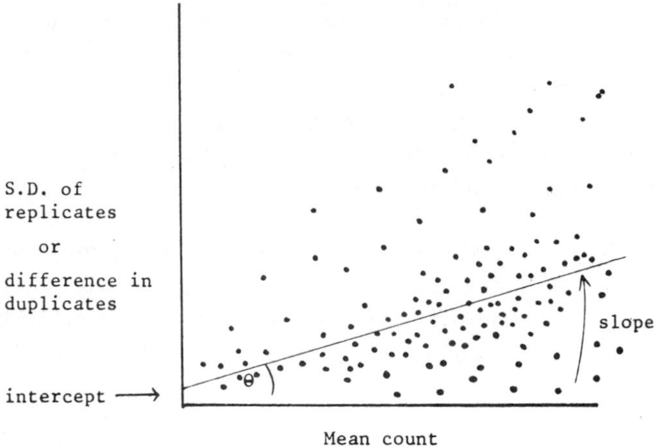

FIG.7. Response-error relationship of an assay. The slope indicates the overall within-assay precision. The intercept is usually small and can be fixed at zero if required.

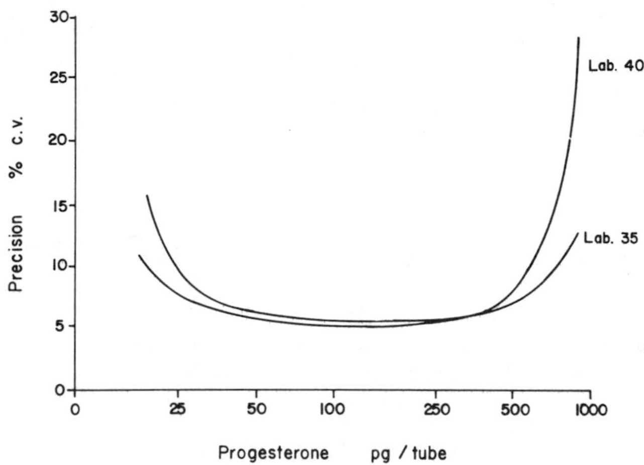

FIG.8. Precision profiles for progesterone obtained by two laboratories (3 000 miles apart) participating in the WHO Matched Reagent Programme.

4. BIAS OR SYSTEMATIC ERRORS

These can occur:

(a) *Between replicates,* as a result, for instance of one probe being partially blocked in a double-probe automatic dispensing system, so that replicate A will consistently be different from replicate B.

(b) There can also be *drift within an assay* (or bias across an assay) for instance as a result of a charcoal separation procedure which has not been carefully optimized.
(c) There can also be bias *from assay to assay.*
(d) Finally, there is the bias *between laboratories* arising from differences in environment and methodologies.

Drift across an assay can only be assessed by including tubes within the assay which are capable of detecting it, by for example setting up B_0 tubes, NSB tubes or QC tubes at different points in the assay and then plotting the counts against the position of the assay and testing the line for its slope (Fig.10).

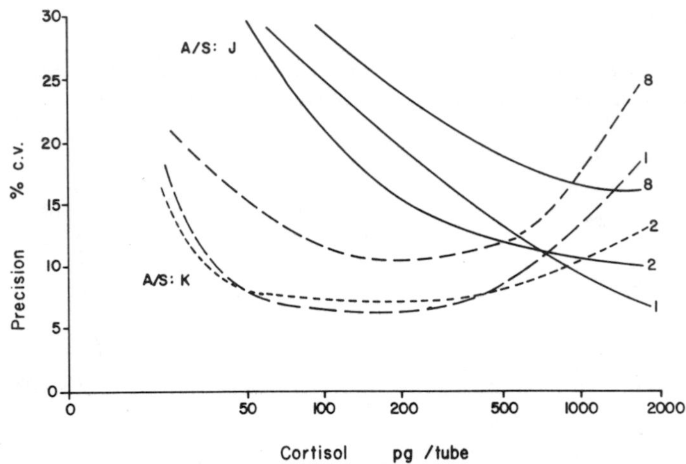

FIG.9. Precision profiles for cortisol obtained by three laboratories (1, 2 and 8) testing two antisera (J and K) in the WHO Matched Reagent Programme.

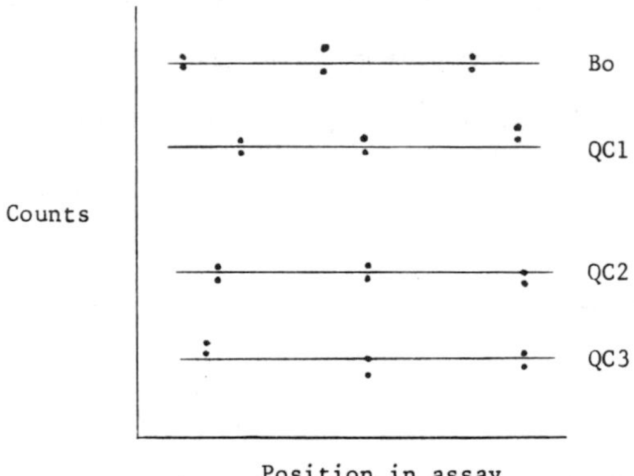

FIG.10. Within-assay drift control in an assay. Plotting the counts of 'drift-control tubes' against their position should give a line with zero slope.

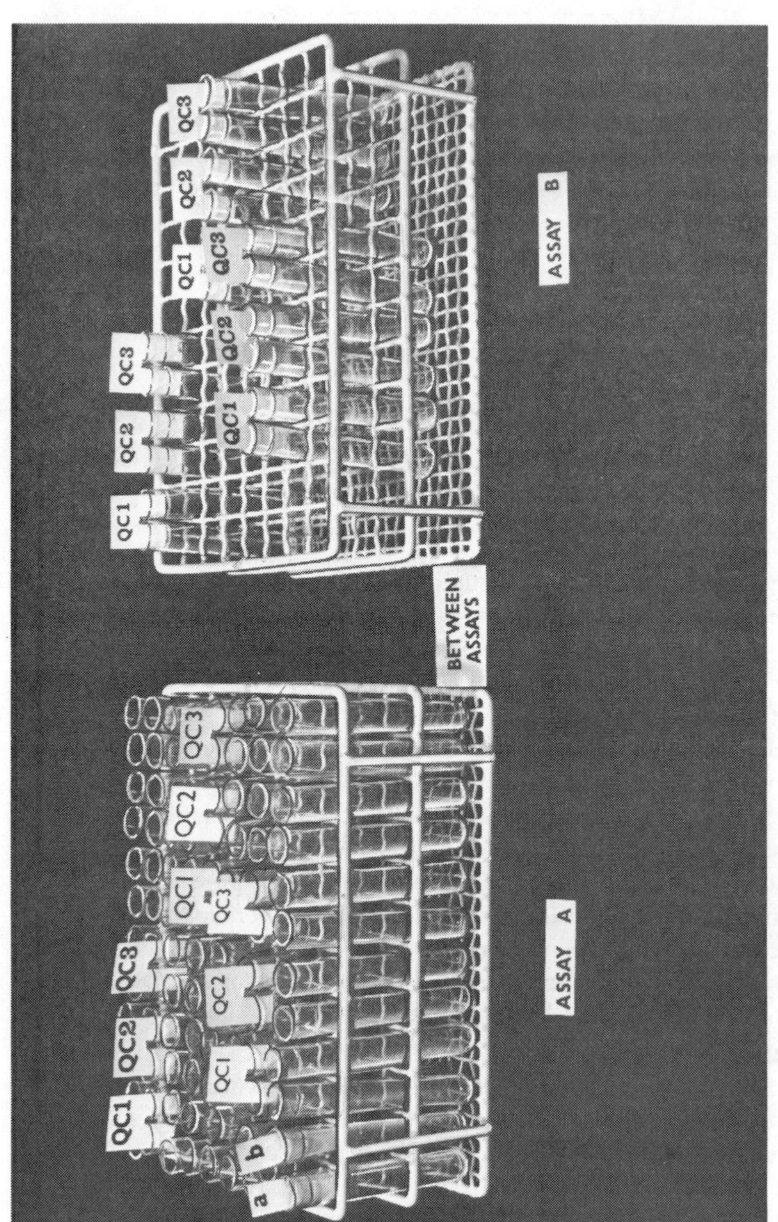

FIG.11. Use of quality-control pools in every assay to check between-assay reproducibility.

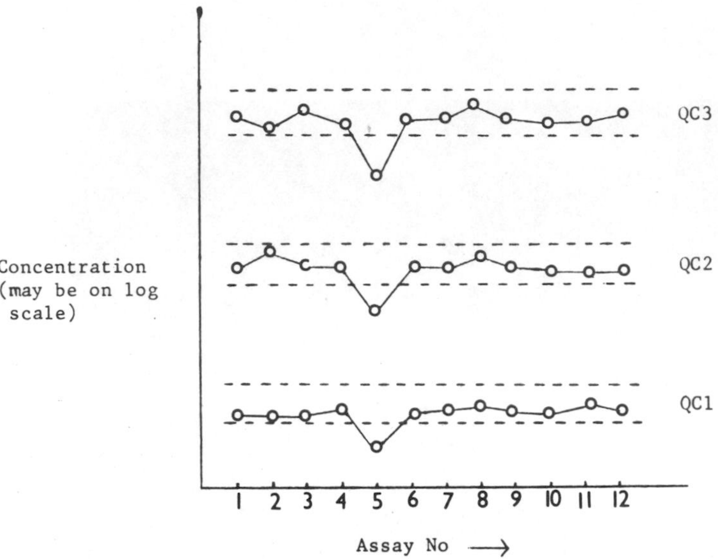

FIG.12. Between-assay reproducibility as shown by a control chart.

There are ways of normalizing all these data so that the information can be pooled, Comparing the middle of the assay with each end, or one end with the other, will check on any drift occurring within the assay. All these procedures are best carried out as part of an automated calculation package; this can be done with a small desk-top calculator.

When comparing the results from one assay with those of another within a laboratory, quality-control tubes must be set up on each occasion on each assay (Fig.11). Again, high, middle and low QC pools are preferable and by comparing the potency estimates from one assay to another, a check can be made on the assay-to-assay reproducibility. Control charts can be plotted (Fig.12) and after a number of assays (at least ten), the mean, and perhaps confidence limits, for each of these three pools can be estimated. There are many different variants on this, e.g. using 'cusum' (cumulative sum) charts or normalizing the data so that information can be pooled. Looking now at the assay-to-assay precision of those same three pools, a crude three-point precision profile can be drawn (Fig.13). The between-assay precision includes the within-assay precision, or lack of it, of the two assays and, in addition, there will be an element of imprecision which is occurring because the assay is being done on a different day, with a different batch of buffer or a different technician. Figure 14 shows schematically the precision profiles obtained using all the information in an assay, not just the three quality-control pools. The gap between the two profiles represents the assay-to-assay bias. Note how the concepts of precision and bias overlap.

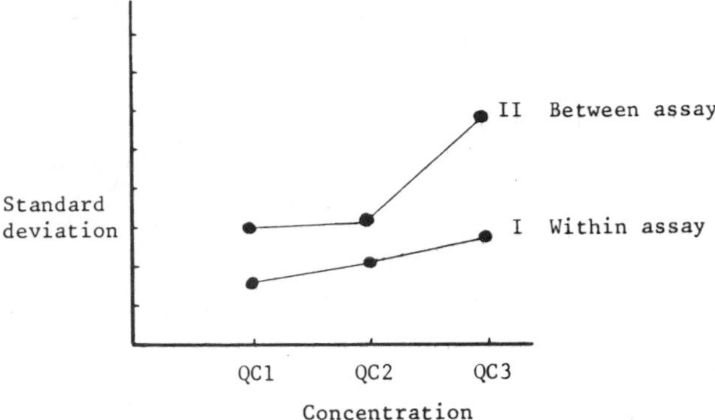

FIG.13. Precision profiles obtained with samples of three quality-control pools showing the within-assay and between-assay reproducibility at three different concentrations. The gap between the two profiles represents the between-assay component of the total variation.

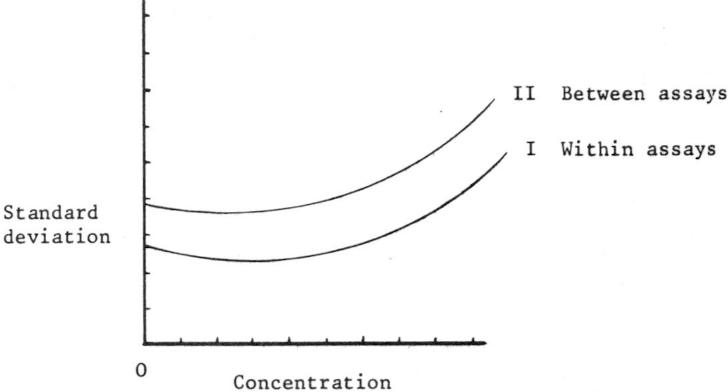

FIG.14. Within-assay and between-assay precision profiles derived from all assay results (see also Fig. 13).

When looking at between-laboratory precision (Fig.15) there will be a third tier, expressing differences in methodology or environment in different laboratories. The between-laboratory precision again reflects the bias of the individual members. Note also that a bias profile can be plotted (Fig.16) showing that the bias of a method (or a laboratory) may be dose-related.

5. HOW TO USE QUALITY CONTROL

Quality control in RIA is used for two separate purposes. The longer-term one is to monitor and improve the overall design of the assay (as discussed by Prof. Ekins elsewhere in this symposium). The more immediate function is to

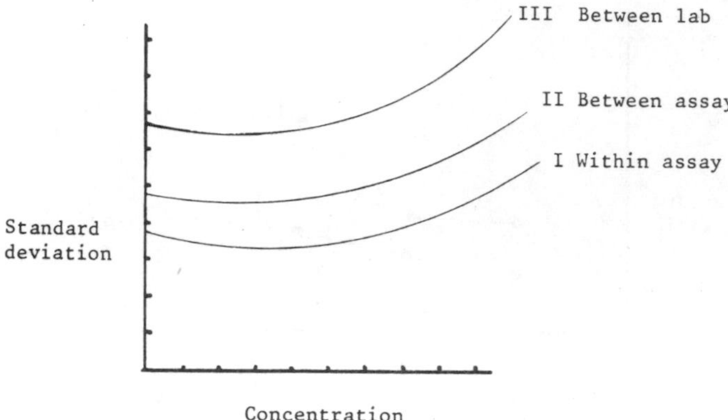

FIG.15. Within-assay, between-assay and between-laboratory precision profiles. The gap between profiles II and III represents the between-laboratory component of the total variation (due to differences in reagents, methods, etc).

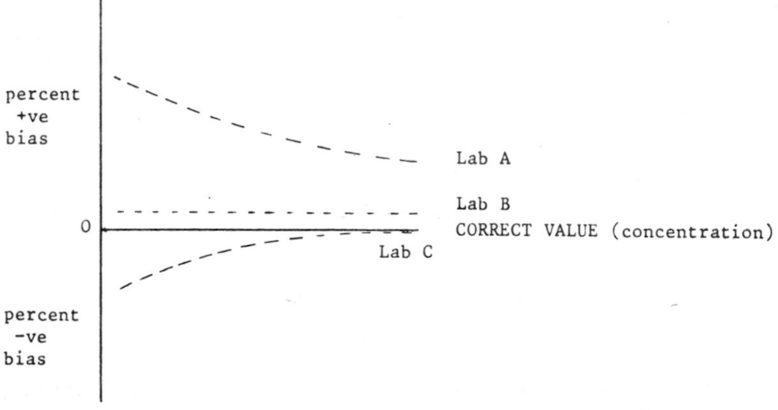

FIG.16. Bias profiles for three laboratories, showing the relationship between correct value of measured concentration and per cent bias.

identify individual samples in the assay or in some instances, complete assays, in which quality is so bad that the results are unreliable and have to be rejected. The establishing of criteria for rejection on the basis of the quality-control procedures is a difficult and neglected topic. An initial proviso is that the rejection criteria cannot and should not be inflexible, each laboratory deciding them for itself for each particular assay – and being prepared to bend the criteria in certain situations. For example, rather strict rejection criteria may be required if the level needs to be known accurately, or if the differences between samples before and after treatment, or between physiological and pathological levels are narrow.

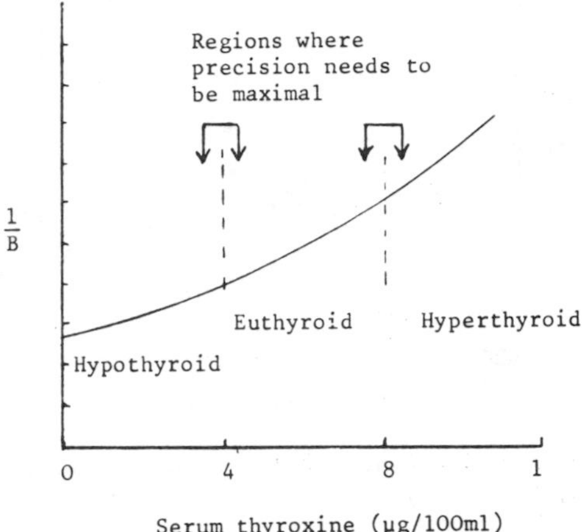

FIG.17. Regions of maximum clinical interest in which scrutiny of samples for rejection needs to be more strict.

Thus, if the rise in plasma progesterone in the luteal phase of the cycle is being used as an index of ovulation, where there might be a rise from 0.3 to 18 ng/ml, a less precise assay may be acceptable. There might be some situations where the rejection criteria are varied even within an assay, as illustrated in Fig.17 for a thyroxine assay where the rejection criteria are more strict in the region of maximal clinical doubt.

(a) Criteria for rejection

For many years we have used a simple rule of thumb for individual samples: any duplicates whose difference is more than 10% of the mean should be scrutinized and considered for rejection on the basis of imprecision. Figure 18 shows this schematically the differences in counts being plotted against the mean count. The RER of the whole assay is shown as the solid line. Any samples over a slope of 0.1 (shown by the dotted line) are considered for rejection. This is one arbitrary criterion, others might prefer different criteria.

Rejection of complete assays might be considered because of poor overall precision (e.g. a change in the slope of the response-error relationship) or significant bias. Figure 19 illustrates a particular assay which has been run a number of times (n) and a mean RER slope for these n assays obtained. Suddenly in the next assay (n+1) something has happened to the slope – it might be due to a change of buffer or the tracer having deteriorated or the technician having emotional problems, but something has happened to assay precision. When this occurs the assay should be considered for complete rejection on the basis of

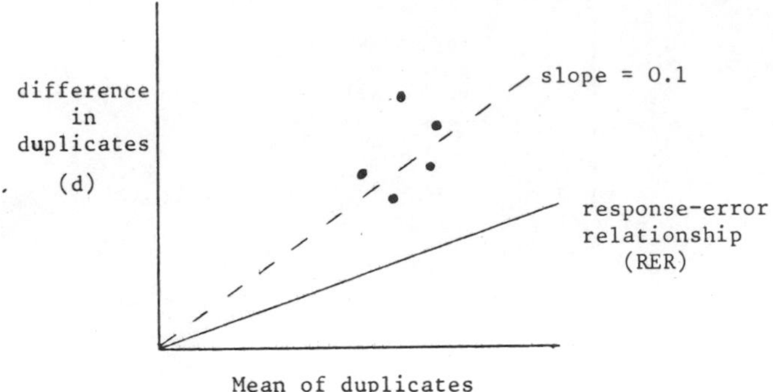

FIG.18. Rejection of samples with discrepant duplicates. In this case, three duplicates differ by more than 10% of their mean.

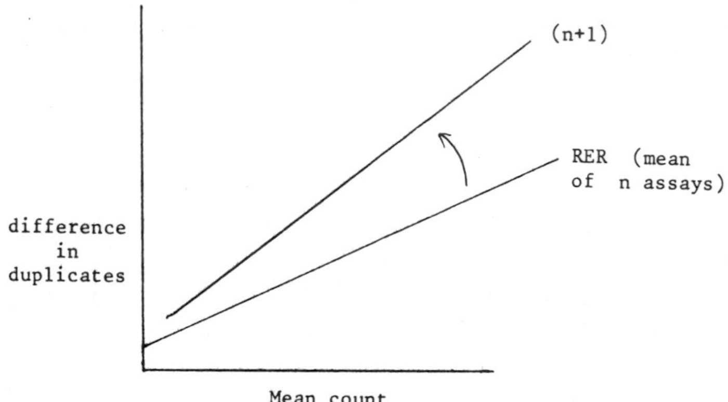

FIG.19. Use of slope of response-error relationship to indicate when on-assay is unacceptably imprecise.

unacceptable precision. However, there is an important point to be made here: that a change in this RER slope should be taken not so much as a reason for rejection of assays, although it may be used for that purpose, but more as a stimulus to seek the possible causes of deterioration within the laboratory.

Finally, the difficult question of the rejection of assays on the basis of bias in results between assays. Assaying quality-control samples in every assay may reveal that the QC samples are on occasion giving results which are significantly different from the results expected for those pools. What does one do with such assays? Again it is unwise to establish rigid criteria. The following are some that we have considered using in our laboratory. If two out of the three QC samples are more than two standard deviations in the same direction from the expected (correct) value, then we consider rejecting that assay on the basis of bias. If all

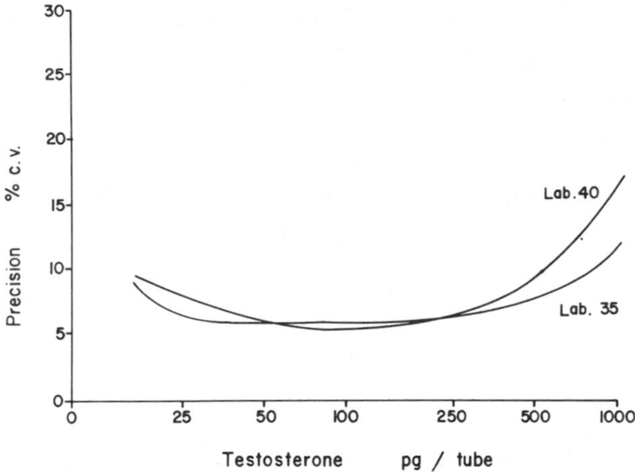

FIG.20. Benefits of assay standardization. Precision profiles for testosterone obtained by two laboratories (3 000 miles apart) participating in the WHO Matched Reagent Programme (see also Fig. 8).

three of them are more than one standard deviation, again all in the same direction from the expected (correct) value, then we consider rejecting that assay. This is at the moment only an experimental set of criteria, we are not sure yet how it is going to work in practice – we may find that we are rejecting too many assays. As for precision, marked bias between assays should not be taken so much as a reason for rejecting an assay but more as a stimulus to develop assays which are less susceptible to variations between assays. Such assays are called **robust** or **rugged** assays. These are assays which are not susceptible to changes from assay to assay in buffer or technician or quality of the label, etc.

(b) Development of high-quality assays

There are three ways in which high quality assays can be developed and maintained. The first is a result of staff education and an improvement in the laboratory environment and equipment. The second is the development of assays which are rugged, and the third is the concept of standardization both of reagents and methodology. I want to introduce this concept briefly here. Figure 20 shows one of the results of standardization. When the same two laboratories as in Fig.8 assayed testosterone, using the same methodology, the same materials and method manual, they obtained identical precision profiles. This can be achieved by providing laboratories with reagents which have been carefully characterized and matched together in an assay kit. As Prof. Ekins pointed out elsewhere in this symposium, this is the only way we are going to achieve comparability of results in assays which are, to use his terminology, analytically invalid.

D.K. HAZRA: As you have pointed out, standardized reagents are a prerequisite for high-quality assays. All laboratories in the world obviously cannot be supplied with reagents from the same source. Can you envisage standardized reagents being used in a two-tiered or multi-tiered system?

S.L. JEFFCOATE: Yes, I think we must envisage a multi-tiered system. This is already happening in the United Kingdom, where we have a national reagents scheme and a national quality-control scheme, below these a number of developing regional schemes, and below these even a number of developing smaller schemes. Now these schemes cannot all use exactly the same reagents. But if they inter-digitate, we can ensure comparability of results.

S.A. SIDDIQUI: Dr. Jeffcoate, you have touched upon some very important aspects of quality control in routine laboratories, and you have talked about various sources of bias which lead to imprecision in radioimmunoassay. However, you have not mentioned one source of bias, namely the human tendency to record a result, especially where the visual means are used, that is nearest to the known mean. Such bias may arise from the repetitive and tedious nature of radioimmunoassay. We have observed this effect in measurements on pooled sera in our own laboratory. I wonder whether you have any solution?

S.L. JEFFCOATE: Yes, I think this is a very real point. With the best will in the world, whether consciously or unconsciously, people tend to get the results that they are supposed to get. The advantages of automation are clear, here, because a machine cannot know what results it is supposed to get.

D. RODBARD: May I comment on this point as a statistician? Quality-control samples should be randomized and measured 'double blind'. Indeed this is about the only way in which you can treat them if, for example, you are a clinician and want to decide to which laboratory to send your samples. If a laboratory knows that its performance is being tested, it may give very special care to the samples in question.

R.M. LEQUIN: It seems to me that good precision is more important than freedom from bias in assay. May I invite Dr. Jeffcoate's comments on this point.

S.L. JEFFCOATE: It is obviously true that a laboratory which is precise but biased with respect to other laboratories will provide results which are internally consistent and valuable. Whether it is essential for a group of laboratories to get results in very close numerical agreement depends on their functions. If they are engaged in a multi-centre research project, it is clearly essential that they do so. There are other advantages in freedom from bias. Clinicians often move from hospital to hospital and difficulties may arise if they have to adjust to different normal ranges in different laboratories. You have, however, touched upon two very important points, namely that the group mean for a quantity measured by a group of laboratories may not be the true value and that any individual laboratory may be expected to show some bias.

R.P. EKINS: In comparing possibly invalid methods, one must also be aware of the fundamental problem that the bias may change from one sample to another depending on the spectrum of substances present in the sample.

D. FULD: For the past two years we have developed and employed a computerized quality-control system in our laboratory. The samples are analysed in a 'double blind' fashion: the samples are submitted in such a manner that the technicians do not know which samples are the quality-control samples. As a general rule, we use samples derived from the collaborative programme of The American College of Pathologists. Accordingly, it is possible to compare our results with those coming from more than 100 different laboratories and to analyse bias both within laboratories and between laboratories. In my opinion, one, two, or even three quality-control samples are not sufficient to enable one to say whether or not an assay has been performed 'correctly'. One should have a much larger number of observations (degrees of freedom) in order to make reliable statements of this type. Accordingly, we rely very heavily on the analysis of the variance of y versus $\bar{y}$ (σ_y^2 versus $\bar{y}$). By analysing the distribution of the ratio $\sigma_v^2/\bar{y}$, we are able to detect outliers, and reject them in comparison with the chi-square distribution. While we utilize the between-laboratory study as a means to detect bias, we utilize the data generated within any given assay as the basis to detect large random errors. Thus, we are able to perform a very thorough analysis and make reliable statements as to whether a sample or assay is 'in line' with previous results. While I do not maintain this is the only way to perform these analyses, it has certainly proven to be satisfactory in large-scale use in practice.

D. RODBARD: I would agree that the use of a chi-square test in the context of an analysis of σ_y^2 versus y provides an objective, statistically valid basis for rejecting an individual point, or for rejecting an entire assay as being out of control with regard to the magnitude of the random errors in the response variable. This test is objective, and the only arbitrary decision is the choice of the probability level selected to reject outliers under the 'null hypothesis'. In other words, we must decide how many samples we are willing to reject as presumptive outliers, when in fact we are simply dealing with random sampling error. As a general rule, I would suggest the use of either 'one in 200' ($P = 0.005$) or 'one in 1000' ($P = 0.001$). This means that in a 1000-sample assay, we might expect (on the average) to reject either five samples or one sample (respectively) as subject to unsatisfactory agreement between duplicates, if indeed the samples had been in control and we were simply dealing with a 'bad luck' situation. Once the probability of this type of error has been specified, then the analysis of σ_y^2 versus y provides an objective basis for rejecting an individual point or for rejecting an entire assay. Personally, I prefer to utilize an 'F-test' rather than a chi-square test, but this is simply a matter of convention, and the two approaches are nearly interchangeable. I would like to compliment Dr. Fuld for being one of the first, if not the first, person to utilize this type of analysis on a large-scale routine basis.

A. MALKIN: As a clinical biochemist, involved for years in quality-control procedures on a local, a provincial and an international level, I am sceptical as to the practicability of imposing standardized procedures such as those described by Dr. Jeffcoate on a broad scale.

R.P. EKINS: The problem that you mention is one that we faced in the United Kingdom some two or three years ago following the establishment there of the Supraregional Assay Service. It was obvious to one or two of us then that the only way we were going to bring the participating laboratories into numerical agreement was by complete replication, in each laboratory, of reagents and procedures. Clearly, if one has a situation in which a clinician can send his sample to any one of a number of laboratories, it is absolutely imperative that these laboratories should be producing identical results. Initially there was a lot opposition to the concept of common procedures, but the results of external quality-control schemes, which consistently revealed wide disagreements between participating laboratories, gradually persuaded them of the necessity of its adoption. At the present time, the laboratories concerned with providing assay services within the United Kingdom are attempting to establish 'packaged' reagents and procedures for their common use. This takes considerable time because, apart from overcoming the psychological resistance of the users, one must identify in some objective manner the most 'rugged' available procedure, that is, the one that displays the least variability in within- and between-batch and between-laboratory precision profiles. There is also, of course, the problem of ensuring a fairly long-term supply of the relevant reagents. Whether or not we shall succeed in this quest I do not know, although I am hopeful. If we do not achieve agreement in these matters, we shall have something approaching chaos in the field of measurement of hormones and similar substances, and it will be totally impossible for the clinician to interpret assay results reliably except by establishing a particular and stable relationship with a single laboratory. The latter may be the only solution, but it is a precarious one. We have witnessed assay results obtained in one laboratory being interpreted entirely erroneously in the light of ranges obtained in another, a situation which at best reduces the clinical value of the data and at worst makes them even dangerous.

A. MALKIN: Even in Toronto, where we have seven major university-affiliated teaching hospitals, with about 5 000 beds, we cannot agree among ourselves as to the best assay procedure for a given substance so I do not see how such agreement could ever be reached on a world-wide scale.

R.P. EKINS: There are proper statistical procedures for the evaluation of assay procedures applicable to the results of a group of collaborating laboratories. I agree that the problem is to persuade the laboratories to collaborate.

P.E. HALL *(Chairman):* It is noteworthy that both in the United Kingdom Supraregional Assay Service and in the WHO Special Programme of Research, Development and Research Training in Human Reproduction, after a period of time laboratories have started to collaborate in this respect. It is necessary, though, to demonstrate that a quality-control programme is of use to the investigator, in order to obtain such collaboration.

D. RODBARD: I am somewhat pessimistic, and much closer to Dr. Malkins' opinion, regarding the acceptance of 'universal' reagents, 'universal' standards and 'universal' assay systems. There are great difficulties in achieving such standardization and, indeed, non-standardized assays are essential for many research purposes. For instance, one antiserum may detect the amino-terminal end of parathyroid hormone, while another one detects the carboxy-terminal end. Both assay systems may be needed to obtain certain physiological insights. Hence, we must retain and foster the variability in assay methods for research purposes. However, in the context of routine clinical applications, we do seek the elusive goal of attempting to standardize the method, and hence (hopefully) the normal ranges and the physiological interpretation of results. In this context, we do need to strive for the 'universal' method insofar as possible. However, we must compromise between long-term stability within a given laboratory and uniformity between laboratories. A given antiserum with a given titre might be usable in one laboratory for 100 years, or in 100 laboratories for one year each. All of our reagents are present in finite supply. Hence, it is impossible for all laboratories in the world to utilize exactly the same reagents for radioimmunoassays. Long-term stability within a laboratory or within a small cluster of laboratories may be more important than uniformity of results among a large number of laboratories, if the latter leads to rapid depletion of reagents. The compromise between these two approaches will depend on the mobility of the patient population and the relative needs for reproducibility within an institution and reproducibility between institutions.

R.P. EKINS: Can I make just one added point, which stems directly from my first presentation in this round-table discussion, namely that we must also strive towards valid analytical methods. Only when methods are valid in the sense that we have been discussing will it be possible for assayists – in Canada or elsewhere – to carry out their own procedures and hope to reach agreement. While we are struggling with invalid assay methods, the only means of replicating each other's results is by the adoption of common procedures.

W.G. WOOD: I agree fully with what Prof. Ekins has said. It is important to differentiate between a centralized health service such as that in the United Kingdom, where the Supraregional Assay Service undertakes the more difficult assays, and a decentralized service such as that in the Federal Republic of Germany, where there are many small laboratories carrying out assays but lacking means to label antigens or to raise or characterize antisera, and therefore depending on kits, on their protocols and on the reproducibility of their components. This situation generates great competition between commercial enterprises which would like to capture the market and it is essential to make a careful selection between available kits, ensuring that those giving unacceptable results are rejected and those giving acceptable results are adequately standardized. I may refer particularly to the spate of 'same-day' TSH kits which have recently appeared on the market – I currently have information on five such – and which, in my eyes, have little or no value. We have tested such kits in our laboratory against the International Reference Preparation No. 68/38 and found them to give completely false results. Although the quality of commercial kit components has improved greatly over the past two years, the protocols are often far from satisfactory. A further problem is that commercial firms may change their protocols, so that the results of assays carried out today may not be comparable with those obtained three, six or nine months hence. This may be less likely in the centralized British system than in our decentralized one.

P.E. HALL (*Chairman*): One of the messages that should have come out of this round-table discussion is that there are methods of comparing kits. As you have inferred, what is required is the establishment and publication of appropriate criteria for what constitutes a good or bad kit. This would assist users in choosing kits as well as aiding professional or governmental bodies in kit selection.

R.P. EKINS: I would just like to add that I sympathize greatly with Dr. Wood, because I find it very necessary to have some degree of stability in assay procedures if the clinician is to learn to interpret the results that they yield. It may for this reason be necessary to continue to use a relatively inferior assay system for longer than one might wish in order not to totally disorientate the clinician in his interpretations. Certainly, it would seem to me very dangerous to switch kits or procedures every six months, and even more dangerous if a kit manufacturer changes one of the key reagents, such as the antibody, without notifying the user. Ideally, for maximal clinical benefit, I think that all laboratories within a given region or country should agree to adopt a common kit or procedure for a period of a year or two. The present situation, in which we have a multiplicity of kits all yielding different results, even in the case of simple chemical substances such as thyroxine, seems to me totally against the interests of the patients, and only in the interests of the kit manufacturers and those who, in countries unlike the United Kingdom, are paid a fee for each assay they perform.

R.J. BAYLY: Involved as I am with a commercial supplier, I agree entirely with Dr. Wood and would emphasize that the remedy is in the hands of the users, who should apply the sort of methods that Prof. Ekins has indicated to verify kit performance. I should like also to refer to quality-control schemes using distributed samples, such as are carried out by The American College of Pathologists. These are very valuable, but my great worry about them is that the samples distributed may not be representative of the samples actually measured. As ... reminded us, many of our assays are analytically invalid. This ...d difficulty when, for example, animal sera are distributed for ... instead of human sera.

K. PAINTER: Prof. Ekins has suggested that ideally the antibody concentration should approach zero, while Dr. Rodbard has suggested that each sample should be measured in as many as 30 replicates. But if the antibody concentration approaches zero, the counting rate also approaches zero so that for our 30 replicates we need 30 counters each with an infinite counting time. Under such circumstances we shall need a 3002-sample rather than a 302-sample kit and, what is more, we shall never get a result!

D. RODBARD: Dr. Painter has used a reductio ad absurdum. The major purpose of quality-control schemes such as the one I described is to obtain a reliable estimate of precision based on a minimal number of samples and at a minimal cost. Simply by analysing one sample in duplicate in each of ten assays gives us an estimate of within-assay variability based on ten degrees of freedom and an estimate of between-assay variability based on nine degrees of freedom. Thus, the schemes proposed here are extremely practical, simple, and actually reduce the amount of work and expenditure for the laboratory. I never advocated analysing every sample 30 times. In a previous reply to Dr. Fuld, I did agree that in order to obtain a reliable estimate of the standard deviation, the more observations the better. Twenty or 30 measurements are obviously better than two or three. When we need a very precise estimate of the standard deviation (as when we attempt to utilize a Studentizing transformation to achieve uniformity of variance to combine results from several different quality-control samples), then we need to have a larger data base.

Likewise, increasing counting time does result in a decrease in the counting error, but, of course, we rapidly encounter a region of diminishing returns.

D. FULD: I have been very pleased to see that Prof. Scriba and his group have proposed an approach to quality control of commercially available kits. While this approach is extremely useful, it is still vulnerable to the problem of instability of reagents. It is well known that radioimmunoassay products are unstable. Antisera are subject to degradation. The standard material may also be degraded or deteriorate during storage. The radioactively labelled ligand is rarely stable for more than four to six weeks. Thus, we encounter the problem that a kit which has initially performed well, may rapidly deteriorate. This is something which must be monitored by every individual radioimmunoassay laboratory. This problem is not readily accessible to analysis by an outside organization. It emphasizes the need for careful, on-going quality control within each laboratory.

S.L. JEFFCOATE: I think a very important point has been made here. The assessment and control of kits must be an on-going activity, because of possible variations in reagents with time, and it is best done within the laboratory and not by an external agency. That is why we encourage laboratories to carry out their own within-laboratory quality control.

R.P. EKINS: One should add the comment that, for the reasons you have given, it takes a long time to assess the performance of a kit. One must not only evaluate the within-batch precision profiles, as we have been discussing, but also the between-batch precision profiles as a function of time. This kind of examination really does demand a lot of effort. For this reason, I frankly feel that the evaluation of kit performance is beyond the possibility of most 'small' users – particularly if they are faced with a wide range of different kits. It would be very helpful if an organization, or a group of collaborating laboratories, were able to carry out and publish independent evaluations of kit performance along the lines we have been discussing.

D.K. HAZRA: It appears that the precision profile offers the best method to check the quality of one's assay results. The data base for this method is the measurement of replicates. Could I ask for a working rule as to how many replicates one needs to measure in order to get a sufficiently reliable data base?

R.P. EKINS: We would normally construct a within-assay precision profile on not less than 100 incubation tubes. These might comprise 10 replicates at each of 10 dose values, or 50 duplicate tubes along the range covered by the standard curve. The resulting profile would not be very exactly defined, but would give a reasonable indication of a major change in assay performance resulting, for example, from a change in assay protocol.

D. RODBARD: There are two ways to construct a precision profile, an empirical approach and one based on analysis of variance of y versus y, combined with a quantitative analysis of the shape of the dose-response curve. In the first approach, one can simply analyse three quality-control samples in duplicate in each of ten assays. These data permit one to evaluate within-assay and between-assay variability at three dose levels. This is adequate for many purposes. The second approach, which is more efficient from a statistical point of view, is to analyse all of the standards and the unknowns in duplicate. One then constructs a graph of σ_y^2 versus y for both the standards and the unknowns, and describes this in quantitative terms by a straight line, parabola, or power function. Such analyses can then be compared and combined with previous assays, thus rapidly establishing an enormous data base characterizing the random error in the response variable. This information can be combined with the shape (slope) of the dose-response curve, in order to calculate a predicted, smoothed estimate of the standard deviation (or coefficient of variation) of the potency estimate for any position on the dose-response curve. This permits one to verify the validity of the empirical approach, for estimation of within-assay variability, but provides no information regarding the between-assay variability.

J. GRENIER: I am surprised that we refer so much to precision and sensitivity and so little to reference methods. At least for steroids, if not for proteins, accurate reference methods such as mass fragmentometry, which all people must accept, can be devised and used for the standardization of kits.

P.E. HALL *(Chairman):* Certainly there are not reference methods available for protein hormones. Even for the steroids, I don't think that methods have been as available as has been assumed. Dr. Breuer has now developed isotope dilution – mass fragmentography methods for several steroids and is assisting us in obtaining 'true' values for the sera used in the WHO External Quality Control Programme.

P.G. MALAN: What can be done to assist laboratories which are out of control to improve their performance? Is it feasible for such laboratories to obtain advice and help after submitting complete assay results to a centre for analysis in terms of precision profiles?

P.E. HALL *(Chairman):* We are actually about to undertake a 10-laboratory study under the WHO Programme of Research, Development and Research Training in Human Reproduction in which we shall obtain all the raw data for every assay undertaken over a period of four to five months and assess performance in terms of the principles discussed in this round-table discussion. The object of this study is exactly as you have suggested, to identify parameters that should be examined in the evaluation of assay performance, good or bad.

EXTERNAL QUALITY-CONTROL SURVEYS OF PEPTIDE HORMONE RADIOIMMUNOASSAYS IN THE FEDERAL REPUBLIC OF GERMANY

*The present status**

H. BREUER[2], D. JUNGBLUTH[2], I. MARSCHNER[1],
G. RÖHLE[2], P.C. SCRIBA[1], W.G. WOOD[1]
[1] Medizinische Klinik Innenstadt
der Universität München,
Munich
[2] Institut für Klinische Biochemie
der Universität Bonn,
Bonn,
Federal Republic of Germany

Abstract

EXTERNAL QUALITY-CONTROL SURVEYS OF PEPTIDE HORMONE RADIO-IMMUNOASSAYS IN THE FEDERAL REPUBLIC OF GERMANY: THE PRESENT STATUS.

Two types of quality-control survey (QCS) of hormone assays are performed in the Federal Republic of Germany. In the one survey, the participating laboratories are requested to determine seven or eight different hormones in two lyophilized sera that are distributed several times a year. Because of the lack of reference methods for peptide hormones, the statistical evaluation of the results indicates only whether they are "correct" or subject to systematic or nonsystematic errors with respect to the findings of the other participants. In the other survey, the participating laboratories are requested to assay only one given hormone in some 20 deep-frozen sera (including standards in hormone-free sera for derivation of a standard curve) that are distributed at relatively long intervals. The statistical analysis of the data derived from these QCSs allows – together with the methodological inquiry form – detection of probable causes for discrepancies in the results.

During recent years a system has been introduced in the Federal Republic of Germany (FRG) for internal and external quality control of quantitative clinical chemical analyses. This quality control is conducted according to the guidelines of the Bundesärztekammer (Medical Association of the FRG) [1]. The guidelines are based on the Calibration Act of 1969, which requires that if the instruments used for the determination of volume are not officially calibrated, the accuracy of analytical results has to be demonstrated by means of continuous monitoring with the methods of statistical quality control.

* Supported by the Bundesministerium für Forschung und Technologie.

TABLE I. COEFFICIENTS OF VARIATION OF THE RESULTS OF THE THIRD AND FOURTH QUALITY-CONTROL SURVEY FOR HORMONE DETERMINATIONS (BONN)

Survey	Compound	T_3	T_4	TSH	Prolactin	LH	FSH	hGH	Insulin
3	Number of results	66	71	50	32	44	41	29	28
	CV(%) (Sample A)	23	18	53	28	–	38	39	42
	CV(%) (Sample B)	27	18	54	31	53	33	58	51
4	Number of results	63	68	47	31	45	40	29	33
	CV(%) (Sample A)	25	24	43	42	38	34	44	49
	CV(%) (Sample B)	25	23	32	38	28	32	37	28

Results lying beyond the double value of the median were omitted.

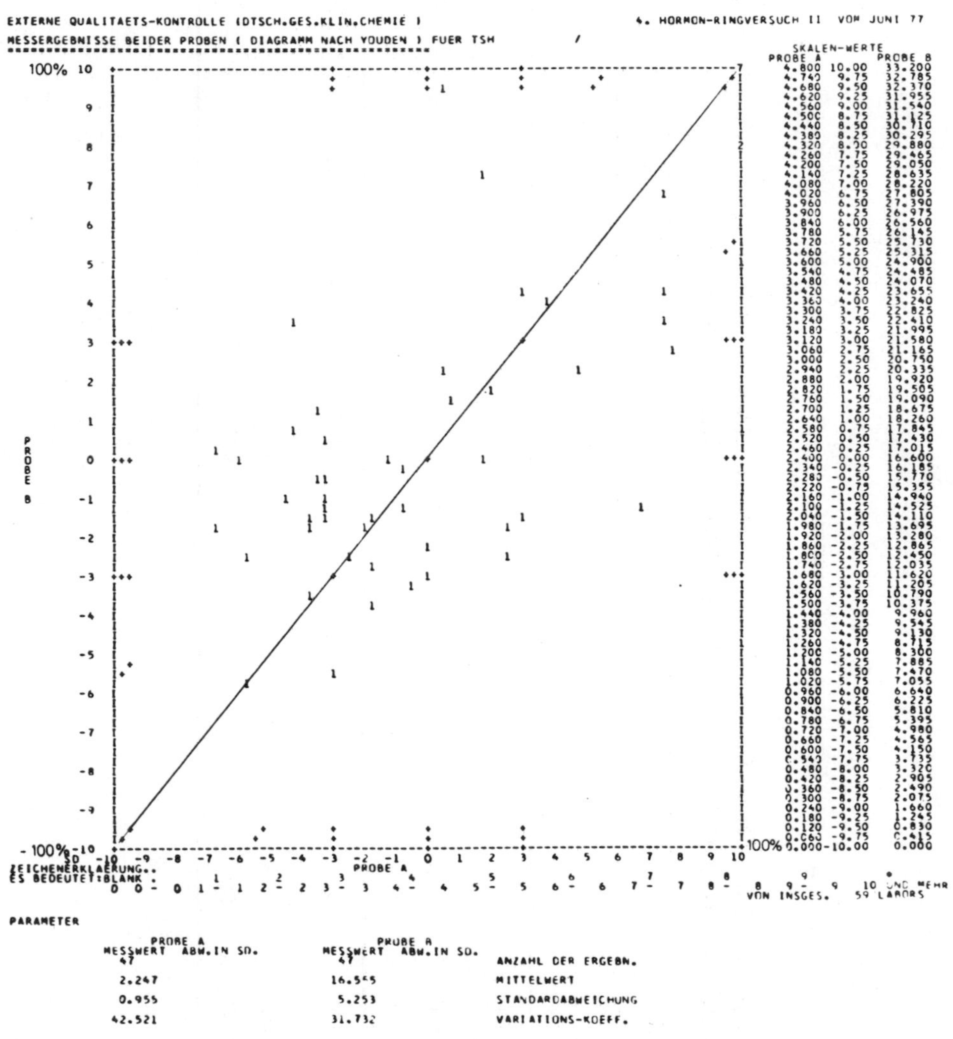

12 LABORS LAGEN MIT IHREN WERTEN AUSSERHALB DES BEREICHS

FIG.1. Youden plot of a QCS of TSH assays with two sera. The x-axis shows the results of sample A, the y-axis those of sample B. The expected value lies in the middle of the 45° line. Deviations along the line show systematic errors, deviations away from the line show random errors.

TABLE II. 50%, 16% AND 84% PERCENTILES (mU/litre) OF TSH DETERMINATIONS DIVIDED ACCORDING TO COMMERCIAL KITS USED BY THE PARTICIPANTS OF THE FOURTH SURVEY (BONN)

	Kit (No.)	1	4	5	6	7	8	9	10
	Number of results	9	6	7	2	10	5	3	2
SAMPLE A	50% percentile (median)	2.9	7.9	2.8	3.2	2.2	2.0	1.9	2.3
	16% percentile	1.0	1.8	1.4	–	1.4	–	–	–
	84% percentile	11.1	27.2	3.4	–	4.2	–	–	–
SAMPLE B	50% percentile (median)	16.6	27.5	22.4	13.8	16.9	12.0	13.5	13.3
	16% percentile	10.9	11.8	16.7	–	13.9	–	–	–
	84% percentile	49.6	55.8	27.2	–	29.1	–	–	–

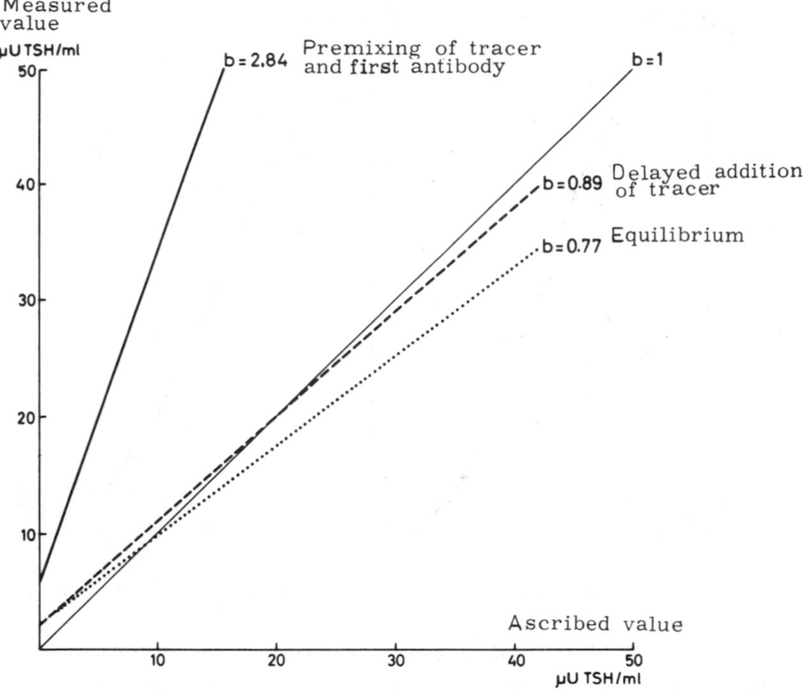

FIG.2. QCS of TSH assays. Mean regression of all assays (separated according to incubation mode) between ascribed values and measured values in the dose range between 1.8 and 26 µU TSH/ml.

The system of external quality control for routine clinical chemical analyses is now well established [2]. In each quality-control survey (QCS) at least two specimens, differing in concentrations of the various constituents, are to be analysed by the participating laboratories. The results are evaluated on the basis of assigned values and the standard deviations, as calculated from the results of reference laboratories. A single result meets the requirements provided it lies between the limits of the assigned value plus or minus three times the interlaboratory standard deviation of the reference laboratories. The participant receives a certificate to this effect which is valid for 12 months.

In the Federal Republic of Germany there are two institutions officially authorized and acknowledged by the Bundesärztekammer that carry out external quality surveys in the field of clinical chemistry, namely the Institut für Klinische Biochemie der Universität Bonn (supported by the German Society for Clinical Chemistry) and the Institut für Standardisierung und Dokumentation, Düsseldorf.

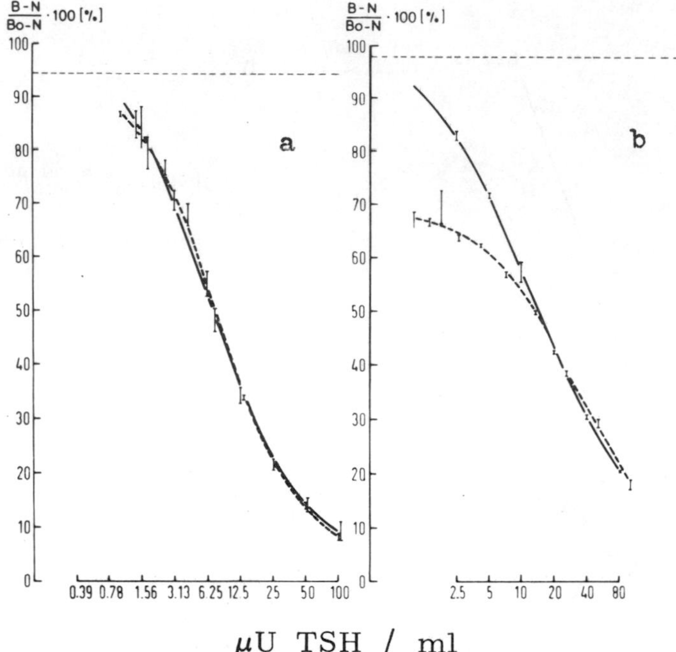

FIG.3. Graphs from a QCS of TSH assays showing four typical relationships between the standard curves of the participating laboratories (——) and the recovery curves (– – –). The abscissa is logarithmic and shows the TSH concentrations (μU/ml) of the participants' standard curves.
(a) Laboratory-developed assay (non-kit) (cold preincubation, double-antibody separation). Both curves show perfect agreement.
(b) Kit assay (equilibrium, cellulose-bound second antibody separation). Good agreement only in the high dose range. High blanks.

As far as hormone assays are concerned, the legal regulations can only be partly met because of a number of technical difficulties. Thus, there are numerous techniques for the measurement of hormones in biological fluids. Although some of these methods may give satisfactory levels of precision, many of them yield unsatisfactory results, particularly with respect to accuracy and specificity.

For steroid hormone assays, however, it may be possible in the not too distant future to find a way to carry out QCSs according to the legal guidelines. The true values of the concentrations can, on the one hand, be obtained by adding defined quantities of steroids to plasma samples from which endogenous steroids have been removed; on the other hand, these low molecular hormones can be determined by a definitive method (isotope dilution-mass fragmentography). Four pilot QCSs performed on this basis by the Bonn study group have proven the practicability of this system.

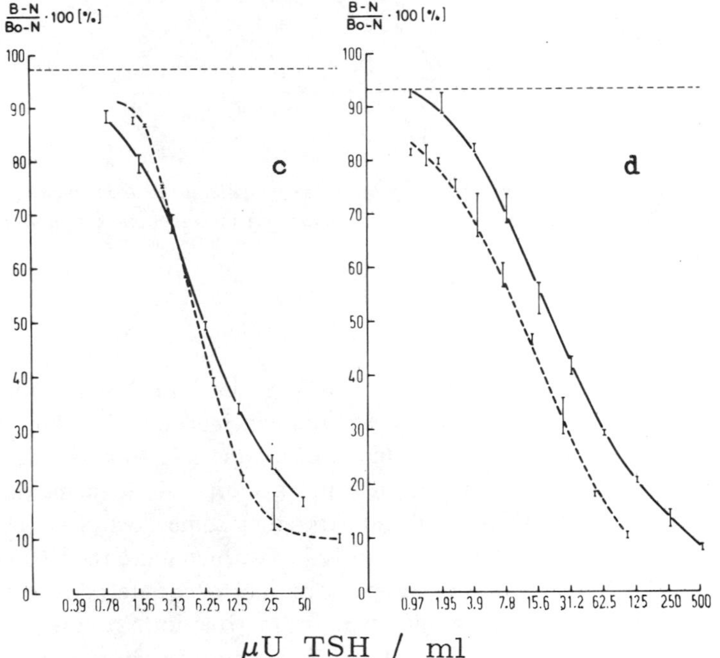

(c) Kit assay (equilibrium, double antibody). Different slope of standard and recovery curve (standards in buffer instead of in hormone-free serum).
(d) Kit assay (mixing of tracer and first antibody before pipetting to save one pipetting step; second antibody separation). False high values over the whole range.

It seems to be much more difficult to create an equivalent basis for the evaluation of results of QCSs for peptide hormones. At present, no possibility exists to determine the true concentrations of peptide hormones; as long as no agreement has been reached on standardized analytical methods, values obtained by reference laboratories cannot reasonably be used for the evaluation of the results.

The efforts of the two institutions at Bonn and at Munich are directed to establish the conditions for an optimalization and standardization of the determinations of peptide hormones. Up to now, the Bonn group has included six peptide hormones in their QCSs which are offered about three times a year; the form of organization of these QCSs follows the legal rules set up for clinical chemical determinations. The results of each of these surveys yield information [1] on the extent to which the analytical values of the various laboratories are comparable to each other, and [2] whether there is a relation between the

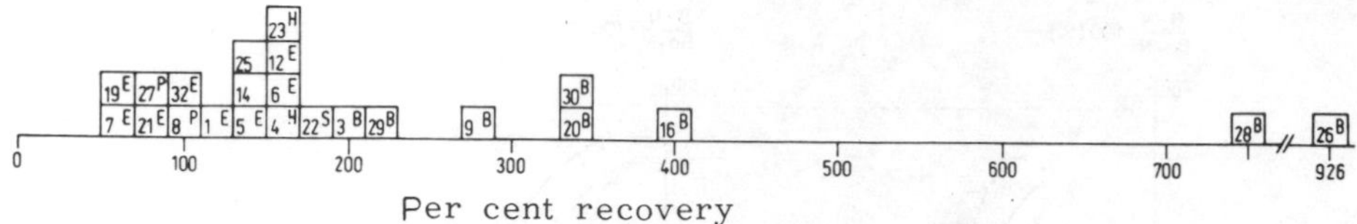

FIG.4. QCS of TSH assays. Mean recovery of all participants in the dose range between 1.8 and 26 μU TSH/ml. Each box contains the participant's number and a symbol indicating the method or kit used.

differing results and the reagents used. The QCSs performed by the Munich group are concerned with only one compound which is determined by the participating laboratories in a large number of samples. In this way, detailed information may be obtained about the sources of errors influencing the results.

The findings of the QCSs are demonstrated by some examples. In two surveys carried out by the Bonn group in 1977 in which more than 100 laboratories participated, the following peptide hormones were determined: TSH, prolactin, LH, FSH, hGH and insulin; in addition, tri-iodothyronine (T_3) and thyroxine (T_4) were analysed. Table I shows the interlaboratory imprecision – given as coefficients of variation – of the participants' results for each compound.

Whereas T_3 and T_4 were determined with relatively good precision, the coefficients of variation for the peptide hormones were rather high. In some cases, an improvement from the third to the fourth survey was noticed. With LH, the increase in precision was probably due to the fact that the samples of the fourth survey were supplied together with the same standard material of this hormone.

The results for each compound in each survey were analysed as a Youden plot, all pairs of results within the range of zero and the double value of the median being included. Figure 1 demonstrates this for TSH from the fourth survey. From Table II it can be speculated that the scatter of the results may depend, at least to some extent, on the origin of the kits. Laboratories that used kit No. 4 measured significantly higher values than most of the other participants. An interpretation of this phenomenon will only be possible when more information becomes available.

A second and more complex form of QCS has been carried out by the Endocrinological Study Group of the University Clinic in Munich. Here, approximately 20 serum samples are sent express in dry-ice to each participant. In these sera, a concealed standard curve in hormone-free serum, including a zero value, serves as a control to check the method and standards in use in the participants' laboratory. The remaining tubes contain interfering substances, serum from function tests, e.g. OGTT in an insulin quality control survey,

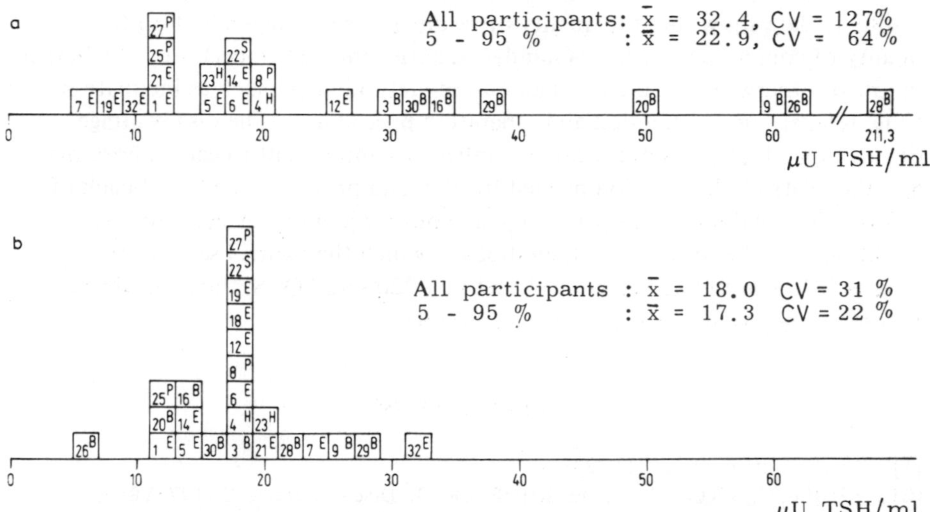

FIG.5. QCS of TSH assays.
(a) Histogram of the results for one pooled serum (17.5 μU TSH/ml) taken from each laboratory standard curve (x̄ = mean value, CV = coefficient of variation).
(b) Histogram of the results for the same pooled serum taken from the recovery curves.

TRH test in TSH, an intra-assay precision control where three tubes contain the same serum (in the normal range), and sera below, within and above the expected normal range. The 20 sera are randomly numbered to keep anonymity. All sera used are human sera from volunteer blood donors. Hormone-free serum is obtained either from donors who have undergone suppression therapy (e.g. T_4 dosage to suppress TSH secretion) or from donors in whom the hormone is not present, e.g. hGH-free serum from hypophysectomised patients. All participants are asked to assay each serum at least in duplicate, and all count-rates as well as the standard curve values and test serum values obtained. A comparison of values obtained using the participants' standard curves and the hidden standard curves (recovery curves) allows a thorough evaluation of the methodology and the pin-pointing of the probable sources of error (Fig. 2). From the recovery curve, the concentrations of the participants' standard curves can be checked, and dilution errors of differences in immunoreactivity of standards detected (Fig. 3). The interfering substances show the specificity of the participants' antisera.

The results from completed QCSs of this type (three surveys for insulin, two for TSH and one each for T_3, T_4, hGH and cortisol) [3–5] show that it allows the causes of methodological errors to be stated with greater probability than does the aforementioned type using only two sera (Figs 4 and 5). The results to date show that the quality of results is far less dependent on the quality of component reagents (standards, antiserum and tracer) used – whether in kits or otherwise obtained – than on the methodology, such as incubation time, temperature, extraction and separation procedures. The disadvantage of this type of QCS lies in the large number of samples sent to each laboratory and the relatively long period needed for the data-processing and feed-back of information, making it impossible to carry out frequently. A compromise might be a combination of both methods in which the control sera for the "2-sera" QCS would be determined first in a "20-sera" QCS, thus allowing a better-assigned value to be put on each sample.

REFERENCES

[1] Dtsch. Ärztebl. **68** (1971) 2228.
[2] RÖHLE, G., BREUER, H., OBERHOFFER, G., Dtsch. Ärztebl. **72** (1975) 883.
[3] MARSCHNER, I., BOTTERMANN, P., ERHARDT, F., LINKE, R., LOEFFLER, G., MAIER, V., SCHWANDT, P., VOGT, W., SCRIBA, P.C., Horm. Metab. Res. **6** (1974) 293.
[4] MARSCHNER, I., ERHARDT, F.W., SCRIBA, P.C., J. Clin. Chem. Clin. Biochem. **14** (1976) 345.
[5] HORN, K., MARSCHNER, I., SCRIBA, P.C., J. Clin. Chem. Clin. Biochem. **14** (1976) 353.

DISCUSSION

D. FULD: I must emphasize that external quality control has no meaning if the different laboratories are not asked or required to carry out internal quality control. Furthermore, a minimum of sensitivity should be required for each product. The problem of preparing good quality-control samples is quite a difficult one. Frozen samples should be avoided because they don't have enough stability in the range we have covered.

H. BREUER: I fully agree that good internal quality control is a prerequisite for successful external quality control. Moreover, I believe the results of surveys reflect the qualification of the participant only to a certain extent. Precision and accuracy also depend on the quality of the kit used and the experimental procedure.

K.-D. DÖHLER: You demonstrated, in the case of TSH, that the best agreement of results was achieved in assay systems with delayed addition of tracer. Did this apply to the other hormones tested or was this a specific feature of the TSH assay?

I. MARSCHNER: I think that the reason why delayed addition of tracer gives the best results in peptide hormone assays is the increased sensitivity and reproducibility of this approach, when compared with those based on equilibrium conditions. The poor results of methods using premixing of tracer and the first antibody are attributable to the binding kinetics.

MISE EN PLACE ET PREMIERS RESULTATS D'UN PROGRAMME DE CONTROLE DE QUALITE NATIONAL FRANÇAIS EN RADIOIMMUNOLOGIE

Ch.-A. BIZOLLON, R. COHEN, D. FROGET
Service de radiopharmacie et de radioanalyse,
Centre de médecine nucléaire des
Hospices civils de Lyon,
Hôpital neuro-cardiologique,
Lyon, France

Abstract–Résumé

ESTABLISHMENT OF AND FIRST RESULTS FROM A FRENCH NATIONAL QUALITY-CONTROL PROGRAMME IN RADIOIMMUNOLOGY.

The considerable development that has taken place in radioimmunology has led to the need for a programme for checking the quality of the results obtained. Various systems of control have been set up throughout the world, some of them in Europe. Certain systems are the business of official or public bodies and others come under private initiative. The paper describes the quality-control programme which has been in effect in France since February 1977 and which has been proposed to all French hospital departments specializing in radioimmunology. It is intended to be simple, inexpensive, fast and anonymous. It applies to 16 hormones or substances and is based on the use of untitrated, lyophilized human sera which come from pools made up in the Radiopharmacology and Radioanalysis Department of the authors and whose concentrations for the different parameters cover the range of normal and pathological values. The paper is divided into two distinct sections: the first deals with the interlaboratory investigation, by means of which each laboratory can compare its results with those of different laboratories using the same technique and assess the results obtained by the use of different techniques; the second is concerned with permanent intralaboratory control, by means of which each laboratory can evaluate the reproducibility of its results (inter-laboratory and intralaboratory reproducibility – interassay). For this first year there have been 32 participants in the interlaboratory investigation and 20 in the permanent control. The paper describes the first results achieved. Modifications and improvements are planned.

MISE EN PLACE ET PREMIERS RESULTATS D'UN PROGRAMME DE CONTROLE DE QUALITE NATIONAL FRANÇAIS EN RADIOIMMUNOLOGIE.

Le développement considérable de la radioimmunologie a fait apparaître la nécessité d'un contrôle de qualité des résultats. Différents systèmes de contrôle existent dans le monde, et plus près de nous en Europe. Certains appartiennent à des organismes officiels ou publics, d'autres relèvent d'initiatives privées. Le mémoire décrit le programme de contrôle de qualité mis en place en France depuis février 1977 et proposé à l'ensemble des services hospitaliers français spécialisés en radioimmunologie. Il se veut simple, peu onéreux, rapide et anonyme. Ce contrôle porte sur 16 hormones ou substances. Il s'effectue à l'aide de sérums humains, non titrés, lyophilisés, provenant de pools confectionnés dans le Service de radiopharmacie et radioanalyse et dont les concentrations pour les différents paramètres couvrent la gamme des valeurs normales et pathologiques. Il comporte deux parties bien distinctes: 1) l'enquête interlaboratoire, qui permet à chaque laboratoire de comparer les résultats qu'il obtient avec ceux des différents laboratoires qui utilisent la même technique et de situer les résultats obtenus à l'aide de différentes techniques; 2) le contrôle permanent intralaboratoire, par lequel chaque laboratoire peut apprécier la reproductibilité de ses résultats (reproductibilité interlaboratoire et intralaboratoire (interessai)). Le nombre de participants pour cette première année est de 32 pour l'enquête interlaboratoire et de 20 pour le contrôle permanent. Le mémoire expose les premiers résultats obtenus. Des modifications et améliorations sont envisagées.

INTRODUCTION

Le développement considérable de la méthode radioimmunologique, son application au dosage d'un nombre de plus en plus important de substances sur des prélèvements de plus en plus nombreux ont fait apparaître la nécessité d'un contrôle de qualité des résultats obtenus par cette méthode.

C'est pour répondre à cette nécessité que nous avons proposé en octobre 1976 un programme de contrôle à l'ensemble des laboratoires hospitaliers français spécialisés en radioimmunologie. Celui-ci est opérationnel depuis février 1977. Nous voudrions dans cet exposé décrire l'organisation de ce contrôle et livrer les premiers résultats.

1. GENERALITES

La conception de ce contrôle repose sur quelques principes simples: peu onéreux il doit être suffisamment souple pour convenir à l'ensemble des services intéressés, quelles que soient leur structure ou leur importance. Il doit de plus permettre à chaque laboratoire d'apprécier rapidement la valeur de ses résultats (exactitude, précision, etc.). Enfin, chaque laboratoire doit conserver la connaissance exclusive de ses propres résultats.

Le contrôle porte sur les 16 substances suivantes: insuline, hGH, ACTH, IgE, TSH, T_3 RIA, thyroxine, rénine-angiotensine, aldostérone, cortisol, FSH, LH, prolactine, testostérone, œstradiol, progestérone.

Les sérums humains de contrôle, non titrés, lyophilisés, proviennent de «pools» confectionnés dans notre service et dont les concentrations pour les différents paramètres couvrent la gamme des valeurs normales et pathologiques.

CENTRE DE CONTROLE		LABORATOIRE
- EXPEDITION DES SERUMS DE CONTROLE NECESSAIRES POUR UNE CAMPAGNE (20 QUINZAINES)	→	- RECEPTION
- EXPEDITION DU PLANNING D'UTILISATION POUR 5 QUINZAINES	→	- DOSAGE  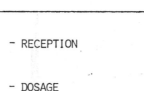
- RECEPTION ET TRAITEMENT DES RESULTATS	←	- ENVOI DES RESULTATS DE LA QUINZAINE
- CONFECTION DU COMPTE-RENDU-ENVOI	→	- VERIFICATION DE LA PLACE DU RESULTAT DANS LA DISTRIBUTION

FIG.1. Organisation de l'enquête interlaboratoire.

L'absence de l'antigène B de l'hépatite virale a été vérifiée par dosage radio-immunologique.

La période de contrôle est fixée à un an, plus précisément 40 semaines. Elle est découpée en 4 parties égales de 10 semaines.

2. MISE EN ŒUVRE DU PROGRAMME DE CONTROLE DE QUALITE

Le programme de contrôle de qualité comprend deux parties bien distinctes: l'enquête interlaboratoire et le contrôle permanent intralaboratoire.

2.1. Enquête interlaboratoire

2.1.1. Principe (fig. 1)

A chaque laboratoire qui participe à l'enquête, nous envoyons au début de celle-ci l'ensemble des sérums nécessaires au contrôle pendant les 40 semaines, et au début de chaque période de 10 semaines, les indications pour l'utilisation de chaque sérum de contrôle.

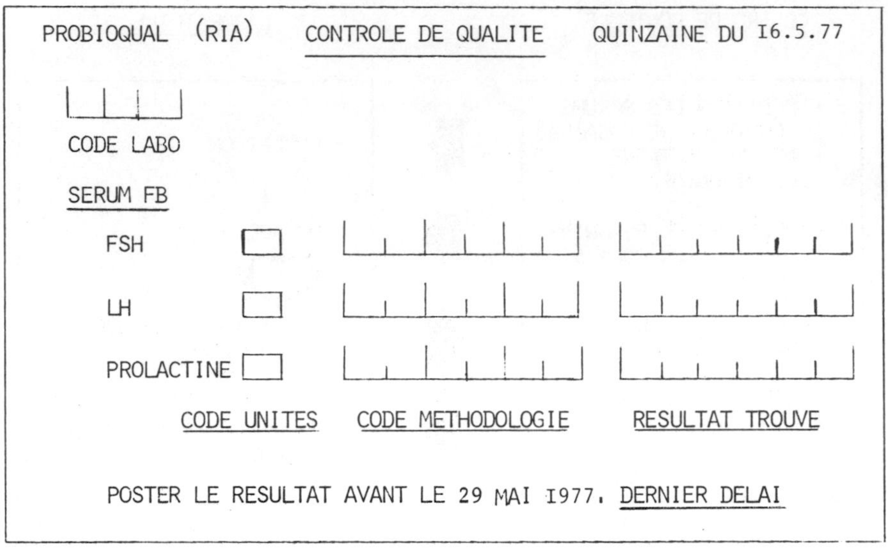
PROBIOQUAL (RIA) CONTROLE DE QUALITE QUINZAINE DU 16.5.77

CODE LABO

SERUM FB

FSH

LH

PROLACTINE

CODE UNITES CODE METHODOLOGIE RESULTAT TROUVE

POSTER LE RESULTAT AVANT LE 29 MAI 1977. DERNIER DELAI

FIG. 2. Exemple de feuille pour l'envoi des résultats de l'enquête interlaboratoire.

Les résultats obtenus par les laboratoires participants sont envoyés à la fin de chaque quinzaine au Centre de contrôle, qui en fait une étude statistique. Celle-ci est envoyée aux laboratoires participants.

2.1.2. Applications

Les 16 hormones ou substances à doser sont réparties en 5 groupes:

I	insuline, hGH, ACTH, IgE
II	TSH, T_3RIA, T_4
III	FSH, LH, prolactine
IV	aldostérone, cortisol, rénine-angiotensine
V	testostérone, œstradiol, progestérone

Les hormones appartenant à un groupe sont dosées en 15 jours (2 semaines). Ceci signifie que le dosage de l'ensemble des paramètres nécessite $5 \times 2 = 10$ semaines. Ceci signifie également que chaque paramètre sera dosé 4 fois pendant la durée de la période de contrôle. Nous donnons à titre d'exemple (fig. 2) un modèle de feuille qui assure la liaison aller-retour entre le Centre de contrôle et le laboratoire participant au contrôle.

µU U/ML	CODE TECHNIQUE	INCUBATION SIMULTANEE	SATURATION SEQUENTIELLE
IO - +	AA	I	
-			
9 -			
-			
8 - ++	AA-XX	2	
-			
7 - +	EA		I
- ++	GX-XX	I	I
6 - ++	AA-AB	2	
- ++	EA-EA		2
5 - ++++	AX-FB-GX-YX	I	3
- ++	FB-AB	I	I
4 - +	FB		I
- +	AB	I	
3 -			
- +	FX		I
2 -			

N	I9	9	IO
MOYENNE	5,7	6,4	5,0
ECART-TYPE	I,8	2,0	I,3
MOY. TRONQUEE A 2 ET	5,4		
INTERVALLE DE CONFIANCE DE LA MOYENNE (95%)	4,8-6,6	4,9-7,9	4,I-5,9

FIG. 3. Enquête interlaboratoire: tableau récapitulatif. Sérum TA: TSH

Sur ce document, on note la nature des hormones (FSH, LH, prolactine) qui doivent être dosées dans le sérum de contrôle FB pendant la quinzaine commençant le 16 mai 1977 et dont les résultats doivent parvenir au Centre de contrôle avant le 29 mai 1977.

A chaque substance correspond un code à 7 lettres; la première lettre représente le code unités, les six autres représentent le code méthodologie qui se divise de la façon suivante: deux lettres pour la technique utilisée, deux lettres pour l'appareillage, deux lettres pour l'étalonnage.

Chaque feuille, une fois remplie, sera *envoyée anonymement* au Centre de contrôle par le laboratoire, qui mentionnera seulement son numéro de code (3 chiffres).

Le traitement des résultats reçus pour un groupe de substances aboutit à la confection d'histogrammes dont nous donnons un exemple (fig. 3). On note:

– la distribution des résultats obtenus à l'aide de l'ensemble des méthodes utilisées par les participants (moyenne $\overline{x}$, écart-type s, intervalle de confiance de la moyenne);
– la distribution des résultats obtenus par groupes de méthodes analogues (incubation simultanée par exemple ou saturation séquentielle).

Si les résultats obtenus à l'aide d'une seule méthode sont suffisamment nombreux, il sera possible d'établir une telle distribution statistique pour chaque méthode.

2.2. Contrôle permanent intralaboratoire

2.2.1. Organisation (fig. 4)

Nous fournissons au laboratoire participant au contrôle, pour chaque hormone ou substance, autant de sérums de contrôle qu'il envisage de séries de dosages dans l'année. Les résultats obtenus nous sont communiqués à la fin de chaque mois et ceci jusqu'à obtention pour chaque paramètre de ce que nous appelons la valeur «cible».

En effet, à partir de l'ensemble des résultats cumulés sur 1, 2 ou éventuellement 3 mois, il nous est possible de calculer pour chaque groupe de méthodes ou, si l'information est suffisante, par méthode:

– la valeur moyenne de la concentration ($\overline{x}$);

– l'écart-type global qui tient compte à la fois de la variabilité interlaboratoire et de la variabilité intralaboratoire

$$S_G = \sqrt{\frac{\sum_{i=1}^{N} X_i^2 - T_G^2/N}{N-1}}$$

T_G = totalité des résultats, N = nombre total des résultats;

– l'écart-type intralaboratoire ou résiduel représentant uniquement la variabilité intralaboratoire

$$S_R = \sqrt{\frac{\sum_{i=1}^{N} X_i^2 - \sum_{j=1}^{n} T_j^2/n_j}{N-n}}$$

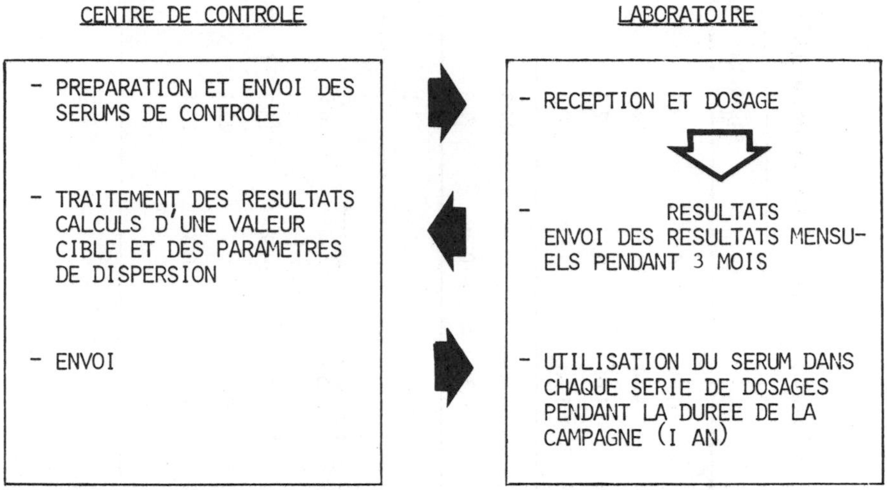

FIG.4. Organisation du contrôle permanent.

T_j = total des résultats du jième laboratoire, n_j = nombre de résultats du jième laboratoire, n = nombre de bulletins récapitulatifs envoyés à la fin de chaque mois par chaque laboratoire;

– le coefficient de variation (C.V.) calculé en faisant le rapport $S_R/\bar{x}$.

2.2.2. Résultats

A titre d'exemple nous donnons dans le tableau I, pour un certain nombre d'hormones, les résultats cumulés sur trois mois de contrôle, et dans le tableau II, l'évolution des résultats (moyenne et coefficient de variation) cumulés sur 1, 2 et 3 mois pour le dosage de la TSH.

Nous constatons que ces résultats donnent déjà à la fin du premier mois une bonne idée de la valeur cible pour chaque groupe de méthodes et que cette valeur s'affine lors des mois suivants sans changer sensiblement.

Ceci montre que les valeurs obtenues à la fin du premier mois peuvent être considérées comme très proches de la valeur cible et permettre dès lors à chaque laboratoire de s'y rapporter pour apprécier l'exactitude de ses résultats.

TABLEAU I. CONTROLE PERMANENT INTRALABORATOIRE: RESULTATS CUMULES SUR TROIS MOIS, SERUM I

Paramètre	Technique	N	$\bar{x}$	S_G	S_R	$S_R/\bar{x}(\%)$
Insuline (μUl/ml)	Charbon Dextran	16	20,8	4,06	4,14	19,9
	AC anti-insuline sur Séphadex	89	18,6	4,74	2,62	14,1
	Double AC	157	20,9	4,65	3,70	17,7
	AC anti-insuline fixés sur verre	28	25,7	5,68	4,99	19,4
hGH (ng/ml)	Double AC	123	3,75	0,93	0,92	24,5
	AC anti-hGH sur papier	13	4,71	0,35	0,36	7,6
IgE (U/ml)	AC sur Séphadex	62	225	30,7	29,4	13,1
TSH (μU/ml)	1) Incubation simultanée					
	Double AC	98	7,15	1,56	1,21	16,9
	2) Saturation séquentielle					
	AC anti-TSH sur Séphadex	53	5,43	1,09	0,99	18,3
	Polyéthylène glycol	45	3,23	0,73	0,72	22,4
	Double AC	15	5,45	1,31	0,57	10,4
	Double AC sur support solide	3	10,1			

TABLEAU II. EVOLUTION DES MOYENNES ET DES COEFFICIENTS DE VARIATION INTRALABORATOIRE AU COURS DES TROIS PREMIERS MOIS DU CONTROLE PERMANENT POUR LA TSH (μUI/ml)

Technique	1er mois			1er + 2^e mois			1er + 2^e + 3^e mois		
	N	Moyenne	C.V. intralabo (%)	N	Moyenne	C.V. intralabo (%)	N	Moyenne	C.V. intralabo (%)
1) Incubation simultanée									
Double AC	35	7,14	17,5	62	7,19	18,3	98	7,15	16,9
2) Saturation séquentielle									
AC anti-TSH sur Séphadex	20	5,31	16,4	34	5,29	18,6	53	5,43	18,3
Polyéthylène glycol	24	3,18	22,6	41	3,25	22,7	45	3,23	22,4
Double AC	2	5,10	–	10	6,20	10,0	15	5,45	10,4

3. DISCUSSION

Le programme de contrôle de qualité que nous venons de décrire n'a débuté qu'en février 1977 et il est peut-être un peu tôt après 6 mois d'expérience d'en tirer des conclusions définitives.

Il est néanmoins possible, à l'heure actuelle, d'établir un premier bilan et d'envisager éventuellement des modifications ou améliorations pour l'avenir.

3.1. Enquête interlaboratoire

Précisons tout d'abord que la réalisation des dosages sur les sérums de ce type de contrôle doit comporter le maximum de soins, car son but n'est pas de mettre en évidence des défaillances humaines.

D'autre part, les laboratoires participant à notre programme de contrôle de qualité sont ceux qui en ont exprimé le désir; ils n'ont été l'objet d'aucune sélection de notre part.

Ces points étant précisés, nous pensons que l'intérêt de l'enquête interlaboratoire dans son fonctionnement actuel est double:

- elle permet à chaque laboratoire de comparer les résultats qu'il obtient avec ceux des différents laboratoires utilisant la même technique;
- elle permet de situer les résultats obtenus à l'aide des différentes techniques.

Dans l'avenir, il nous paraît souhaitable d'effectuer pour chaque paramètre le contrôle à plusieurs niveaux de concentrations, ce qui permettrait de simuler par exemple les tests au TRH, au LH RH, etc. De plus, en réalisant le dosage en double ou en triple sur chacun de ces sérums, il serait possible pour chaque laboratoire par des calculs simples [1–3] d'estimer la reproductibilité intraessai. Enfin, de cette manière nous pensons approcher le contrôle de la spécificité des antisérums: il suffirait pour cela de prévoir le dosage d'un «pool» avant et après surcharge avec le composé dont on veut étudier la réaction croisée.

Ce contrôle étant ponctuel – nous avons vu précédemment que le dosage du même paramètre revenait seulement quatre fois par période de quarante semaines – il nous a semblé indispensable, pour compléter ce programme, d'introduire des vérifications au sein de chaque série de dosages. C'est le but du contrôle permanent intralaboratoire.

3.2. Contrôle permanent intralaboratoire

Dans ce cas, les sérums de contrôle doivent être traités de la même façon que ceux des malades. L'utilisation de sérums non titrés a pour inconvénient de ne rendre ce contrôle efficace qu'au bout d'un certain temps, celui nécessaire à l'obtention de la valeur cible. Ce temps peut être réduit à quelques semaines si le nombre d'observations est suffisant. D'autre part, jusqu'à maintenant, le

TABLEAU III. NOMBRE DE LABORATOIRES PARTICIPANT AU PROGRAMME DE CONTROLE DE QUALITE

	Enquête interlaboratoire	Contrôle permanent
Insuline	19	14
hGH	16	11
ACTH	4	4
IgE	7	6
TSH	25	16
T_3 RIA	23	13
T_4	22	14
FSH	14	9
LH	16	10
Prolactine	11	10
Cortisol	11	9
Aldostérone	10	7
Rénine	11	9
Progestérone	9	7
Œstradiol	8	7
Testostérone	8	4
Nombre total	32	20

contrôle s'est effectué sur un seul niveau de concentration. Dans ces conditions, il permet:

– à chaque laboratoire, comme cela était possible avec l'enquête interlaboratoire, de vérifier sa position par rapport à la valeur cible de la technique qu'il utilise;
– d'avoir une idée assez précise de la reproductibilité interlaboratoire et de la reproductibilité intralaboratoire (interessai).

Il est certain que l'utilisation d'un sérum de contrôle à un seul niveau de concentration n'offre pas suffisamment de garanties en vue de la validation d'une série de dosages. C'est pourquoi nous envisageons lors des prochaines campagnes d'effectuer ce contrôle à trois niveaux de concentrations, ce qui, de plus, permettrait d'accéder à la reproductibilité intraessai [1–3]. Enfin, il faut noter que, ce programme reposant sur l'utilisation de sérums non titrés, son intérêt est directement lié au nombre de participants (tableau III); actuellement, leur nombre est de 32 pour l'enquête interlaboratoire et de 20 pour le contrôle permanent.

CONCLUSION

A nos yeux, le contrôle de qualité doit avoir pour but:

- de faciliter le choix de la technique de dosage pour un laboratoire nouveau venu dans le domaine de la radioimmunologie; il doit donc permettre d'apprécier les qualités des différentes techniques;
- d'aboutir à une harmonisation des résultats rendus dans les différents laboratoires;
- d'améliorer la qualité des résultats au sein d'un laboratoire.

Seule une organisation nationale ou internationale regroupant un nombre important de participants peut atteindre ce triple but.

REMERCIEMENTS

Nous tenons à remercier Mademoiselle S. Breysse pour son excellente collaboration technique.

REFERENCES

[1] BIZOLLON, Ch.A., FAURE, A., Critères et contrôle de la qualité d'un dosage radioimmunologique, Lyon Pharm. 27 (1976) 134.

[2] RODBARD, D., RAYFORD, P.L., COOPER, J.E., ROOS, G.T., Statistical quality control of radioimmunoassay, J. Clin. Endocrinol. Metab. 28 (1968) 1412.

[3] VALLERON, A.J., «Méthodes statistiques en radioimmunologie», Techniques radioimmunologiques (C.R. Coll. INSERM, 1972), INSERM, Paris (1972) 149.

DISCUSSION

D. FULD: Have you enough values for an intercomparison of commercial kits?

Ch.-A. BIZOLLON: No, not at present. On this subject I should like to make two comments. First, certain procedures suggested in different kits are very similar to each other in regard to the labelled hormone, standard, buffer, separation process, etc. For an initial analysis, these procedures can be grouped. Second, the 100–150 hospital services in France at present specializing in radioimmunoassay use a fairly restricted number of methods, thus facilitating our task.

D. FULD: So you have a heterogeneity within your sub-groups?

Ch.-A. BIZOLLON: Yes, but subject to the restriction I have just mentioned.

P.Y. CATHOU: Do you intend to include manufacturers of kits in your programme and, if so, to send them samples ahead of time to ensure that the target value is established in accordance with their recommended protocol?

Ch.-A. BIZOLLON: We do not exclude manufacturers from our quality-control system. They can join the system on the same footing as hospital services, and participate both in the external and internal quality control and thus in the determination of target values. For each method, the larger the number of participants the more rapid will be the determination of their values and the greater will be their precision.

AN ELEMENTARY COMPONENTS OF VARIANCE ANALYSIS FOR MULTI-CENTRE QUALITY CONTROL

P.J. MUNSON, D. RODBARD
National Institute of Child Health and
Human Development,
National Institutes of Health,
Bethesda, Maryland,
United States of America

Abstract

AN ELEMENTARY COMPONENTS OF VARIANCE ANALYSIS FOR MULTI-CENTRE QUALITY CONTROL.

The serious variability of RIA results from different laboratories indicates the need for multi-laboratory collaborative quality-control (QC) studies. Simple graphical display of data in the form of histograms is useful but insufficient. The paper discusses statistical analysis methods for such studies using an "analysis of variance with components of variance estimation". This technique allocates the total variance into components corresponding to between-laboratory, between-assay, and residual or within-assay variability. Components of variance analysis also provides an intelligent way to combine the results of several QC samples run at different levels, from which we may decide if any component varies systematically with dose level; if not, pooling of estimates becomes possible. Problems with RIA data, e.g. severe non-uniformity of variance and/or departure from a normal distribution violate some of the usual assumptions underlying analysis of variance. In order to correct these problems, it is often necessary to transform the data before analysis by using a logarithmic, square-root, percentile, ranking, RIDIT, "Studentizing" or other transformation. Ametric transformations such as ranks or percentiles protect against the undue influence of outlying observations, but discard much intrinsic information. Several possible relationships of standard deviation to the laboratory mean are considered. Each relationship corresponds to an underlying statistical model and an appropriate analysis technique. Tests for homogeneity of variance may be used to determine whether an appropriate model has been chosen, although the exact functional relationship of standard deviation to laboratory mean may be difficult to establish. Appropriate graphical display aids visual understanding of the data. A plot of the ranked standard deviation versus ranked laboratory mean is a convenient way to summarize a QC study. This plot also allows determination of the rank correlation, which indicates a net relationship of variance to laboratory mean.

INTRODUCTION

The importance of large-scale multi-centre collaborative studies has become increasingly apparent in view of the continuing problem of serious variability of results from RIAs from different laboratories. Several such studies have been undertaken and have started to produce substantial quantities of data. Statistical analysis of such data has typically been fairly limited, e.g. construction of histograms, calculation of means, and standard deviations for each laboratory. In some cases, two-sample Youden plots have been used [1]. While important, these simple analyses do not extract all the information available in the data base. For instance, they do not provide a **quantitative** and reliable measure of the intrinsic degree of variability among laboratories over and above the between-assay variability for a typical laboratory. Ideally, results of multi-centre studies should allow us to answer the questions: How much additional variability is observed by sending samples to different laboratories? How much is this variability reduced by the use of common reagents and methods? Are some laboratories or groups of laboratories significantly more precise than others?

A two-sample Youden plot can provide a graphical indication that there is significantly more between-laboratory than within-laboratory variability. However, we wish to estimate how **much** more variability in quantitative terms. While the standard deviation of the mean values obtained in different laboratories provides a measure of between-laboratory variability, it is not sufficient. Its magnitude is influenced by how many replicates have been sent to each laboratory, and thus depends on study design. Accordingly, it would be inappropriate to compare standard deviations from two studies unless their designs are identical.

We have adopted a method of analysis for inter-laboratory collaborative studies which can provide precise, statistically well-defined answers to the questions posed above. The method is based on analysis of variance (ANOVA) with special attention to estimation of "**components of variance**". This analysis may be used to quantify within- and between-laboratory reliability, and may be used to provide a hierarchical analysis of components of variance arising between-methods, between-reagents, between-laboratory, between-assay, and within-assay.

By using components of variance estimation, we may also combine the results of several studies using different quality-control (QC) samples, while allowing a flexible study design. We may further investigate the question of uniformity of variance among laboratories. Are some laboratories more precise than others? Does the ratio of between-assay to within-assay variability itself vary among laboratories?

Although this is a conventional and classical statistical approach [2], its application to RIA has so far been restricted to only a few laboratories [3, 4] and requires special study. Specifically, the underlying assumptions of normality (Gaussian distribution of errors), uniformity of variance, and additivity of effects are usually violated. Problems arising due to missing observations and lack of balanced study design complicate the analyses. Outliers or spurious observations can seriously bias or even completely invalidate a study unless they are detected and removed before analysis.

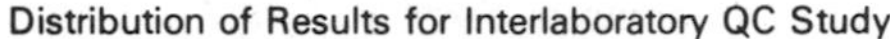

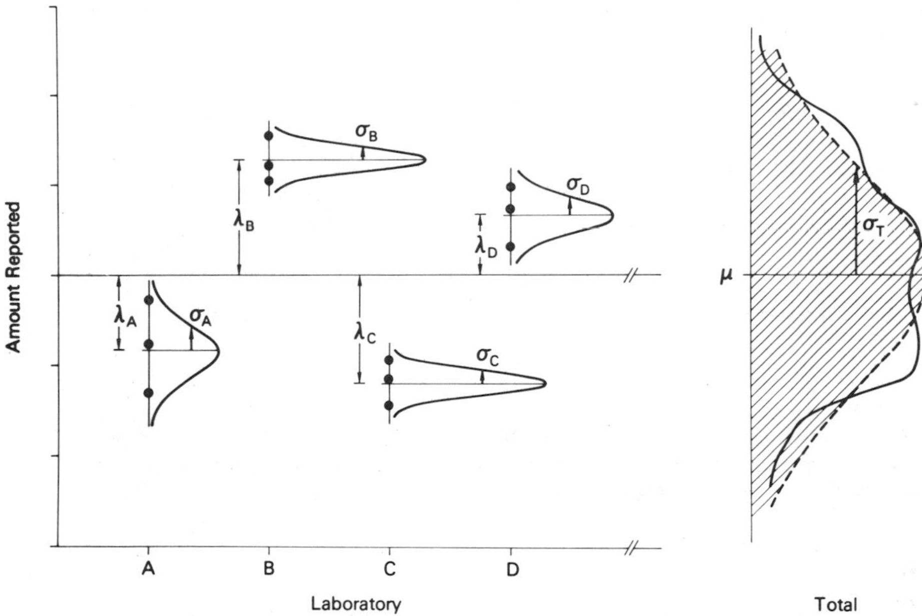

FIG.1. Schematic representation of the results of a collaborative study. The four small curves are distributions of results for each laboratory. μ is the true value of the QC sample, λ is the bias introduced by each laboratory, and σ_A, σ_B, etc. are the standard deviations for each laboratory. σ_T is the overall standard deviation. The curve on the extreme right represents the distribution for all laboratories combined. The shaded area is the theoretical distribution of combined results from an "infinite" number of laboratories.

MODELS OF SOURCES OF VARIABILITY

A simple breakdown of the variability of results of a collaborative study is shown schematically in Fig. 1. The X-axis shows the amount reported by any given laboratory. The upper curve represents the theoretical distribution of results if a sample were analysed by an "infinite" number of laboratories. The overall or total variability is denoted by σ_T, i.e. the standard deviation of all the measurements. The "true" value is denoted by μ. The four narrower distributions schematically represent the theoretical distributions of results for four separate laboratories. Notice that the standard deviation, σ, for each laboratory, is usually much smaller than the overall σ_T. In general, the σ's for each laboratory (e.g. σ_A, σ_B, σ_C and σ_D) will differ. Laboratory C has better between-assay precision than laboratory D. However, laboratory D's results

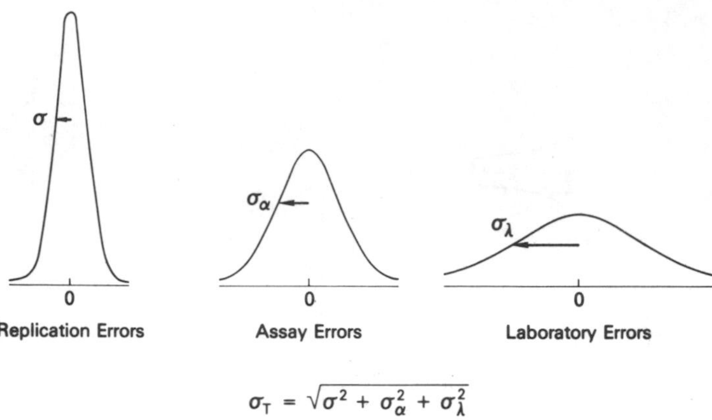

FIG.2. Distribution of components of total variance showing approximate relative size of σ_λ, σ_α and σ. Total variance is a combination of the components of variance due to laboratory, assay and replication.

tend to be much closer to the true value. Thus, good reproducibility, as indicated by a small σ, does not certify that the results from a given laboratory are near the "true" value. The mean for each laboratory is biased by an amount λ from the "true" value for the sample. We may regard these λ values as a series of constants for each laboratory. This is the "fixed effects" model. Alternatively, we may regard λ as a "random variable", itself subject to an underlying Gaussian distribution. This is the "random effects" model. The philosophical choice between these two models leads to subtle but important differences in subsequent analyses. λ values indicate the effects of the differences in technique between laboratories. The total variability is the sum of the variability within-laboratory plus the variability due to the laboratory "shift" of bias λ.

Figure 2 shows distributions for three components of error with a slightly more complicated error breakdown. The first, σ, is the within-laboratory, within-assay error. This error results from "tube to tube" variability during the course of a single assay (e.g., counting errors, pipetting errors, and misclassification errors). The next component, σ_α, is the between-assay error within laboratories and results from possible instability of reagents, use of different batches of iodinated antigen, changes of technician, temperature, incubation time, and other variables within any given laboratory. Finally, the term σ_λ, the component of variability due to differences among several laboratories is often two or three times larger than σ_α. The observed total error for a single observation is given by:

$$\sigma_T = (\sigma_\lambda^2 + \sigma_\alpha^2 + \sigma^2)^{1/2} \qquad (1)$$

Within Laboratory Precision *vs* Dose

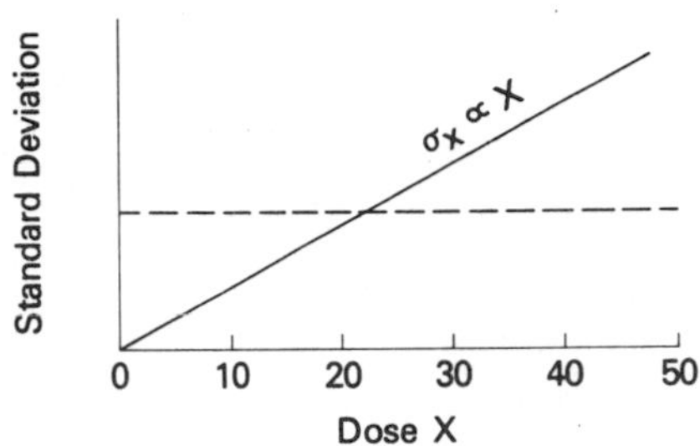

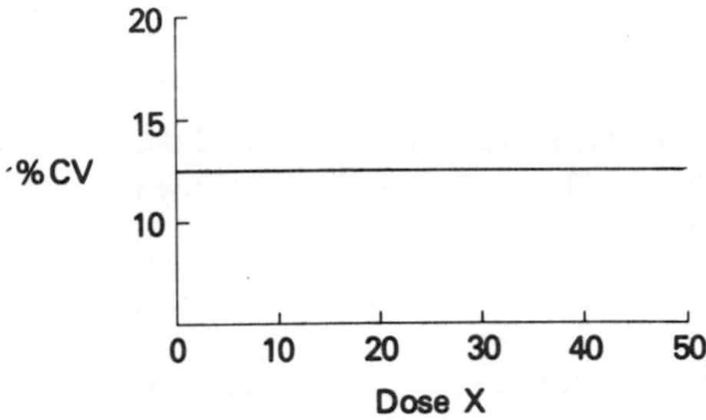

FIG.3. Within-laboratory precision versus dose expressed as standard deviation (upper panel) or per cent coefficient of variation (% CV) (lower panel). This shows the hypothetical relationships of a constant standard deviation (dashed line) or of a standard deviation proportional to dose.

Within Laboratory Precision *vs* Dose

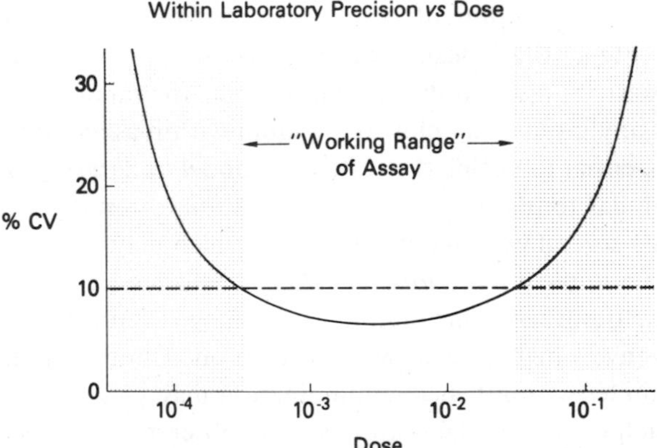

FIG.4. Within-laboratory precision versus dose on log scale. A constant %CV (dashed line) and a more realistic relationship (solid line) are indicated. Outside of the "working range" of an assay, the %CV "blows up".

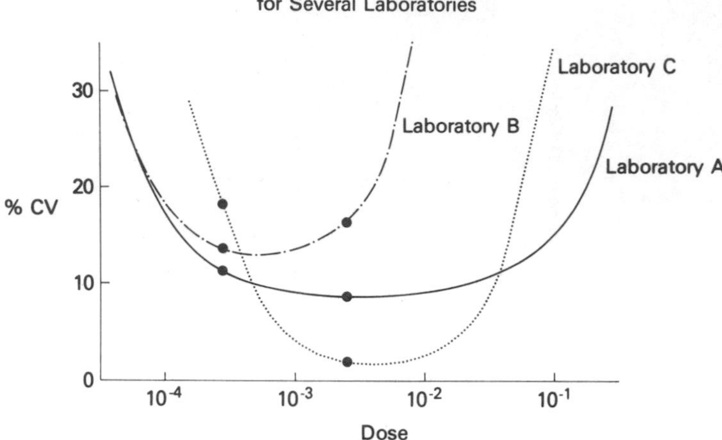

FIG.5. Within-laboratory precision versus dose for several laboratories showing complex error structure. QC samples at two dose levels will be analysed with different relative errors (%CV) by different laboratories.

We assume that all errors are random and Gaussian. Then, a single replicate k for a given tube in assay j in laboratory i can be written as:

$$x_{ijk} = \mu + \lambda_i + \alpha_{ij} + \epsilon_{ijk} \quad (2)$$

where λ_i, α_{ij} and ϵ_{ijk} are random variables, each with a population mean of zero and expected standard deviations of σ_λ, σ_a and σ, respectively.

Equation (2) is the formal statement of the statistical model corresponding to Fig. 1. The term x_{ijk} represents a single measurement from laboratory i on assay j for replicate k. Statistically, x is equal to the sum of the true value μ plus the error λ attributable to the laboratory, plus the random error α associated with any given assay plus the random within-assay, within-laboratory error, ϵ. It is essential to define the statistical model underlying any analysis of variance formulas to permit proper interpretation of results. For this reason, we shall examine several variants of this model which may be applicable to RIA.

Laboratory-sample interaction: If two laboratories are utilizing reagents of differing specificities, then some samples containing certain cross-reacting substances may give a higher result when sent to one laboratory than when sent to another. Samples without such contamination may yield the same result when sent to each of the two laboratories. The observed result is then not simply the sum of the "laboratory effect" plus the "sample effect"; there is also an effect termed "laboratory-sample interaction". One can expand the statistical model to include this component (see Appendix II of Ref. [5]).

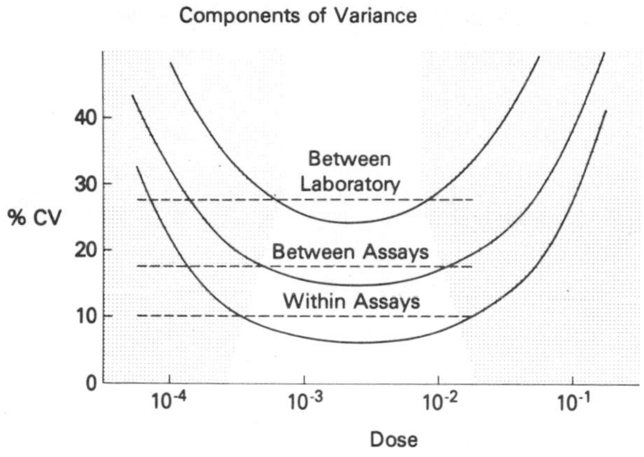

Components of Variance

% CV

Dose

FIG.6. Components of variance expressed as %CV versus dose on log scale, showing relative sizes of components. Also shown is the shrinking "working range." of an assay as we move from within-assay to between-assay to between-laboratory components of variance.

The assumptions of an underlying Gaussian distribution with uniformity of variance is usually violated in most RIA applications if one uses "raw data". However, by use of suitable transformations, one can provide satisfactory "normality" and "uniformity of variance". Figure 3 shows schematic representations of standard deviation or coefficient of variation versus dose. In the upper panel the assumption of uniform variance is indicated by the horizontal line. Usually, it is more reasonable to assume that the standard deviation is proportional to dose, ($\sigma_X \propto X$), corresponding to a constant percentage error, or coefficient of variation ($\%CV = 100\sigma/\mu$).

Figure 4 shows another view of the within-laboratory precision as a function of dose, on a logarithmic scale. There is a central region (working range) wherein the %CV is nearly constant, but the curve "blows up" at both extremes. This relationship can readily be derived from the sigmoidal nature of the RIA dose-response curve versus log dose. Figure 5 is a schematic illustration of within-laboratory precision for several different laboratories. Laboratory A has fairly good precision over a fairly broad range. Laboratory C has a much better precision than laboratory A, though over a much narrower range. Laboratory B has uniformly worse precision than laboratory A, but may have better precision than laboratory C at some dose levels. Thus, the random variability in results for a QC sample sent to each laboratory depends on the dose level of the sample, and on the shape of the standard curve for each laboratory and assay. This complex interaction creates problems in the application of conventional analysis of variance.

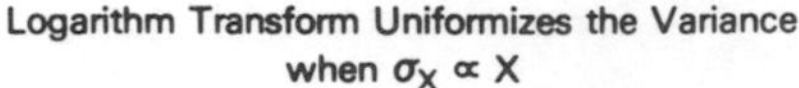

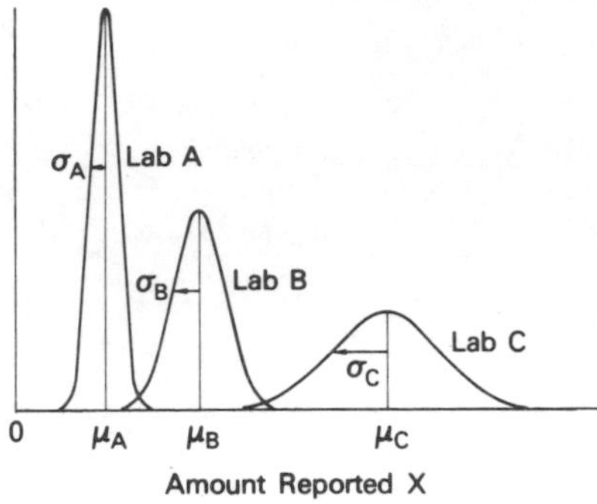

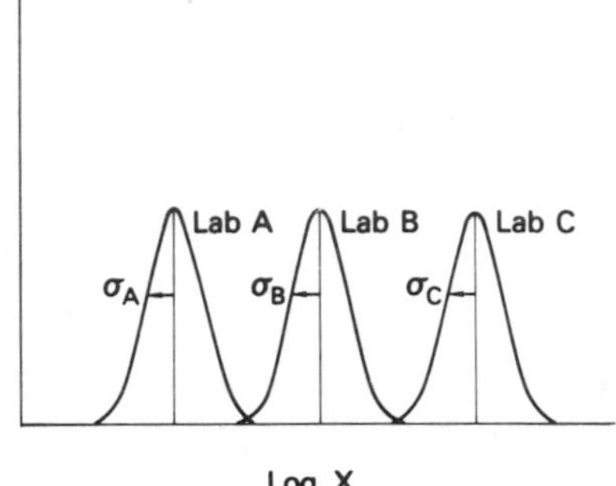

FIG. 7. A logarithmic transformation will stabilize the variance when the standard deviation for each laboratory is approximately proportional to the laboratory mean. Lower panel shows distribution of transformed results.

If we combine estimates of within-assay precision from several laboratories whose inherent precision is widely diverse, we may obtain a meaningless average value, not representative of the precision of any one of the laboratories. Moreover, the statistics associated with this average will be complex. However, if the within-laboratory precision is not too heterogeneous, this average may still be useful.

Figure 6 shows the theoretical relationship for the pooled within-assay, between-assay and between-laboratory components of variance as a function of the dose of the QC sample, expressed as %CV. For a typical RIA the within-assay variability is ≈ 5%, the between-assay ≈ 10%, while the between-laboratory variability component may range from 15% and up. Note that the "working range" for an assay shrinks as additional sources of error are considered.

Before we begin a conventional ANOVA, we attempt to stabilize the variance by applying an appropriate transformation to the data. If the standard

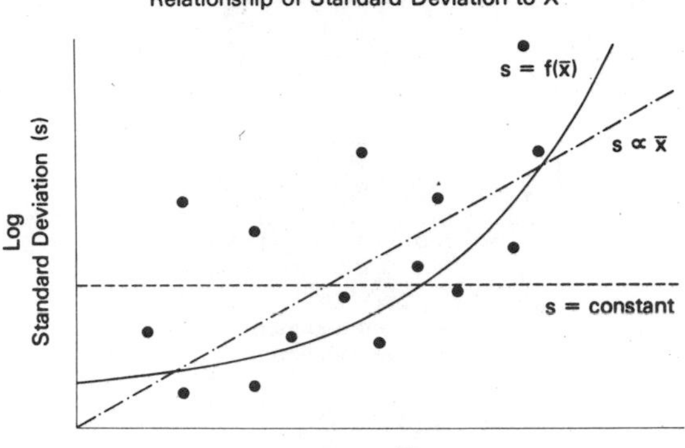

FIG.8. Schematic representation of relationships of standard deviation to the laboratory mean $\bar{x}$, on a log-log scale. Constant standard deviation (dashed); constant %CV (dot-dashed); a polynomial or power function f (solid) fit to the data. Logarithmic transform of the standard deviation helps to normalize their otherwise severely skewed distribution, and allows least-squares fitting.

deviation increases roughly in proportion to X (Fig.7), then a log transformation should result in nearly perfect uniformity of variance (lower panel). Depending on the nature of the relationship of variance to the dose X, other transforms, such as square root, may be suitable [6]. The logarithmic transform has the additional virtue that it will change a positively skewed log-normal distribution into a normal one. Most RIA samples are more nearly log-normally distributed. This is a consequence of the nearly linear relationship between response and log dose over about two-thirds of the usual dose-response curve.

Figure 8 shows some other candidates for functional relationships of the standard deviation to the laboratory mean value, e.g. when the standard deviation is a polynomial or power function of $\bar{X}$. The latter two functions may be fitted if sufficient data are available [7].

For any assumed relationship of standard deviation to dose, we may write the underlying statistical model. We consider the case when both within-assay and between-assay variability (within any given laboratory) are directly proportional to the laboratory mean, i.e. both show a constant %CV. Thus any one observation is the sum of the true value (μ) plus the laboratory bias (λ) plus the within-laboratory errors multiplied by the laboratory mean:

$$x_{ijk} = \mu + \lambda_i + (\mu + \lambda_i) \cdot (\alpha_{ij} + \epsilon_{ijk}) \quad (3)$$

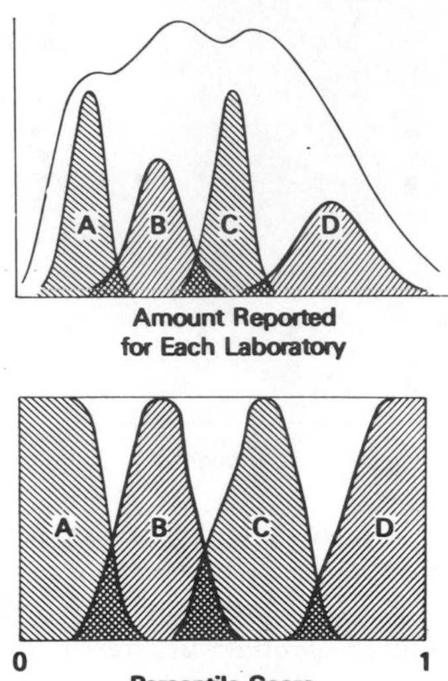

FIG.9. Four laboratories A,B,C and D with differing variances (upper panel) have approximately the same variance in the percentiled results (lower panel). The overall distribution of results is forced into a rectangular, uniform distribution.

where α and ϵ are normally distributed with means equal to zero and standard deviations of σ_α and σ. The laboratory error λ_i may be considered to be a random normal deviate with standard deviation σ_λ, or, in the "fixed effect model", as a constant bias, subject to the constraint that the mean value of λ_i is zero, i.e. $\Sigma\lambda_i = 0$. Equation (3) can be rewritten to illustrate that the model is no longer linear in the parameters λ, α, and ϵ.

$$x_{ijk} = (\mu + \lambda_i) \cdot (1 + \alpha_{ij} + \epsilon_{ijk}) \tag{4}$$

While it is possible to analyse a non-linear model such as Eq. (4), conventional ANOVA is restricted to linear models. By the use of log transformations, we can convert this non-linear model into an essentially linear one, more readily amenable to conventional analysis.

$$\begin{aligned} \log(x_{ijk}) &= \log(\mu + \lambda_i) + \log(1 + \alpha_{ij} + \epsilon_{ijk}) \\ &\approx \log(\mu + \lambda_i) + \alpha_{ij} + \epsilon_{ijk} \qquad (5) \\ &\text{when } |\alpha_{ij} + \epsilon_{ijk}| \ll 1 \end{aligned}$$

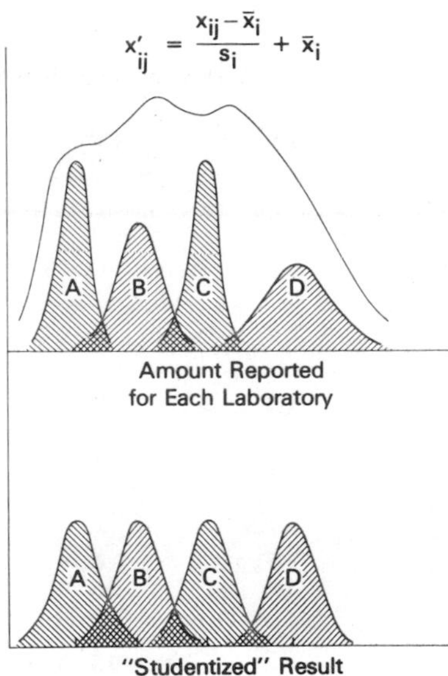

FIG.10. The "Studentizing" transform forces each laboratory to have a standard deviation of unity, by dividing each deviation from the laboratory mean ($\bar{x}_i$) by the estimated laboratory standard deviation (s_i). If the standard deviation is estimated precisely (high degrees of freedom) then the distributions for the transformed results for each laboratory will have identical variances, and be centred on each laboratory mean.

If, as in Fig. 1, the standard deviation varies among laboratories in a very complicated or arbitrary manner, we may use an ametric approach such as rank, percentile, or "RIDIT" transformations [8]. In Fig. 9 we display the effect of a percentile transformation on some hypothetical data. These transformations provide uniformity of variance but have the undesirable effect of losing information in terms of the original measurement scale: only ordinal information is preserved. However, for answering certain questions, this may be just the information required.

Another approach to achieving uniformity of variance is illustrated in Fig. 10. If we have sufficient replicates, e.g. 50 to 100, we may obtain reliable estimates of precision for each laboratory. We can then Studentize the data from any laboratory by subtracting its mean and dividing by its overall standard deviation. This results in a transformed variable with an expected variance and standard deviation of unity. This can be helpful, but is limited by the requirement for a high degree of replication to obtain sufficiently reliable estimates of σ_i.

ANOVA Table for Ranked
Within-laboratory Standard Deviation

		Laboratory Number				
		I	II	III	IV	V
	1	10	14	1	11	16
Assay	2	7	9	8	17	13
Number	3	2	12	6	15	19
	4	5	4	3	18	20
Mean	Rank	6.	9.75	4.5	15.25	17.

$s^2 = 30.4$

FIG.11. ANOVA table on the rank transformation of within-assay standard deviation of results from 5 laboratories on 4 trials. Average rank for each laboratory is shown in the bottom row, and the variance (s^2) of these averages is computed. Then a chi-square statistic is calculated (see text). Here the results are "significant" at the $P < 0.01$ level, indicating that the laboratories differ in their precision.

One statistical model for this problem is given by:

$$x_{ijk} = \mu + \lambda_i + \kappa_i(\alpha_{ij} + \epsilon_{ijk}) \quad (6)$$

Here κ_i represents the "precision factor" for any given laboratory i. Although this model is non-linear, it is still possible to estimate values for precision, κ_i, relative to that of a reference laboratory κ_1. This model assumes that there is a constant ratio of true between-assay to true within-assay errors for each laboratory. However, we may also consider the more general case where the ratio of between-assay to within-assay variability is itself variable, at the cost of a marked increase in the number of parameters to be estimated:

$$x_{ijk} = \mu + \lambda_i + \xi_i\alpha_{ij} + \zeta_i\epsilon_{ijk} \quad (7)$$

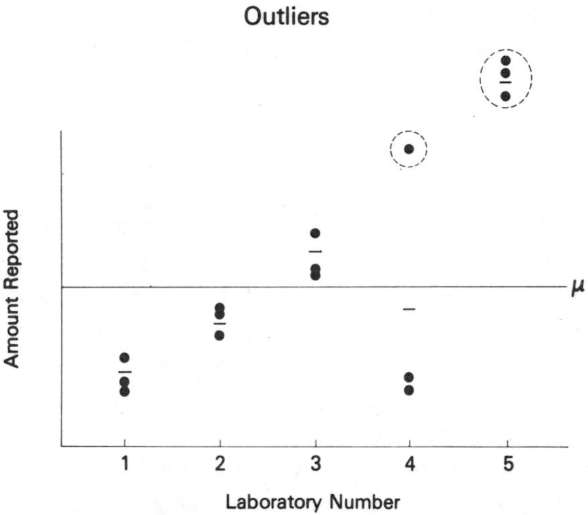

FIG.12. Results of QC study plotted versus laboratory number showing the "true" value μ. The mean for each laboratory is indicated with a dash. Even though the mean for laboratory 4 is near μ, its relatively high within-laboratory variance indicates the presence of an outlier (circled). Laboratory 5 contributes excessively to the overall estimate of between-laboratory variance, indicating that its entire set of results (circled) may be questionable.

Here λ, α, and ϵ are normally distributed with means of zero and standard deviations of σ_λ, σ_α and σ, respectively. We now define ξ_i as the between-assay precision factor, and ζ_i as the within-assay precision factor for a laboratory i. Equation (7) involves twice as many parameters as Eq. (6). We would therefore need at least twice as much data to obtain meaningful estimates of the components of variation.

In an appropriately designed study, we should be able to determine whether different laboratories have different degrees of precision. One can use an ANOVA for this purpose, based on the standard deviation (or other measure of dispersion) rather than the measured result [9]. Figure 11 illustrates such an analysis, using a rank transformation on the standard deviation in order to stabilize its inherent non-normality. Here the within-laboratory standard deviation has been estimated in several assays for each of five different laboratories. The bottom row shows the mean rank (over assays) for each of the laboratories. If all of the laboratories were to have the same inherent measurement error, then the mean ranks should be equal, except for random sampling error. One can test if there is a significant heterogeneity of ranks simply by computing the variance of the five entries in the bottom row (s^2), and comparing it to its expected value (cf. Fig. 11, bottom) by use of an approximate chi-square statistic:[1]

$$\chi^2 = \frac{s^2(L-1)\cdot 12}{L(M\cdot L+1)}$$

where M = number of assays and L = number of laboratories. This χ^2 statistic may be compared with tabulated values for (L − 1) degrees of freedom. Use of the **ranks** of the original standard deviations in Fig. 11 allows us to use a chi-square statistic instead of an F ratio. This example illustrates that ranking may be usefully applied, not only to the original data, but to derived values such as standard deviations. This kind of analysis requires a substantial amount of data before one can determine whether there is a significant variability of standard deviation among laboratories. We would require at least ten trials in duplicate from each laboratory before we could determine whether there was even modest heterogeneity in standard deviation among laboratories.

Another approach to evaluate homogeneity of variance is the use of Bartlett's test [10]. This classical test utilizes the log of the variance estimates for each laboratory, computes the standard deviation of these transformed estimates, and compared the result to the expected value.

It is often desirable to combine the results from several QC samples analysed in different studies. One could do this by adding another level to the ANOVA, at the cost of increased complexity. The components of variance approach provides a simple method for presenting results. In Fig. 6, we plot each component (expressed as a standard deviation) versus sample mean. After the components for each sample have been calculated, we may test whether the components represent a constant %CV with changing $\overline{X}$. If so, we might then take the median as the best estimate.

DETECTION OF OUTLIERS

ANOVA is extremely sensitive to the presence of outliers. In an internal quality-control setting, the technician is likely to be able to detect and remove unreasonable values before they enter the QC calculations. However, in the context of an automated, computerized external QC program, outliers are much more difficult to detect.

---

[1] Approaches chi-square asymptotically with M, L large.

Figure 12 illustrates two kinds of outliers: laboratories 1, 2 and 3 are apparently "well behaved". However, in laboratory 4, a single outlying replicate has caused an anomalously high within-laboratory standard deviation. We may calculate an F-test for the ratio of within-laboratory standard deviation for laboratory 4 compared to the within-laboratory standard deviation of other laboratories, 1, 2, 3 and 5 to evaluate the statistical significance of this suspected outlier:

$$F_{\nu_1,\nu_2} = \frac{SSW_1/\nu_1}{SSW_2/\nu_2} \qquad (8)$$

where SSW_1 is the sum of squared deviations for laboratory 4 with ν_1 degrees of freedom, and SSW_2 is the within-laboratory sum of squares for the remaining laboratories, with ν_2 degrees of freedom.

Laboratory 5, in Fig. 12, also has measurements which appeared to be aberrant. This can be tested by noting that laboratory 5 contributes appreciably more than the average to the overall estimate of between-laboratory variability. Again, this may be evaluated with an F-test of the local between-laboratory variability for laboratory 5 versus the between-laboratory variability for all other laboratories:

$$F_{1,\nu-1} = \frac{SSB_1 - SSB_2}{SSB_2/(\nu-1)} \qquad (9)$$

where SSB_1 is the between-laboratories sum of squares for all laboratories with ν degrees of freedom, and SSB_2 is the between sum of squares for all laboratories except the suspected outlier.

The significance level for these F-tests must be adjusted since we are implicitly making multiple comparisons, i.e. we are simultaneously testing each laboratory for extreme values. We can approximately compensate by multiplying the P level by the number of laboratories [11].

The tests for outliers and for homogeneity of variance are very similar. One laboratory may appear to be an outlier because its underlying variance is very much higher than for the other laboratories.

Another classical test for detection of outliers is Dixon's gap test [12]. This test compares the gap or difference between the most extreme and next most extreme values to the overall range of the observations. Both outlier detection rules are derived on the assumption that the observed data have been sampled from a normal distribution. Departure from normality may invalidate or at least change the effective P level for an outlier test. Statistical outlier detection rules are generally quite insensitive. However, appropriate graphical analysis of the data can be very useful for this purpose.

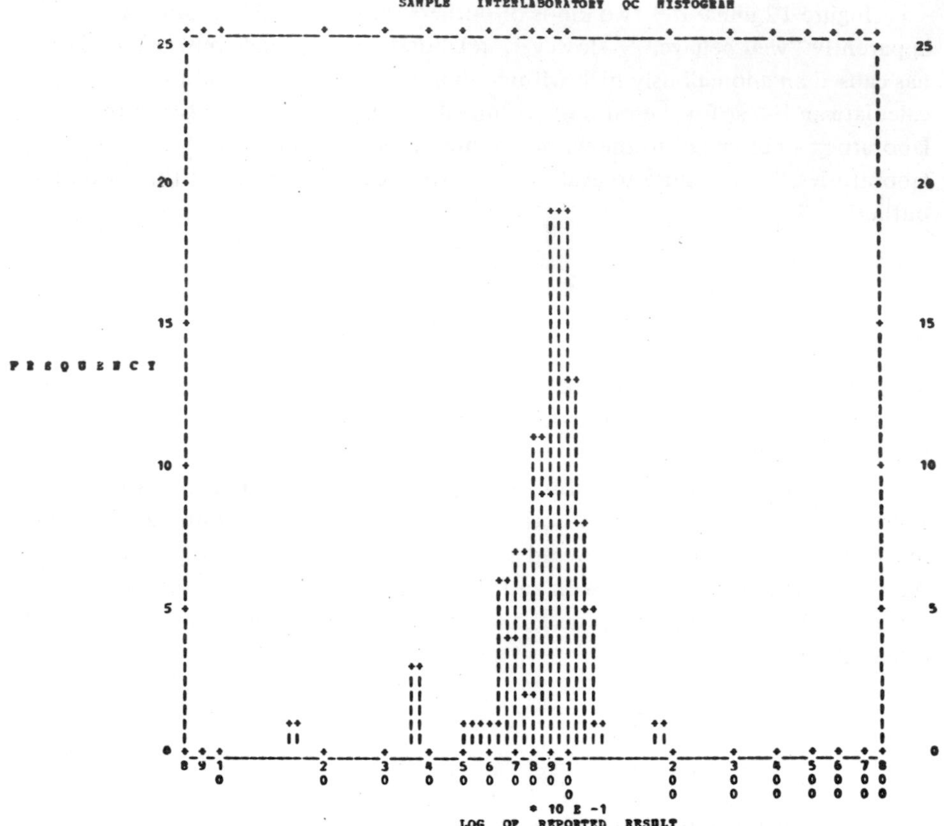

FIG.13. Computer output histogram of results of QC study on log scale gives summary of results and provides visual check for outliers and for the approximate log-normality of the distribution.

GRAPHICAL DISPLAY

Graphical display of the data remains highly desirable. The first step in any multi-laboratory QC analysis is a simple histogram of all the results (Fig. 13). A logarithmic scale is useful, since the results often span more than one order of magnitude. The histogram provides a general idea of the magnitude of the total variability. Display of results from individual laboratories in small histograms or as ranges of a fixed number of replicates permits immediate comparison of within- and between-laboratory variability. Figure 14 shows a plot of laboratory standard deviations versus laboratory means, using a percentile transformation on the raw data. This transformation protects from the undue influence of

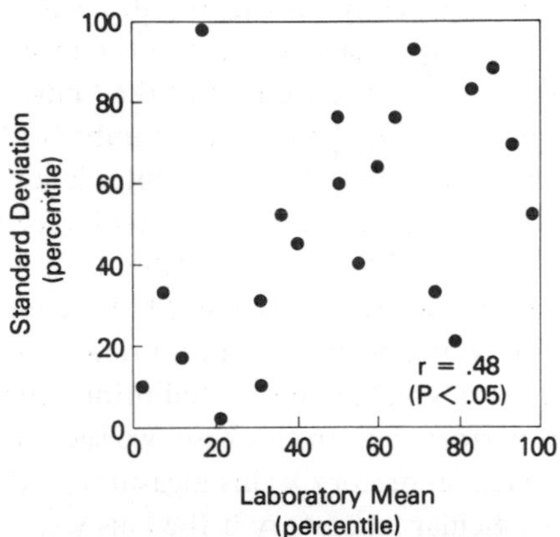

FIG.14. Laboratory standard deviation versus laboratory mean, both on a percentile scale. The percentile transformation protects against the undue influence of outlying observations and provides a convenient compact plotting format which may be compared across several successive QC studies or across samples. A significant positive correlation indicates that standard deviation increases with mean, and that a preliminary transformation of the data is needed.

outliers, and accordingly may be preferable to the plot of the raw data itself. The Spearman rank correlation of 0.49 for this data is just significant at the 0.05 level. One might conclude that there is an association between standard deviation and mean. However, to improve the reliability of the statement, one should pool results over several assays (and/or QC samples) to increase the number of degrees of freedom.

We may also use a graphical analysis shown in Fig.14 as a convenient summary of the data. If the median value for laboratory mean were near the true value for the given QC sample, then the ideal laboratory would appear on the graph at the 50th percentile in laboratory mean and the zeroth percentile for standard deviation. Thus, we have assigned a simple two-dimensional score to each of the participating laboratories. Figure 14 can also be used to determine whether we have selected an appropriate transformation of the data to obtain uniformity of variance. The rank correlation between laboratory mean and standard deviation should be indistinguishable from zero if we have selected an appropriate transformation. In most small-scale inter-laboratory quality-control studies, there will be insufficient data to distinguish between the various transformations with regard to their stabilization of the variance. Until a large data base becomes available, one may use the logarithm transformation as a first approximation.

INTERPRETATION OF RESULTS

As with any statistical calculation, the estimated components of variability must be interpreted in the perspective of the intentions of the original study. The component σ_λ^2 is ordinarily interpreted as the variance of the error introduced by each laboratory, in the context of the "random effects" model. If we estimate σ_λ^2 by randomly sampling a small number of laboratories from a much larger population, we can then predict the inter-laboratory component for that larger group. We can expect the average results from 95% of these laboratories will be within $2\sigma_\lambda$ of the true result, in the long run.

We might also consider the errors introduced by each laboratory to be fixed rather than random, which would be appropriate when we are dealing with a small number of laboratories and are interested primarily in how well each individual laboratory is performing. In this case, we seek to estimate the laboratory bias, λ_i, for each laboratory. This measurement could be used to correct results from a particular laboratory if the bais were shown to be uniform for all samples. It is likely that the bias observed during one study period would change with time, so it would be inappropriate for another period. Correction factors, if they are applied to laboratory results, should only be applied while the laboratory is monitored in a QC study, and when statistical consultation provides the necessary controls built into experimental design.

Interpretation of results also depends on the assumption of appropriate sampling techniques. Laboratories included in a collaborative study are seldom, if ever, selected according to a randomization scheme. Often the sample is biased to preferentially include larger, more competent laboratories with a resulting bias in the reported inter-laboratory component of variance; this effect can be both severe and misleading.

Whenever one uses a preliminary transformation of the data before analysis, the results should be transformed back into the original scale. With logarithmic, square-root or other continuous transforms, it is a simple matter to take the inverse transform (i.e. antilog, square, etc.) to obtain estimates of the mean, μ, or of the laboratory means $(\mu + \lambda_i)$. Likewise, we can obtain approximate estimates of the standard deviations in terms of the original measurement scale by multiplying the standard deviation in the transformed units by the derivative of the inverse transform function evaluated at the mean. In the case of logarithmic transformation:

$$s_x \approx \text{antilog}\{\text{mean } \log(x)\} \cdot s_{\log(x)} \tag{10}$$

Thus, many statements about the data in the original coordinates can be made **verbatim** about the data transformed by a continuous function.

If we have used an ametric transformation, such as percentile or ranking, special care must be taken in interpreting the results. The mean of ranked data may be reported as the median. However, since the variance of a set of n ranks is theoretically fixed at n(n + 1)/12, any components of variance analysis must obey this constraint. The components may be treated as somewhat arbitrary indices of precision, but are at best only approximately proportional to measures of precision using the original metric scale.

DESCRIPTION OF COMPUTER PROGRAM

A computer program package has been prepared to implement some of the types of ANOVA with components of variance analysis discussed here. It is written in PL/I for the IBM 370/168 at the computer installation at National Institutes of Health in Bethesda, Md., USA. Typical running costs are approximately $5 per run, using about 8 seconds of machine time. This package consists of a main program and three subroutines, and utilizes standard statistical subroutines in the International Mathematical and Statistical Libraries program library. This program package is available directly from the first author on request.

NOMENCLATURE

%CV	per cent coefficient of variation
ν	degrees of freedom
F	Fisher's F ratio of two sample variances
σ_T^2	total variance of a set of observations
σ_λ^2	component of variance due to laboratories
σ_α^2	component of variance due to assays
σ^2	variance of replicates (residual)
x_{ijk}	individual measurement made by i^{th} laboratory in the jth assay, and the kth replicate
μ	expected or population (true) mean
λ_i	bias due to laboratory i
α_{ij}	bias or effect due to assay j in laboratory i
ϵ_{ijk}	random error effect in replicate k, assay j, laboratory i
κ_i	precision factor for laboratory i
ξ_i	between-assay precision factor for laboratory i
ζ_i	within-assay precision factor for laboratory i
s	sample or estimated standard deviation
s^2	sample variance
X	generic dose variable

REFERENCES

[1] YOUDEN, W.J., STEINER, E.H., Statistical Manual of the Assoc. of Official Analytical Chemists (Association of Official Analytical Chemists), Washington, DC (1975).
[2] HARRIS, E.K., DEMETS, D.L., Clin. Chem. **18** (1972) 244.
[3] RODBARD, D., Clin. Chem. **20** (1974) 1255.
[4] RUSSELL, C.D., DE BLANC, H.J., WAGNER, H.N., Johns Hopkins Med. J. **135** (1974) 344.
[5] McDONAGH, B.F., MUNSON, P.J., RODBARD, D., Computer Programs in Biomedicine **7** (1977) 179.
[6] BARTLETT, M.S., Biometrics **3** (1947) 39.
[7] RODBARD, D., LENOX, R.H., WRAY, H.L., RAMSETH, D., Clin. Chem. **22** (1976) 350.
[8] BROSS, I.D., Biometrics **14** (1958) 18.
[9] FRIEDMAN, M., J. Am. Stat. Assoc. **32** (1937) 675.
[10] BENNETT, C.A., FRANKLIN, N.L., Statistical Analysis in Chemistry and the Chemical Industry, J. Wiley and Sons, New York (1954).
[11] COCHRAN, W.G., Biometrics **3** (1947) 22.
[12] DUNCAN, A.J., Quality Control and Industrial Statistics, 4th Edn, Richard D. Irwin, Homewood, Ill. (1974).

DISCUSSION

P.G. MALAN: Your paper gives a very clear description of the methods which can be applied to the analysis of quality-control results. There are several laboratories around the world which are now applying these techniques in order to obtain more information about the detailed performance of individual laboratories, rather than to make a more general assessment in which a single, usually relatively meaningless, overall coefficient of variation is quoted. In our experience, the distribution of quality-control samples is carried out at relatively infrequent intervals – fortnightly or monthly – and this does not generate sufficient data within a reasonably short time to yield detailed statistical information or to obtain precision-dose profiles. The only way to obtain the necessary information appears to be to take complete data from each assay in order to determine within- and between-assay variations of individual laboratories. May I ask you to comment on this difficulty.

D. RODBARD: Unfortunately, in contrast to your remarks, the use of the analysis of variance approach to analysis of multi-laboratory studies has been woefully neglected and is missing from many studies where it should have been applied. Furthermore, a component of variance approach has scarcely ever been applied to such studies. The use of such analyses by Peter Munson and myself in studies sponsored by WHO and the United Kingdom may have represented the first occasion on which such analyses were used in this area (cf. Refs [2–5] of the paper).

I agree that the use of quality-control samples, by itself, does not generate all the desired information within a reasonable period of time. It is essential for each laboratory to have its own, on-going internal quality-control programme.

In this manner, we can obtain very reliable estimates of within-assay and between-assay variance for several dose levels. Knowledge of the ratio of between- to within-assay variance and the relationship between these and the laboratory mean can enable us to simplify the analysis of variance and reduce the number of parameters which must be estimated.

Lastly, the quality control pools used in the internal quality-control programmes cannot provide all the desired information. These can be used to "check" or "verify" the results generated as part of the routine data-processing programme. By simple analysis of the relationship between the standard deviation of the response and the response level, together with the shape of the dose-response curve, we can predict the relationship between the within-assay standard deviation or coefficient of variation and the dose level, with reliability corresponding to hundreds of degrees of freedom (cf. Refs. [1], [12], [19] and [24] of paper SM-220/58). The analysis of the quality-control sample data can verify these results (objectively evaluated by an F-test) and validate their application. However, the analysis of individual assays can provide no information regarding the between-assay variance. For this purpose the quality-control programmes, both internal and external, are essential.

R.J. BAYLY: As you are aware, it is essential to treat individual laboratories as part of a continuum of laboratories in order to apply the component of variance approach. Provided this can reasonably be done, this approach is evidently a most valuable one. However, you mentioned interaction between laboratories, which in practice is not surprising. I am interested in how you remove these interaction elements before applying the component of variance approach to the remaining "random effect" model.

D. RODBARD: Actually, the analysis of variance with a component of variance breakdown can be applied to studies involving a small number of laboratories; in this case, the use of a "fixed effects" model appears to be more appropriate. The problem of "laboratory-sample interaction" certainly complicates the analysis. Approaches to this problem are discussed in Refs [1] and [5]. Use of percentile transformations or other ametric methods is sometimes of help. Likewise, we can combine the results from different samples only after the ANOVA is completed. If various groups of laboratories are using different methodologies (e.g. steroid assays with and without preliminary chromatography), then we can anticipate that there will be varying degrees of cross-reactivity (e.g. between testosterone and dihydrotestosterone), and hence the increased likelihood of laboratory-sample interaction. Accordingly, we can restructure the analysis in an attempt to minimize these effects. Finally, despite the fact that we can never satisfy all the assumptions underlying the theoretical analysis of the statistical method, we still have a simple, pragmatic informative approach to data reduction, which provides a number of meaningful and useful statistical parameters.

THE NEED FOR STANDARDIZATION OF METHODOLOGY AND COMPONENTS IN COMMERCIAL RADIOIMMUNOASSAY KITS*

W.G. WOOD, I. MARSCHNER, P.C. SCRIBA
Medizinische Klinik Innenstadt
der Universität München,
Munich, Federal Republic of Germany

Abstract

THE NEED FOR STANDARDIZATION OF METHODOLOGY AND COMPONENTS IN COMMERCIAL RADIOIMMUNOASSAY KITS.

The problems arising from the increasing use of commercial kits in radioimmunoassay (RIA) and related fields are discussed. These problems differ according to the substance under test. The quality of individual reagents is often good, but the methodology is often not optimal and may contain short-cuts which, although commercially attractive, can lead to erroneous values and poor sensitivity and precision. Minor modifications in the methodology often lead to big improvements in sensitivity and precision. This has been demonstrated in three digoxin kits employing antibody-coated tube techniques and in four kits for thyrotropin (TSH) using different techniques. It has also been noted that with many quality-control sera imported from the USA no values are ascribed to European kits for the components listed, thus reducing these sera to the function of precision control. The study underlines the need to standardize kit components and assay methods to enable the results obtained by different laboratories with different kits to be compared.

The decentralized nature of health care in the Federal Republic of Germany (FRG) has contributed to the rapid increase in the use of commercial kits in RIA and associated techniques. The problems arising from the extended use of kits are many and they are not only concerned with methodology. The differing results obtained for certain substances with kits from different manufacturers may lead to a false diagnosis when only the absolute values are compared without reference to the given normal range. This problem arises particularly with the proteohormones.

Table I is an excerpt from the values ascribed to digoxin, TSH and insulin in different kits of commercial quality-control sera. For each component the control sera are at three concentrations with the aim of controlling low, middle and high ranges of the standard curve. For the drug digoxin, which is not normally present in serum, it can be seen from Table I that the measured values

* Supported by the Bundesministerium für Forschung und Technologie.

TABLE I. VALUES ASCRIBED TO DIFFERENT KITS FOR DIGOXIN, TSH AND INSULIN IN COMMERCIAL QUALITY-CONTROL SERA
(Taken from manufacturers' data)

Test (units)	Kit	Level 1 mean ± 2 SD	Level 2 mean ± 2 SD	Level 3 mean ± 2 SD
Digoxin (ng/ml)				
	Abbott	0.6 ± 0.16	1.7 ± 0.28	3.0 ± 0.54
	Amersham/Searle	0.7 ± 0.04	1.8 ± 0.12	3.0 ± 0.24
	Beckman	0.9 ± 0.12	1.9 ± 0.16	3.1 ± 0.38
	Burroughs Wellcome	0.8 ± 0.10	1.8 ± 0.12	3.1 ± 0.32
	Clinical Assays	0.8 ± 0.16	2.0 ± 0.24	3.0 ± 0.22
	Corning	0.8 ± 0.12	1.9 ± 0.26	2.9 ± 0.40
	Curtis	1.0 ± 0.26	2.0 ± 0.36	3.2 ± 0.28
	Kallestad ^{3}H	0.8 ± 0.24	1.8 ± 0.50	2.8 ± 0.54
	Kallestad ^{125}I	0.8 ± 0.06	1.8 ± 0.22	3.0 ± 0.24
	Micromedic	0.8 ± 0.16	1.9 ± 0.24	3.1 ± 0.48
	Dade	0.8 ± 0.08	2.0 ± 0.16	3.2 ± 0.20
	NEN ^{125}I	0.8 ± 0.18	1.8 ± 0.12	3.0 ± 0.20
	NEN ^{125}I Solid Phase	0.7 ± 0.08	1.7 ± 0.12	3.0 ± 0.30
	Radioassay Systems	0.6 ± 0.14	1.6 ± 0.20	3.0 ± 0.46
	Schwarz-Mann	0.8 ± 0.10	2.0 ± 0.28	3.4 ± 0.60
	Squibb	0.8 ± 0.20	1.6 ± 0.20	2.5 ± 0.40

TABLE I (cont.)

Test (units)	Kit	Level 1 mean ± 2 SD	Level 2 mean ± 2 SD	Level 3 mean ± 2 SD
TSH (μU/ml)				
	Abbott	5.3 ± 1.28	15.2 ± 3.10	47.3 ± 16.20
	Diagnostic Products	8.7 ± 0.76	19.6 ± 1.20	38.6 ± 2.82
	Nichols Institute	4.6 ± 0.75	15.7 ± 1.64	32.3 ± 2.90
	Radioassay Systems	4.4 ± 1.86	13.6 ± 1.62	29.9 ± 1.96
	Beckman	6.1 ± 0.72	15.5 ± 3.84	38.1 ± 13.24
Insulin (μU/ml)				
	Amersham/Searle	15 ± 3.1	39 ± 3.5	101 ± 11.1
	Corning	17 ± 4.4	38 ± 8.0	112 ± 12.3
	Curtis	6 ± 0.6	32 ± 8.0	87 ± 11.7
	Schwarz-Mann	13 ± 2.2	34 ± 4.1	105 ± 21.7
	Pharmacia	24 ± 7.5	50 ± 8.5	115 ± 27.1

TABLE II. VALUES ASCRIBED TO DIFFERENT KITS FOR T_3, CORTISOL AND T_4 IN COMMERCIAL QUALITY-CONTROL SERA
(Taken from manufacturers' data)

Test (units)	Kit	Level 1 mean ± 2 SD	Level 2 mean ± 2 SD	Level 3 mean ± 2 SD
T_3 RIA (ng/dl)				
	Beckmann	61.1 ± 11.54	163.6 ± 26.56	390.0 ± 80.46
	Abbott	107.0 ± 32.00	250.0 ± 72.00	530.0 ± 190.0
	Ames	85.4 ± 13.72	196.0 ± 21.48	428.3 ± 59.74
	Amersham/Searle	65.0 ± 8.00	170.0 ± 22.0	444.0 ± 46.00
	Corning	45.5 ± 7.84	147.6 ± 28.52	328.9 ± 60.94
	Curtis	72.4 ± 30.62	195.3 ± 31.76	384.4 ± 35.72
	Diagnostic Products	78.1 ± 8.44	165.5 ± 11.60	356.6 ± 42.16
	Maloy Laboratories	101.6 ± 10.16	245.6 ± 41.30	536.6 ± 53.40
	Nichols Institute	71.1 ± 10.58	173.8 ± 20.84	402.9 ± 34.01
	Radioassay Systems	43.9 ± 17.46	147.9 ± 20.82	349.8 ± 29.34
Cortisol (μg/dl)				
	Amersham/Searle	6.4 ± 0.60	24.3 ± 3.38	>41
	Clinical Assays ^{3}H	4.6 ± 1.88	21.4 ± 5.16	57.8 ± 14.12
	Clinical Assays ^{125}I	5.3 ± 1.48	21.6 ± 6.96	51.7 ± 16.76
	Diagnostic Products	5.6 ± 0.62	23.4 ± 2.74	52.1 ± 4.80
	NEN	5.0 ± 0.82	21.5 ± 4.38	51.3 ± 7.32
	Micromedic Autopak	5.2 ± 0.84	18.0 ± 1.34	34.9 ± 3.22
	Micromedic	5.4 ± 1.02	20.6 ± 2.28	40.7 ± 9.04
	Radioass. Syst.	4.8 ± 1.32	17.8 ± 3.00	51.6 ± 6.89
	Schwarz-Mann	4.7 ± 1.46	17.3 ± 5.48	39.5 ± 11.00
T_4 (μg/dl)				
	Dade CPB	4.2 ± 1.08	9.3 ± 1.54	16.1 ± 1.68
	Abbott CPB	2.9 ± 1.31	10.2 ± 1.35	20.7 ± 3.70
	Abbott RIA	3.4 ± 0.60	8.3 ± 0.74	15.5 ± 2.32
	Abbott RIA-PEG	3.6 ± 0.54	8.3 ± 1.02	15.3 ± 2.32
	Ames CPB	3.6 ± 0.84	8.5 ± 1.22	16.5 ± 1.22
	Amersham/Searle CPB	4.1 ± 0.34	11.3 ± 1.04	>19.2
	Amersham/Searle RIA	3.8 ± 0.82	9.3 ± 0.96	17.7 ± 1.56

TABLE II (cont.)

Test (units)	Kit	Level 1 mean ± 2 SD	Level 2 mean ± 2 SD	Level 3 mean ± 2 SD
	Curtis CPB	4.0 ± 1.12	8.4 ± 1.46	14.7 ± 1.48
	Curtis RIA	4.4 ± 0.64	8.7 ± 1.08	14.9 ± 2.24
	Curtis RIALIQUA	5.5 ± 0.92	10.4 ± 0.90	16.1 ± 1.38
	Oxford STAT 4	2.9 ± 0.96	5.4 ± 0.62	10.0 ± 0.84
	Oxford Column	2.2 ± 0.36	5.2 ± 0.92	9.0 ± 2.30

are relatively constant, especially at higher concentrations. Other small molecules such as T_3, T_4 and cortisol, which occur naturally in serum together with metabolites of similar structure and must first be separated from a binding protein before assay, give a different range of values, as shown in Table II. Here, the values from different kits are not so constant; in some cases the highest value is more than twice that of the lowest one for the same component in the same serum. Another point that is brought out here is that the results and precision of different kits produced by the same manufacturer for the same component may differ markedly.

Larger proteohormones show even more anomalous results, as can be seen in Table I. These anomalies are due to the assay systems used as well as to the reference preparation against which the standards are calibrated.

Many kits are delivered with methodological weaknesses which give rise to far from optimal performance. Often minor changes in the protocol give rise to major improvements in performance. Table III shows the results of such modifications in three antibody-coated tube assays for digoxin. The danger of such assays is the poor precision at low concentrations because of non-specific binding sites. Non-specific binding can be minimized by pre-incubation before labelled tracer is added. In fact, the procedure for the Clinical Assays kit includes such a pre-incubation step and good precision is achieved over the entire range of the standard curve. When this step is omitted, precision and sensitivity are poor. The Schwarz-Mann AbTRAC kit provides not only antibody-coated tubes but also lyophilised tracer already in the tubes. Here, the protocol states that first serum and then buffer should be added to each tube in turn. If, however, buffer is added to all the tubes followed by serum, then precision is achieved at lower concentrations. The Boehringer-Mannheim kit combines the tracer and buffer, thus obviating the need for pre-incubation. If, however, the tracer and buffer from the Clinical Assays kit are used with the Boehringer tubes and standards, and a pre-incubation step is included, the precision improves markedly

TABLE III. RESULTS FROM ORIGINAL AND MODIFIED METHODS FOR THREE DIGOXIN ANTIBODY-COATED TUBE KITS

Kit	Sensitivity*		50%**	Precision			CV
	$\%B_0$	ng/ml	intercept	No.	Mean	SD	
1. Clinical Assays			ng/ml				
(a)	89.8	0.24	1.09	30	1.40	0.06	4.93
				30	3.62	0.29	7.97
(b)	85.6	0.41	1.76	19	1.30	0.21	16.0
				19	3.90	0.16	4.00
2. Schwarz-Mann AbTRAC							
(a)	98.0	0.05	2.23	20	0.81	0.09	10.6
				20	3.44	0.11	3.17
(c)	95.2	0.06	1.28	22	0.78	0.06	7.27
				22	3.83	0.28	7.28
3. Boehringer-Mannheim							
(a)	99.2	0.02	2.06	20	0.84	0.23	28.5
				20	4.05	0.20	4.96
(d)	96.6	0.14	1.69	20	0.93	0.06	6.92
				20	4.24	0.17	4.15
(e)	90.4	0.40	2.64	14	0.72	0.12	16.5
				14	3.93	0.14	3.63

* Sensitivity is defined here and in Tables IV, V and VI as the value on the standard curve, 3 standard deviations from the zero standard.

** All data here and in Tables IV, V and VI were obtained from standard curves plotted using a spline function.

(a) Assay performed according to protocol.
(b) Without pre-incubation.
(c) Buffer added before serum.
(d) Boehringer Ab-coated tubes and standards, Clinical Assays buffer and label, with pre-incubation.
(e) As for (d) but without pre-incubation.

A further Boehringer-Mannheim digoxin kit of a different batch has been tested and has been found to give the following results under the conditions in (a). Sensitivity $\%B_0 = 97.0$ or 0.16 ng/ml, 50% intercept = 1.80 ng/ml, CV (1) n = 19, mean = 0.91 ng/ml, SD = 0.05 ng/ml, CV = 5.56%; (2) n = 14, mean = 2.89 ng/ml, SD = 0.23 ng/ml, CV = 8.03%.

TABLE IV. DIGOXIN STANDARDS FROM FIVE KITS MEASURED IN THE CLINICAL ASSAYS KIT

Standard (ng/ml)	Kits				
	Abbott	Schwarz-Mann	Squibb	Boehringer-Mannheim	Corning
0	0.05	0.08	0	0.05	0.10
0.5	0.70	0.58	0.44	0.50	0.45
1.0	1.14	1.14	0.85	1.00	0.94
1.5	–	1.60	–	–	–
2.0	2.14	2.04	1.74	2.04	–
2.5	–	–	–	–	2.35
3.0	–	2.79	2.89	3.14	–
4.0	4.80	–	–	–	–
5.0	–	5.14	4.70	5.29	5.00

at low concentrations. Omission of the pre-incubation step immediately lowers the precision. Pre-incubation has little or no effect at higher digoxin levels. This is to be expected because of the excess of unlabelled digoxin present. Pre-incubation increases the slope of the standard curve, as seen in the reduced values of the 50% intercept. The results in Table III are taken from the assay in which intra-assay precision was measured.

The reagents of the kits are often of very high quality, as shown in Table IV: the standards from five different digoxin kits were measured by the Clinical Assays kit (standard curve range 0–8 ng/ml). The question of quality is further highlighted by the results from the Boehringer kit in which the coated tubes were tested with the Clinical Assays reagents. The problems arising from proteohormone assays, which usually require a longer pre-incubation period before labelled tracer is added to increase sensitivity, concern methodology and kit components to a greater extent than in the digoxin kits. The use of standards in hormone-free serum instead of buffer for derivation of a standard curve has been described elsewhere [1, 2]. Such a curve is more realistic and gives better results, especially at lower hormone concentrations.

Four TSH kits were tested and modified to check their performance; the results are given in Tables V and VI. Table V gives the incubation details, the assay sensitivity and the 50% intercept together with the medium in which the standards were dissolved. The performance of the Kabi kit could have been improved greatly by pre-incubation before addition of the label, as shown by the sensitivity and 50% intercept values. The Schwarz-Mann kit was improved by

TABLE V. EFFECTS OF INCUBATION PROCEDURES ON SENSITIVITY AND 50% INTERCEPT IN FOUR TSH KITS

Kit	Pre-inc. (h)	Temp. (°C)	Main inc. (h)	Temp. (°C)	2nd Ab (h)	Temp. (°C)	Sensitivity ($\%B_0$)	Sensitivity (μU/ml)	50%-intercept (μU/ml)	Kit standards
Kabi*										
(a_1)	–	–	96	4	24	4	92.9	2.89	20.9	Buffer
(b_1)	72	4	24	4	24	4	92.8	0.66	5.18	(A)**
Schwarz-Mann										
(a_1)	2	37	3	37	1.5	37	95.1	0.77	9.35	Buffer
(b_1)	18	RT	3	RT	1.0	RT	92.0	0.59	4.61	(A)
Diagnostic Products										
(a_1)	3	37	2	37	0.25	37	92.4	2.58	26.1	Protein
(b_1)	3	37	2	RT	0.75	RT	92.8	2.85	25.9	based
(b_2)	18	RT	2	RT	0.75	RT	95.9	0.96	13.7	(B)
Henning										
(a_1)	2	37	2.5	37	0.17	37	86.2	3.06	14.6	In TSH-free
(a_2)	18	RT	2	RT	0.50	RT	92.9	0.81	6.92	serum (A)

* (a_x) = Original method given with kit
(b_y) = Modified methods
** (A) = Calibrated against MRC 68/38 Standard
(B) = Calibrated against WHO 1st IRP 1974

RT = Room temperature
Pre-incubation = Incubation without labelled hormone
Main incubation = After addition of labelled hormone
2nd Ab = Incubation after addition of precipitating antiserum

TABLE VI. PERFORMANCE OF TSH KITS WITH COMMERCIAL CONTROL SERA, PATIENT SERA AND MRC 68/38 IN TSH-FREE SERUM
(Assay notation is as in Table V)

Quality control sera	Kit								
	Kabi assay		Schwarz-Mann assay		Diagnostic Products assay			Henning assay	
	a_1	b_1	a_1	b_1	a_1	b_1	b_2	a_1	a_2
RIACON 1 (7.48*)	7.48	6.27	8.39	10.27	4.59	4.46	4.79	5.72	6.51
2 (41.0)	32.0	30.1	42.4	45.3	23.5	23.6	25.7	26.6	20.5
Patient sera									
801 – 0 min TRH test	2.89	2.09	3.36	3.34	4.13	4.24	3.97	3.06	2.00
801 – 30 min	13.9	14.4	23.2	27.7	17.3	15.3	16.0	12.8	12.7
815 – 0 min TRH test	< 2.89	0.65	0.77	1.09	< 2.58	< 2.85	< 0.96	< 3.06	< 0.81
815 – 30 min	< 2.89	0.64	0.93	0.59	< 2.58	< 2.85	< 0.96	< 3.06	< 0.81
TSH Standard MRC 68/38									
0.39 μU/ml	< 2.89	0.73	1.66	1.63	3.56	3.45	2.49	< 3.06	0.84
0.78	< 2.89	1.01	1.81	2.07	4.65	3.19	3.26	< 3.06	0.98
1.56	2.83	1.65	3.11	2.94	5.81	3.89	3.76	3.52	1.74
3.12	4.57	3.05	4.17	4.94	6.99	5.70	5.19	3.66	3.04
6.25	6.91	6.43	8.85	10.1	9.05	9.19	7.97	5.44	6.08
12.5	11.72	13.3	18.2	19.2	14.5	15.5	13.2	11.0	12.6

TABLE VI (cont.)

Quality control sera	Kit: Kabi assay a_1	Kabi assay b_1	Schwarz-Mann assay a_1	Schwarz-Mann assay b_1	Diagnostic Products assay a_1	Diagnostic Products assay b_1	Diagnostic Products assay b_2	Henning assay a_1	Henning assay a_2
25.0	23.83	28.7	29.7	29.2	26.4	29.1	24.5	24.0	22.2
50.0	61.29	51.2	>50	>50	65.9	61.0	55.8	47.2	48.0
Normal range given by kit manufacturer mean ± 2 SD	1.5–8.0		0.4–9.2		3.1–9.6			0.5–4.0	

* Mean of 4 kits listed by manufacturer (Dr. Molter, Heidelberg, FRG).
All values in μU/ml.

overnight incubation at room termperature instead of for a shorter time at 37°C, as were the Diagnostic Products and Henning kits.

The values obtained from the patient sera, control sera and MRC Standard 68/38 dissolved in TSH-free serum differ only at lower concentrations when the sensitivity for each kit is improved. The introduction of "Quick-Tests" for TSH that require a total incubation time of only 5 or 6 hours are a commercial innovation with no clinical advantages. Although the incubation time is short and the protocol states that the results are ready the same day, the realistic assay time is somewhat different. In addition to the assay time, the patients must be attended to, the TRH tests performed and the assay tubes and kit components prepared. In addition, the tubes must be counted, the assay data analysed and the results written up. This is only possible when all the patients present themselves very early in the morning and there are enough staff on hand to perform all the required tests! With an overnight pre-incubation a hectic morning is avoided and the results are available within a few hours, with better sensitivity and precision.

The different absolute values obtained from different TSH kits often make it difficult for laboratories to compare results, and these comparisons are necessary when a patient transfers from one clinical practice to another. In such cases, false diagnoses can arise when the results are not compared with the normal range given for each method.

A final observation is that with many commercial quality-control sera imported from the United States of America, values for the components listed are ascribed to American kits but none are ascribed to European kits. This means, at best, that such sera, which take up the largest part of the market for RIA in the Federal Republic of Germany, can only be used in precision control.

The clear need for standardization of reagents and methods in kits has been stressed because of the importance of achieving inter-laboratory comparisons similar to those already achieved by the Deutsche Gesellschaft für Klinische Chemie (German Society for Clinical Chemistry) for other routine clinical chemical parameters.

REFERENCES

[1] ERHARDT, F.W., MARSCHNER, I., PICKARDT, R.C., SCRIBA, P.C., J. Clin. Chem. Clin. Biochem. **11** (1973) 381.

[2] MARSCHNER, I., ERHARDT, F.W., SCRIBA, P.C., J. Clin. Chem. Clin. Biochem. **14** (1976) 345.

DISCUSSION

D. FULD: Don't you think that making recoveries on each sample would be better than extracting the standards, as you suggest?

W.G. WOOD: This would be better in the case of big laboratories.

D. RODBARD: I was interested in the patient sample resulting in 155 $\%B/B_0$. This increase in binding could be due to the presence of endogenous antibodies to TSH (thyrotropin). At the 1967 meeting of the American Thyroid Association and subsequently in the Journal of Clinical Endocrinology and Metabolism, M. Hays et al.[1] reported that injection of bovine TSH into human subjects could result in antibody formation with some biological neutralizing properties. Therefore, I would like to ask whether any of your subjects had previously received bovine TSH.

I would also point out that even in the case of a double-antibody radioimmunoassay, the presence of endogenous antibodies to an antigen may result in either parallel displacement and a false positive or a false negative (and elevated $\%B/B_0$), depending on the specificity of the second antiserum used (cf. PEETERS et al. Endocrinology (1977)[2]).

W.G. WOOD: This point is at present under investigation in our laboratory as well as in laboratories in Sweden and the USA. Our view is the same as yours, and until we hear anything to the contrary, we think that the "rogue factor" is either an antibody to bovine or perhaps human TSH.

As the sera were pooled from more than 100 patients according to TSH content, and not according to names, we have unfortunately no data as to whether any patient had undergone prior treatment with bovine TSH.

Your comment on the possibility of false values with the double-antibody assays in this case is very important and should be borne in mind when such cases arise. As we have not yet fully analysed the results of the TSH quality-control survey in which these two sera were assayed, we have not yet been able to assess whether the different methods or kits using double-antibody methods give different results, which would support your theory!

K. PAINTER: One can see that your results on coated-tube digoxin assays would lead you to believe that the pre-incubation step is necessary in coated-tube assays. However, you are seeing an effect, rather than a cause, of the problem. There are coated-tube digoxin assays on the market which do not behave in this way. The problem lies in the chemical structure of the iodinated digoxin derivative and in components added to the tracer buffer. The relevant studies of structure-function relationship will be published shortly. They contradict your conclusion that the reagents are good but the methodology is not.

---

[1] HAYS, M.T., SOLOMON, D.H., BEALL, G.N., Suppression of human thyroid function by antibodies to bovine thyrotropin, J. Clin. Endocrinol. Metab. **27** (1967) 1540.

[2] PEETERS, S., FRIESEN, H.G., RODBARD, D., Growth hormone binding factor in serum of pregnant mice, Endocrinology **101** (1977) 1164.

W.G. WOOD: I can only reiterate that our experience with coated-tube assays, not only for digoxin, but for digitoxin, T_4, cortisol and phenytoin, shows the same effect of pre-incubation on precision at low dose levels. Therefore I must stick to the results we have obtained and the logical explanation which we have derived from them. I should add that the coated tubes tested came from several different producers.

PERFORMANCE OF RADIOIMMUNOASSAYS FOR DIGOXIN AS EVALUATED BY A GROUP EXPERIMENT

A. DWENGER, R. FRIEDEL, I. TRAUTSCHOLD
Medizinische Hochschule Hannover,
Hanover, Federal Republic of Germany

Abstract

PERFORMANCE OF RADIOIMMUNOASSAYS FOR DIGOXIN AS EVALUATED BY A GROUP EXPERIMENT.

To gather information on the performance of routinely employed test systems for the radioimmunological determination of digoxin in serum, a group experiment was set up in which 36 laboratories in the Federal Republic of Germany took part. They were asked to determine the digoxin content in 24 specimens including specimens of known concentration providing a recovery curve, sera with pathological composition and known concentrations of digoxin, sera from a pharmacokinetic study and commercial control sera. The identity of the specimens was withheld from the participants. The accuracy and precision of the results reported for a total of 54 assays were better than those obtained in group experiments on radioimmunological determinations of hormones. Recovery ranged from 90% to 110% in 57% of the assays and from 80% to 120% in 85%. Reproducibility in the series expressed as coefficient of variation was better than 5% in 54% of the assays and better than 10% in 85%. Considerable differences were found for the cross-reactivities of antibodies with digitoxin and metabolites of spironolactone. Dysproteinaemia seems to be an unsolved problem, whereas moderate haemolysis and hyperlipaemia did not lead to severe errors. Improvements, especially in inter-laboratory variances, can be expected mainly from a further standardization of standard preparations.

1. INTRODUCTION

So far, group experiments for the evaluation of the performance of radioimmunoassays have been devoted to the determination of hormones [1–3]. Their results gave only limited information on the special problems of radioimmunological determinations of drugs because not only the plasma concentrations of the drug administered may be of interest but also the concentrations of its pharmacologically active metabolites. Moreover, in the radioimmunoassay for digoxin the following problems are evident:

(a) The patients are usually treated with other drugs too, some of which may influence the results of the assay, as is known for spironolactone and its metabolites.

(b) In patients treated with glycosides, disturbances in the concentration and pattern of plasma proteins are common, as is the incidence of hyperlipaemia.

(c) The patients may have had previous treatment with glycosides other than digoxin.

(d) The sera to be analysed frequently show slight to moderate haemolysis.

The aim of this study was first to obtain data on the intra- and inter-laboratory and the intra- and inter-method variances of the results of digoxin assays and second to document the different behaviour of kits or test systems should some of the problems mentioned above arise.

2. MATERIALS AND METHODS

2.1. Participants and test systems

Thirty-six laboratories in the Federal Republic of Germany took part in the experiment. They reported data on 54 assays (some of the laboratories ran several different test systems). In four of the assays the tracer was tritiated digoxin and in the remaining 50 assays, ^{125}I-labelled tracer was used. Two assays were based on individual test combinations and in 52 assays, 13 different commercially distributed test combinations were used. For the evaluation of the results the participants were divided into the following groups:

Group A: 13 participants who used the test kit from Amersham/Buchler (^{125}I, charcoal separation)
Group B: 13 participants who used the test kit from Schwarz/Mann (^{125}I, charcoal separation)
Group C: 8 participants who used the test kit from Boehringer-Mannheim (^{125}I, coated tube)
Group D: 4 participants who used tritiated digoxin as tracer and charcoal separation
Group O: all participants

2.2. Origin and preparation of specimens

Ten milligrams of digoxin purissimum ("Digoxin reinst", Boehringer-Mannheim Corp.) were weighed to an accuracy of 10 μg, dissolved in 100 ml of 70% ethanol and diluted with barbital buffer, pH 7.4, containing 0.5% bovine serum albumin, to a concentration of 1 μg/ml. This stock solution was diluted with pooled serum from healthy male blood donors to give nine specimens with

TABLE I. CHARACTERISTICS OF ABNORMAL SPECIMENS

Type and degree of abnormality		Digoxin added (ng/ml)
Haemolysis	1.23 mg haemoglobin/ml	2
Dysproteinaemia	Total proteins 70 g/l 48% albumin, 52% globulins	2
Hyperlipaemia	Triglycerides 10.2 mmol/l	2
Treatment with spironolactone	150 mg/d	0
Addition of digitoxin	20 ng/ml	0

TABLE II. MEAN RECOVERY AND REPRODUCIBILITY OF DIFFERENT TEST SYSTEMS FOR THE RADIOIMMUNOLOGICAL DETERMINATION OF DIGOXIN

For explanation of groups, see Section 2.1

Group	Recovery ($\bar{x}$ ± SD) concentration range 0.5 – 4 ng/ml	Reproducibility CV (%)	
		Range	Mean
A	95.4 ± 12.3%	1.2 – 18.3	5.7
B	93.9 ± 10.3%	0.9 – 10.4	4.8
C	108.4 ± 11.2%	2.3 – 11.7	5.5
D	112.5 ± 17.3%	6.6 – 12.4	9.3
O	101.5 ± 13.3%	0.6 – 18.3	5.4

different concentrations ranging from 0 to 6 ng/ml (recovery curve). Two specimens were commercially controlled sera with expected digoxin concentrations of about 1 ng/ml and 4 ng/ml. Six specimens originated from a pharmacokinetic study; the samples were collected before and up to 24 hours after the last administration of digoxin. The specifications of abnormal sera are listed in Table I. The specimens were frozen and sent to the participating laboratories which were asked to determine the digoxin content by their routine procedures. The results were reported as count rates and as concentrations calculated by the participant from his own calibration curve. In addition, the data for the calibration curve and some technical information on the test system were reported.

TABLE III. MEAN DIGOXIN CONCENTRATIONS (ng/ml; $\bar{x}$), COEFFICIENTS OF VARIATION (CV) AND RANGES OF VALUES (ng/ml) IN ABNORMAL SPECIMENS REPORTED FOR DIFFERENT GROUPS OF TEST SYSTEMS

For explanation of groups see Section 2.1.: degree of abnormality is explained in Section 2.2

Type of abnormality		System				
		A	B	C	D	0
Haemolysis	$\bar{x}$	2.03	1.91	2.30	2.76	2.10
	CV(%)	19.0	13.9	14.0	33.4	19.3
	range	1.73 – 3.08	1.30 – 2.19	1.84 – 2.80	1.70 – 3.37	1.25 – 3.37
Dysproteinaemia	$\bar{x}$	2.36	2.51	3.14	3.01	2.70
	CV(%)	15.5	16.5	19.9	23.0	20.8
	range	1.90 – 3.05	1.55 – 3.08	2.55 – 4.60	2.18 – 3.66	1.35 – 4.60
Hyperlipaemia	$\bar{x}$	2.13	2.01	2.64	2.36	2.29
	CV(%)	22.9	12.2	18.6	19.6	19.4
	range	1.70 – 3.50	1.60 – 2.34	2.38 – 3.00	1.90 – 2.84	1.20 – 3.50
Spironolactone	$\bar{x}$	0.51	0.05	0.28	0.31	0.43
	CV(%)	20.3	158.2	80.4	89.9	104.2
	range	0.33 – 0.70	0 – 0.21	0 – 0.55	0 – 0.57	0 – 2.53
Digitoxin	$\bar{x}$	0.72	1.72	0.98	0.88	1.12
	CV(%)	18.2	19.0	37.8	41.0	55.9
	range	0.50 – 1.00	1.20 – 2.24	0.59 – 1.50	0.42 – 1.22	0.27 – 3.00

TABLE IV. MEAN DIGOXIN CONCENTRATIONS (ng/ml; $\bar{x}$), COEFFICIENTS OF VARIATION (CV) AND RANGES OF VALUES (ng/ml) IN SIX SPECIMENS FROM A PHARMACOKINETIC STUDY REPORTED FOR DIFFERENT GROUPS OF TEST SYSTEMS

For explanation of groups see Section 2.1

Serum sample		System				
		A	B	C	D	O
1	$\bar{x}$	0.44	0.33	0.56	0.60	0.52
	CV(%)	25.5	31.7	23.9	44.5	45.5
	range	0.27 – 0.68	0.21 – 0.54	0.35 – 0.80	0.20 – 0.75	0.20 – 1.33
2	$\bar{x}$	0.65	0.52	0.83	0.81	0.71
	CV(%)	23.6	30.4	18.0	34.5	33.5
	range	0.42 – 1.00	0.24 – 0.80	0.68 – 1.10	0.40 – 1.02	0.24 – 1.45
3	$\bar{x}$	1.51	1.39	1.82	1.77	1.64
	CV(%)	14.1	10.7	11.0	28.9	19.9
	range	1.25 – 1.90	1.12 – 1.59	1.54 – 2.12	1.30 – 2.26	1.12 – 2.67
4	$\bar{x}$	1.23	1.12	1.50	1.47	1.32
	CV(%)	16.4	12.8	11.3	27.2	22.8
	range	1.00 – 1.63	0.91 – 1.40	1.28 – 1.77	0.97 – 1.84	0.69 – 2.18
5	$\bar{x}$	0.62	0.46	0.76	0.70	0.67
	CV(%)	23.4	30.1	13.6	32.7	36.8
	range	0.51 – 0.93	0.25 – 0.74	0.63 – 0.90	0.37 – 0.89	0.25 – 1.42
6	$\bar{x}$	0.23	0.15	0.43	0.35	0.33
	CV(%)	36.5	74.5	33.5	63.7	75.6
	range	0.13 – 0.40	0 – 0.33	0.30 – 0.70	0.04 – 0.53	0 – 1.16

3. RESULTS

3.1. Recovery and reproducibility

The results for the specimens providing the recovery curve are listed in Table II. Since the specimen containing 2 ng/ml was distributed in triplicate, the reproducibility (inter-laboratory variance) within the series could be calculated for each participant. These data are also summarized in Table II.

3.2. Effects of abnormal serum composition

The results for the five abnormal specimens (see Section 2.2 and Table I) are summarized in Table III. Moderate haemolysis showed only minor effects in groups A, B and C, whereas two members of group D reported results which were more than 50% too high. In the dysproteinaemic specimen all groups found mean concentrations significantly higher than 2 ng/ml. Hyperlipaemia affected groups C and D only. Marked differences between the groups were found for the cross-reactivities of digitoxin and metabolites of spironolactone.

The inter-laboratory variances of all these results were markedly higher than those found for the specimens of the recovery curve.

3.3. Pharmacokinetic study

As shown in Table IV, differences between the groups were found mainly in the mean concentrations. The kinetics (slopes of increase and subsequent decrease of digoxin concentrations) were almost identical for all groups. Again the inter-laboratory variances of the results were considerably higher than those found for the specimens of the recovery curve.

3.4. Control sera

The results reported for the two control sera ranged from 0.51 to 1.45 ng/ml (expected value about 1.0 ng/ml) and from 2.5 to 7.05 ng/ml (expected value about 4.0 ng/ml).

4. DISCUSSION

Compared with the results of group experiments for the evaluation of radioimmunological hormone analyses [1–3], the data reported here reveal several peculiarities. First, it can be stated that accuracy as well as reproducibility of radioimmunoassays for the determination of digoxin in serum are considerably better than those of radioimmunoassays for insulin [1, 2] or triiodothyronine and thyroxine [3]. From 31 out of 54 assays included in this evaluation a recovery between 90% and 110% was reported for the concentration range 0.5–4 ng/ml. For only eight assays the recovery was found to be lower than 80% or higher than 120%. The reproducibility (inter-laboratory variance) within the series, expressed as coefficient of variation for the specimen with 2 ng/ml distributed as unknown triplicate, was better than 10% in 46 assays; in more than 50% of the assays (29 out of 54) the coefficients of variation were lower than 5%.

From the results reported in Table II it is obvious that the comparatively high inter-laboratory variances found for the abnormal specimens (Table III) and those from the pharmacokinetic study (Table IV) can, for the most part, be traced back to the differences in the recovery between the assay systems. By and large it can be stated that systems employing antibody-coated tubes show a tendency to measure concentrations slightly too high, whereas for both systems based on charcoal separation the mean recoveries were slightly less than 100%. For all other separation systems employed by the participants (ion-exchange resin, solid-phase antibody, double antibody, polyethylene glycol precipitation), no such consistent deviations from the ideal recovery were observed. Although no definite conclusions can be drawn as to whether the differences in the recovery are specific for the separation system or whether they are due to differences in the standard preparations, it should nevertheless be noted that inter-laboratory variances could be lowered considerably if the calculation of the results was based on the recovery curve (identical standards for all participants).

As can be seen from the results reported for the specimens from the pharmacokinetic study, possible differences in the reactivity of the antibodies with digoxin metabolites seem to play only a minor role as far as the inter-laboratory variances of the kinetics are concerned; more severe sources of error were found to be the cross-reactivities of the antibodies with digitoxin and metabolites of spironolactone and differences herein. The "digoxin" concentrations reported ranged from 0.27 to 3.00 and 0 to 2.53 ng/ml, respectively. Moderate haemolysis as well as hyperlipaemia affected the results to a minor extent only. For the dysproteinaemic specimen (total proteins normal, globulins elevated) all groups reported results significantly too high. Since only one specimen of this type was included in the study, no conclusions can be drawn as to whether this error is due to the elevation of globulins or to the lowering of albumin. This specimen originated from a patient with cirrhosis of the liver, so it is possible that another pathological component of the serum influenced the results.

The use of a uniform calculation procedure (spline approximation) did not result in any significant deviations of the concentrations from those individually calculated by the participants nor did it give a significant lowering of the inter-laboratory variances.

In the final judgement of the results it should be remembered that the digoxin assay is not representative of the majority of radioimmunoassays. Firstly, the standard, which is chemically well defined, can be obtained absolutely pure and can be dissolved in antigen-free serum. One of the main problems in radioimmunoassay, the discrepancy in the slope of standard curves obtained with buffer and antigen-free serum [4], can easily be avoided. Secondly, for clinical diagnostics there are no problems as regards sensitivity. The concentrations relevant to diagnostic use are spread over the most sensitive part of the standard curve.

In our opinion, the results of this group experiment document that, under favorable circumstances, radioimmunoassays can be performed with an accuracy and precision equal to those of other quantitative biochemical tests. In the special case of digoxin, an improvement is to be expected mainly from a further standardization of standard preparations.

REFERENCES

[1] MARSCHNER, I., et al., Group experiments on the radioimmunological insulin determination, Horm. Metab. Res. **6** (1974) 293.

[2] MARSCHNER, I., et al., Bericht über den Insulin-Ringversuch der Deutschen Diabetes-Gesellschaft 1974, Informationsblatt der Deutschen Diabetes-Gesellschaft **3** (1975) 1.

[3] GORDON, A., GROSS, J., An inter-laboratory comparison of total serum triiodothryonine determination, Acta Endocrinol. **83** (1976) 539.

[4] ERHARDT, F., et al., Verbesserung und Qualitätskontrolle der radioimmunologischen Thyreotropin-Bestimmung, Z. Klin. Chem. Klin. Biochem. **11** 9 (1973) 381.

DISCUSSION

T.C. SMEATON: During a survey of digoxin kits our laboratory considered five RIA kits and an EMIT enzyme-coupled system. Do you have any experience with the latter kit?

A. DWENGER: EMIT was not included in our survey.

IAEA-SM-220/115

QUALITY CONTROL IN RIA
A preliminary report on the results of the World Health Organization's programme for external quality control

M.A. CRESSWELL*, P.E. HALL+, B.A.L. HURN*
* Wellcome Research Laboratories,
Beckenham, Kent,
United Kingdom
\+ World Health Organization,
Geneva, Switzerland

Abstract

QUALITY CONTROL IN RIA: A PRELIMINARY REPORT ON THE RESULTS OF THE WORLD HEALTH ORGANIZATION'S PROGRAMME FOR EXTERNAL QUALITY CONTROL.

A continuing interlaboratory quality-control survey should be specially valuable in radioimmunoassay because of problems of standardization in this field. Nevertheless, there are particular difficulties associated with such surveys related to the provision of suitable assay samples, the timely return of assay results from participating laboratories and the methods of processing the combined data. The WHO Special Programme of Research, Development and Research Training in Human Reproduction brought together investigators from throughout the world to work on many aspects of new and improved methods of fertility regulation. Within this group it has been necessary to institute a programme for the standardization and quality control of radioimmunoassay for seven hormones (luteinizing hormone, follicle stimulating hormone, prolactin, progesterone, estradiol, testosterone and cortisol). As part of this programme, WHO introduced an interlaboratory survey covering all seven assays which ran for an experimental six-month period ending in August 1976. Many laboratories had initial difficulty with the routine but their reporting rate rose steadily throughout the six months. The organizers encountered several problems in collation and presentation of RIA data. The survey was re-started with minor modifications in June 1977, on this occasion including a total of nearly 150 laboratories. Sixty of the participating laboratories will be receiving matched sets of reagents provided as part of the WHO Special Programme of Research in Human Reproduction. The survey will thus permit a detailed study of the benefits of common methodology in a major group of RIA laboratories.

INTRODUCTION

The concept of analytical quality control has taken a surprisingly long time to become established in RIA laboratories in view of the importance attached to it in routine clinical chemistry. The reasons for this delay are complex, but two factors are of major importance. Firstly, RIA began primarily as a research tool in the hands of endocrinologists and immunologists, and the increasing demand from practising physicians was for many years just added to the burden of laboratories with little previous experience of the problems of routine assay work in large volume. Secondly, many of the assays show a marked interlaboratory bias, possibly related to the use of different, inadequately characterized reagents and standards as well as the inherently poor precision of methods pushed to their maximum possible sensitivity. Such numerical anarchy has, in the past, been felt to place great difficulties in the way of systematic comparison between laboratories, especially as most of the latter have believed themselves to be yielding clinically useful information based on their local "normal range" data and resented the suggestion that they were "inaccurate". Remarkably few formal interlaboratory trials of RIA have been published, in fact, and the extent to which variation in results could be attributed to variation in methodology and reagents remains unclear; "accuracy", too, is very difficult to define for many of the analytes measured by RIA.

In the past six years there has been a major expansion of the activities of WHO in the field of research in human reproduction because of the establishment of the Special Programme of Research, Development and Research Training in Human Reproduction. The Programme was established at the request of member states of the Organization to investigate the safety and effectiveness of existing methods for fertility regulation, and to undertake research on new and improved methods. Many of the projects supported by the Programme, particularly clinical trials of fertility regulating methods, are undertaken on a multi-centre collaborative basis in many parts of the world. Thus, to ensure comparability of results in such multi-centre trials and in other collaborative studies, a major effort has gone into standardization and quality control of laboratory procedures. For clinical chemistry, well proven methods, both manual and automated, have been selected and a quality-control scheme instituted. However, for the radioimmunoassay of hormones a large number of methods exist for the measurement of any particular substance with every laboratory making modifications to these methods. Moreover, many individual investigators and commercial organizations make their own antisera with greatly varying characteristics; laboratories use different antigens and standards.

Thus, a strategy has been evolved which includes: the monitoring of assay performance by external quality-control programmes; the monitoring of assay performance by various internal quality-control procedures; the provision of matched assay reagents; and the organization of training courses. To date, the programme has concentrated on the following seven hormones: luteinizing hormone (LH), follicle stimulating hormone (FSH), prolactin, estradiol, testosterone, cortisol and progesterone.

It was apparent from the start that, for the results emanating from laboratories collaborating in the Programme to be of more than local significance, an effective programme of internal quality control must be established in each laboratory and a system for the central monitoring of the performance of the whole group would be equally essential. In addition, for the purposes of reducing method/reagent related variance and of controlling costs, WHO, after a lengthy testing phase, commenced the distribution of "kits" of reagents to be used with specified methodology for each of the seven radioimmunoassays.

The purpose of the present paper is to describe the organization and results of the interlaboratory quality-control programme.

ORGANIZATION OF THE PROGRAMME

Interlaboratory surveys of this type involve quite complex arrangements. In the interest of early introduction, therefore, it was decided to adapt the organization and methods of data handling from an existing, commercial scheme operating in the field of clinical chemistry (Group Quality Control Programme, Wellcome Reagents Ltd.).

The principal features of the Wellcome scheme were:

1. To have regular assays, once a fortnight, of coded samples of composition unknown to the participant. Results of analyses to be reported by post to to the computer unit, by a specified date.
2. To report the collated results for each assay back to all participants by post as soon as possible (in the UK, so as to arrive before the next sample was due for analysis).
3. To relate analytical results to methods of analysis, both in the regular reports to participants and in the data bank, so that method comparisons could be made.
4. To carry out these operations with all reasonable care for the confidentiality of reported results, yet to have the facility to identify and separately report a group of specified participants' results to a regional (or other) quality-control supervisor, with the consent of all concerned.
5. To incorporate a degree of replication with the coded samples for assay, so that information could be derived concerning long-term reproducibility of the results of each participant.
6. To minimize cost and inconvenience to participants by dispatching samples for six-months' analyses (12 samples) at the beginning of the period.

It was felt that these major objectives of the programme were suitable to the requirements of WHO. Some residual details of the operation remained to be solved, however:

TABLE I. AVERAGE NUMBER OF PARTICIPANTS REPORTING RESULTS IN TIME FOR THE FORTNIGHTLY COMPUTER RUNS

	FSH	LH	Prolactin	Cortisol	Estradiol	Progesterone	Testosterone
Trial survey:							
First two occasions	28	30	16	25	35	32	34
Next two occasions	33	37	22	27	42	44	43
Last two occasions	43	46	43	29	48	50	46
Current survey:							
First two occasions	29	34	20	31	38	41	45
Next two occasions	41	38	28	38	53	53	53

(a) *Size of the laboratory group.* It is a truism to suggest that the more participants, the more information will become available. For this reason it was felt desirable to include in the survey as many laboratories collaborating with WHO as possible, although only approximately 60 laboratories are receiving the reagent "kits". The total number of participating laboratories now stands at around 150, many of which are very experienced and could be regarded as reference centres. This will allow the assessment of the benefits of method and reagent standardization in comparison with a group of laboratories using a variety of assay procedures.

(b) *Materials for assay.* The value of an interlaboratory survey is heavily dependent on the properties of the material being assayed, which should neither introduce variables not caused by clinical samples nor disguise sources of error which exist normally. Control materials for RIA are particularly difficult to formulate because of the pronounced "matrix" effects seen in such assays and the dissimilarity of many of the purified antigens from their corresponding forms existing in plasma. For these reasons it was felt desirable to prepare assay samples from human serum collected from selected donors (e.g. post-menopausal females, normal males) so as to enable levels of target antigens to be varied without addition of extraneous material. This idealistic approach proved complex to operate and was not capable of offering a practicable method for adjusting prolactin levels. As a result, the current programme cycle, which commenced in June 1977, uses serum pools in which a certain amount of variation achieved by selective pooling has been further adjusted by addition of exogenous steroids and pituitary hormone preparations.

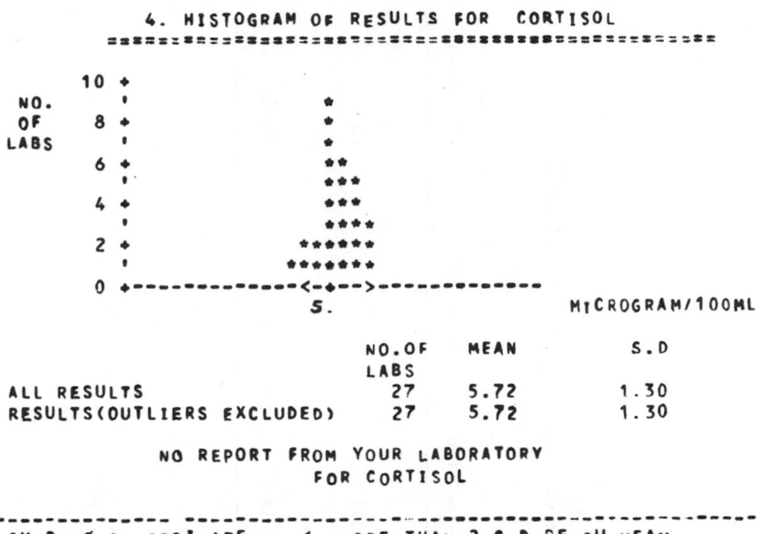

FIG.1. Part of one of the fortnightly reports to participants in the first survey, showing the results reported for cortisol. On this occasion the participant to whom the report was sent had not sent in a result for this assay.

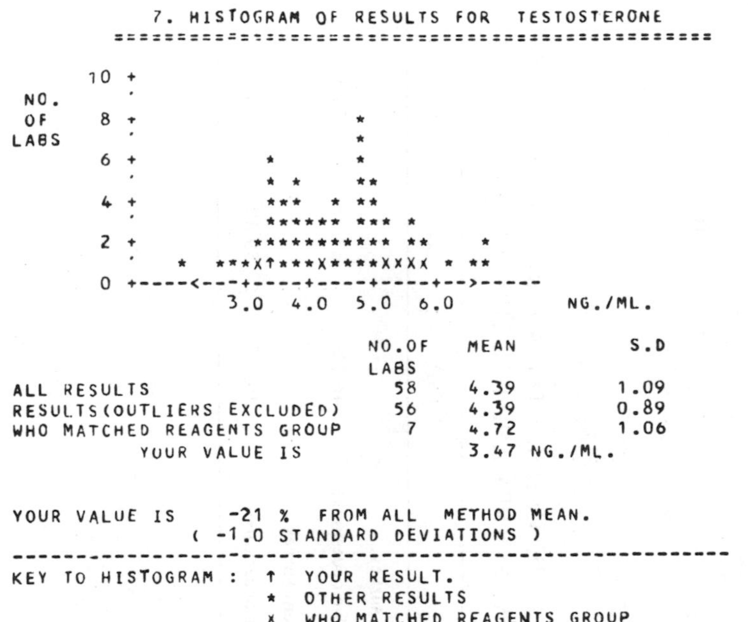

FIG.2. Part of a fortnightly report from the current survey. The participant's own result is shown by the upward arrow on the bottom line of the histogram. Crosses are results reported by users of the WHO "kit" methods.

TABLE II. UNWEIGHTED AVERAGE IMPRECISION (CV) FOR THE ASSAY OF EACH HORMONE DURING THE TRIAL SURVEY AND FOR THE FIRST FOUR SAMPLES OF THE CURRENT SURVEY

	FSH	LH	Prolactin	Cortisol	Estradiol	Progesterone	Testosterone
Trial survey:							
(twelve occasions)	46.1%	63.9%	37.1%	23.9%	48.1%	69.6%	40.8%
Current survey:							
(four occasions)	39.1%	59.5%	43.2%	23.5%	43.6%	58.8%	35.2%

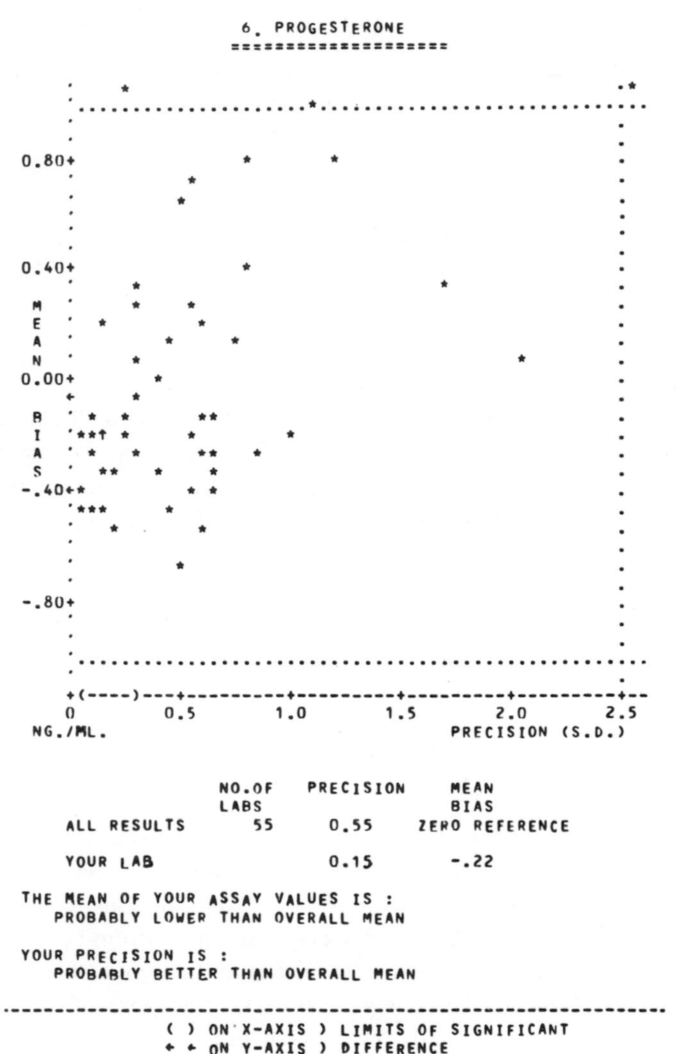

FIG.3. Part of the end-of-period summary report from the first survey. Average precision is shown on the horizontal axis and average bias on the vertical (the reference point for bias on each sample is the mean of all results reported for that sample).

(c) *Methods of handling and presenting data.* A key feature of the existing clinical chemistry programme was the facility to catalogue incoming data on the basis of analytical method used and to calculate and display the performance of participants separately for the different methods. In RIA, however, "methods" are very much less clearly defined than they are in clinical chemistry, largely because of the important variations in the reagents used. Before the start of the survey, information about analytical methods was sought from participants: although the organizers have retained this information in case it should later prove useful, at the time it was obviously impractical to place the methods used in any rational grouping. This unsatisfactory state of affairs has improved with the gradual increase in numbers of those using the WHO "kit" methods, which can be regarded as relatively well-defined procedures separable from the larger, heterogeneous group of other assays.

(d) *Variation due to use of different standards.* In view of the use of relatively poorly characterized standards for the three protein hormones all participants were requested to submit results for these hormones in terms of common standards supplied at the beginning of the survey. The standards supplied were the International Reference Preparation 69/104 for FSH and LH and the MRC standard 71/222 for prolactin. It was left to the discretion of individuals whether these preparations were used as routine working standards in every assay or merely employed to calibrate secondary in-house standards.

RESULTS

The Programme was first run for a trial cycle of six months starting in March 1976 and ending in the following August. Many of the participants were slow to send in their first results, and there were several reasons for this. Apart from delays in getting the Programme package through customs authorities and into the right hands, many of the laboratories found the rigour of regular fortnightly analyses difficult to cope with at first. It is apparent that radioimmunoassay systems are inherently less reliable and less easily scheduled than routine chemistry tests and this led to a high proportion of the control results being missed or posted too late for inclusion in the computer run. This situation improved steadily until an average of 45–50 laboratories were reporting regularly and on time by the end of the trial cycle (Table I). Similar difficulties have been seen in the subsequent programme cycle, albeit with a rather improved response rate overall.

Another minor difficulty was caused by the reporting of undefined values ("less than" values) when samples gave results below the cut-off point of a user's assay. Such results cannot be incorporated into a strictly numeric format and have had to be excluded by instructions to participants and to the staff preparing data for the computer.

The presentation of collated results (Figs 1 and 2) in the form of computer-generated histograms with statistical information, generated uniquely for each participant, appeared to be well liked and understood. "Outlying" values were excluded on the basis of commonsense limits to the acceptable analytical range as well as by the usual processes of truncation at ± 3 SD and re-calculation. The spread of results was, as expected, very substantial even after removal of wild values (Table II). Performance in the prolactin assay was surprisingly good by comparison with the gonadotrophins, especially as all samples in the trial survey period had values toward the bottom of the measurable range and this assay is known to suffer from problems of sensitivity and specificity. A possible explanation is the relatively restricted availability of reagents for the assay, which may therefore be less heterogeneous than the other assays. No obvious explanation appears to account for the fact that performance for LH was markedly worse than for FSH, and progesterone assays were similarly worse than either estradiol or testosterone assays, both in the trial survey and later.

After the completion of the six-month trial period an attempt was made to assess the average bias and precision of each participant, the latter being derived from comparison of results obtained from "hidden" duplicates amongst the twelve coded samples assayed during the relevant period (Fig.3). The statistical procedure, which works well in the routine clinical chemistry field, has proved to be of rather limited use for RIA, mainly because of the much wider range of concentrations represented in the assay samples. Variance is related to dose level in most assay systems and it is therefore not acceptable to add together absolute (as distinct from proportional) error levels at different concentrations when preparing "average" precision data. The various possible methods of performance assessment were extensively discussed at a recent WHO consultative meeting as a result of which certain changes will be made to the statistical procedures to be used at the end of the present and subsequent six-monthly survey periods.

The current series of control assays started in June 1977 and, up to the time of writing, the results from four samples have been reported. These results to date are not markedly dissimilar from those observed in the trial run, although it could be argued that average performance has improved slightly for most of the assays (Table II). Insufficient data have been accumulated as yet to say whether the use of the WHO "kit" methods will reduce interlaboratory errors. A relatively small number of laboratories have so far reported results by these methods since they have only recently started to establish and validate them, but the numbers of users is rising fairly rapidly and should allow certain conclusions to be drawn by the end of the next six-month cycle in 1978.

DISCUSSION

D. RIAD-FAHMY: At the Tenovus Institute for Cancer Research at Cardiff we run the United Kingdom external quality-control scheme for plasma estradiol. In the early part of this programme we saw a similar wide scattering of results about consensus mean values as shown in your figures. Despite several meetings between assayists in participating laboratories, little improvement occurred.

However, with the development of high-resolution mass-fragmentographic gas chromatographic methods for plasma steroids we were able to provide more "absolute" values for estradiol in external quality-control plasmas (Wilson, D.W., et al., J. Endocrinol. **74** (1977) 503). This resulted in an alignment of methodologies and subsequent closer agreement within the external quality-control scheme. Have you had a similar experience?

P.E. HALL: We have not experienced this grouping of results following provision of absolute values; however Professor Breuer is currently analysing WHO specimens by the isotopic dilution mass fragmentography technique.

Whilst we would like to have target values, our matched reagent programme is very much a pilot one. Most of the participants in the programme are in developing countries and have just started work.

B.A.L. HURN: I agree that it is always interesting to know what the right answers should be. But I doubt whether disagreement as to the true values contributes significantly to the overall difficulty in getting individuals to agree in their findings. There is no evidence in clinical chemistry to show that that is the case. In this sort of situation, it is enough to make people aware of the differences between their values for the outliers to come under considerable pressure.

Ch.-A. BIZOLLON: Looking at the results obtained on inter-laboratory reproducibility for different hormones, I do not observe a significant difference in the reproducibility of the results obtained by methods using commercial kits and by "matched" methods.

Have you made a statistical study of the results obtained on inter-laboratory reproducibility by the group of 90 participating laboratories and the group of 60 reference laboratories? Could you please say a few words on this study?

P.E. HALL: Data are being accumulated and will be analysed in depth in the near future. At present, the data base is insufficient for drawing any conclusions on the performance of the reagents being distributed by WHO or for any comparison with other methods used by other participants in the external quality-control programme.

ROUND-TABLE DISCUSSION ON EXTERNAL QUALITY CONTROL

Chairman

P.E. Hall	(World Health Organization)

Panel Members

Ch.-A. Bizollon	(France)
H. Breuer	(Federal Republic of Germany)
A. Dwenger	(Federal Republic of Germany)
R.P. Ekins	(United Kingdom)
B.A.L. Hurn	(United Kingdom)
S.L. Jeffcoate	(United Kingdom)
P.G. Malan	(United Kingdom)
I. Marschner	(Federal Republic of Germany)
D. Rodbard	(United States of America)
W.G. Wood	(Federal Republic of Germany)

P.E. HALL *(Chairman):* We have exactly half an hour for this short round-table discussion. Who would like to ask the first question?

D. FULD: I should first like to propose a relation between the WHO and the producers of kits. The WHO has reference products which could be used by the producers to calibrate their kits and this should lead to very interesting results. Secondly, I should like to suggest that, since the quality of kits varies widely at present, as has been demonstrated in the case of TSH, we should select tests, glucose tolerance tests for example, which are less dependent on kit quality. These should give clinically useful results to the pathologist, for the moment. Thirdly, I should like to point out a danger in external quality control. As you know, pathology laboratories are under attack in many countries and not, I think, without reason. External quality control should be aimed at helping laboratories and not providing fuel for such attack. Finally, I should like to point out that whereas the producers try to make kits which are as simple as possible, simplicity and quality are not always compatible, as has been illustrated by the different results of assays carried out with and without chromatography.

P.E. HALL *(Chairman):* Thank you, Dr. Fuld. You have brought up several issues. Let us start by discussing the first of these, that is, the question of how one assesses kits, be they commercial or non-commercial, and whether any organization can undertake overall monitoring or at least put down guidelines as to requirements. I think that certain international organizations such as WHO might have a rôle here, although I am not sure how this might be organized or how it might be funded. I should like to open the discussion on this question by calling on four persons at the table, Dr. Malan, Dr. Breuer, Dr. Wood and Dr. Rodbard. I call first on Dr. Malan.

P.G. MALAN: I should like to describe some results illustrating our experiences of the Supraregional Assay Service in the United Kingdom. When this service was started, we knew that virtually the only way to obtain some uniformity of results was to introduce reference methods: some of the reasons underlying this view have already been outlined in the review lecture by Professor Ekins. An attempt was made to do this locally with a T_4 assay developed in our laboratory. The participating laboratories after an initial period of interest, did not in general regard the use of such a method with favour and most reverted to their "own" T_4 assays. Since the introduction of national quality control schemes, however, there has been an active demand for such reference methods, as we have already heard; the upsurge in interest presumably arises when a yard-stick is available against which performance can be judged.

Turning now to between-laboratory assessment, I wish to show some results obtained in the digoxin quality control scheme which is organized by Dr.G. Mould at Guildford, United Kingdom, and for which we provide data-processing facilities. For a variety of reasons, including the relatively high cost of obtaining or preparing large batches of quality control sera, any one quality control pool was distributed on only two occasions to approximately 40 participating laboratories; in one or two cases sufficient material was available for three distributions. We were therefore forced to use the Youden X-Y analysis [1] to assess the performance of laboratories in this scheme. Figure A shows a typical Youden X-Y plot for a particular QC pool assayed on two separate occasions. The large cross at the centre of the diagram indicates the consensus mean of all laboratories, with ± 1 SD limits. Results of laboratories whose estimates of digoxin on the two occasions were identical should lie on the dashed 45°-line through the consensus mean, and their distance from this mean is a measure of the bias of their results from the mean. Such an identity of results implies that a laboratory has a high precision. An index of precision, or random error component, may be obtained by the perpendicular distance of any point from the 45°-line. The "accuracy" of a laboratory may then be considered as the mean square combination of the precision and bias components, i.e. the distance of any point from the consensus mean. Numbers at the top of the plot are participating laboratory code-numbers, while the alphabetic letters indicate different assay methods or reagent combinations used.

Approximately 15 different methods or combinations of methods were used: these included five commercial kits and a variety of combinations of different antisera and separation procedures. In Fig.A, "R" and "Y" are two commercial kits which are seen to form groups of points with mean values (+) close to the 45°-line. Thus, kit "R" has a slight negative bias, while "Y" has a slight positive bias; this bias relationship was found at all digoxin concentrations over the range examined in the scheme. The dotted ellipses show the ± 1 SD limits for each group. No such grouping of results was observed when laboratories using the same antisera were compared, but those laboratories using coated charcoal appeared to achieve more consistent results when albumin, rather than dextran, was used in the separation mixture. In order to accumulate information on the performance of different laboratories we have had to examine closely the results obtained by the Youden X-Y analysis, with eight different QC pools distributed separately over an eight- or nine-month period on two (or more) occasions each.

Assessment of laboratory performance was judged by Youden's criteria (Ref. [1]), and "reasonable" performance was assumed if the results of a particular laboratory were rejected in less than 20% of the analyses (i.e. 0 or 1 out of 8 occasions). Of the ten laboratories using kit "R", seven performed reasonably on the above criteria, while only three of the six laboratories using kit "Y" managed to maintain some sort of stability. It was impossible to obtain any reasonable evaluation of the performance of the heterogeneous combinations of reagents in the hands of different laboratories, as no clear clustering of the results occurred.

As a result of this analysis, and similar analyses of variance in other schemes, it has become clear that a "rugged" or stable reference-method is required for the evaluation and monitoring of laboratory performance. This is so because the large variations seen in quality control schemes could be due either to the use of "non-rugged" assay systems or to poor laboratory performance. Once "ruggedness" of an assay system has been demonstrated, it is possible to monitor laboratory performance and also make reasonable assessments of bias due to slightly different methodologies or reagents.

H. BREUER: As you have heard, we have set up a study group to deal with the assessment of kits for the determination of steroid hormones. The major advantage we have here is that we can determine the true values of standards by reference of definitive methods, which permits us, at least to some extent, to assess the kits. The major problem we encounter is that in the Federal Republic of Germany, as indicated by Dr. Wood, there are maybe as many as ten kits offered for any one constituent, so on the one hand we support the Federal system and on the other hand we want to encourage the development of kits which fulfil the requirements of optimal kits. Even while we can offer standards for which the true values are known, we believe that it will be at least three or four years before we have good kits for the determination of steroids. As far as peptide

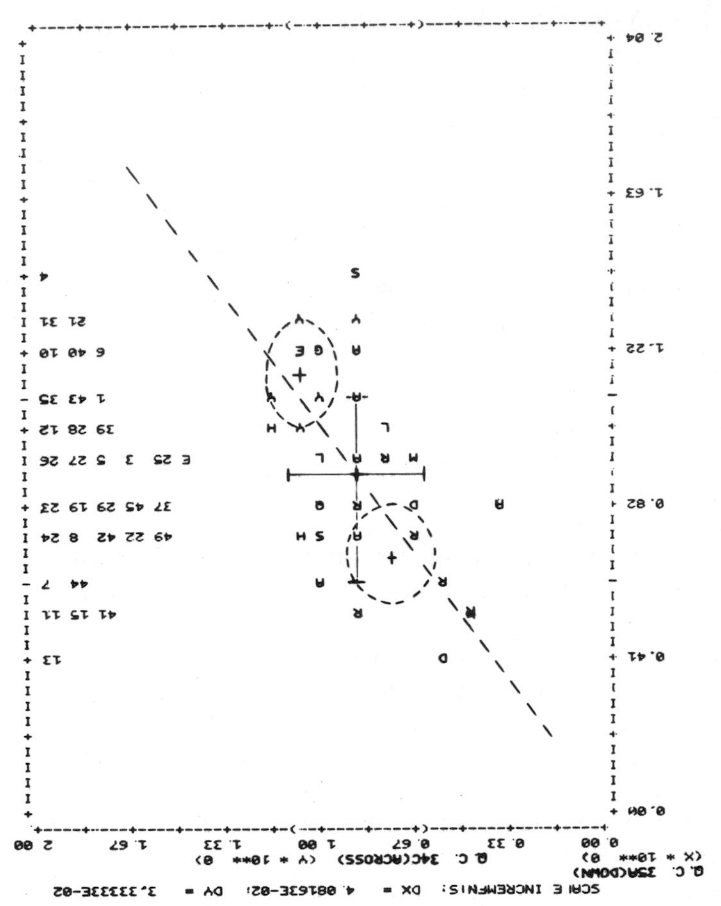

FIG.A. A Youden X-Y plot of results obtained on the same digoxin quality-control pool on two separate occasions by participating laboratories. Numbers at the top of the plot are laboratory code numbers, and alphabetic letters indicate different assay methods or reagent combinations used. See text for a further discussion.

hormones are concerned, the present situation is horrible, as we have shown, and there we rely very much upon the activities of the WHO.

P.E. HALL *(Chairman):* I agree that, theoretically, steroid assays should be easier to control, and I think, however, that Dr. Fuld was referring to assays for protein hormones. For these substances, standards are available, for example, from the National Institute of Biological Standards and Control in London. However, since in the case of say gonadotrophins, the standards are rather heterogeneous preparations, when we assay these standards with different kits, we don't know what the different antibodies are seeing in them. I think we are rapidly coming to a point at which we may well question the whole concept of isolated protein hormone standards and we will have to provide a defined "standard" set of reagents for reference purposes. Dr. Wood, could I bring you into this discussion?

W.G. WOOD: I think there are three ways of testing a kit. First of all you can test the components; we have done this and, as I said before, the components in kits are usually very good. Secondly, one can test the methodology; we have also done this and the methodology is, more often than not, somewhat lacking. Thirdly, one can test both components and methodology as in the Munich system of quality control surveys. In these, as Professor Breuer described earlier, we send out twenty sera for analysis including standards giving a hidden standard curve. We are able in the Federal Republic of Germany to test the kits which are used for the determination of any single constituent. We have this year carried out quality control surveys for cortisol and TSH. In the TSH quality control survey, we had 72 returns of a rather detailed questionnaire, in which we ask for details of methodology and raw data, so that we can derive the precision profile for every participant as well as his performance with, in the case of protein hormones, a human hormone-free serum to which has been added one of the international reference preparations. For TSH, for example, we used the MRC standard 68/38. Since over 85% of our participants used kits, this gives a method both of assaying laboratory performance and of comparing kits, though unfortunately it gives no indication of between-assay variation.

P.E. HALL *(Chairman):* Dr. Rodbard, would you care to comment?

D. RODBARD: I think that the problems with kits are both the responsibility of the manufacturers and the users. Both have been negligent. The manufacturers provide a kit and tell the user how to use it, but they almost never give the validation data. I believe that no kit should be distributed to anyone without the user getting information regarding the within – and between – assay variability in the manufacturer's laboratory, the results of tests of parallelism, the cross-reactivity, and in the case of steroids or drugs, a comparison with an independent method. This gives the user a basis for judging the validity of the kit. Beyond this, one can not expect to buy anything from anyone and be sure that it will meet the specifications. Hence it is the responsibility of the user to

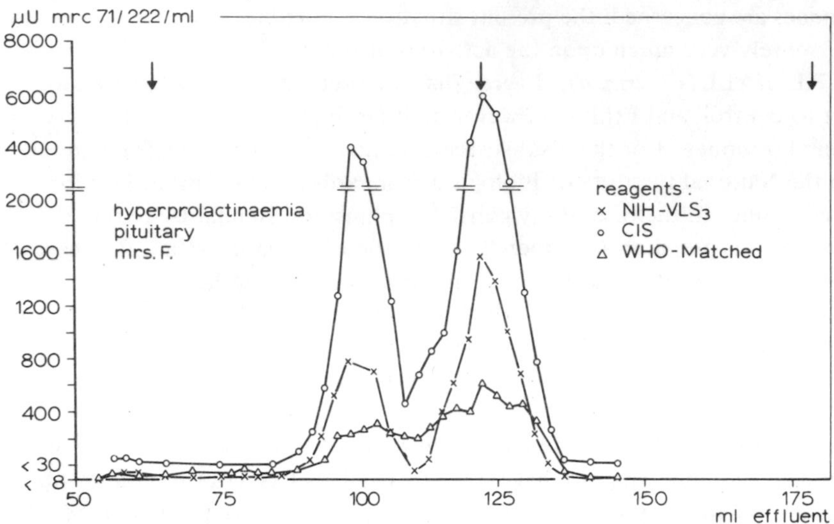

FIG.B. Assay of chromatographic fractions of serum for prolactin with different sets of reagents in a case of hyperprolactinaemia.

attempt to validate the kit in his own laboratory, above all by comparison with an independent method, as noted by Dr. Breuer, Dr. Fuld, Dr. Riad-Fahmy and many others. If both manufacturer and user co-operate and fulfil their responsibilities, then I think that the situation, if not entirely corrected, will at least be much improved.

Ch.-A. BIZOLLON: It is not possible for each laboratory to check all the kits on the market; it would take several years for one laboratory to achieve this, by which time newer and better kits might have appeared and precious time been lost. I believe that it is rather the rôle of the WHO, for example, or the IAEA, to define the specifications which each manufacturer should follow in order to provide the optimum performance.

R.M. LEQUIN: As a spin-off of the quality control which we have done over the past two years in the Netherlands, we have done a rather simple laboratory experiment relating to prolactin assays in which we subjected serum samples to chromatographic fractionation and assayed the effluent from the column with different sets of reagents.

Figure B shows the results obtained – prolactin concentration expressed in terms of Medical Research Council standard 71/222 plotted against chromatographic fraction expressed in terms of millilitres of effluent – with three different sets of reagents, first with set VLS_3 from the National Institutes of Health, second with a commercially available set from CEA-IRE-SORIN and third with a WHO matched-reagent set. You see that the patterns with the three sets of reagents are very different. As is generally known, gel filtration separates prolactin into roughly two components. From the areas under the two peaks, it appears that with the CIS set of reagents the first component accounts for a substantially larger percentage of the total response. Although these results should not be taken in absolute terms, this is a good example which shows how difficult it is to do quality control in protein hormone assays and that, in fact, we should go back to the bench and find out what we are measuring.

A. MALKIN: I should just like to make two or three brief comments. First, the problems of quality control that arise in radioimmunoassay are not basically different from problems of quality control in other analytical procedures which those of us who are professional analytical chemists have been facing for a good part of our professional lives. Other problems have been resolved and I believe that these will be resolved likewise. Second, I believe that laboratories participating in quality-control programmes will themselves take the necessary steps to correct their mistakes. Third, I want to emphasize the importance of choosing procedures offering high precision, both within an assay and between assays, within the individual laboratory. Only on such a basis can procedures giving erroneous results be identified and rejected.

P.E. HALL *(Chairman):* Thank you, Dr. Malkin. I should like to return later to this question of the relative importance of bias and precision. May I first return to Dr. Fuld's points, in particular the desirability of choosing dynamic or other tests which are less dependent on kit quality and the question whether those organizing quality-control schemes should be "policemen" or "teachers".

S.L. JEFFCOATE: I should like to make a very general comment on the latter point and illustrate it with respect to what we have been doing in the United Kingdom. I think it most important that external quality control should be purposefully directed towards the improvement of performance. We in the United Kingdom have a rather special system. We have a number of quality-control laboratories, each with expertise in a particular assay, and each forming a nucleus round which cluster all the other laboratories in the country doing that particular assay. An important aspect of this system is intercommunication by telephone or mail or at meetings between the associated laboratories and the central laboratory, whereby methodology is discussed and components of the assay leading to good performance or bad performance are gradually identified, it being equally important to identify both of these. As a result, we develop recommended reagents and procedures, identify those laboratories which are performing badly and attempt to help them to perform better. There is thus an important trouble-shooting element. Such quality control must be continuous. I should like to add that external quality control must never be a substitute for a laboratory's own internal quality control and that a most important function of a quality-control laboratory is to advise associated laboratories on how best to do their own internal quality control.

P.E. HALL *(Chairman):* Such a system may not be applicable in countries which have legislated for control of laboratories, where the "policing" rôle may assume greater importance.

D. RIAD-FAHMY: A further aspect of the quality-control system in the United Kingdom is that if a particular assay, e.g. for estradiol, in one laboratory is out of control, or has broken down for some reason, the laboratory may transfer its work load to another laboratory. It is therefore vital that all laboratories in the country carrying out estradiol assays have standardized techniques. The external quality-control linkup is of paramount importance here, because it is the only factor which makes laboratories bring their techniques into alignment.

P.E. HALL *(Chairman):* Thank you. I should like now to return to Dr. Malkin's question regarding the relative importance of bias and precision.

D. RODBARD: I agree with Dr. Malkin that indeed the within-assay precision is the limiting factor in the sense that no matter how much we do to reduce the variability within laboratories, we are still going to have more variability between laboratories than within them. We may reduce the between-laboratory variability from ± 50% to ± 25%, or even to ± 15%, but there will still be more variability between laboratories than within a given assay in a given laboratory, so that both clinicians and researchers must whenever possible make all relevant comparisons within a given assay. When we do glucose tolerance tests, insulin tolerance tests, thyrotropin release tests, etc., we are using the other samples in the same test as controls. Likewise, if we wish to measure testosterone levels after vasectomy, it is important to keep the samples in the freezer so that they can all be analysed in the same assay. I should add that in large-scale multi-centre studies, where it is indeed necessary to carry out assays in several different laboratories, the effects of between-laboratory variability can be minimized by an optimal experimental design for allocation of samples to assays and to laboratories, which then assumes great importance.

S.L. JEFFCOATE: We have found in the United Kingdom that the adoption of a standardized assay protocol leads not only to improvements in between-laboratory variability, but also in within-laboratory variability – in other words, the laboratories are usually provided with better assays than those which they were carrying out previously. Such measures may thus lead to improvements in both bias and precision.

B.A.L. HURN: I agree that within-laboratory precision is primary, but I think one should see the external quality-control programmes, at least in part, as devices for identifying those laboratories with problems and so needing assistance which they may then be given. I don't think any laboratory wilfully has poor within-laboratory precision, but some laboratories cannot achieve adequate precision unaided and some may even be unaware that they need help.

These are our aims in the clinical chemistry external quality-control programme which we run. The organizational basis of such programmes must obviously depend on the circumstances.

P.G. MALAN: We have discussed assay design, reference methods and the use of kits, and there has been comment about the poor performance of certain kits. I should like to point out that the assay designs and reference methods used in external quality-control programmes may also be open to criticism.

J. INGRAND: In this regard, I should like here to make a comment on quality control carried out by those possessing automatic assay equipment. As was established in paper SM-220/203, the design of automatic equipment is not always adequate with respect to assay design. There is no certainty, for example, that data on total activity and non-specific bound activity are presented. The question of replicate measurements is not always treated satisfactorily. Guidance on these matters should be made available to the manufacturers.

P.E. HALL *(Chairman):* I think that there is a need for general guidance on quality-control procedures which can be applied whatever type of assay, whether manual or automated, is being carried out.

I give the floor to Dr. Painter who has a brief announcement.

K. PAINTER: I should like to mention that there is in the United States of America a Clinical Radioassay Society, concerned with education, quality control and research, mainly in relation to clinical radioassay techniques. The society holds meetings usually in conjunction with those of the Society of Nuclear Medicine. I or other members of the society will be pleased to provide further information about its activities on request.

P.E. HALL *(Chairman):* I should like to thank the participants in this round-table discussion and to apologize to anyone who wished to put further questions to them but could not because of time limitations

REFERENCE

[1] YOUDEN, W.J., STEINER, E.H. Statistical Manual of the AOAC (1975), Association of Official Analytical Chemists, P.O. Box 540, Benjamin Franklin Station, Washington, DC, 20044, USA.

Session VI, Part 2

APPLICATIONS

Assays for vitamins

Chairman

R.P. EKINS
United Kingdom

A NOVEL RADIOASSAY FOR THE DETERMINATION OF FOLATE IN SERUM AND RED CELLS AND NEW OBSERVATIONS ON THE STABILITY OF SERUM FOLATE

E.P.J. LYNCH, K.C. TOVEY, H. GUILFORD
The Radiochemical Centre,
Amersham,
United Kingdom

Abstract

A NOVEL RADIOASSAY FOR THE DETERMINATION OF FOLATE IN SERUM AND RED CELLS AND NEW OBSERVATIONS ON THE STABILITY OF SERUM FOLATE.

A competitive protein-binding assay for the determination of folate in serum and red cells has been developed. The assay has been fully validated in hospital trials and comparisons have been made with the microbiological assay. We have based the standardization of the radioassay on N^5-methyltetrahydrofolate (N^5-MTHF) as this is the predominant folate derivative in serum samples. At about pH 9.5, pteroylglutamic acid (PGA) and N^5-MTHF demonstrate the same affinity for folate-binding proteins. Therefore, many folate assays have adopted PGA largely because of the popular belief that N^5-MTHF is highly unstable. However, we have demonstrated that N^5-MTHF in serum standards is surprisingly stable at $-20^\circ C$. All the reagents for the assay (including the N^5-MTHF standards) have shown perfectly acceptable stability, permitting their storage for at least three weeks at $-20^\circ C$ and one week at $4^\circ C$. Evidence is presented to support the use of N^5-MTHF as being the more appropriate standard. Moreover, we have observed that folate in human serum samples is stable even at room temperature in the presence of 0.1% sodium azide. It is common practice for some laboratories to send samples at room temperature to centres for analysis without taking the precaution of adding preservative. Erroneous results may be obtained under these conditions which would negate the value of the test. The simple addition of azide makes possible the non-refrigerated transfer of samples between laboratories without alteration in folate values.

A competitive protein-binding assay for the determination of folate in serum and in red cells has been developed. The method is based on the use of a novel selenofolate-^{75}Se label and porcine serum as folate binder with the naturally occurring (DL)-N^5-methyltetrahydrofolate (N^5-MTHF) as standard. The assay has been fully validated in hospital trials for the measurement of both serum [1] and red cell [2] folate. Comparisons with the microbiological assay were made and the radioassay results provided a similar discrimination between patients of normal folate and folate-deficient status in both serum and red cells.

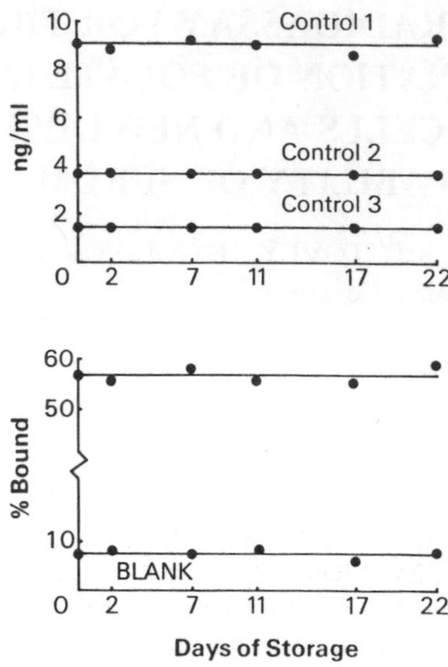

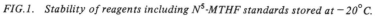

FIG.1. Stability of reagents including N^5-MTHF standards stored at −20°C.

TABLE I. REAGENTS STORED AT −20°C FOR THREE WEEKS COMPARED WITH FRESH UNSTORED REAGENTS

Control parameter	Reagents stored/fresh	Mean	Standard deviation
		Folate concentration in ng/ml	
Control serum 1	Stored	8.7	0.9
	Fresh	7.7	1.0
Control serum 2	Stored	3.3	0.2
	Fresh	3.2	0.1
Control serum 3	Stored	1.6	0.1
	Fresh	1.6	0.1
		% bound	
C_0	Stored	54	2.7
	Fresh	52	1.6
Blank	Stored	7.0	0.3
	Fresh	7.1	0.5

TABLE II. REAGENTS STORED AT 4°C FOR ONE WEEK COMPARED WITH FRESH UNSTORED REAGENTS

Control parameter	Reagents stored/fresh	Mean	Standard deviation
		Folate concentration in ng/ml	
Control serum 1	Stored	6.6	1.0
	Fresh	5.6	0.6
Control serum 2	Stored	3.8	0.3
	Fresh	3.4	0.1
Control serum 3	Stored	2.0	0.1
	Fresh	1.8	0.2
		% bound	
C_0	Stored	49	1.8
	Fresh	45	1.9
Blank	Stored	6.7	1.4
	Fresh	6.0	1.2

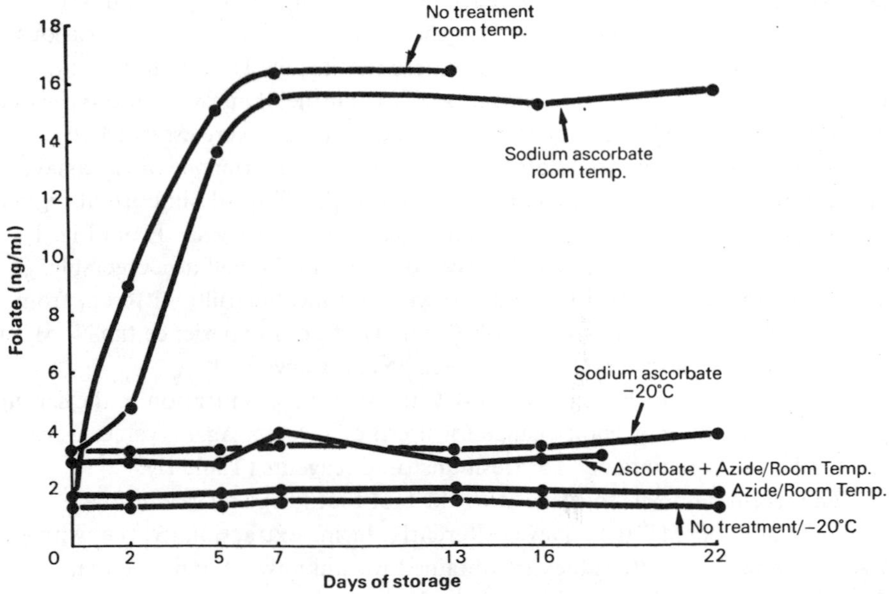

FIG.2. Stability of N^5-methyltetrahydrofolate in serum.

TABLE III. STORAGE OF DILUTED BLOOD SAMPLES AT − 20°C

Blood sample	Days of storage						Mean	Standard deviation
	0	2	7	11	16	22	Folate concentration in ng/ml	
1	3.3	3.3	3.7	2.9	3.5	3.4	3.4	0.3
2	7.1	6.2	8.7	5.5	8.9	6.9	7.2	1.4
3	6.7	6.8	11.8	5.4	9.1	8.6	8.1	2.3

Some authors [3] have strongly suggested that pteroylglutamic acid (PGA) is the more suitable substance for standardization in folate radioassay. At about pH 9.5, PGA and N^5-MTHF demonstrate the same affinity for folate-binding proteins [3, 4]. Therefore, the use of PGA for standardization has proved an apparent practical alternative. This has arisen largely because of the belief that the predominant circulating form of folate, i.e. N^5-MTHF is highly unstable. However, we have shown that N^5-MTHF in serum is surprisingly stable at − 20°C (Fig. 1 and Table I). Preparations of each reagent, including batches of standards, were stored at − 20°C for three weeks. The concentration of folate was measured in fresh control sera 1, 2 and 3 (Fig. 1) using these reagents at intervals spanning the storage period, as shown. In addition, the concentration of folate was measured in the control sera on the same occasions using fresh reagents as a control to the experiment (Table I). The per cent binding at the lowest folate concentration (C_0) and the blank were also measured with both fresh and stored reagents. The values obtained were essentially unchanged. With respect to determining the clinical performance of the assay, control sera 2 and 3 have folate concentrations at the clinically important region, close to the interface between normal and folate-deficient levels. From Fig. 1 the folate concentrations measured in the control sera showed no detectable change over the entire storage period and were not meaningfully different from the values obtained with fresh controls (Table I). In our experience the N^5-MTHF standards can also withstand repeated freezing and thawing.

When the reagents were stored at 4°C the folate concentration in the serum controls showed no important change for up to one week. Again, values were very similar to those obtained for fresh unstored reagents (Table II).

The recent findings, together with the fact that PGA and serum folate (predominantly N^5-MTHF) behave differently during extraction [5] (i.e. with PGA standards low folate values are obtained for unknowns), indicate that N^5-MTHF is the more appropriate standard to use. Moreover, preliminary results have shown that folate in human serum samples is stable even at room temperature when the samples are stored under the appropriate conditions (Fig. 2). Previous authors [6] have suggested that the addition of ascorbate is necessary to maintain the stability of serum folate. We have shown (Fig. 2) that ascorbate does not stabilize serum folate when samples are stored at room temperature. At the moment it is common practice for some laboratories to send samples at ambient temperature to centres for analysis without taking the precaution of adding preservative. Clearly, erroneous results will be obtained under these conditions which will negate the value of the test. We have demonstrated that serum folate levels in the presence of 0.1% sodium azide (Fig. 2) remain constant even when the samples are kept at room temperature for at least three weeks. The simple addition of azide makes possible the non-refrigerated transfer of samples between laboratories without alteration in folate values.

As previously implied, many published methods for both folate bioassay [7–9] and radioassay [10, 11] have recommended the addition of ascorbate previous to assay. It has been recently noted by Lindemans et al. [12] that the addition of ascorbate caused a non-specific increase in folate values. We have noted a similar effect (Fig. 2) which occurred with fresh or stored (−20°C) samples. Moreover, the magnitude of the increase (a factor of approximately 2) appears to be constant for a range of samples. Where expected ranges have been established from assays which include ascorbate, clearly all clinical samples must be similarly treated.

It is now considered by many that an estimate of the amount of folate in the red cells provides a more reliable index of a patient's folate status. Blood samples for the determination of red cell folate may be stored for up to three weeks at −20°C (Table III). The blood may be stored suitably diluted for direct use in the assay. Here again, the use of azide may permit the transportation of samples at ambient temperature and guarantee valid results in possibly the same way as with serum samples.

REFERENCES

[1] JOHNSON, I., GUILFORD, H., ROSE, M., J. Clin. Pathol. **30** (1977) 645.
[2] JOHNSON, I., ROSE, M., J. Clin. Pathol. (in press).
[3] GIVAS, J.K., GUTCHO, S., Clin. Chem. **21** 3 (1975) 427.
[4] LONGO, D.L., HERBERT, V., Clin. Res. **22** (1974) 701 A.
[5] MITCHEL, G.A., POCHRON, S.P., SMUTNY, P.V., GUITY, R., Clin. Chem. **22** 5 (1976) 647.
[6] LEONARD, J.P., BECKERS, C., J. Nucl. Med. Biol. **2** (1975) 89.
[7] HERBERT, V., J. Clin. Invest. **40** (1961) 81.
[8] WATERS, A.H., MOLLIN, D.L., J. Clin. Pathol. **14** (1961) 335.
[9] CHANARIN, I., BERRY, V., J. Clin. Pathol. **17** (1964) 111.

[10] MINCEY, E.K., WILCOX, E., MORRISON, R.T., Clin. Biochem. **6** (1973) 274.
[11] ROTHENBERG, S.P., SHELDON, P., da COSTA, M., LAWSON, J., ROSENBERG, Z., Blood **43** (1974) 437.
[12] LINDEMANS, J., VAN KAPEL, J., ABELS, J., Clin. Chim. Acta **65** (1975) 15.

DISCUSSION

R.D. PIYASENA: Your finding that folate in blood is stable in the presence of sodium azide is of great practical value, especially for those of us who work in situations where samples for folate assay may have to be sent by post to the laboratory.

What tracer did you use, and how did you prepare your MTHF standards? Did you make a spectrophotometric correction for the MTHF standard, since it does not dissolve easily?

E.P.J. LYNCH: We used a selenofolate label, which is a pteroylmethyl-selenocysteine analogue. The N^5-methyltetrahydrofolate solid is added to the serum and then the individual standards are prepared by calibration against a primary standard. We don't need the spectrophotometric correction because we treat each batch of the standard exactly in the same way with respect to preparation and indeed to quality control. Thus we guarantee the consistency of results.

R.D. PIYASENA: Would you please give some details about the nature of the pig serum binding agent used? Was any purification process performed and, if so, was it relatively simple or complicated?

E.P.J. LYNCH: The porcine serum preparation is made by diluting the natural serum in a phosphate buffer and then it is freeze-dried. The procedure is reasonably simple.

STUDIES ON FOLATE BINDING AND A RADIOASSAY FOR SERUM AND WHOLE-BLOOD FOLATE USING GOAT MILK AS BINDING AGENT

R.D. PIYASENA, D.A. WEERASEKERA,
N. HETTIARATCHI, T.W. WIKRAMANAYAKE
University of Sri Lanka,
Peradeniya Campus,
Sri Lanka

Abstract

STUDIES ON FOLATE BINDING AND A RADIOASSAY FOR SERUM AND WHOLE-BLOOD FOLATE USING GOAT MILK AS BINDING AGENT.

Preparations of cow, goat, buffalo and human milk in addition to pig plasma were tested for folate binding properties. Of these, only pig plasma and goat milk showed sufficient binding to enable them to be used as binding agents in a radioassay for serum and whole-blood folate. The binding of folate by cow milk preparations in particular was found to be very poor. Goat milk was preferred to pig plasma as a binder for folate radioassay for reasons of convenience, economy and greater stability, and because pteroylglutamic acid (PGA) can be used both as tracer and standard. Where pig plasma is used with the inclusion of folate-free serum in the standard tubes, differences were observed between the standard and serum blanks which themselves varied from sample to sample. By contrast, with goat milk, all blank readings were normally 3% or less. Five out of eight samples of goat milk were seen to contain 'releasing factor' necessary to liberate folate from endogenous binder (FABP). Where present, the factor was found to be stable for at least three months when the partially purified milk was stored freeze dried at 4°C. Goat milk binder was found unable to distinguish between PGA and methyltetrahydrofolic acid (MTFA) at pH9.3. This enabled PGA rather than the more unstable MTFA to be used as tracer and standard. The assay employs a one-step incubation procedure at room temperature. It is sensitive to about 0.1 ng of PGA and is reproducible to less than 5% variation. The mean % recovery of inactive added folate was 101 ± 4%.

Radioassays for folate in blood have commonly employed preparations of liquid or powdered cow milk [1, 2], milk extracts [3, 4], pig plasma [5] or extract of hog kidney [6] as binding agent. Major problems encountered by previous workers appear to have been (a) irreproducible folate binding from batch of binder, (b) endogenous binding of folate to natural folic acid binding protein (FABP) in serum or plasma, and (c) lower affinity of binder for methyltetrahydrofolic acid (MTFA) than for pteroylglutamic acid (PGA).

The position was considerably eased by two observations: firstly, that untreated (but not purified) cow milk contained a 'releasing factor' that separates folic acid from FABP, thus obviating the necessity for an extraction step or heat inactivation of the native binder; secondly, that at the critical pH of 9.3 milk binder exhibits identical affinity for MTFA and PGA, thus making a two-step incubation with MTFA standard and PGA tracer unnecessary [1]. However, the problem of batch to batch variation remained, added to which was the observation that not all available powdered or skim-milk preparations contained the necessary 'releasing factor'.

The present paper presents the results of a study on serum and whole-blood folate with the above-named agents (with the exception of pure lactoglobulin and hog kidney) and with human, buffalo and goat milk.

MATERIALS AND METHODS

An amount of 10.0 mg of PGA (Sigma Chemicals) was dissolved in 10 ml of 0.1N NaOH and 50 ml of distilled water was added. The pH was adjusted to 7.0 with 0.1N HCl and the volume made up to 100 ml. Aliquots of the PGA solution of strength 100 μg/ml were stored at −20°C. Working solutions were prepared in lysine buffer in the concentration range 0–20 ng PGA per ml.

An amount of 10.0 mg of MTFA (Sigma Chemicals) was dissolved in 10 ml of absolute ethanol containing 5% ascorbic acid. The solution was stored at −20°C in the dark in tubes covered with aluminium foil.

^{3}H-PGA of specific activity 47 Ci/mm (Radiochemical Centre, Amersham) was stored at −20°C in aliquots of strength 25 μCi/ml (235 ng per ml) in lysine buffer under the same conditions as the MTFA solution. Working tracer solutions were prepared fresh each day to contain 4.0 ng PGA per ml.

Pig plasma

Pig plasma was obtained by venepuncture from pigs weighing around 300 lbs and was stored in aliquots at −20°C.

Cow milk

Fresh, pasteurized, sterilized, and fat-free locally available milk was tested in batches together with commercially available preparations of powdered whole milk (Lakspray) and skim milk (Bonlac) for folate binding properties.

Buffalo milk

Buffalo milk was taken from the local buffalo as distinct from imported 'Murrah' and 'Surti' varieties. Only fresh milk preparations were obtainable.

Human milk and colostrum

Human milk and colostrum were obtained fresh from three subjects.

Goat milk

Twelve batches were tested; each was obtained fresh from 'Jamnapari' goats found locally.

Lysine buffer pH9.3

Each litre of lysine buffer contained 9.08 g of lysine monohydrochloride, 1.00 g of sodium azide and 1.00 g of gelatin.

The pH was adjusted to 9.3 ± 0.05 with 0.1N NaOH and the solution stored in an amber glass bottle at 4°C. Fresh buffer was prepared every two weeks and the pH was adjusted before use when necessary.

Albumen-coated charcoal

Albumen-coated charcoal was prepared from equal volumes of 2.5% solution of activated charcoal (Norit A) in normal saline and a 1.75% solution of salt-poor human albumen in normal saline.

Folate-free serum

Folate-free serum was prepared by heating serum to 100°C for 15 min in a water bath, treating with 5 mg of Norit A charcoal per ml for 10 min and then centrifuging.

Blood samples

Serum was stored at −20°C with added ascorbic acid, 5 mg per ml. For measurement of whole-blood folate, blood was deep frozen immediately on collection and the haemolysate diluted 1:20 with lysine buffer. Aliquots were stored at −20°C and 100 μl were taken for assay, as in the case of serum.

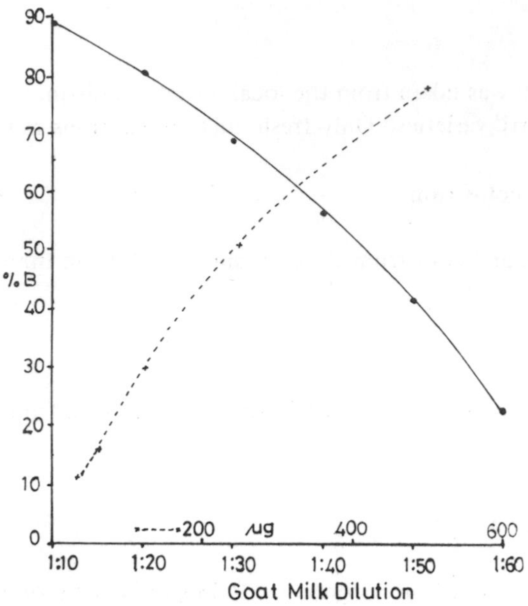

FIG.1. Binding of 0.4 ng of ^{3}H-PGA to goat milk: dilution curves. x - - - x *Dilution curve of 3-month-old dried skimmed goat milk.*

RESULTS

Pig plasma

The assay protocol of Mantzos et al. [5] was followed, 0.8 ng of ^{3}H-PGA per tube and MTFA standard being used. A binding of over 50% tracer with 100 μl of undiluted pig plasma was observed and a satisfactory standard curve constructed within the range 0.1 to 0.8 ng of MTFA standard. However, the standard curves obtained in the presence and absence of folate-free serum were widely different, necessitating the addition of folate-free serum to each standard tube. It was found that although the non-specific binding (serum blank) was then constant in the standards, it differed from that of the test samples which also showed considerable variation between samples. A serum blank had therefore to be determined for each test sample. The MTFA standard showed poor stability and had to be freshly prepared for each assay. Moreover, the binding properties of the pig plasma showed considerable deterioration within 2 weeks when stored at −20°C.

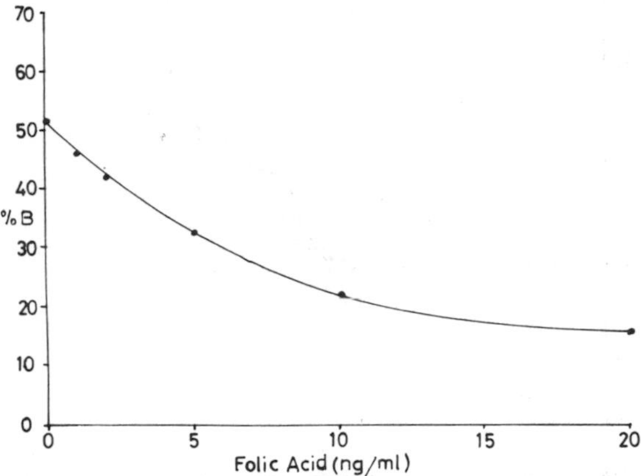

FIG.2. Standard curve for radioassay of serum folate using goat milk, at a dilution of 1:40. The tracer was 0.4 ng of ^{3}H-PGA.

With the above modifications, the assay yielded a sensitivity of 0.11 ± 0.07 (measurements in quadruplicate of folate-free serum in each of three assays). The precision of determination of 0.25 ng of MTFA added to folate-free serum (n = 8) was 0.29 ± 0.08 and that of 0.5 ng of MTFA was 0.52 ± 0.10.

Cow milk

Binding (dilution) curves were constructed in lysine buffer by using 0.4 ng of ^{3}H-PGA per tube and albumen-coated charcoal as separating agent. No available preparation was found satisfactory as a folate binding agent. In several batches tested, the maximum binding obtained from fresh cow milk was only 8%. Pasteurized, sterilized, and sterilized fat-free milk yielded similarly poor binding. Powdered whole milk (Lakspray) did not bind folate. Powdered skim milk (Bonlac) showed less than 1%, 3% and 10% binding when, respectively, 2, 10 and 50 mg of powder in 100 μl of buffer were used.

Buffalo milk

Maximum binding was 64% with undiluted milk, falling to 26% at a 1:8 dilution.

Human milk and colostrum

The folate binding properties of human milk were similar to those of buffalo milk. Colostrum appeared to be somewhat superior, 40% binding being obtained at a dilution of 1:10.

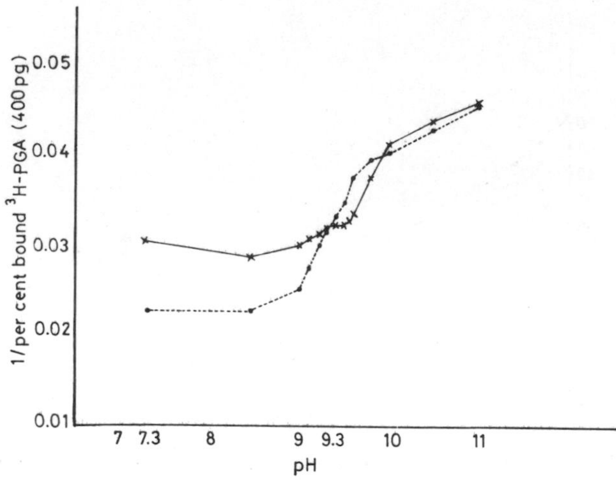

FIG.3. Effect of pH on binding of 2.0 pmole PGA (x —— x) *and 2.0 pmole MTFA* (● - - - ●) *to goat milk.*

Goat milk

Twelve batches of goat milk were tested. A typical binding curve is shown in Fig. 1. A 50% binding was obtained at a dilution of 1:40. The partial removal of fat, as described later, increased the percentage bound at this dilution by about 5%.

The goat milk was beaten in a homogenizer at 4°C for 15 min and then centrifuged at 4°C at 3000 rev./min for 30 min. The thicker upper layer was removed and discarded. The lower layer, which contained the binding agent, was freeze dried and stored at 4°C. It was found to be stable for at least 3 months.

In the typical case to which Fig. 1 relates, 70 ml of partially purified milk yielded 7.5 g of powder freeze dried: 35 mg dissolved in 10 ml would be equivalent to a 1:40 dilution of the original milk.

A typical standard curve is shown in Fig. 2.

Effect of pH

The relative binding of PGA and MTFA to goat milk binder within a pH range of 7.3 to 11.3 was studied according to the method of Longo and Herbert [1]. Equimolar solutions were prepared by dissolving 0.0440 g of PGA and 0.0600 g of MTFA barium salt in 1 litre of water (0.1 micromolar

TABLE I. KNOWN MTFA CONCENTRATION CALCULATED FROM A STANDARD CURVE CONSTRUCTED WITH PGA

Added MTFA (ng/ml)	Calculated MTFA (ng/ml)	Percentage recovery
0.31	0.36	116.1
0.62	0.68	109.6
1.25	1.33	106.4
2.50	2.60	104.0
5.0	4.4	88.0
		Mean = 104.82
		SD = 10.4

TABLE II. ADDITIVE EFFECT OF PGA AND MTFA WHEN MEASURED TOGETHER AT pH9.3 USING PGA STANDARD AND TRACER

Added folate		Assay result (ng/ml)	Percentage recovery
PGA (ng/ml)	MTFA (ng/ml)		
0.125	1.0	1.16	103.1
0.25	1.0	1.30	104.0
0.50	1.0	1.55	103.3
1.0	1.0	2.10	105.0
2.0	1.0	2.90	96.6
4.0	1.0	4.80	96.0
			Mean = 101.33
			SD = 3.9

solutions). One millilitre of each solution was diluted 1:5 and 100 μl (= 0.88 ng of PGA and 1.18 ng of MTFA respectively) incubated with 0.4 ng of ^{3}H-PGA and 100 μl of a 1:40 dilution of milk binder for 30 min. The results are shown in Fig. 3.

It is seen that the binding of MTFA to goat milk binder increases with rise in pH until it equals that of PGA at pH9.3.

The fact that goat milk binder does not exhibit a different affinity for PGA than for MTFA at pH9.3 was further confirmed by an experiment in which known amounts of MTFA added to folate-free serum were assayed using PGA for constructing the standard curve. The results are shown in Table I.

TABLE III. EFFECT OF HEAT INACTIVATION (BOILING) OF NATIVE BINDER OF GOAT MILK BINDING AGENT ON MEASURED FOLATE CONCENTRATION

Milk sample	Folate concentration (ng/ml)	
	Boiled	Unboiled
1	4.4	4.2
2	6.2	6.0
3	4.5	2.2
4	7.8	7.5
5	5.4	2.6
6	7.6	7.9
7	3.9	4.1
8	6.5	3.1

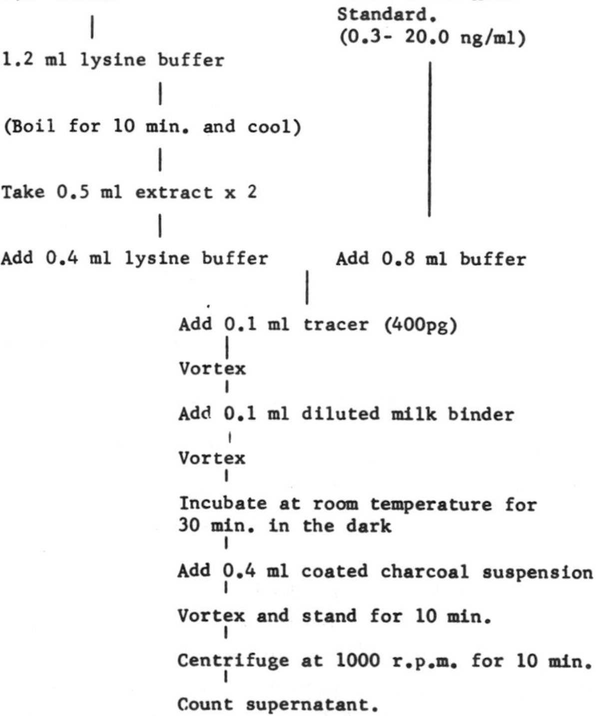
0.3 serum
1.2 ml lysine buffer
(Boil for 10 min. and cool)
Take 0.5 ml extract x 2
Add 0.4 ml lysine buffer
0.1ml Folic Acid Standard.
(0.3- 20.0 ng/ml)
Add 0.8 ml buffer
Add 0.1 ml tracer (400pg)
Vortex
Add 0.1 ml diluted milk binder
Vortex
Incubate at room temperature for 30 min. in the dark
Add 0.4 ml coated charcoal suspension
Vortex and stand for 10 min.
Centrifuge at 1000 r.p.m. for 10 min.
Count supernatant.

FIG.4. Protocol for radioassay of serum folate using goat milk binding protein.

The % recovery of inactive added MTFA is seen to range from 88 to 116%, with a mean of 105 ± 10%.

In a further experiment, 1.0 ng of inactive MTFA was added to folate-free serum together with varying quantities of PGA, and the total folate concentration was measured using PGA standard as before. The results are illustrated in Table II.

An additive effect of PGA and MTFA is seen irrespective of PGA concentration. The % recovery of inactive added folate ranges from 96 to 106%, with a mean of 101 ± 4%.

The above data suggest that an assay employing PGA as standard and tracer would measure both PGA and MTFA in a system run at pH9.3.

Effect of endogenous folate binding protein in serum

Eight samples of fresh goat milk were tested for the presence of a releasing factor that would liberate folate from FABP. 1.2 ml of lysine buffer was added to 0.3 ml of serum and the mixture boiled for 15 min in a water bath. 0.5-ml aliquots were removed from the cooled mixture for assay. A further 0.3 ml of the same serum sample was diluted in buffer as before and aliquots taken for assay using the same milk binder, with the boiling step omitted. The results are shown in Table III.

Of the eight samples tested, five seemed to possess the 'releasing factor' necessary to liberate folate from FABP so that comparable results were obtained with and without the heat inactivation step. In three of the samples, boiling of the diluted serum yielded a folate concentration about twice that obtained from the unboiled samples. This would indicate that, if the boiling step is to be avoided, the batches of goat milk should first be investigated for presence of 'releasing factor' and a batch in which the factor is found should then be chosen for use in the assay.

Where the 'releasing factor' has been found to to be present, it remains stable for at least 3 months when the milk preparation is prepared and stored as described.

The assay protocol is shown in Fig. 4 and the composition of the incubation mixture is given in Table IV.

Figure 5 shows a 'Scatchard plot' from which values for an equilibrium constant (K) under the conditions of the assay of 2.42×10^8 litres per mole and a binding capacity for goat milk of 2.26 ng per ml at a 1:40 dilution have been obtained.

The sensitivity of the assay as precision of determination of zero serum folate is less than 0.1 ng per incubation tube, enabling a folate concentration of 1.0 ng per ml to be determined in a 100-μl serum sample. The precision of determination of 4 ng PGA per ml added to folate free serum (n = 12) was 3.8 ± 0.75 and of 8.0 ng per ml it was 7.8 ± 0.96. Non-specific binding is

TABLE IV. FOLATE RADIOASSAY INCUBATION MIXTURES

Tube No.	Identification	Lysine Buffer ml	Standard or unknown sample, ml	Tracer ^{3}H-PGA ml	Diluted milk Binder ml
1 , 2	Total count	1.4	0	0.1	0
3 , 4	Reagent Blank (NSB)	1.0	0	0.1	0
5 , 6	Std 0 ng pml	0.9	0	0.1	0.1
7 , 8	0.5 "	0.8	0.1	0.1	0.1
9 , 10	1.0 "	0.8	0.1	0.1	0.1
11 , 12	2.0 "	0.8	0.1	0.1	0.1
13 , 14	5.0 "	0.8	0.1	0.1	0.1
15 , 16	10.0 "	0.8	0.1	0.1	0.1
17 , 18	20.0 "	0.8	0.1	0.1	0.1
19 , 20	Serum Blank	0.5	0.5	0.1	0
21 , 22	Unknown Serum	0.4	0.5	0.1	0.1

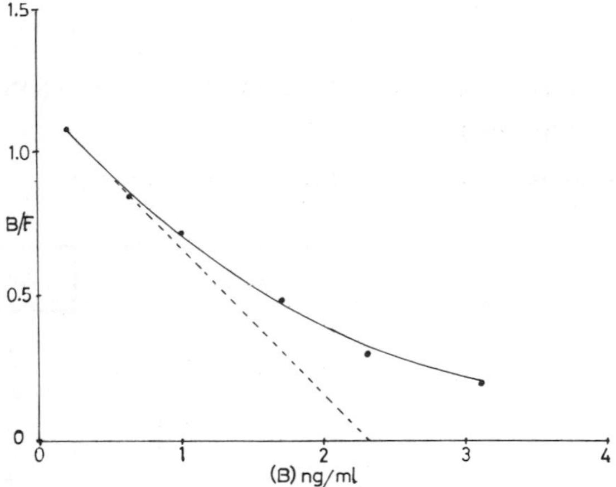

FIG.5. Radioassay of serum folate. Scatchard plot relating counts of bound/free (B/F) to total bound hormone concentration. $q = 2.26$ ng/ml at a 1:40 dilution; $K = 2.42 \times 10^8$ litres per mole.

normally less than 3%. Within- and between-assay variation were determined by assaying ten replicates of the same serum sample (stored in four aliquots at $-20°C$ with ascorbic acid) in four runs at weekly intervals. The results are shown in Table V. There is no significant difference between the mean values obtained. Within-assay variation is less than 7%.

Comparison with microbiological assay

Twenty-three samples of serum were assayed in parallel by the radioassay described and by a microbiological assay using *Lactobacillus casei.* The results are given in Fig. 6.

The correlation coefficient, 0.988, is significant at $p < 0.001$.

Cross-reactivity

Incubation mixtures were prepared containing 0.4 ng of ^{3}H-PGA, milk binder, and 5, 10, 15 and 20 ng of methotrexate with no inactive PGA. On charcoal separation, no significant displacement of tracer PGA from milk binder was observed.

TABLE V. WITHIN- AND BETWEEN-ASSAY VARIATION IN RADIOASSAY OF SERUM FOLATE

Four assays at weakly intervals on the same serum sample

Sample No.	Assay 1	Assay 2	Assay 3	Assay 4
1	6.6	7.6	6.4	6.8
2	7.0	6.8	6.9	6.8
3	6.9	6.7	7.6	6.5
4	7.3	7.0	7.2	6.6
5	6.4	7.0	7.4	7.2
6	6.8	6.7	6.4	6.5
7	7.1	6.9	6.9	6.9
8	6.2	6.6	7.1	6.5
9	7.1	6.9	7.1	7.1
10	6.8	6.2	6.2	6.9
Mean	6.82	6.84	6.92	6.78
S.D.	0.34	0.36	0.46	0.26
S.E.M.	0.11	0.11	0.15	0.09
% Coeff. of variation.	4.98	5.30	6.6	4.0

Whole-blood folate

Identical 'total counts' were obtained when incubation mixtures were prepared in buffer only and when 100 μl of a 1:20 dilution of whole-blood haemolysate were included, indicating no significant colour quenching. Dilution of the haemolysate 1:20 enabled whole-blood folate to be measured off the same standard curve as for serum without constructing a quench curve. However, in contrast to the case of serum, the test sample blank was sometimes found to be high (between 5 and 10%). This was reduced when 50 μl rather than 100 μl of diluted haemolysate was used, but the problem of variable test sample blanks remains in the case of the whole-blood folate assay.

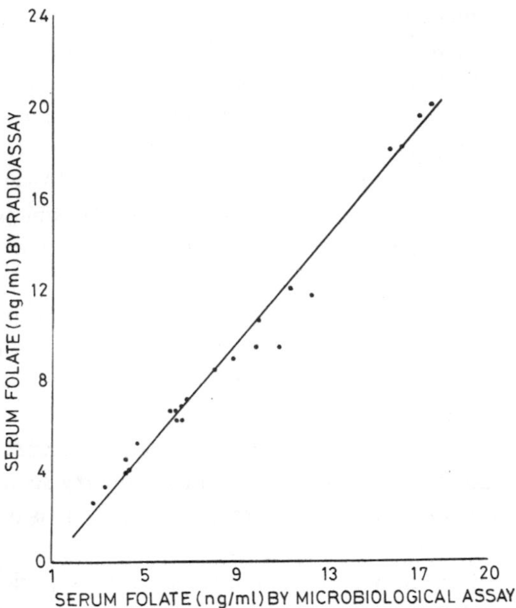

FIG.6. Correlation between radioassay and microbiological assay of serum folate. Correlation coefficient = 0.988; Regression coefficient = 1.2.

DISCUSSION

For radioassay of folic acid, antisera have been relatively little used and are reported to be specific for PGA only [7]. Current methods employ a number of naturally occuring binding agents, or purified extracts, as in the case of hog kidney extract and pure β-lactoglobulin. Where hog kidney extract, pig plasma, or *L. casei* cultures are used in a radioassay, one of the main drawbacks is that endogenous serum binding of folate has to be corrected for by special means. The degree of endogenous binding and consequently the amount of folate unavailable to the assay binding agent used depends on the concentration of FABP present in serum which is itself dependent on serum folate concentration, being increased in folate-deficiency states [4]. Heat inactivation of FABP by autoclaving [8] or boiling of the test serum/buffer mixture is a more satisfactory way of overcoming this problem than the processing of serum blanks to estimate endogenous binding, on the assumption that total binding equals exogenous plus endogenous binding has been shown to be incorrect [1].

An observation made in the assay employing *L. casei* [8] that heat-treated folate-free serum needed to be included in all standard tubes was also found to apply when pig plasma was used as binding agent. Furthermore, any method employing MTFA as standard suffers from a marked disadvantage in the instability of this compound when stored at −20°C with ascorbic acid (storage at −70°C with 2-mercaptoethanol [1] was not possible). However, within these limitations, added to which should be the fact that pig plasma was also relatively unstable when stored at −20°C, the assay was found workable and sensitive to about 0.1 ng MTFA.

Attempts to use cow milk as binding agent for folic acid produced results completely at variance with those of numerous other workers. Patent powdered milk preparations available in the tropics are not identical to those sold in the West under the same trade name and this may account for the difference in the case of milk powder. That no locally available fresh, pasteurized or sterilized cow milk possessed any significant folate binding property seems to be a unique finding for which no ready explanation can be adduced. It is possible that dietary factors may be responsible.

Buffalo milk, human milk and also colostrum were superior to cow milk as folate binders but the maximum obtained, even at dilutions of 1:8 or 1:10, was insufficient to enable any of them to be of practical use in a radioassay of folate because they produce a milkiness of the incubation mixture which is not removed by treatment with charcoal in the separation step. The similarity of human milk to buffalo milk is perhaps worthy of note in view of a previous observation that human milk was similar to cow milk in folate binding ability [2].

Goat milk as a folate binder has shown many advantages over the other agents discussed here. A binding of over 50% ^{3}H-PGA has been consistently obtained at 1:40 dilution with no deterioration when stored freeze dried at 4°C for 3 months. This, considered with the fact that goat milk is readily obtainable, constitutes a distinct advantage over pig plasma which was the only other agent encountered in the present study as a suitable binder for folate assay.

Cow milk is said to possess two binders for PGA, one of which binds with MTFA as well [9]. The affinity of cow milk binder for MTFA increases with rise in pH until at pH9.3 identical binding is exhibited towards both PGA and MTFA [1]. The results presented confirm this finding for goat milk. The effect has been reported to be due to an increase in binding affinity rather than to the capacity for MTFA [1]. This has not been investigated in the present study but the results demonstrating the measurement of known amounts of MTFA by itself and the additive effect with PGA when the latter was used for constructing the standard curve suggest that goat milk as binder is similar to cow milk in that it does not distinguish between the two substances at pH9.3.

'Releasing factor' was found in five out of eight samples of goat milk. The fact that it has been reported to be present in six out of ten preparations of cow milk [1] suggests its incidence in cow and goat milk to be similar. The reason for this inconsistency is not known but preliminary work (no results presented) suggests there is no relation to the period of lactation. Where found, it remains unchanged for 3 months when stored freeze dried.

The assay appears to be valid by standard criteria. Similar precision, sensitivity, and within- and between-assay variation of less than 10% have been reported by workers using other binding agents in the case of serum folate [2, 3, 9], but when red cell folate was measured the variation appeared to be greater [2]. In the present study, validity criteria have not been investigated in the case of whole-blood folate measurement as the problem of test-sample blanks is yet to be overcome.

From the stands of convenience, reliability and ease of operation, the method described is at least as satisfactory as others available for folate assay. It has advantages in that goat milk as binder shows greater stability and more reproducible binding from batch to batch in the absence of serum blank. Also, there is no interference from endogenous binding of folate to FABP. This is specially so in circumstances such as those encountered in the present study where no preparation of cow milk was found suitable as a folate binder.

ACKNOWLEDGEMENTS

The authors would like to thank Dr. S. Senthi Shanmuganathan, Head, Department of Biochemistry, Medical Research Institute, Colombo, for kindly performing the microbiological assays.

The counting equipment and the radioactive equipment used in this work were provided through technical assistance projects of the International Atomic Energy Agency.

REFERENCES

[1] LONGO, Dan L., HERBERT, V., J. Lab. Clin. Med. **87** 1 (1976) 138.

[2] MINCEY, E.K., WILCOX, Eileen, MORRISON, R.T., "Estimation of serum and red cell folate by a simple radiometric technique", Radioimmunoassay and Related Procedures in Medicine (Proc. Symp. Istanbul, 1973) **2**, IAEA, Vienna (1974) 205.

[3] LEONARD, J.P., TAYMANS, F., BECKERS, C., "A radioassay for serum folate using milk protein as ligand-binding system", Radioimmunoassay and Related Procedures in Medicine (Proc. Symp. Istanbul, 1973) **2**, IAEA, Vienna (1974) 221.

[4] WAXMAN, S., SCHREIBER, C., Blood **42** 2 (1973) 281.

[5] MANTZOS, J., ALEVIZOU-TERZAKI, V., GYFTAKI, E., Acta Haemotol. **51** (1974) 204.

[6] KAMEN, B.A., CASTON, J.D., J. Lab. Clin. Med. **83** (1974) 164.

[7] ROTHENBERG, S.P., Metabolism **22** (1973) 1075.

[8] McCALL, Mary S., WHITE, Jerry D., FRENKEL, Eugene P., Proc. Soc. Exp. Biol. **134** (1970) 536.
[9] WAXMAN, S., SCHREIBER, C., HERBERT, V., Blood **38** (1971) 219.

DISCUSSION

G. ODSTRCHEL: As regards the lack of binding in milk mentioned by Dr. Piyasena, we have found in our laboratory tremendous variability not only between the different lots of whole or of powdered milk but also within the same lot, i.e. there is a large variability in milk presumably processed in the same manner. We can only speculate as to the reason for this.

R.D. PIYASENA: I am inclined to think the lack of binding may be due to differences in the vitamin content.

ESTIMATION OF FOLATE BINDING CAPACITY (UNSATURATED AND TOTAL) IN NORMAL HUMAN SERUM AND IN β-THALASSAEMIA*

S. MOULOPOULOS, J. MANTZOS, E. GYFTAKI,
M. KESSE-ELIAS, V. ALEVIZOU-TERZAKI,
E. SOULI-TSIMILI
The University of Athens Medical School,
"Alexandra" Hospital,
Athens, Greece

Abstract

ESTIMATION OF FOLATE BINDING CAPACITY (UNSATURATED AND TOTAL) IN NORMAL HUMAN SERUM AND IN β-THALASSAEMIA.

A method is described for measuring the total serum folate binding capacity (TBC) after treating the serum with urea at pH5.5, the unsaturated serum folate binding capacity (UBC) being determined without treatment with urea. The method was applied to 50 normal controls and 20 patients with homozygous β-thalassaemia. The results show an increase in folate binding capacity after treating the serum with urea in all cases studied. There is no correlation between serum folic acid level and total or unsaturated folate binding capacity or per cent saturation. The method described is a simple and rapid one for screening the different groups studied for saturated and unsaturated specific folate-binding proteins.

1. INTRODUCTION

The binding capacity of human serum for a certain substance is of importance because the transport and availability of the substance is mainly dependent on the binding proteins. Therefore, disturbances in binding capacity may be reflected in disturbances in the metabolism of the substance.

As for folates, studies have shown that a large proportion of the circulating folates in human serum is bound to non-specific proteins [1, 2]. Also, different investigators have found specific binding proteins for added radioactive pteroylglutamic acid (^{3}H-PGA) in normal controls [3] and in various conditions [4–6].

In this investigation we studied the serum folic acid binding capacity (FABC) (unsaturated and total) for added ^{3}H-PGA in normal controls and in patients with β-thalassaemia in whom the serum folate is lower than normal because of the increased consumption due to the increased haemopoiesis.

---

* This work has been carried out under a Research Contract with the University of Athens.

With the method, which was developed in our laboratory, and is described here, we determined (1) the FABC for ^{3}H-PGA of untreated serum, which is considered to represent the unsaturated folate binding capacity (UFBC), and (2) the total folate binding capacity after treating the serum with urea.

2. MATERIAL AND METHOD

For determining the total folate binding capacity, urea was used to release the binders from the endogenous folates.

The method briefly is as follows: 10 μl of human serum is added to 300 μl of a solution containing 8M urea in 0.15M phosphate buffer at pH5.

Urea is allowed to act upon the folate binder complex for 2h at room temperature. A quantity of phosphate buffer (0.15M, pH 7.8) and 0.2 ng of ^{3}H-PGA is added to bring the volume to 2 ml and the mixture is incubated at room temperature for 15 min. After incubation, 0.5 ml of a suspension of 0.25% charcoal in 0.15M phosphate buffer, pH 7.8, containing 0.025% dextran of average molecular weight 70 000 is added, the tubes are shaken and the charcoal is removed by centrifuging.

An aliquot of the supernatant is added to the scintillation solution for counting.

For determining the unsaturated folate binding capacity, the same procedure is followed but without treating the serum with urea.

A supernatant control to measure non-absorbable radioactivity was prepared as described for the samples, but without human serum. The counts of this control, which represent impurities of ^{3}H-PGA, were subtracted from the counts of each sample. The results in both experiments are expressed in ng PGA/ml.

The saturated folate binding capacity is the difference between the total and unsaturated binding capacities.

With the method described, samples from 50 normal controls and from 20 patients with homozygous β-thalassaemia were studied. In all the subjects, the total and unsaturated folate binding capacities and the serum folic acid levels were measured. None of the studied subjects was under folic acid therapy and the normal controls had a normal blood picture.

3. RESULTS

As shown in Table I, the mean value of the TFBC from 50 normal controls is 91 ± 7.8 pg/ml and of the UFBC, 50 ± 7.7 pg/ml. The mean percentage saturation for the same group is 52.1 ± 4.1%.

TABLE I. VALUES FOR TFBC, UFBC AND PERCENTAGE SATURATION FOR CONTROLS AND PATIENTS WITH β-THALASSAEMIA

Cases	TFBC pg/ml	UFBC pg/ml	% saturation
Normal (50)ˣ	91 ± 7.8• 23 −491▪	50 ± 7.7• 0 −247▪	52.1 ± 4.1• 3.1 − 100▪
β-Thalassaemia (20)ˣ	107 ± 11• 38 − 220▪ $p > 0.1$	67 ± 10• 8 − 197▪ $p > 0.1$	41.4 ± 4.4• 2 − 82▪ $p > 0.05$

TFBC = Total folate binding capacity

UFBC = Unsaturated folate binding capacity

ˣ = Number of cases studied

• = Standard error

▪ = Range

The corresponding values for the thalassaemic group (20 subjects) are 107 ± 11 pg/ml (TFBC) and 67 ± 10 pg/ml (UFBC), and the mean percentage saturation is 41.4 ± 4.3%.

It is clear from the results that there is an increase in the binding capacity after treating the serum with urea.

There is no correlation between folic acid level and total or unsaturated folate binding capacity or per cent saturation for both groups.

4. COMMENTS

In the method described, dissociation of endogenous folate from the binders was achieved by urea at pH5.5.

The freed folate was not removed from the medium containing the binders, the binding capacity being estimated in the presence of the endogenous folate.

This was done because the error due to rebinding of endogenous folate to the binders in the presence of urea must be small because the ratio of the exogenous radioactive folate to the endogenous folate bound by the specific folate binding protein is very high.

Even if the affinity of endogenous folate is the same as that of the added radioactive folate, the error thus introduced is small, being less than 5%, which does not alter the diagnostic value of the results.

On the other hand, the results of samples examined by our method and by that of Colman and Herbert [7], who remove endogenous folate before assay, were comparable.

The method was applied to normal subjects and to patients with β-thalassaemia, a disease known to be associated with low folate levels. No difference was noticed in saturation between normal and thalassaemic subjects. The results show that unsaturated binding capacity tends to be higher in thalassaemia, although not statistically significant, and this finding is in agreement with the findings of other investigators who noticed an increase of unsaturated binding capacity in folate deficiency [5, 8]. The increase in unsaturated binding capacity may be caused by the protein disturbances present in thalassaemia [9].

To summarize, the presented method is simple and rapid for screening the different groups studied for saturated and unsaturated specific folate binding proteins.

REFERENCES

[1] MARKANEN, T., PETROLA, O., Carrier proteins of folic acid activity in human serum, Acta Haematol. **45** (1971) 106.

[2] RETIEF, F.P., HUSKISSON, Y.J., Folate binders in body fluids, J. Clin. Pathol. **23** (1970) 703.

[3] ROTHENBERG, S.P., DaCOSTA, M., Further observations on the folate binding factor in some leukemic cells, J. Clin. Invest. **50** (1971) 719.

[4] DaCOSTA, M., ROTHENBERG, S.P., Appearance of a folate binder in leukocytes and serum of women who are pregnant or taking oral contraceptives, J. Lab. Clin. Med. **83** (1974) 207.

[5] WAXMAN, S., SCHREIBER, C., Measurement of serum folate levels and serum folic acid-binding protein by ^{3}H-PGA radioassay, Blood **42** (1973) 281.

[6] HINES, J.D., KAMEN, B., CASTON, D., Abnormal folate binding protein(s) in azometic patients, Blood **42** (1973) 997.

[7] COLMAN, N., HERBERT, V., Total folate binding capacity of normal human plasma, and variations in uremia, cirrhosis and pregnancy, Blood **48** (1976) 911.

[8] WAXMAN, S., SCHREIBER, C., Characteristics of folic acid binding protein in folate-deficient serum, Blood **42** (1973) 291.

[9] NECHELES, T.F., ALLEN, D.M., FINKEL, H.E., Clinical Disorders of Hemoglobin Structure and Synthesis, Appleton-Century-Crofts, NY (1969) p. 141.

DISCUSSION

R.D. PIYASENA: Have you any information on the efficiency with which urea can release folate from endogenous binders in plasma?

E. GYFTAKI: We used different concentrations of urea and found the greatest dissociation at 6M.

A. MALKIN: What is the normal folate-binding protein? Is its folate-binding capacity influenced by the administration of naturally occurring substances such as steroids?

E. GYFTAKI: The precise nature of the folate binders in human serum has not been fully elucidated, although many papers have been published on the subject. All that is known so far is that the greater part of the circulating folic acid (MTHFA) is free or weakly bound (non-specific binding) to a wide range of plasma proteins.

In spite of this finding, there is strong evidence to suggest that a protein or proteins with the properties of a specific folate binder occur in small quantities in normal sera. This can be explained by the assumption that the binder has lower affinity for reduced folic acid.

The folate-binding capacity of the specific binders cannot be influenced by other substances.

T.A. WILKINS: Laboratories carrying out thyroid hormone measurements often perform the calculation:

$$\text{(FTI) Free thyroxine index} = \frac{\text{(total thyroxine)}}{\text{(unsaturated thyroxine binding protein capacity)}}$$

to improve discrimination between the clinical categories. I wonder if you have analysed the analogous parameter for folate studies, viz.

$$\text{Free folate index} = \frac{\text{(total folate)}}{\text{(unsaturated folate binding protein capacity)}}$$

If you have, does this improve the discrimination between normals and patients with β-thalassaemia?

E. GYFTAKI: No, we did not estimate a free folate index.

ASSAY OF 25-OH VITAMIN D_3

Ph. De NAYER, M. THALASSO, C. BECKERS
Centre de médecine nucléaire,
Ecole de médecine,
Université de Louvain,
Brussels, Belgium

Abstract

ASSAY OF 25-OH VITAMIN D_3.

A simplified version of the competitive protein-binding assay for 25-OH vitamin D_3 (25-OH D_3) derived from the method of Belsey et al. is presented. The procedure does not include a chromatographic step, and it is performed on an alcoholic extract of 0.1 ml plasma or serum. Normal rat serum (1 : 20 000) was used as binding protein. No β-lipoproteins were added to the assay buffer. A 10% displacement of the tracer was observed at 0.04 ng/tube and a 50% displacement at 0.15 ng/tube, allowing for the measurement of 25-OH D_3 concentrations between 2 ng/ml and 200 ng/ml. Mean values in a normal group were 23.1 ± 6.5 ng/ml (range 16–37 ng/ml, n = 11).

1. INTRODUCTION

Vitamin D_3 needs to undergo two hydroxylations before it acquires its final active form. The first hydroxylation occurs in the liver and yields the 25-OH vitamin D_3 (25-OH D_3). This metabolite undergoes a further hydroxylation in position 1, in the kidney, to form the biologically active derivative 1,25-OH vitamin D_3 (1,25 di-OH cholecalciferol, 1,25-$(OH)_2D_3$). Plasma levels of 25-OH D_3 give a good index of the overall vitamin D_3 status, provided that the renal hydroxylase activity is normal.

A radio-competitive binding assay for 25-OH D_3 that is derived from the method of Belsey et al. [1] is presented here.

In addition to meeting the requirements for sensitivity and reproducibility it is essential that: (a) the method uses minimal amounts of serum or plasma to make it suitable for pediatric studies; (b) the assay is convenient and can handle a large number of samples in a routine procedure.

2. MATERIALS

2.1. Tracer

The 25-OH [26(27)-methyl-^{3}H] cholecalciferol was obtained from The Radiochemical Centre, Amersham, UK (specific activity: 7 Ci/mmol, 17 mCi/mg).

The benzene was evaporated under a stream of N_2, and the dry material redissolved in 95% ethanol to a dilution of 2.5 μCi/ml. The tracer was stored in aliquots of 0.5 ml at -20°C. Before use, the content was diluted 10 times with 95% ethanol.

2.2. Standards

The 25-OH D_3 was purchased from Philips-Duphar, Amsterdam, The Netherlands. A starting solution was made up in 95% ethanol at a concentration of 1 μg/ml. Aliquots of this solution were kept at -20°C. Before use, 25 μl of this solution was dissolved in 1 ml of 95% ethanol, and standards were prepared by serial dilutions to yield a range of 2.5 ng to 0.04 ng per tube in the assay (addition of 100 μl per tube, see later). The actual concentration was verified by spectrophotometry.

2.3. β-lipoproteins

β-lipoproteins were prepared according to Belsey et al. [1] and stored in aliquots at -20°C.

2.4. Dextran-coated charcoal

This solution, made up in assay buffer, contained 2.5 g% charcoal (Norit A, Serva, Heidelberg) and 0.25 g% dextran (dextran, grade C, BDH, Poole, UK). It was used as such or in a 1 : 5 dilution.

2.5. Assay buffer

The assay buffer was prepared according to Belsey et al. [1]. The stock solution of barbital acetate contained 9.7 g of sodium acetate and 15.74 g of barbital per litre. Before use, 50 ml of this stock solution was diluted with 0.9% NaCl, adjusted to pH 8.6 with 0.1 M HCl and made up to 1 litre. When added to the buffer, the β-lipoproteins were at a concentration of 1 : 100 to 1 : 200.

2.6. Binding protein

Serum was obtained from adult rats on a regular diet. The serum (1 : 1000 dilution) was kept at -20°C in small aliquots. In this assay, it was used at dilutions ranging from 1 : 10 000 to 1 : 40 000 (see later).

3. METHOD

All manipulations were performed at 4°C. Glass tubes (12 mm × 75 mm) were used in the assay.

3.1. Samples

0.1 ml of serum was added to 0.9 ml of 95% ethanol. The mixture was briefly stirred on a vortex and centrifuged for 20 min at 2000 × g in a Sorvall RC3. After centrifuging, 0.450 ml of the supernatant was pipetted off and mixed with 50 μl of the ^{3}H-25-OH D_3. For each sample, four assay tubes were prepared:

1 tube with 0.9 ml of assay buffer (tube D)
2 tubes with 0.9 ml of rat serum at a suitable dilution in the assay buffer (tubes B and B′)
1 tube for the measurement of total radioactivity added in the assay (tube T).

In each of these tubes, 100 μl of the extracted and labelled serum was added and the content mixed.

3.2. Standards

50 μl of the ^{3}H-25-OH D_3 was added to 450 μl of each dilution of standard. From each of these dilutions, 100 μl was pipetted in four assay tubes, as for the samples, and incubated for 16 h at 4°C.

After incubation, 0.4 ml of ice-cold dextran-coated charcoal was added. The tubes were stirred and left at 4°C for 15 to 45 min (see later). Phase separation was performed by centrifuging at 2000 × g for 20 min. The supernatant was decanted into a counting vial and 8 ml of scintillation fluid were added (Aquasol, New England Nuclear Co., Federal Republic of Germany, or Aqualuma, Lumac A.G., Switzerland).

The results were calculated using the following formula for expressing the bound-to-free ^{3}H-25-OH D_3 ratio:

$$\frac{B}{F} = \frac{B - D}{T - (B - D)}$$

As mentioned later, other expressions of the data were also used: B/B_0, B/T, (B–D)/T. The results are expressed in per cent.

TABLE I. SURVEY OF 25-OH VITAMIN D_3 COMPETITIVE BINDING ASSAYS

Authors and reference	Extraction	Solubilizer	Chromatography	Binding-protein	Values (ng/ml) $\bar{x} \pm SD$	Country and year
Belsey et al. [1]	Ethanol	β-lipo-protein	–	Vit. D-deficient rat serum	35.2 ± 3.6 (SEM)	USA (1974)
Bayard et al. [2]	Dichloromethane methanol	–	Silica gel	Osteomalacic patient serum	15.0 ± 4.2	France (1972)
Bouillon et al. [3]	Dichloromethane methanol	β-lipo-protein	Sephadex LH20	Rat serum	13.4 ± 4.1	Belgium (1976)
Edelstein et al. [4]	Chloroform methanol	–	Sephadex LH20	Rat serum (fraction)	15.2 ± 5.6	UK (1974)
Ellis and Dixon [5]	Ethanol	Triton X405	Silicic acid	Human serum	12.6 ± 5.1	UK (1977)
Garcia-Pascual et al. [6]	Ethanol	–	–	Vit. D-deficient rat serum	39.5 ± 9.3	Switzerland (1976)
Haddad and Chyu [7]	Ether	–	Silicic acid	Vit. D-deficient rat kidney cytosol	27.3 ± 11.8	USA (1971)
Justova et al. [8]	Toluene	–	–	Osteomalacic patient serum	28.8 ± 5.3	Czechoslovakia (1976)
Mason and Posen [9]	Ethanol	–	Silicic acid	Vit. D-deficient rat kidney cytosol	28.5 ± 7.7	Australia (1977)

TABLE I (cont.)

Morris and Peacock [10]	Ethanol	–	–	Osteomalacic patient serum	26.9 ± 17.7	UK (1976)
Offermann and Dittmar [11]	Ethanol	–	–	Vit. D-deficient rat kidney cytosol	36.7 ± 16.5	FRG (1974)
Offermann et al. [12]	Chloroform methanol	–	Silicic acid	Vit. D-deficient rat kidney cytosol	37.8 ± 16.5	FRG (1974)
Okano et al. [13]	Ether	–	–	Vit. D-def. rat serum (fraction)	28.9 ± 2.9 (SEM)	Japan (1976)
Pettifor et al. [14]	Ethanol	Albumin	–	Vit. D-deficient rat serum	30.7 ± 9.9	South Africa (1976)
Preece et al. [15]	Chloroform methanol	Albumin	Silicic acid	Vit. D-deficient rat serum	11.9 ± 5.7	UK (1974)

4. RESULTS AND DISCUSSION

Several methods for measuring 25-OH D_3 based on competitive-binding assay have been published. They differ mainly in the nature of the binding protein, the extraction procedure, the presence of a "solubilizer" such as β-lipoproteins and the use or omission of a chromatographic step. A survey of data published during the past few years is given in Table I.

Here, we present and discuss our experience with an assay based on the method proposed by Belsey et al. [1].

4.1. Extraction procedure

95% ethanol was used for extraction. There seems to be good reason to consider this method as efficient as the use of other lipid extractants in terms of the recovery of 25-OH D_3 [1, 6, 9–11].

4.2. Binding-protein

Normal rat serum was chosen: indeed, it appears, there is no need to use vitamin-D-deficient serum from humans or rats, or rat kidney cytosol [3,9]. The dilution of the binding protein was 1 : 20 000. This yielded a binding of 15 to 20% in the assay with β-lipoproteins and 40% without β-lipoproteins using the (B-D)/T –(B-D) formula. These percentages were, respectively, 25% and 45% using the B/T expression. This dilution was selected because the 50% displacement of the tracer was obtained at a 30 ng/ml concentration of 25-OH D_3. In the assay using rat serum (1 : 20 000), β-lipoproteins (1 : 100), and the formula of Belsey et al. [1], a value of 26.0 ± 7.76 (SD) was obtained in a group of 15 normal subjects.

4.3. Addition of a solubilizer

The addition of a solubilizer, such as β-lipoproteins, has been advocated by Belsey et al. [1]. Others have recommended albumin [14,15] or Triton X405 [5]. However, the inclusion of a solubilizer does not seem to be required since the ethanol present in the assay would assure the solubility of the 25-OH D_3 [10]. The inclusion of β-lipoproteins has been studied by Garcia-Pascual et al. [6], Mason and Posen [9] and Pettifor et al. [14]. Their conclusion was that the inclusion of the solubilizer did not improve the performance of the assay, and even could induce a greater variability. Our experience was that the addition of β-lipoproteins did affect the binding in the standard curve because the "D" tubes (no rat serum added) exhibited a high radioactivity, thus affecting significantly the computation of the results, especially at low values of 25-OH D_3. This is probably due to an artefact resulting from the absence of binding protein in the "D" tubes modifying the equilibrium and increasing in a non-proportional way the fixation of the tracer to the β-lipoproteins in the tubes containing only buffer. Moreover, when expressing the same data as B/T, low values (1 to 10 ng/ml) were less erratic, without affecting the values in the mid-range.

Assays were therefore performed without the inclusion of β-lipoprotein in the buffers. At this point, however, it appeared that the dextran-coated charcoal (DCC) concentration was critical. The B_0 (in %) values, expressed as (B - D)/T, were:

With β-lipoproteins	with β-lipoproteins	without β-liporoteins
DCC (1 : 1)	DCC (1 : 5)	DCC (1 : 5)
13.8%	20.7%	29.9%

The assay thus devised does not include a solubilizer. With normal rat serum (1 : 20 000) as binding protein and using DCC at 1 : 5 of the initial concentration, the following results were obtained. In a group of normal subjects a mean value of 23.1 ± 6.5 (SD) ng/ml was recorded. The normal range was between 16 to 37 ng/ml. Displacement of 10% of the tracer occurred at 4 ng/ml and 50% at about 30 ng/ml. Comparison of values in the normal range within the same run gave a CV of 8.1% and between runs of 12.8%.

As this assay does not involve a chromatographic step, we would like to comment on this debated point.

4.4. The chromatographic step

The need for a chromatographic step – either on silicic acid or Sephadex LH20 – in the assay is also questionable. A preference for Sephadex LH20 has been expressed because of leakage from the silicic acid of material that interferes in the assay [4]. In most cases, assays that include a chromatographic step yield lower values, but when they are compared directly this difference is not apparent: 35.2 ± 3.6 (SE) without versus 33.3 ± 3.6 (SE) with chromatography on silicic acid [1], and 36.7 ± 16.5 (SD) versus 37.8 ± 16.5 (SD) in a study by Offerman and Dittmar [11]. Differences have been attributed to the presence of 24,25-$(OH)_2$ D_3 in non-chromatographic assays, this derivative being equipotent in displacing ^{3}H-25-OH D_3 from its binding-protein [18]. However, in a detailed study by Taylor et al. [19] it was shown that this hydroxylated derivative is not likely to amount to more than 10% in the total assay, as is also true for vitamin D_3 [9]. Mason and Posen [9] suggest that an error could be due to the presence of an incompletely separated

TABLE II. ASSAY OF 25-OH VITAMIN D_3 WITH NON-COMPETITIVE BINDING METHODS

Authors and reference	Method	Extraction	Chromatography	Values (ng/ml)	Year	Country
Björkhem and Holmberg [16]	Mass fragmentography	Chloroform methanol	Sephadex LH20	27.0 ± 10.0 (SD)	1976	Sweden
Eisman et al. [17]	High-pressure liquid chromatography	Chloroform methanol	Sephadex LH20	31.9 ± 1.7 (SE)	1977	USA

protein during the initial extraction that would interfere with the assay. However, one has to consider the fact that non-competitive protein-binding assays give values that are close to 30 ng/ml (Table II), leaving the debate open as to the real role of the chromatographic steps in this context.

5. CONCLUSION

The critical evaluation of some of the aspects of the non-chromatographic method for assaying 25-OH D_3 proposed by Belsey et al. [1] indicates that: (a) β-lipoproteins are not required; (b) the dextran-coated charcoal concentration has to be checked; (c) the 25-OH D_3 binding ability of normal rat serum is satisfactory; (d) the results obtained under these conditions (B-D/T), 23.1 ± 6.5 ng/ml, are close to the values reported by others using the same assay, but are higher than in the assays using a chromatographic step.

This study emphasizes the need for standardized control sera with 25-OH D_3 levels assessed by independent methods.

REFERENCES

[1] BELSEY, R.E., DE LUCA, H.F., POTTS, J.T., A rapid assay for 25-OH-vitamin D_3 without preparative chromatography, J. Clin. Endocrinol. Metab. **38** (1974) 1046.

[2] BAYARD, F., BEC, P., LOUVET, J.P., "Measurement of plasma 25-hydroxycholecalciferol in man, Europ. J. Clin. Invest. **2** (1972) 195.

[3] BOUILLON, R., van KERKHOVE, P., de MOOR, P., Measurement of 25-hydroxyvitamin D_3 in serum, Clin. Chem. **22** (1976) 364.

[4] EDELSTEIN, S., CHARMAN, M., LAWSON, D.E.M., KODICEK, E., Competitive protein-binding assay for 25-hydroxycholecalciferol, Clin. Sci. Mol. Med. **46** (1974) 231.

[5] ELLIS, G., DIXON, K., Sequential-saturation-type assay for serum 25-hydroxyvitamin D, Clin. Chem. **23** (1977) 855.

[6] GARCIA-PASCUAL, B., PEYTREMANN, A., COURVOISIER, B., LAWSON, D.E.M., A simplified competitive protein-binding assay for 25-hydroxycalciferol, Clin. Chim. Acta **68** (1976) 99.

[7] HADDAD, J.G., CHYU, K.J., Competitive protein-binding radioassay for 25-hydroxycholecalciferol, J. Clin. Endocrinol. **33** (1971) 992.

[8] JUSTOVA, V., STARKA, L., WILCZEK, H., PACOVSKY, V., A simple radioassay for 25-hydroxycholecalciferol without chromatography, Clin. Chim. Acta **70** (1976) 97.

[9] MASON, R.S., POSEN, S., Some problems associated with assay of 25-hydroxycalciferol in human serum, Clin. Chem. **23** (1977) 806.

[10] MORRIS, J.F., PEACOCK, M., Assay of plasma 25-hydroxyvitamin D, Clin. Chim. Acta **72** (1976) 383.

[11] OFFERMANN, G., DITTMAR, F., A direct protein-binding assay for 25-hydroxycalciferol, Horm. Metab. Res. **6** (1974) 534.

[12] OFFERMANN, G., von HERRATH, D., SCHAEFFER, K., Serum 25-hydroxycholecalciferol in uremia, Nephron **13** (1974) 269,

[13] OKANO, K., NAKAI, R., GOTO, H., YOSHIKAWA, M., Effects of age and diseases on human serum 25-hydroxycholecalciferol determined by competitive protein-binding assay, Endocrinol. Jpn. **23** (1976) 265.

[14] PETTIFOR, J.M., ROSS, F.P., WANG, J., A competitive protein-binding assay for 25-hydroxyvitamin D, Clin. Sci. Mol. Med. **51** (1976) 605.

[15] PREECE, M.A., O'RIORDAN, J.L.H., LAWSON, D.E.M., KODICEK, E., A competitive protein-binding assay for 25-hydroxycholecalciferol and 25-hydroxyergocalciferol in serum", Clin. Chim. Acta **54** (1974) 235.

[16] BJÖRKHEM, I., HOLMBERG, I., A novel specific assay of 25-hydroxyvitamin D_3, Clin. Chim. Acta **68** (1976) 215.

[17] EISMAN, J.A., SHEPARD, R.M., DE LUCA, H.F., "Determination of 25-hydroxyvitamin D_2 and 25-hydroxyvitamin D_3 in human plasma using high-pressure liquid chromatography, Anal. Biochem. **80** (1977) 298.

[18] HADDAD, J.G., MIN, C., WALGATE, J., HAHN, T., Competition by 24, 25-dihydroxycholecalciferol in the competitive protein-binding radioassay of 25-hydroxycalciferol, J. Clin. Endocrinol. Metab. **43** (1976) 712.

[19] TAYLOR, C.M., HUGHES, S.E., de SILVA, P., Competitive protein binding assay for 24, 25-dihydroxycholecalciferol, Biochem. Biophys. Res. Comm. **70** (1976) 1243.

DISCUSSION

Ch.-A. BIZOLLON: In preparing your reagents, including the tracer and reference solutions, and in performing your assay, did you not experience difficulties due to the degradation of 25-OH vitamin D_3 under the action of light and air? How do you get round these difficulties?

Ph. De NAYER: In preparing the reagents, we try to take account of these difficulties by using nitrogen to drive off oxygen from the solutions. We keep the standards and solutions in the dark. Incubation itself is performed away from light.

D.K. HAZRA: How useful is the method you have described for measuring the biologically active 1,25-dihydroxy form of D_3?

Ph. De NAYER: This assay does not measure the 1,25-dihydroxy form of vitamin D_3. It gives an estimate of its precursor. The assay is useful in two respects: (a) except in renal diseases and possibly in a few other situations the 25-hydroxy form seems to be a good index of vitamin status, corresponding to the active 1,25 dihydroxy form; and (b) since no method is available for a routine assay of the 1,25 dihydroxy form, we have to rely on measurement of the 25-hydroxy form.

J. GRENIER: Describing your operating procedure, you said you started from a plasma volume of 100 μl. Did you eliminate the possibility of an effect of the plasma sample volume on the calculated 25-OH vitamin D_3 value?

Ph. De NAYER: This point was not verified although we have always operated by this procedure. May I ask you whether an effect will be observed even if the extraction is performed from variable volumes of serum, the ratio between serum and the ethanol solution used in extraction remaining the same?

J. GRENIER: The volume effect takes the form of variation in the calculated value inversely proportional to the initial sample volume. This phenomenon is encountered in non-chromatographic RIA methods, as I have shown for example in the case of estradiol in paper SM-220/72. In the absence of a volume-effect test, it is impossible to know whether the value observed for a given volume is accurate.

Ph. De NAYER: Our method does not involve a radioimmunological technique but displacement by competition. It would be interesting to verify whether this concept also applies to this case.

Session VII

APPLICATIONS

Assays for steroids and other small molecules

Chairman

R.D. PIYASENA
Sri Lanka/IAEA

IAEA-SM-220/205

Invited review paper

RECENT ADVANCES IN STEROID RADIOIMMUNOASSAY

S.L. JEFFCOATE
Chelsea Hospital for Women,
London, United Kingdom

Abstract

RECENT ADVANCES IN STEROID RADIOIMMUNOASSAY.

The advances since 1974 in the techniques of measuring steroid molecules by radioimmunoassay are reviewed. They are considered under the following headings: preparation and use of antisera; preparation and use of tracers; preparation of biological samples before assay; dispensing of the reagents in the assay; separation of free and bound radioactivity; counting and data processing; quality control and standardization.

INTRODUCTION

The rapid progress of steroid radioimmunoassays since their introduction in 1969 has resulted in their widespread application to mammalian physiology and experimental and clinical medicine. The technical aspects of this progress up to the middle of 1974 have been covered in a number of books and reviews (see, for example, Abraham [1, 2], James and Jeffcoate [3], Cameron, Hillier and Griffiths [4] and Gupta [5]. This review is a somewhat personal assessment of current developments (up to mid-1977) and their possible place in the future.

1. STEROID ANTISERA

In the past 3 years, there have been no significant developments in the production, assessment or treatment of antisera for steroid RIA (apart from separation methods, see Section 5). It was established by mid-1974 that the nature of the immunogen, i.e. the steroid hapten, the chemistry, site and number of linkages, and the nature of the protein carrier, governed the properties of the resulting antisera. The site of linkage to the steroid nucleus was found to be particularly important and chemists were induced to try all the possible sites. For testosterone, for instance, virtually every carbon atom has been tried in an attempt to limit the cross-reaction with 5α-dihydrotestosterone (DHT). Even the most specific antisera for testosterone still show, however, a 15% cross-reaction with DHT which is little improvement on the antisera raised against the easily prepared 3-linked conjugates.

Grover and Odell [6] have recently reviewed the effects of substitution and the stereochemistry of the steroid-protein conjugates on the resulting specificity of the antisera. They have proposed a theory that steroid derivates, in which the coplanarity of the steroid molecules is maintained, tend to give more specific antisera.

One point that needs to be stressed in the preparation of steroid antisera (and this has received little attention since the pioneering studies of Liebermann and his colleagues over 20 years ago) is the need to purify and characterize steroid derivatives before conjugation. In this way the production of several populations of antibodies, for instance, against steroids linked at different points on the steroid skeleton or against cis and trans isomers, can be avoided, or at least reduced.

Affinity chromatography has been used in attempts to improve the specificity and affinity of steroid antisera. In my view, these attempts are doomed to failure, primarily because the cross-reaction from closely related steroids is not the result of a separate population of antibodies which can be removed, but is an inherent property of the binding site of the antibody. As regards the selecting out of the high affinity antibodies, this is made difficult by the fact that it is these antibodies that bind most avidly to the solid-phase ligand and are the most difficult to elute without damage.

2. STEROID TRACERS

Tritium-labelled steroids are most widely used as tracer ligands in the assay and also for recovery checks. Indeed, other tracers cannot be used for the latter purpose since they will not behave identically to the unlabelled steroid in partition and chromatographic systems. With the move toward less preparation of the sample before assay (see Section 3) the use of (^{3}H)steroids will become less necessary. The advantages and disadvantages of (^{3}H)steroids have been discussed elsewhere (Jeffcoate, Edwards, Gilby and White [7]) and are summarized in Table I. The need to ensure radiochemical purity is most important; it should not be taken for granted that manufacturers have provided the correct steroid in the stated amount and with the desired degree of purity. In one study, wide ranges of purity were found (Manlimos and Abraham [8]) and attributed to the shipment of the steroids from the manufacturer in solution at ambient temperatures. Stability was improved by shipping in the dry state after addition of carrier cholesterol (1 μg/1μCi) which should not cross-react with the antiserum. Purity should be checked frequently, e.g. every 3 months.

TABLE I. A COMPARISON OF THE ADVANTAGES AND DISADVANTAGES OF ^{3}H- AND ^{125}I-LABELLED TRACERS

^{3}H	^{125}I
Advantages	
1. Available commercially	1. Easier counting
2. Chemically defined	2. Higher specific activity
3. Long half-life	3. Higher affinity
Disadvantages	
1. Expense	1. Preparation
2. Lower specific activity	2. Higher affinity
3. Isotope effects	3. Cost of iodine

The need to check the radiochemical purity of (^{3}H)steroids to some extent negates the main disadvantages of ^{125}I-labelled tracers, the short half-life and the need for frequent preparation. The use of ^{125}I-labelled tracers has been reviewed elsewhere (Jeffcoate [9]) and in my view their advantages outweigh their disadvantages. The routine plasma testosterone assay at St. Thomas's Hospital has utilized a testosterone-histamine-^{125}I tracer without trouble for the past 3 years and the results are comparable to those obtained using (^{3}H)labels when collaborative assays are carried out between laboratories (M.J. Wheeler, personal communication). Another gamma emitter, ^{75}Se with a half-life of 120 days, has been used in a competitive protein-binding assay for cortisol (Chambers, Glover and Tudor [10]), but this isotope has not yet been used successfully in an RIA. At present the specific activity of ^{75}Se is low compared with that of ^{125}I.

One development in the field of steroid tracers is in the use of non-isotope tracers. Enzymes have been the most widely used and the prospect of cheap automation is the main attraction. At present these non-isotopic methods are less sensitive than the radioimmunoassays and it is hard to see how any tracer could be measured with the same ease and precision as radioactivity is measured with modern equipment.

3. SAMPLE PREPARATION

The extent to which a biological sample has to be purified before steroid RIA is proportional to the amount of error (losses, blanks, transcriptional) introduced and inversely proportional to the number of samples that can be

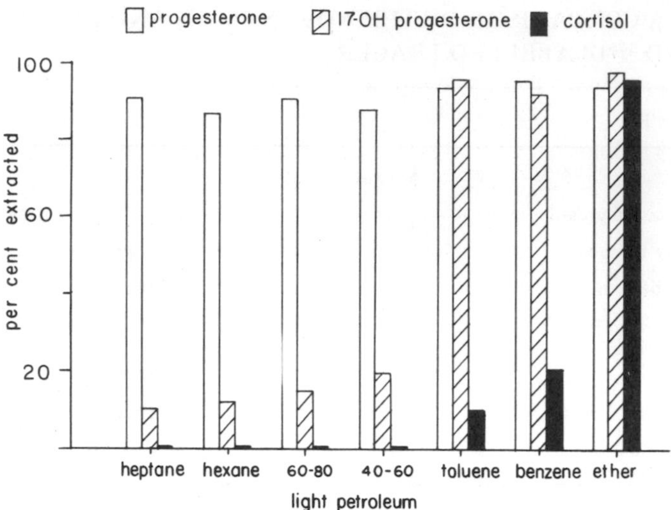

FIG.1. Selecting a solvent to add specificity to a steroid radioimmunoassay. Extraction of three steroids of increasing polarity (progesterone, 17-hydroxyprogesterone, cortisol) from plasma by solvents of increasing polarity (heptane → ether). Note that a non-polar solvent like heptane will extract over 90% of the progesterone but almost no cortisol. For a steroid of intermediate polarity like 17-hydroxyprogesterone, a solvent of intermediate polarity like toluene is required to extract it without extracting too much cortisol.

processed in unit time. For both these reasons, there is a gradual move to less and less pre-assay preparation. This approach obviously carries its own potential danger, that of loss of specificity because of the presence in the sample of cross-reacting steroids or other interfering, 'non-specific' substances.

The ultimate goal, that of no sample treatment at all, is only possible for steroids present in biological fluids in very high concentration (μmol/l), e.g. cholesterol and cholesterol esters, dehydro-epiandrosterone (DHA) sulphate or steroid glucuronides (Kellie [11]).

For steroids like cortisol, which are present in moderate concentration (nmol/l), non-extraction methods are also possible but in this case only after cortisol-binding globulin has been inhibited. This can be done by (a) heating to 60°C for 15 min, (b) treatment with ANS (8-anilino-haphthalene sulphonic acid) as used in thyroid hormone assays or (c) precipitation of plasma proteins with ethanol. These methods could also be applied to sex hormone-binding globulin (SHBG).

For most steroids a solvent extraction is required. Although there has been little recent development in this area, four points are worth making. First, the purity of the solvent should be initially high and frequently checked: a few millilitres evaporated and run as a sample in the RIA will soon reveal whether pseudosteroid 'blank' material is being added. Secondly, the choice of solvent can add specificity to the assay. This can be illustrated with respect to progesterone (Fig.1). It is unnecessary to extract with a polar solvent like ether when a much 'cleaner' extract can be obtained with a less polar solvent, such as hexane, with a minimum reduction in recovery. The logical extension of this view is that each steroid has its own extraction recipe tailored to its polarity so as to produce the cleanest extract with maximal recovery.

This conclusion does, however, militate against the third consideration, that of assay standardization (see also Section 7). The more solvents in use in a laboratory and within a group of laboratories, in which attempts are being made to achieve comparability of assay results, the more difficult it is to control the quality of the reagents. It may thus be best to select one (e.g. ether) which will extract all the steroids of interest, and to specify its purity and mode of use in as much detail as possible.

Finally, there have been developments in speeding up the rate-limiting step in steroid RIA, the separation and drying of the organic phase. A neat method of separation is to freeze the aqueous subnatant either in solid CO_2/acetone or with a cryoprobe (use of a deep-freeze is not recommended if ether is the solvent) and then to decant the organic supernatant without fear of contamination with the water phase. Evaporation machines are becoming commercially available. These will hold up to 100 tubes and will shake or warm them in a flow of nitrogen or air.

Chromatographic separation of steroids from biological fluids has been a traditional approach of steroid assayists, but with the gradual improvement of reagents and the increasing pressure of sample numbers, it is becoming less necessary and less popular. It still has two important places. First, non-chromatographic methods need to be validated against those in which chromatography has been used. The second application is in obtaining multiple steroid analyses of a single sample. This may be of value when several related steroids are of pathophysiological interest in a specific situation. Although other systems have been used, Abraham has developed this approach using extracts of 1 ml plasma on celite columns, e.g. for four androgens (Abraham, Manlimos, Solis and Wickman [12] or for four progestins (Abraham, Manlimos, Solis, Garza and Margoulis [13]). Celite column chromatography was also used by Parker, Ellegood and Mahesh [14] for assay of seven steroids of interest in reproductive endocrinology after separation (in < 2 h) from a single 1–2 ml sample of plasma.

Some other examples of multiple steroid assays using automated column techniques are presented elsewhere in these Proceedings.

4. REAGENT DISPENSING

The move toward increased mechanization of steroid RIA is occurring within the context of increasing automation of RIA and clinical chemistry in general. There has been a rash of dilutors, dispensers and pipetting stations on the market in addition to the relatively simple hand-held repeating pipettes. All these have their place, as do the completely automated machines under development which take in a sample at one end and, after a suitable delay, push out an answer at the other end.

In my view these machines have not yet reached a stage of development where they can replace the older more labour-intensive methods. They may never do so.

5. SEPARATION OF FREE AND BOUND RADIOACTIVITY

After the incubation of the reagents for an appropriate time the next important phase in steroid RIA is the separation of free from bound radioactivity. Many methods have been used (Ratcliffe [15]) and perhaps the aims of these methods should be stated before discussing how developments might advance steroid RIA. These are: no mis-classification error (i.e. all the bound and none of the free is in the bound fraction); cheapness and simplicity; potential for automation; ability to be standardized within and between laboratories.

Adsorption of the free fraction onto activated charcoal, uncoated or coated with dextran, albumin or gelatin is the most widely used method in steroid RIA. It has the advantage of cheapness and simplicity and can be fairly well standardized: one large batch of charcoal can be purchased to serve a number of laboratories for many years. Its disadvantages are (i) the dependence on time between addition and centrifugation; there is an increase in the radioactivity adsorbed to the charcoal caused either by dissociation of the bound complex and adsorption of the freed tracer or, more likely, adsorption of the bound complex itself, and (ii) the difficulty of using charcoal in automatic equipment.

Polyethylene glycol (PEG) is easier to handle in several respects (Schiller and Brammall [16, 17]) and recently has been widely used. One disadvantage of PEG is the need for higher centrifugation speeds (at least 1500 × g) compared with dextran-coated charcoal (500 × g). This may limit its universal applicability.

The double-antibody methods widely used in peptide assays can also be applied to steroids but they seem to be unnecessarily expensive and time-consuming when other techniques are available.

Although the first steroid RIA published was a solid-phase (coated-tube) method, these techniques have been slow to gain ground. They appear to have many advantages particularly in terms of cost, ease and potential automation.

The routine plasma testosterone RIA at St. Thomas's Hospital mentioned previously has employed antibody-coated tubes for several years. Temperature control at the coating stage is the only critical factor.

Other solid-phase methods that seem to be increasingly used are those in which antibody is covalently bound to particles which can be easily centrifuged for separation (e.g. Sepharose or glass beads). A novel approach is the use of antibodies coupled to magnetic particles which can be simply and automatically removed from the incubation medium with a magnet.

In summary, developments in this area of steroid RIA are in the direction of methods that are either cheap, automated or easily standardized and preferably all three.

6. COUNTING AND DATA PROCESSING

The counting of the radioactivity in either the antibody-bound or free fractions (or both) requires automatic counters. These machines are expensive and becoming more so. Two tendencies are discernible however: first, in the direction of more complicated counters that will do a certain amount of data processing in addition to counting; and second in the direction of cheaper, simpler bench-top counters with, for example, a single channel and limited sample capacity. Different users will have different needs and this will govern the choice of counter. Counters are also being developed with small computers (microprocessors) built into them which actually control the counting so that each tube is counted only for as long as is necessary to achieve a predetermined precision in the assay. It is undoubtedly true that many assayists count for far longer than their assays deserve in an effort to reduce counting errors at a time when other errors are far greater and receiving no attention.

Computers are used in RIA for two other purposes: optimal assay design and the calculation and evaluation of results. The theoretical basis and practical application of these have been extensively discussed. In 1974, Rodbard wrote that "the literature on RIA statistics and data processing is large and growing rapidly". This is still true in 1977. The reviews of Rodbard [18] and Cook [19] summarize the situation admirably. As regards standard curve-fitting, the logit-log linear transform appears to have gained widest currency and this and other programmes are readily available for use on relatively simple programmable calculators. It is an inefficient use of resources to have an on-line computer system for data calculation.

Scintillation-counting of β-emitters such as (^{3}H)steroids has been advanced by the use of polypropylene inserts which are produced by several manufacturers. The sample plus scintillation fluid is put in the insert which is then placed in a standard counting vial. Three benefits accrue: less scintillant is used; the waste scintillant and the insert can be easily disposed of by incineration thus reducing the health hazard; washing of counting vials is reduced to a minimum.

7. QUALITY CONTROL AND ASSAY STANDARDIZATION

Although it is the least glamorous aspect of steroid RIA, in my view this is the area in which the most significant developments were taking place in 1976. It has been recognized in public health laboratories (and is even permeating into the thinking in 'pure' research laboratories) that the quality of the assays performed is at least as important as the number of assays performed. Many of the principles and practices adopted by bioassayists for decades are only reluctantly used by immunoassayists and yet they are essential if the results are to have any meaning.

Quality control is aimed at two interrelated problems, internal and external. Within a laboratory, the assay needs to be as near 'correct' as possible with errors limited and with a mechanism for detecting real or potential breakdown in the assay. This is done by incorporating relevant samples in each assay. Thus the maximal binding (B_0), minimal (non-specific) binding and slope of the standard curve can be assessed. Quality-control samples can be included and should preferably cover the range to be expected in the unknown samples which they should resemble as closely as possible. Thus, it is better to use the endogenous steroid rather than to 'strip' (e.g. with charcoal) the sample and add known amounts of standard steroid. Cumulative charts showing within-assay and between-assay variance should be kept and make good laboratory wall-paper. Rodbard [18] and Rodbard, Lenox, Wray and Ramseth [20] have summarized the use of internal quality-control schemes.

External quality-control schemes are necessary because (i) many laboratories do not run adequate internal quality-control schemes, (ii) results between laboratories need to be comparable so that, in the first place, clinicians and others can use data from physiological and pathological situations without having to readjust to different normal ranges, and secondly, multi-centre research programmes obtain uniform results.

A number of external quality-control schemes for steroid RIA are under development. In the United Kingdom, a national scheme has arisen out of the work of the Supra-regional Assay Service (SAS) and all the steroids of major biological interest are covered. In general, about four coded samples are sent out at monthly intervals and the results returned and processed centrally. These schemes give information regarding between- and within-laboratory variance and reproducibility. A trouble-shooting element is an essential feature with the organizing quality-control laboratory being able to give advice on reagents, assay protocols, etc.

On a world-wide scale, the Human Reproduction Unit of WHO has instituted an external quality-control scheme for four steroid hormones in an attempt to increase the quality and comparability of the results obtained by the research laboratories participating in its research programmes in fertility control.

Those who have experienced the results of external quality-control schemes for RIA are well aware of the need for assay standardization. International organizations (for example IAEA and WHO) have seen the need for this and laid down guidelines very clearly [21, 22]. The 26th Report of the WHO Expert Committee on Biological Standardization is a milestone in this area and covers the need to provide well-characterized, matched reagents for immunoassay and the organization of hormone assay services at district, regional, national and international levels.

The UK is ahead of the world here with the SAS scheme and a developing network of regional schemes. The standardization of RIA within the SAS and within the WHO programmes involves a package of matched reagents (well-characterized, in sufficient supply to last for 3–5 years and in ampoules available for distribution) plus detailed assay protocols (buffers, incubation and separation procedures, etc.) and an external quality-control scheme. Using such a package, the achievement of the goal of assay standardization and universal comparability of high-quality RIA results is brought immeasurably closer.

REFERENCES

[1] ABRAHAM, G.E., Radioimmunoassay of steroids, Acta Endocrinol. Suppl. **183** (1974) 1.

[2] ABRAHAM, G.E., "The application of steroid radioimmunoassay to gynecologic endocrinology", Progress in Gynecology, Vol. VI (TAYMOR, M.L., GREEN, T.H., Eds), Grune and Stratton, New York (1975) 111.

[3] JAMES, V.H.T., JEFFCOATE, S.L., Steroid radioimmunoassays, Br. Med. Bull. **30** (1974) 50.

[4] CAMERON, E.H.D., HILLIER, S.G., GRIFFITHS, K. (Eds), Steroids Immunoassay (Proc. 5th Tenovus Workshop), Alpha Omega Alpha Publishing Ltd., Cardiff (1975).

[5] GUPTA, D. (Ed.), Radioimmunoassay of Steroid Hormones, Verlag Chemie, Weinheim (1975).

[6] GROVER, P.K., ODELL, W.D., Specificity of antisera to sex steroids. I. The effect of substitution and sterochemistry, J. Steroid Biochem. **8** (1977) 121.

[7] JEFFCOATE, S.L., EDWARDS, R., GILBY, E.D., WHITE, N., "The use of (^{3}H)-labelled ligands in steroid radioimmunoassays", Steroid Immunoassay (CAMERON, E.H.D., HILLIER, S.G., GRIFFITHS, K., Eds), Alpha Omega Alpha Publishing Ltd., Cardiff (1975) 133.

[8] MANLIMOS, F.S., ABRAHAM, G.E., Chromatographic purification of tritiated steroids prior to use in radioimmunoassay, Analyt. Letters **8** (1975) 403.

[9] JEFFCOATE, S.L., "Use of ^{125}iodine tracers in steroid radioimmunoassays", Radioimmunoassay of Steroid Hormones (GUPTA, D., Ed.), Verlag Chemie, Weinheim (1975) 185.

[10] CHAMBERS, V.E.M., GLOVER, I.S., TUDOR, R., "(^{75}Se)-radio ligands in steroid immunoassay", Steroid Immunoassay (CAMERON, E.H.D., HILLIER, S.G., GRIFFITHS, K., Eds), Alpha Omega Alpha Publishing Ltd, Cardiff (1975) 177.
[11] KELLIE, A.E., "Radioimmunoassay of steroid glucuronides", Radioimmunoassay of Steroid Hormones (GUPTA, D., Ed.), Verlag Chemie, Weinheim (1975) 165.
[12] ABRAHAM, G.E., MANLIMOS, F.S., SOLIS, M., WICKMAN, A.C., Combined radioimmunoassay of four steroids in one ml of plasma. II. Androgens, Clin. Biochem. **8** (1975) 374.
[13] ABRAHAM, G.E., MANLIMOS, F.S., SOLIS, M., GARZA, R., MARGOULIS, G.B., Combined radioimmunoassay of four steroids in one ml of plasma. I. Progestins, Clin. Biochem. **8** (1975) 396.
[14] PARKER, C.R., ELLEGOOD, J.O., MAHESH, V.B., Methods for multiple steroid radioimmunoassay, J. Steroid. Biochem. **6** (1975) 1.
[15] RATCLIFFE, J.G., Separation techniques in saturation analysis, Br. Med. Bull. **30** (1974) 32.
[16] SCHILLER, H.S., BRAMMALL, M.A., A radioimmunoassay of plasma estradiol-17β with the use of polyethylene glycol to separate free and antibody-bound hormone, Steroids **24** (1974) 665.
[17] SCHILLER, H.S., BRAMMALL, M.A., Non-chromatographic radioimmunoassay of unconjugated estriol in plasma with polyethylene glycol as precipitant, Clin. Chem. **22** (1976) 359.
[18] RODBARD, D., Statistical quality control and routine data processing for radioimmunoassays and immunoradiometric assays, Clin. Chem. **20** (1974) 1255.
[19] COOK, B., "Automation and data processing for radioimmunoassays", Steroid Immunoassay (CAMERON, E.H.D., HILLIER, S.G., GRIFFITHS, K., Eds), Alpha Omega Alpha Publishing Ltd, Cardiff (1975) 293.
[20] RODBARD, D., LENOX, R.H., WRAY, H.L., RAMSETH, D., Statistical characterisation of the random errors in the radioimmunoassay dose-response variables, Clin. Chem. **22** (1976) 350.
[21] Standardization of radioimmunoassay procedures, Report of an International Atomic Energy Agency panel, Int. J. Appl. Radiat. Isot. **25** (1974) 145.
[22] WORLD HEALTH ORGANIZATION, WHO Expert Committee on Biological Standardization, Twenty-sixth Report, Technical Report Series, No. 565, WHO, Geneva (1975).

DISCUSSION

A. BOSCH: We have compared tritiated estradiol and estradiol labelled via conjugation with radioiodinated histamine. In the latter case, we obtained a much more shallow standard curve and a lower sensitivity. However, applying the same procedure to a synthetic steroid, we found just the opposite. Have you also observed this phenomenon in the assay for estradiol?

The behaviour of these radioiodinated steriods is comparable with that of enzyme-labelled steroids. It is, however, possible to choose the system in such a way that a sensitive and precise assay is achieved. We can, for instance, measure testosterone by enzyme immunoassay with a sensitivity of about 30 pg/ml and an inter-assay variation coefficient of less than 10%.

S.L. JEFFCOATE: I do not think that we can generalize about the behaviour of iodo-histamine tracers in steroid radioimmunoassays. In some cases it works, in others it does not. It is a question of selecting an antiserum and a separation system in which the full benefits of radioiodine-labelled steroids can be realized. Perhaps Dr. Vitins, who I know has much experience with these tracers, would like to comment.

P. VITINS: I will first offer some remarks on the question of "flat" standard curves which are obtained when radioiodinated, as opposed to tritiated, steroid tracers are used. I suggest that this depends on the particular antiserum used. In our experience relating to estradiol and progesterone, for example, using histamine-labelled conjugates, some antisera give very good standard curves, while others do not.

As regards deterioration of assay quality with time, due to decreased tracer binding in the case of polypeptide hormones, this has not been observed in our laboratory with our ^{125}I-labelled steroid tracers. We can confirm Dr. Jeffcoate's comment that binding is stable over periods of at least 3 months; we have in fact used tracer 6 months after radioiodination. A different chemistry, so to speak, governs the decrease observed for polypeptide hormones, and we speculate that it may be due to dissociation of non-specifically bound iodine. We often find that removal of free iodine from old tracers yields a ligand which is as good as the freshly prepared material.

H. MEINHOLD: You mentioned radioiodine-labelled albumin conjugates which can be used as tracers in steroid assays. I would expect that there are also antibodies directed against the albumin part of the conjugate. Are there no interferences in the steroid assay due to binding of the tracer by these albumin-specific binding sites?

S.L. JEFFCOATE: We have looked for antibodies against albumin in our antisera and failed to find them. I think the explanation is that when the albumin molecule has been conjugated with 20–30 molecules of steroid, its structure, and particularly its surface, is quite altered and can no longer be recognized as albumin.

D. FULD: Do you find a difference in quality when you use radioiodine-labelled steroids?

S.L. JEFFCOATE: We have examined a series of quality parameters such as specificity, sensitivity (minimal detectable dose), slope of dose-response curve, and within- and between-assay precision. One cannot draw general conclusions. In some cases the assays are worse, in some others they are substantially unchanged and in still others they are improved. In the testosterone assay for example, specificity and sensitivity are better, while the precision is unchanged.

E. KUSS: I was a little puzzled by the references to the diversity of anti-estrogen-antisera affinity and specificity. Our experience (see paper SM-220/8) indicates that the pattern of cross-reactions is governed strictly by the structure of the immunodeterminant used. We found that the affinity of estrogens for bridge elements never exceeded the affinity of E_2-6-one as expressed by the inhibition potency of ^{3}H-E binding (ID_{50}). Thus, the high affinity of the histamine derivates claimed I think first by Nars and Hunter[1], could not be reproduced in our laboratory, even with lysine derivatives.

So I would like to ask whether you checked the purity of ^{125}I-histamine estrogens and whether there may be another kind of binding of ^{125}I-histamine estrogen as well as an immunochemical one exhibiting high affinity.

S.L. JEFFCOATE: The data I presented were obtained in the testosterone-3-CMO-human albumin system and we have not looked in the same detail as has Dr. Kuss at an E_2 system. The point about purity of tracers is an important one but I cannot imagine what kind of binding might be present in the system that has a higher affinity than the immunochemical one.

M. JOUSTRA: Could you please comment on the use of A-ring radio-iodinated estriol as a tracer in E_3 RIA described in a recent paper?

The use of the so-called direct RIAs of estrogens (without extraction) is based on the assumption that the antibodies used can differentiate between estrogens and their 3-sulphate and 3-glucoronide derivatives. Do you know of any laboratory that has really succeeded in raising such an antibody?

S.L. JEFFCOATE: This confirms what I said about the possibility of A-ring radioiodination of steroids. In spite of the certainty of a loss in the affinity of such label, it could still be used in the assay of E_3 in pregnancy, where high sensitivity is not required.

Many laboratories have prepared estrogen antibodies which show undetectable cross-reaction with estrogen conjugates. The problem is that these cross-reaction studies have usually not been carried out using physiological ratios of estrogen conjugate to unconjugated estrogen. This ratio is very high, of course.

---

[1] NARS, P.W., HUNTER, W.M., J. Endocrinol. **57** (1973) xlvii.

RADIOIMMUNOASSAY OF STEROIDS IN HOMOGENATES AND SUBCELLULAR FRACTIONS OF TESTICULAR TISSUE*

S. CAMPO, G. NICOLAU, E. PELLIZARI,
M.A. RIVAROLA
Centro de Investigaciones Endocrinologicas,
Hospital de Niños,
Buenos Aires, Argentina

Abstract

RADIOIMMUNOASSAY OF STEROIDS IN HOMOGENATES AND SUBCELLULAR FRACTIONS OF TESTICULAR TISSUE.

Radioimmunoassays for testosterone (T), dihydrotestosterone (DHT) and 5-α-androstan--3-α, 17-β-diol (DIOL) in homogenates of whole testis, interestitial tissue and seminiferous tubules as well as subcellular fractions of the latter were developed. Steroids were extracted with acetone, submitted to several solvent partitions and isolated by celite : propylene glycol : ethylene glycol column chromatography. Anti-T serum was used for the assay of T and DTH, and a specific anti-DIOL serum for DIOL. Subcellular fractions were separated by differential centrifugation. The nuclear fraction was purified by centrifuging in a dense sucrose buffer followed by several washings. Losses were corrected according to recovery of DNA. Optimal condition for purification of acetone extracts at minimal losses were established. Validation of the method was studied by testing linear regression of logit-log transformations of standard curves and parallelism with unknowns. T was found to be the steroid present in higher concentrations in all samples studied. It is concluded that the present method for determining endogenous androgen concentrations in testicular tissue is valid and might be useful in studying testicular function.

INTRODUCTION

The assay of steroids is usually carried out in blood serum or in urine. These measurements give information on overall production and metabolism of hormones and have been of great value in assessing glandular function. However, hormones not only need to reach peripheral organs, they also have to be concentrated and retained in target cells. In the case of steroids, they diffuse into the cell, are bound to cytoplasmic receptors and are eventually transferred into the nucleus. Therefore, determination of tissue concentrations, as well as intracellular distribution

* The work was supported by research grants from IAEA (1895/RB), PLAMIRH (57.129.2.76) and CONICET (Argentina).

of these steroids and their metabolites, will certainly be useful in understanding organ response. This is particularly true for the testis where an endocrine secreting tissue, the interstitial compartment, is intimately associated with a target organ, the seminiferous tubules. In this case, the target cells directly receive steroids synthesized by Leydig cells, i.e. without being diluted in the blood, and therefore plasma or urinary levels might not necessarily reflect tissue levels. It must also be kept in mind that dissociation between blood and tissue levels might be found for any target organ, since androgen concentrations depend not only on external supply, but also on metabolic activity, presence of specific receptors and other factors.

The measurement of endogenous tissue concentrations of steroids brings in several technical difficulties, particularly if a large sample has to be processed. They obviously vary with the particular tissue under study.

These difficulties are discussed here where a method is presented designed to assay testosterone (T), dihydrotestosterone (DHT), and 5-α-androstan-3-α, 17-β-diol (DIOL) in rat whole testis and kidney, in testicular interstitial tissue and in seminiferous tubules. In the latter, assays were also carried out in sub-cellular fractions.

MATERIALS AND METHODS

Non-radioactive steroids were purchased from Steraloids, USA and tritium-labelled steroids from New England Nuclear, USA. The specific activity for T was 85, for DHT 40 and for DIOL 40 Ci/mmole. Radioactive steroids were purified by silica-gel thin-layer chromatography before use. Antitestosterone serum, generously provided by Dr.E. Nieschlag (Düsseldorf, FRG) was used for RIA of T and DHT [1]. Antiandrostandiol serum was a gift from Dr. D.L.Loriaux (NIH, USA).

Tissue homogenization

Rats were sacrificed by cervical dislocation. Whole testis, kidney and seminiferous tubules were homogenized at 4°C, in four volumes of 50 mM Tris-HCl, 3 mM $MgCl_2$ and 0.32M sucrose buffer, using an Ultraturrax mixer. Seminiferous tubules and interstitial tissue were separated by teasing as previously described [2]. DNA was determined by the method of Fleck and Munro [3] and proteins by the method of Lowry et al. [4].

Subcellular fractionation

Homogenates, corresponding to approximately 4 g of tissue, were centrifuged at 800 × g for 10 min in a refrigerated centrifuge. Purification of the nuclear fraction was carried out as published by Calandra et al. [5]. The unpurified nuclear fraction was resuspended in a 2M sucrose buffer and spun at 60 000 × g for 60 min in a Beckman L5 65 ultracentrifuge. The pellet was washed with the 0.32M sucrose buffer containing 0.3% Triton-100 and centrifuged at 800 × g. Two additional washings were carried out with the 0.32M sucrose buffer in the absence of Triton-100. The final pellet was resuspended in 1 ml of buffer. The supernatant from the first 800 × g spin was centrifuged at 15 000 × g for 30 min to obtain the mitochondrial fraction. The supernatant was then centrifuged at 100 000 × g for 60 min to obtain the microsomal pellet and cytosol.

Extraction and preliminary purification

Samples were processed in duplicate. Radioactive tracers were added to tissue homogenates or suspensions of cellular fractions. After standing for 10 min in the cold, the steroids were extracted with 5 ml of acetone. The acetone was evaporated and the residue dissolved in 1 ml of distilled water. Acetone precipitation was omitted for cytosol fractions and washes of seminiferous tubules containing the interstitial tissue.

Samples were submitted to several solvent partitions namely, water:ether (1:10) (1:4 in the case of interstitial tissue and cytosol), 70% methanol:hexane (1:1) and 70% methanol:dichloromethane (1:4). The dichloromethane was then evaporated to dryness.

Column chromatography

Micro-glass columns were packed with celite coated with ethylene glycol and propylene in 1 ml of iso-octane. Ten millilitres of iso-octane, run under positive pressure (N_2), was discarded. DHT was eluted with 4 ml of iso-octane: toluene (70:30), T with 4 ml of iso-octane:toluene (60:40) and DIOL with 6 ml of cyclohexane:ethyl acetate (85:15). One-tenth of the sample was used for the assay and 1/4 for estimation of recovery.

Incubation

Phosphate buffer, 0.01M, pH7, with 0.1% (wt/vol.) sodium azide, 0.9% (wt/vol.) NaCl and 0.1% (wt/vol.) gelatine was used for RIA. Antibody, tracer and standards or unknowns were incubated for 15 h at 4°C in a final volume of 0.3 ml.

TABLE I. CONCENTRATIONS OF PROTEINS AND DNA IN HOMOGENATES AND SUBCELLULAR FRACTIONS OF TESTIS AND KIDNEY

Tissue	Proteins (mg/g)	DNA (mg/g)	Protein/DNA ratio
Whole testis homogenate	50.3	3.66	13.7
Interstitial tissue homogenate	17.0	0.67	25.3
Seminiferous tubules homogenate	40.1	2.68	14.9
Seminiferous tubules nuclei	5.52	–	1.62
Seminiferous tubules mitochondria	6.24	–	–
Seminiferous tubules microsomes	2.29	–	–
Seminiferous tubules cytosol	8.16	–	–
Kidney homogenate	109.5	4.50	22.0
Kidney nuclei	18.5	–	3.73
Kidney mitochondria	5.0	–	–
Kidney microsomes	3.3	–	–
Kidney cytosol	24.6	–	–

TABLE II. EXTRACTION AND PURIFICATION

	% Recovery		
	T	DHT	DIOL
Water			
Acetone extraction	84	85	84
Partitions			
H_2O : ether (1 : 10)	100	100	100
70% methanol : hexane (1 : 1)	52	52	52
70% methanol : dichlormethane (1 : 4)	95	99	82
Celite column	97	90	99
Overall recovery	41	39	36
100% methanol – Vortex – add H_2O down to 70%			
Overall recovery	60	44	71
Tissue homogenates			
Overall mean ± SD (n = 24)	35 ± 9.5	34 ± 8.8	32 ± 10.6

TABLE III. METABOLIZATION OF STEROIDS DURING EQUILIBRATION AT 37°C FOR 10 min

	Steroid added (ng)		Steroid measured (ng)	
Tissue	T	DHT	T	DHT
Mitochondria	8	8	1.9	13.3
Microsomes	8	8	2.3	16.0
Cytosol	8	8	1.0	19.0

Bound and free fractions were separated with 0.2 ml of charcoal, 1.25 g/100ml.

Calculations

Logit-log transformation of the data was carried out for evaluation of standard curves and calculation of unknowns. Linear regression was calculated after truncation [4].

RESULTS

Concentration of proteins and DNA in tissue homogenates and subcellular fractions

The concentrations of proteins and DNA in tissue homogenates and subcellular fractions in mg/g of wet tissue are shown in Table I. The amount of DNA in the two testicular compartments added up to 91% of whole testis, seminiferous tubules representing 80%. Losses of nuclei were evaluated by recovery of DNA (20 to 40%) and effectiveness of purification by proteins/DNA ratios (1.6 and 3.7 for seminiferous tubules and kidney respectively).

Evaluation of the method

Purification and recovery

The ^{3}H-tracer recovery of the purification steps was checked by using water and tissue. The recovery of isolated steps is shown in Table II. Considerable loss was found in the 70% methanol: hexane partition which was not accounted for by losses in the hexane phase. This was improved by solubilization of the

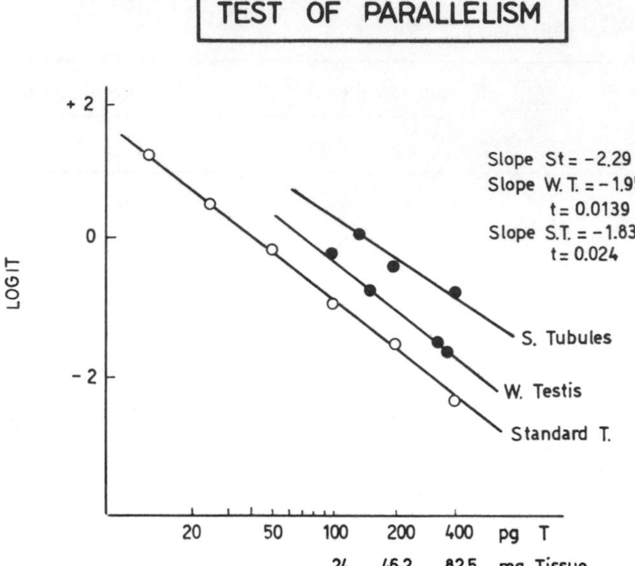

FIG.1. Test of parallelism between T contents in whole testis or seminiferous tubules and standard curve.

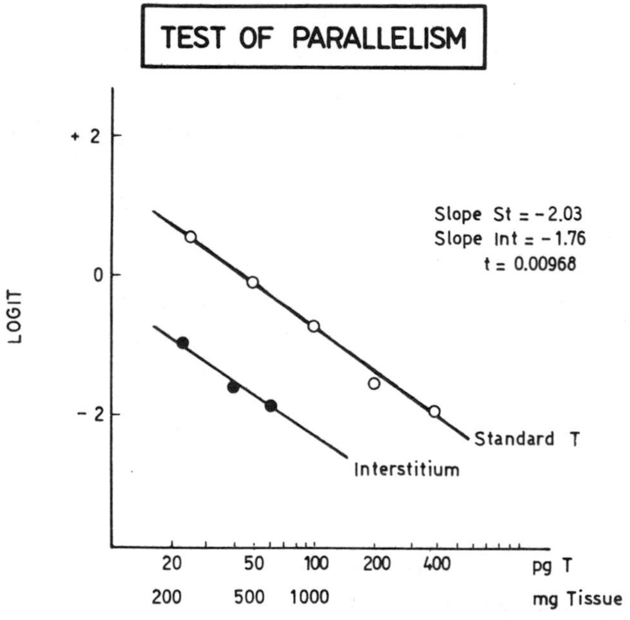

FIG.2. Test of parallelism between T contents in testicular interstitial tissue and standard curve.

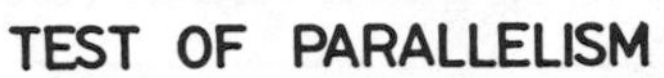

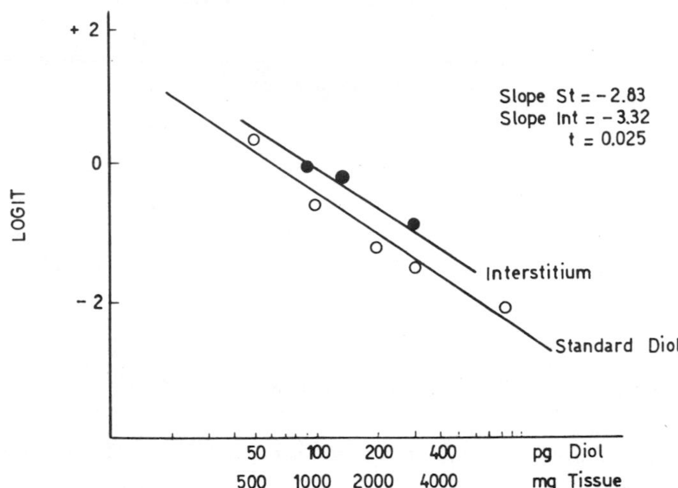

FIG.3. Test of parallelism between DIOL contents in testicular interstitial tissue and standard curve.

dried residue in 100% methanol followed by addition of water down to 70%. Recovery with tissue homogenates was lower than with water.

The mean overall recovery for the three steroids in 24 samples varied from 32 to 35%. Recovery was influenced by the amount of tissue processed and it was much lower when more than 300 mg were used.

Equilibration of tracer with endogenous steroids

Spontaneous metabolism can occur during equilibration of tracers with endogenous steroids at 37°C as evidenced by the experiment shown in Table III. T was converted to DHT during a 10-min equilibration period. This was not seen at 4°C.

Water blanks

Water blanks for DHT and DIOL were significant when 1/5 of the eluate of the column was assayed (50 and 25 pg), but undectable for T. No significant blank was observed when 1/10 of the sample was assayed.

TABLE IV. T, DHT AND DIOL CONTENTS IN TISSUE HOMOGENATES

Tissue	T	DHT (ng/g)	DIOL
Whole testis	27.1	10.1	3.24
Interstitium	4.58	0.89	1.11
Seminiferous tubules	16.4	12.3	N.D.
Kidney	1.63	N.D.	N.D.

Validation of standard curves and parallelism with unknowns

Regression analysis of standard curves for T, DHT and DIOL after logit-log linearization is shown in Figs 1, 2 and 3. Truncation of both extremes at 0.8 and 0.15 levels was employed to reduce variance at both ends. The test of parallelism for T in whole testis and in homogenates of seminiferous tubules and for T and DIOL in interstitial tissue is also shown in Figs 1, 2 and 3. In each case, no significant difference was found between the slopes for standard curves and those for tissues.

Concentrations of T, DHT and DIOL in homogenates of whole testis, seminiferous tubules, interstitial tissue and kidney of 60-day-old rats

Concentrations of the three androgens in ng/g of tissue are shown in Table IV. T was the main androgen present in all tissues. In whole testis, the T/DHT ratio was 2.7 and the T/DIOL ratio 8.4, whereas in seminiferous tubules the relative concentration of DHT was increased (ratio 1.3). The addition of the contents of seminiferous tubules and interstitial tissue amounted to a total similar to the value measured in whole testis.

Concentrations of T, DHT and DIOL in subcellular fractions of seminiferous tubules and kidney

Concentrations of the three androgens in ng/100 mg of proteins is shown in Table V. Approximately 4 g of tissue was processed for separation of subcellular fractions. For this reason, in some cases, steroids could be detected in sub-cellular fractions but not in whole tissue homogenates where only 250 mg was assayed.

TABLE V. T, DHT AND DIOL CONTENTS IN SUBCELLULAR FRACTIONS

Fraction	T	DHT	DIOL
	(ng/100 mg protein)		
Seminiferous tubules			
Nuclei	9.2	9.1	N.D.
Mitochondria	6.3	3.0	N.D.
Microsomes	43.7	36.9	10.2
Cytosol	62.6	11.1	1.3
Kidney			
Nuclei	N.D.	13.9	N.D.
Mitochondria	N.D.	N.D.	N.D.
Microsomes	2.7	N.D.	N.D.
Cytosol	0.4	0.6	N.D.

The cytosol fraction of the seminiferous tubules had the highest concentration of T while the highest values for DHT and DIOL were found in the microsomes. T and DHT were present in similar amounts in nuclei. Kidney nuclei, on the other hand, seemed to be rich in DHT.

DISCUSSION

Several technical problems arise in the determination of the concentration of steroids in tissues. A first major difficulty is the low levels usually present, particularly in target organs. Higher levels are probably present in endocrine secreting tissues but measurements might not be as informative. In the testis, we have quite a unique situation, the endocrine secreting tissue is in close association with one of its targets, the seminiferous tubules. There is some evidence that seminiferous tubules function at high endogenous androgen levels. This is an advantage from the technical point of view, the disadvantage being the difficulty in separating both testicular compartments. As judged by the relative proportions of DNA that we have determined in our compartments of seminiferous tubules and interstitial tissue, separation seemed to be satisfactory. The problem of low endogenous contents of androgens in tissues could theoretically be overcome by increasing the amount of tissue to be processed. However, in our hands there is a serious limitation to it. Increasing the amount of tissue above 250 mg resulted both in poor recovery and loss of parallelism of the assay.

In some instances, steroids could not be detected in this relatively small sample of whole-tissue homogenate, but they were assayed in subcellular fractions obtained from 4 to 5 g of tissue.

Special care should be taken in the collection and manipulation of tissue for steroid assay in order to avoid metabolism in vitro, particularly after homogenization and subsequent release of enzymes. The experiment shown in Table III is an example of this phenomenon. Samples should remain cold during manipulation and solvent extraction should be carried out as soon as possible. Whenever feasible, samples should be homogenized in an organic solvent. However, if subcellular fractions are to be obtained, this is not possible. In this case, spontaneous metabolism in vitro should be ruled out.

Extensive purification of the sample is critical for reproducible assays. Efforts were conducted to get rid of heavy tissue contaminants with minimal steroid losses. The combination of solvent partitions and celite column chromatography gave satisfactory recovery (Table II) and adequate blanks. The test for parallelism of regression between standard curves and unknowns was taken as evidence for absence of interferences in the assays. Tissues were gently homogenized in four volumes of an isotonic buffer before subcellular fractionation. It is accepted that steroids act directly inside the nucleus and, therefore, determination of intranuclear concentrations of androgens was of interest. Several techniques were tried to purify the nuclear fraction, using the protein/DNA ratio as a parameter of purification. With the technique described, we obtained a satisfactory ratio with a recovery of approximately 20 to 40%. Intranuclear contents of androgens were calculated correcting for these losses.

T, DHT and DIOL could be measured in whole-testis homogenate. T and DHT were present in seminiferous tubules in approximately equal concentrations while the relative proportion of DHT was much lower in the interstitial tissue, probably because the reduced androgen is retained in the target tissue. A similar DHT/T ratio was found in the nuclear fraction of seminiferous tubules suggesting that the two androgens might be active in this tissue. Microsomes seem to have high concentrations of androgens, the significance of this finding is not known.

It is concluded that we have developed an assay for the determination of T, DHT and DIOL in whole-tissue homogenates and subcellular fractions of testis that will be useful in the study of testicular function.

ACKNOWLEDGEMENTS

The assistance of Miss S. Malkischer and Mr. R. Bianchi in the statistical evaluation of the data is greatly appreciated.

REFERENCES

[1] NIESCHLAG, E., LORIAUX, D.L., Radioimmunoassay for plasma testosterone, Z. klin. Chem. u. klin. Biochem. **4** (1972) 164.

[2] RIVAROLA, M.A., PODESTA, E.J., Metabolism of testosterone-^{14}C by seminiferous tubules of mature rats: formation of androstandiol-^{14}C, Endocrinology **90** (1972) 618.

[3] FLECK, A., MUNRO, H.N., The precision of ultraviolet absorption measurements in the Schmidt-Thannhauser procedure for nucleic acid estimation, Biochem. Biophys. Acta **55** (1962) 571.

[4] LOWRY, D., ROSENBROUGH, M., LEWIS-FARR, A., RANDAL, R., Protein measurement with the Folin phenol reagent, J. Biol. Chem. **193** (1951) 265.

[5] CALANDRA, R.S., PURVIS, K., HANSSON, V., Appendix IX, Measurement of specific androgen binding protein, In: Techniques of Human Andrology (HAFEZ, E.S.E., Ed.), Elsevier/North-Holland Biochemical Press, Amsterdam (1977).

[6] RODBARD, D., HUTT, D.M., "Statistical analysis of radioimmunoassays and immunoradiometric (labelled antibody) assays: a generalized, weighted, iterative, least-squares method for logistic curve fitting", Radioimmunoassay and Related Procedures in Medicine (Proc. Symp. Istanbul, 1973) **1**, IAEA, Vienna (1974) 165.

DISCUSSION

G.F. READ: Have you obtained any data for DIOL levels in human tissue or do all your results relate to the rat? It would, for example, be interesting to know tissue levels in benign prostatic hyperthropy.

M.A. RIVAROLA: Our data refer only to the rat.

R. VIHKO: We performed a comparable study some years ago[1] but using gas-liquid chromatography and gas chromatography-mass spectrometry. Steroid concentrations were determined from total homogenate and seminiferous tubules, and interstitial cells were separated by the Christensen technique[2]. We found that the highest concentration of testosterone was in the interstitial cells. On the other hand, your recovery for testosterone seems to be low, which you ascribe to the effect of 5α-reductase. Don't you think that there could be a methodological reason for the discrepancy?

M.A. RIVAROLA: It is true that the endogenous contents in interstitial tissue are lower than in the seminiferous tubules in these rats when the values are expressed in ng/g of whole testis. This cannot be attributed to conversion

---

[1] RUOKONEN, A., VIHKO, R., NIEMI, M., Steroid metabolism in testis tissue. Concentrations of testosterone, pregnenolone and 5-androst-16-en-3ol in normal and cryptorchid rat testis and in isolated interstitial and tubular tissue, FEBS Lett. **31** (1973) 321.

[2] CHRISTENSEN, A.K., MASON, N.R., Comparative ability of seminiferous tubules and interstitial tissue of rat testes to synthesize androgens from progesterone-4-^{14}C in vitro, Endocrinology **76** (1965) 646.

to 5α-reduced products during manipulation because (a) we checked this possibility and (b) the values of DHT and DIOL were much lower. It is difficult to prove or disprove that the difference is due to methodological artefacts.

H. BREUER: Why did you use acetone to extract steroids from tissue? It is well known, for instance, that ether-chloroform mixtures yield better results. Furthermore, in some of your experiments the recovery was much more than 100%. Did you arrive at these figures by calculation?

M.A. RIVAROLA: Acetone was preferred in order to ensure extraction of steroids from subcellular particles.

In one case, in the experiment designed to show that metabolism of androgens can take place during manipulation, we appeared to recover 120% of steroids added to samples. This was probably an error of the method.

SENCILLO METODO DE DOSIFICACION DE PROTEINA TRANSPORTADORA DE HORMONAS SEXUALES (PTHS) – SUS VALORES EN HOMBRES, EN MUJERES Y EN EL EMBARAZO

C.A. TAFURT, R. de ESTRADA
Hospital Militar Central,
Servicio de Endocrinología,
Bogotá, Colombia

Abstract–Resumen

A SIMPLE METHOD FOR MEASURING SEX-HORMONE BINDING PROTEIN (SHBP) – TYPICAL VALUES IN MEN AND WOMEN AND IN PREGNANT WOMEN.

Assuming that the binding forces between steroid hormones and their binding proteins are similar to those between antigens and their antibodies, the authors describe how to determine SHBP activity by a dilution method analogous to that used for titration of antisera in radioimmunoassay. The method consists of the following stages: (1) plasma dilution; (2) incubation of the dilution with 20 000 dis/min of 1, 2-^{3}H-testosterone; (3) separation of the fraction of tracer bound to the SHBP by precipitation with ammonium sulphate; (4) centrifugation and measurement of the supernatant; and (5) plotting of the results on a graph where the axis of ordinates represents the quotient given by bound steroid over free steroid (U/L) and the abscissa represents the plasma dilutions. The values are expressed as the 50% bound titre. An advantage of the method is the higher sensitivity of the dilution curves in the steepest part where the 50% bound is encountered; it is thus not necessary to use the saturation part of the curves where sensitivity is lost owing to the steeper slope. A further advantage of the method is that there is no need for costly processes such as dialysis. The SHBP values obtained for healthy subjects were as follows: 1/5 for men, 1/93 for women, and 1/360 in pregnant women. These physiological values showed no overlapping.

SENCILLO METODO DE DOSIFICACION DE PROTEINA TRANSPORTADORA DE HORMONAS SEXUALES (PTHS) – SUS VALORES EN HOMBRES, EN MUJERES Y EN EL EMBARAZO.

Partiendo de la base de que las fuerzas de unión entre las hormonas esteroides y sus proteínas transportadoras son similares a las que ocurren entre los antígenos y sus anticuerpos, se describe en este trabajo la determinación de la actividad de PTHS por un método de dilución análogo al de la titulación de antisueros para radioinmunoanálisis. El método consta de las etapas siguientes: 1) dilución del plasma; 2) incubación de las diluciones con 20 000 des/min de 1, 2-^{3}H-testosterona; 3) separación de la fracción del trazador ligada a la PTHS por precipitación con sulfato de amonio; 4) centrifugación y medición del sobrenadante; 5) Graficación de los resultados en un sistema donde la ordenada representa la fracción esteroide unido sobre esteroide libre (U/L) y la abscisa las diluciones del plasma. Los valores se expresan como el título al 50% de enlace. El método ofrece la mayor sensibilidad que presentan las curvas de dilución en su zona más pendiente, donde se encuentra el 50% de enlace, evitando así el uso de la zona de saturación de las mismas, donde por razones de mayor pendiente se pierde la sensibilidad. El método omite también procedimientos dispendiosos como el de diálisis. Los valores obtenidos de PTHS en sujetos sanos fueron los siguientes: 1/5 para hombres, 1/93 para mujeres y 1/360 en el embarazo. Estos valores fisiológicos no presentaron ningún grado de entrecruzamiento.

INTRODUCCION

La PTHS fue descubierta por Daughaday en 1958 [1]. Es una beta globulina [2] que tiene capacidad de ligar andrógenos y estrógenos [3, 4].

Los métodos usuales para dosificar la PTHS se basan en procedimientos de saturación de la proteína con esteroides sexuales y separación del esteroide libre del ligado por sistemas cromatográficos, electroforéticos o de diálisis de equilibrio [5, 6]. Los valores obtenidos por Rivarola y col. [7], expresados en porcentaje de unión de testosterona a la globulina usando un método de diálisis, son: en hombres 92,8 ± 1,6%; en mujeres 95,1 ± 1,2%; en el embarazo 99,0 ± 0,2%. Los niveles de PTHS encontrados más recientemente por Corvol y col. [5] expresados como microgramos de testosterona necesarios para la saturación de la proteína existente en 100 ml de plasma son: para hombres 0,49 ± 0,04 μg; para mujeres 1,42 ± 0,22 μg y para el embarazo 10,91 ± 0,74 μg.

En base al hecho de que las fuerzas de enlace entre los esteroides y sus proteínas transportadoras son similares a las que ocurren entre los antígenos y sus anticuerpos, fuerzas de Van der Waals y otros tipos de enlaces débiles no covalentes, nos propusimos determinar la actividad de la PTHS por un método de dilución análogo al de titulación de antisueros para uso en radioinmunoanálisis.

En el presente trabajo se describe el método y se presentan los resultados obtenidos en plasmas de 10 hombres, 10 mujeres y 26 embarazadas, todos sujetos normales.

REACTIVOS

Se empleó como reactivos 1,2-^{3}H-testosterona obtenida de la New England Nuclear, actividad especifica 43,5 Ci/mM, en solución alcohólica, de tal manera que 100 μl contengan 20 000 des/min; sulfato de amonio p.a. Merck, Darmstadt, solución saturada; solución centelladora: 4 g de 2,5-difeniloxasol, Sigma; 0,04 g de 1,4-bis-2-(4-metil-5-feniloxasoil)-benceno, Packard; 20 ml de etanol, E. Merck, y tolueno hasta completar 1000 ml.

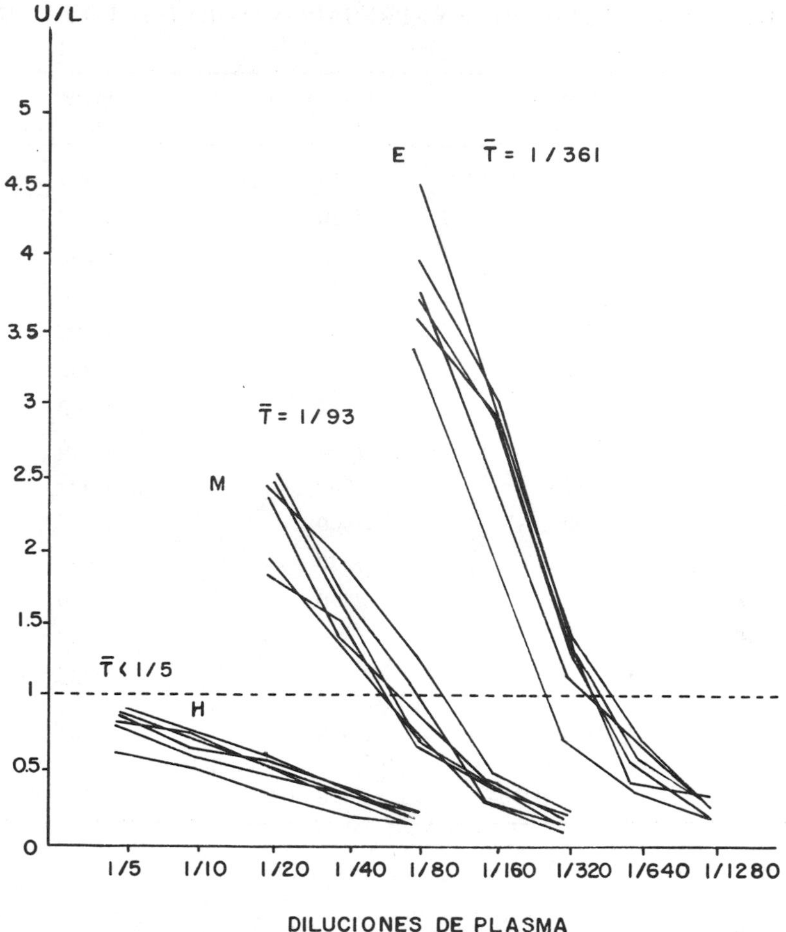

FIG.1. Curvas de titulación de PTHS en plasma de 6 hombres (H), 6 mujeres (M) y 6 embarazadas (E), con sus respectivos títulos promedio al 50% de enlace $\overline{T}$ (U/L = 1).

METODO

En tubos de vidrio de 12 mm × 75 mm se evaporaron 100 μl de la solución de testosterona tritiada. Se agregó a los residuos 0,5 ml de las diluciones de plasma en solución salina, que se efectuaron de la siguiente manera: 1/5, 1/10, 1/20, 1/40, 1/80 para hombres; 1/25, 1/50, 1/100, 1/200, 1/400 para mujeres; 1/100, 1/200, 1/400, 1/800, 1/1600 en el embarazo. Los plasmas maternos fueron tomados en el momento del parto. Los tubos se dejaron en incubación a temperatura ambiente por una hora. Luego se efectuó la separación del esteroide libre

CUADRO I. VALORES DE PTHS EXPRESADOS COMO TITULO AL 50%

Hombres (n = 10)	Mujeres (n = 10)	Embarazos (n = 12) ♂	Embarazos (n = 14) ♀
<1/10	1/110	1/210	1/390
<1/5	1/95	1/330	1/360
<1/5	1/80	1/400	1/330
<1/5	1/115	1/456	1/380
<1/5	1/90	1/536	1/360
<1/5	1/85	1/520	1/352
<1/5	1/85	1/330	1/340
<1/5	1/90	1/400	1/300
<1/5	1/100	1/360	1/435
<1/5	1/90	1/400	1/400
		1/270	1/640
		1/370	1/340
			1/360
			1/335
$\overline{X}$ = <1/5	1/93	1/358	1/368
Rango:	1/83–1/104	1/278–1/502	1/319–1/434

del ligado a la PTHS por precipitación de este último con 0,5 ml de la solución de sulfato de amonio. Se centrifugó a 3000 rev/min durante 15 min a 4°C. Se decantaron los sobrenadantes en frascos de centelleo que contenían 5 ml de solución centelladora, los cuales se midieron en un contador beta, Beckman SL 3100.

Los datos obtenidos se llevaron a un sistema de coordenadas donde la ordenada representa la fracción (U/L) del esteroide unido (U) sobre el esteroide libre (L) como función de las diluciones del plasma (fig. 1). El empleo de la fracción U/L en lugar del porcentaje de enlace, como es usual en la titulación de antisueros, presenta la ventaja de que las curvas de dilución tienden a linearizarse. Como título de actividad se tomó la dilución del plasma que ligó el 50% del trazador o sea la fracción U/L = 1.

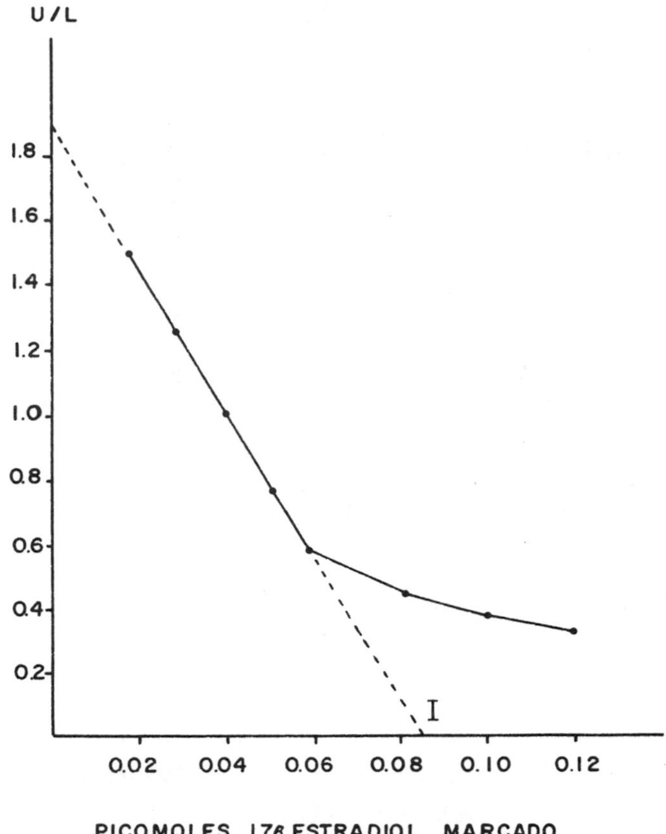

FIG.2. Curva de Scatchard efectuada con citosoles de conejo.

RESULTADOS

La figura 1 representa las curvas de titulación obtenidas en plasmas de 6 hombres, 6 mujeres y 6 embarazadas y el cuadro I muestra los títulos al 50% de unión del trazador en plasmas de 10 hombres, 10 mujeres, 12 embarazadas con feto masculino y 14 embarazadas con feto femenino.

CONCLUSIONES

El método descrito para dosificar la actividad de PTHS es práctico y económico y permite diferenciar ampliamente y sin entrecruzamientos los

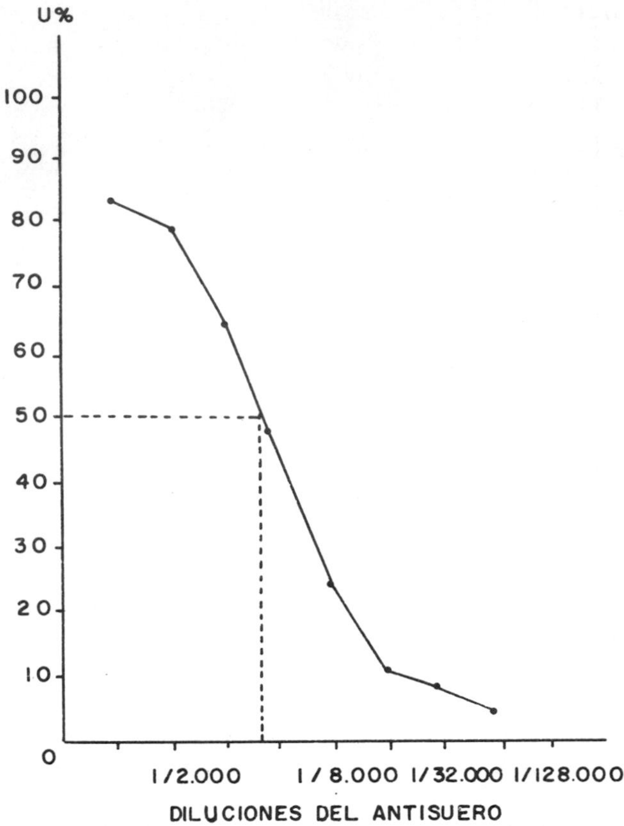

FIG.3. Titulación de un suero antitestosterona.

niveles de esta globulina en hombres, mujeres y en el embarazo con títulos promedio de $< 1/5$, 1/93 para hombres y para mujeres, respectivamente. En el embarazo estos valores fueron de 1/358 para embarazadas con feto masculino y 1/368 para embarazadas con feto femenino; la diferencia de los títulos en el embarazo con relación al sexo del feto no fue significativa al nivel del 5% ($\alpha = 0{,}05$).

Los métodos usuales de determinación de PTHS por medio de su saturación con esteroides sexuales presentan el inconveniente de emplear una región de muy poca sensibilidad, como se aprecia en la curva de Scatchard (fig. 2), que representa una curva de saturación de citosoles de útero de coneja con estradiol tritiado. En esta figura se evidencia claramente cómo el proceso de saturación nunca es completo, teniendo que determinarse el punto de saturación de los sitios de enlace, por extrapolación de la curva en la intersección I con el eje de la abscisa.

En cambio, el método de dilución propuesto en este trabajo emplea la zona más pendiente de la curva de saturación, y por lo tanto más sensible, como se aprecia en la figura 3, que representa la titulación de un suero antitestosterona destacando el punto del 50% de enlace del trazador.

La simplicidad del método propuesto lo hace ampliamente aplicable en el trabajo de rutina y de investigación.

REFERENCIAS

[1] DAUGHADAY, W.H., J. Clin. Invest. **37** (1958) 511.
[2] ROSEMBAUM, S., CHRISTY, N.P., KELLY, W.G., J. Clin. Endocrinol. Metab. **26** (1966) 1399.
[3] MERCIER-BODARD, C., BAULIEY, E.E., C.R. Hebd. Acad. Sci. Paris **267** (1968) 804.
[4] STENO, O., HEYNS, W., VAN BAELEN, H., DE MOOR, P., Ann. Endocrinol. (Suppl.) **29** (1968) 141.
[5] CORVOL, P., CHRAMBACK, A., RODBARD, D., BARDIN, C.W., J. Biol. Chem. **246** (1971) 3435.
[6] VERMEULEN, A., VERDONCK, L., Steroids **11** (1968) 609.
[7] RIVAROLA, M., FOREST, M., MIGEON, C., J. Clin. Endocrinol. Metab. **28** (1968) 34.

DISCUSSION

D. FULD: The sensitivity of your system must depend on the specific activity of your tracer. How do you normalize your results when changing the tracer? Also, do you measure the binding only with SHBG or with SHBG + albumin?

C.A. TAFURT: We use only ^{3}H-testosterone as tracer and add a constant 20 000 dis/min to each tube.

At low titres, as in males, albumin can interfere as a non-specific ligand but at 50% binding titre, as in females and in pregnancy, this interference is negligible owing to the high affinity of PTHS for testosterone.

S. SCHWARZ: May I enquire why you did not use ^{3}H-5α-dihydrotestosterone in your binding studies?

C.A. TAFURT: We have been using ^{3}H-testosterone from the beginning, and since the results were good we did not try ^{3}H-5α-dihydrotestosterone. This compound could be better because of higher affinity.

S. SCHWARZ: Did you measure the sex hormone binding globulin concentration at the beginning or at the end of pregnancy?

C.A. TAFURT: The samples were taken at the time of labour.

A MODEL FOR EVALUATING STEROIDS ACTING AT THE HYPOTHALAMUS-PITUITARY AXIS USING RADIOIMMUNOASSAY AND RELATED PROCEDURES*

J. SPONA, Ch. BIEGLMAYER, R. SCHROEDER, E. PÖCKL

I. Universitäts-Frauenklinik für Geburtshilfe und Gynäkologie, Universität Wien, Vienna, Austria

Abstract

A MODEL FOR EVALUATING STEROIDS ACTING AT THE HYPOTHALAMUS-PITUITARY AXIS USING RADIOIMMUNOASSAY AND RELATED PROCEDURES.

The relative affinity constants for binding of estrone (E_1), estriol (E_3), 17β-estradiol (E_2) and 17α-ethinyl-17β-estradiol (EE_2) to cytosol estrogen-receptors of rat hypothalamus and pituitary were estimated by a radioligand-receptor assay procedure. The relative affinity constants in the hypothalamic system were 6.5×10^{-10} M for E_2, 1×10^{-9} M for EE_2 and 2×10^{-8} M for E_1 and E_3. The affinity constants were 1×10^{-9} M for E_2 and E_3 and 7×10^{-9} M for E_1 and E_3 when pituitary cytosol samples were used. Some discrepancies between biological activity and affinity for the estrogen-receptor were noted. These may be due to differences in the metabolism and cellular uptake of the estrogens. The radioligand-receptor assay procedure may be useful in evaluating the action of estrogens and anti-estrogens acting at the hypothalamic and pituitary level. Sedimentation patterns of cytosol samples labelled with the estrogens used in this study revealed, upon ultracentrifugation, protein moieties sedimenting in the 8 S region. The potency of progesterone and D-Norgestrel to modulate the release of LH and FSH stimulated by luteinizing hormone-releasing hormone (LH-RH) in castrated female rats was found to correlate well with the biological activity of the progestogens. It is concluded that the radioligand-receptor assay procedure for estrogens and the in-vivo model for the evaluation of the central action of progestogens may be valuable tools for testing new steroids to be used in oral contraceptives.

Previously, we and others have shown that the release of gonadotrophins stimulated by luteinizing hormone-releasing hormone (LH-RH) is modulated by sex steroids. This effect was observed in vivo as well as in vitro. Progesterone (P) was found to suppress the response to threshold doses of LH-RH in diestrous rats [1] and in estrous rabbits [2]. In contrast, 17β-estradiol (E_2) enhances the

* This work is part of a co-ordinated program of research under the sponsorship of the IAEA, Research Agreement No. 1357/CF.

response to LH-RH in diestrous rats [3,4] and in ewes [5]. Similarly, different responses to LH-RH were recorded in the female during the menstrual cycle [6]. In addition, changes in the pituitary sensitivity to LH-RH of female and male rats in vitro were reported recently [7–10]. These previous observations, when considered as a whole, suggest that the gonadotrophin release is at least partly controlled by sex steroids at the pituitary level. Subsequently, the interaction of LH-RH with its pituitary receptor was studied [11]. The results of these investigations indicated that sex steroids influence LH-RH receptor interaction [12] and provided a basis for understanding how steroid hormones could affect the relative ratio of follicle stimulating hormone (FSH) and luteinizing hormone (LH) being secreted.

On the basis of these findings we became interested in how 17β-estradiol could be involved in the maturation of the hypothalamus-pituitary axis and studied the ontogeny of estrogen-binding protein in the hypothalamus and anterior pituitary of female [13] and male [14] rats. Additionally, we studied the estrogen-stimulated translocation of the E_2 receptor complex from the cytosol to the nucleus [15] to get more information on the molecular mechanisms involved in the action of E_2 at the pituitary level. The results of these studies suggested that the nuclear translocation process was one of the primary steps involved in the modulatory functions of estrogen.

The aim of the present investigation was to study the interaction of E_2 with its hypothalamic and pituitary cytosol receptors in more detail, and to work out a radioligand-receptor assay procedure by which estrogens with different biological potencies may be tested. Furthermore, an in-vivo model was designed that could be used to correlate the biological activity of progestogens with their potency to modulate the release of gonadotrophins stimulated by LH-RH.

MATERIALS AND METHODS

Female rats of the Sprague Dawley strain (Him: OFA (SD) SPF, Forschungsinstitut für Versuchstierzucht, University of Vienna, Austria) weighing 180–200 g were used throughout the investigation. The animals were housed in a temperature-controlled room that was illuminated 12 h a day and they had unrestricted access to food and water. For the in-vitro experiments, animals were killed by decapitation. The hypothalami and pituitaries were excised and placed in chilled TMK-buffer (0.01M Tris, 0.0015M $MgCl_2$, 0.01M KCl, pH7.2). The posterior lobes of the pituitaries were removed and discarded. All further procedures were done at 0–4°C. Six glands per ml of TMK-buffer were homogenized by 10 strokes at 500 rev./min in a glass-Teflon Potter Elvehjem-type homogenizer. The homogenate was centrifuged at 110 000 × g (av.) for 60 min to obtain the cytosol fraction. The radioligand-receptor assays performed essentially as described previously for binding assays of the cytosol preparations [13]. Briefly, 0.4-ml cytosol samples were incubated in quadruplicate with unlabelled steroids at concentrations ranging from 1×10^{-10} M to 2×10^{-5} M in the presence of either 1nM ^{3}H-E_2 (specific activity 40 Ci/mmole, The Radiochemical Centre, Amersham, UK) or 1nM 17α-ethinyl-17β-estradiol (specific activity 41 Ci/mmole, New England Nuclear, Dreieichenhain, FRG). After incubation overnight, 0.2 ml of a charcoal suspension (0.6% charcoal Norit-A, 0.06% Dextrane T-70, 0.1% gelatine, 0.1M phosphate buffer, pH7.4) was added. The incubation mixture was centrifuged and the radioactivity of the supernatant was determined. Relative apparent affinity constants were calculated at a 50% displacement level.

Analysis of the sedimentation behaviour of the estrogen-binding proteins was carried out according to procedures described previously [13]. In brief, 0.3-ml aliquots of cytosol samples were incubated with ^{3}H-labelled steroids at a concentration of 2×10^{-9} M in the absence or presence of a 1000-fold excess of unlabelled steroids. After 30 min the incubation mixture was layered on a 5–22% linear sucrose gradient prepared with a TE-buffer (0.01M Tris, 0.015M EDTA, pH7.4) in polyallomere tubes. Centrifugation was done in an SW 65 rotor at 145 000 × g (av.) for 18 h (Beckman Spinco LS 2-65 B). Density-gradient fractionation was performed by puncturing the bottoms of the centrifuge tubes in a Beckman Fraction Recovery System. The effluents were collected manually, and sedimentation coefficients were determined by methods reported previously [16].

In-vivo experiments on rats to test the potency of progestogens in modulating gonadotrophin release stimulated by LH-RH were carried out commencing 7 days after ovariectomy. Groups of 20 rats were injected subcutaneously daily for 7 days with 1, 3 or 10 mg of P or 3, 30 or 300 μg of D-Norgestrel (D-Nor), respectively, dissolved in a mixture of 5% benzylbenzoate and 95% castor-oil. Control groups were injected with the solvent containing no steroids. Twenty-four hours after the final injection, 200 ng of LH-RH was injected interperitoneally in 0.1 ml of physiological saline. The animals were anaesthetized with Ketalar (Parke, Davis, Detroit, USA) 15 min later. Blood samples were taken by heart puncture 30 min after the LH-RH injection. After clotting of the blood, serum samples were obtained by centrifugation and then stored frozen at –25°C until required for gonadotrophin estimations. The serum samples were assayed for LH and FSH by radioimmunoassay. Iodination was carried out with 2 mCi of ^{125}I and 2.5 μg of either LH (NIAMD-Rat LH-I-3) or FSH (NIAMD-Rat FSH-I-3) as described in Refs [17] and [18]. The labelled hormones were purified on cellulose columns [19]. 0.4 ml of each of the unknown samples and the standard solutions of either FSH (NIAMD-Rat FSH-RP-1, 6.25–400 ng) or LH (NIAMD-Rat LH-RP-1, 0.55–400 ng) were incubated with 0.1-ml diluted antiserum (NIAMD-Anti-Rat FSHS-7 at 1 : 800) at 37°C for 24 h. Then 1 ml of sheep anti-rabbit γ-globulin

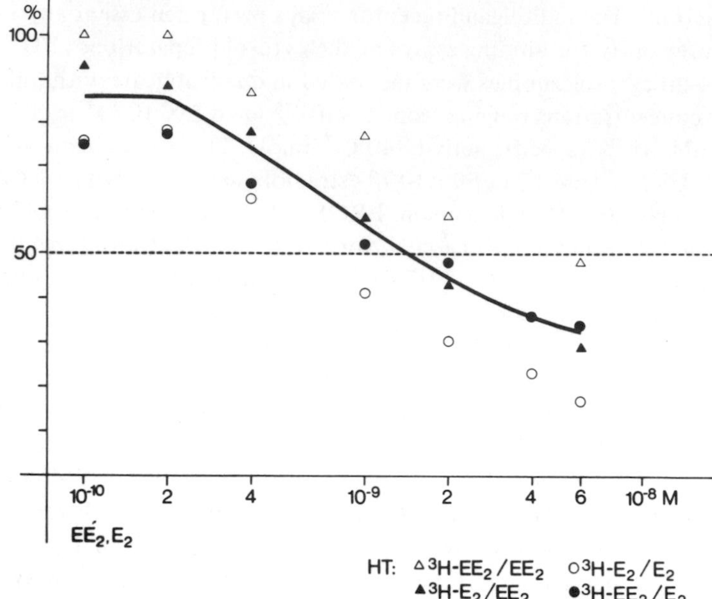

FIG.1. Standard curves of radioligand-receptor assay of E_2 and EE_2 using hypothalamic cytosol samples.

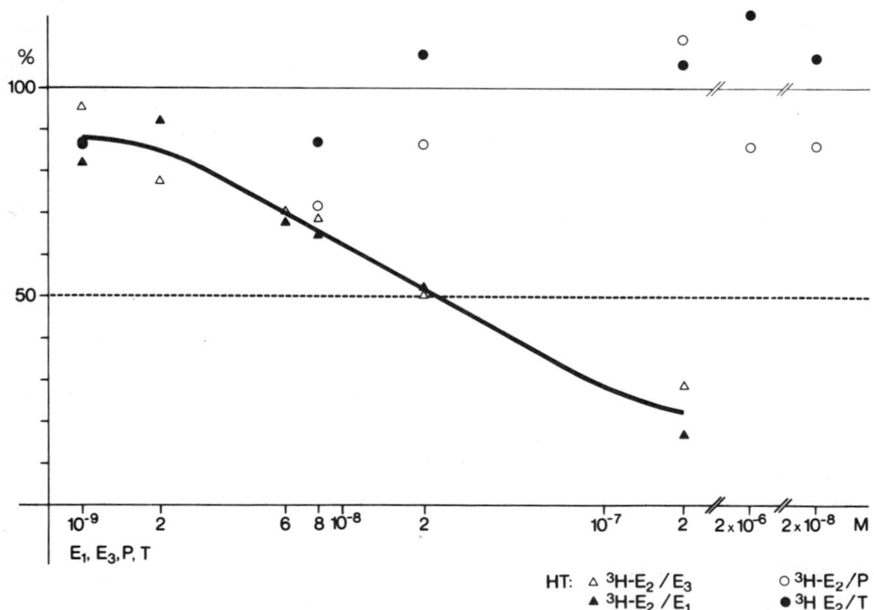

FIG.2. Displacement of ^3H-E_2 from hypothalamic cytosol receptor sites by E_1, E_3, P and T.

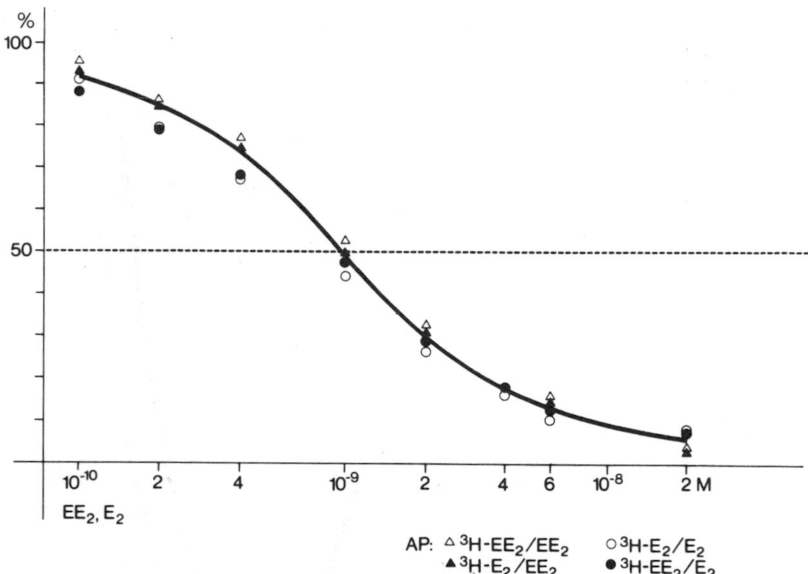

FIG.3. Standard curves of radioligand-receptor assay of E_2 and EE_2 using anterior pituitary cytosol samples.

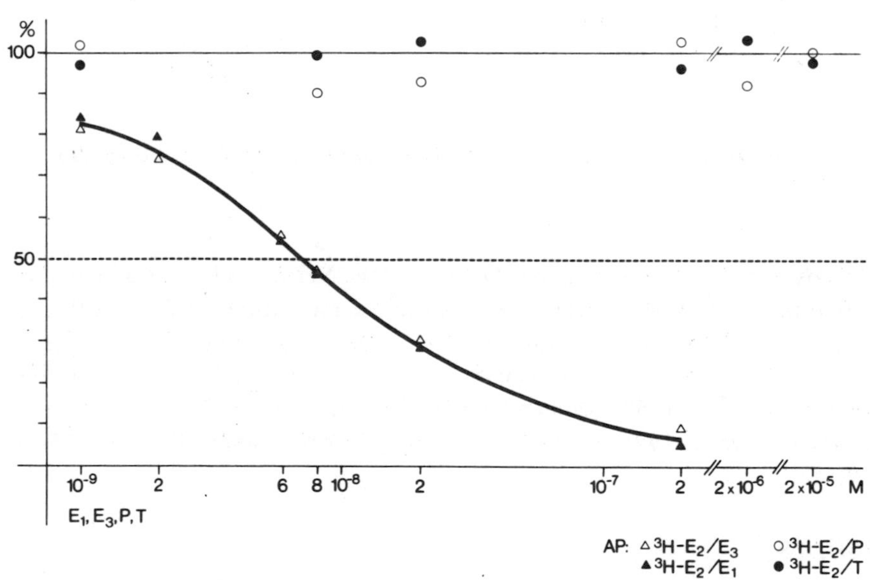

FIG.4. Displacement of ^3H-E_2 from anterior pituitary cytosol receptor sites by E_1, E_3, P and T.

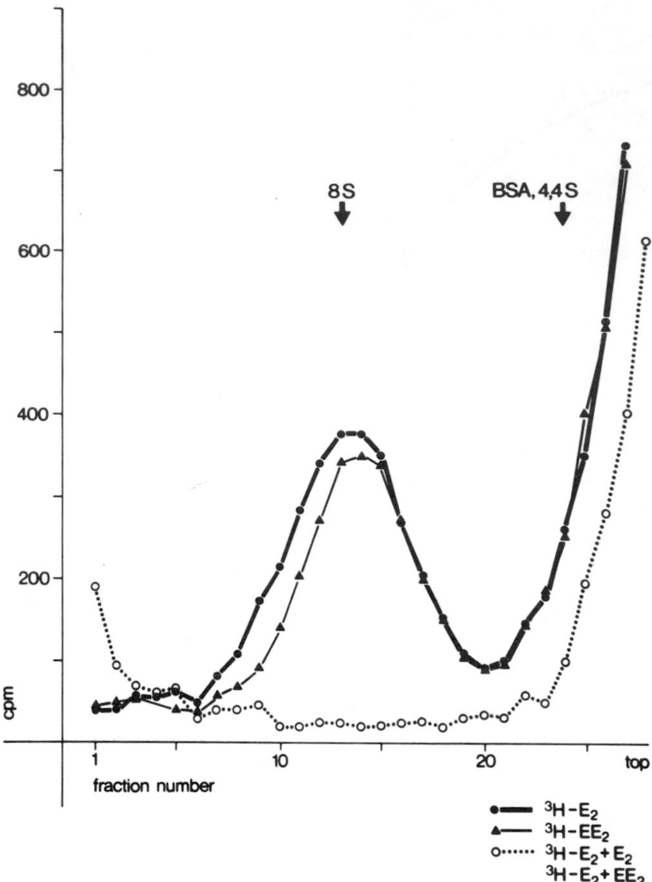

FIG.5. Sedimentation patterns of anterior pituitary cytosol samples labelled with ^3H-E_2 and ^3H-EE_2.

immunosorbent (DASP anti-rabbit, Organon, Oss, Netherlands) was added at a 1 : 10 dilution. The tubes were shaken at room temperature for 2 h and then centrifuged. The supernatant was removed by aspiration. Radioactivity was measured in a Packard Auto-Gamma-Spectrometer, model 5219. The counting efficiency was 57% at 50% gain and a window setting of 70–300. The radioimmunoassay results were evaluated by a computer program [20] on a PDP-8/e computer.

RESULTS

The radioligand-receptor assays that were performed with hypothalamic cytosol samples revealed that significant displacement of ^{3}H-E_2 by the unlabelled

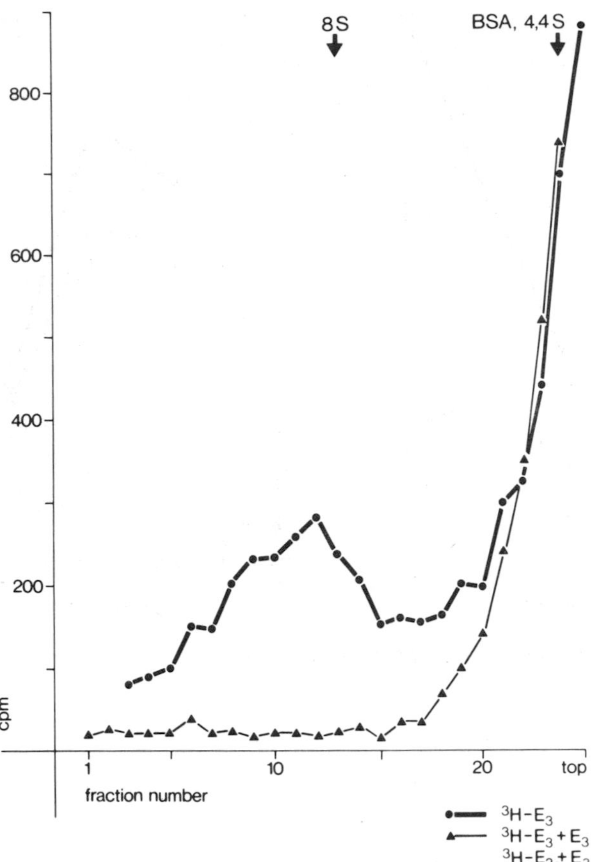

FIG.6. Sedimentation patterns of anterior pituitary cytosol samples labelled with ^3H-E_3 and ^3H-E_2.

hormone occurred at a concentration of 2 to 4 $\times$ 10^{-10} M; a relative affinity constant for the binding protein of 6.5 $\times$ 10^{-10} M was estimated from the displacement curve (Fig.1). Similarly, 17α-ethinyl-17β-estradiol (EE_2) gave significant displacement in a homologous system at a concentration of 4 $\times$ 10^{-10} M, the estimated relative affinity constant being 5 $\times$ 10^{-9} M (Fig.1). The two displacement curves in the homologous systems were found to be parallel. Displacement curves for ^{3}H-E_2 and unlabelled EE_2 and for ^{3}H-EE_2 and unlabelled E_2 were found to be essentially identical (Fig.1), the estimated relative affinity constants being 1 $\times$ 10^{-9} M.

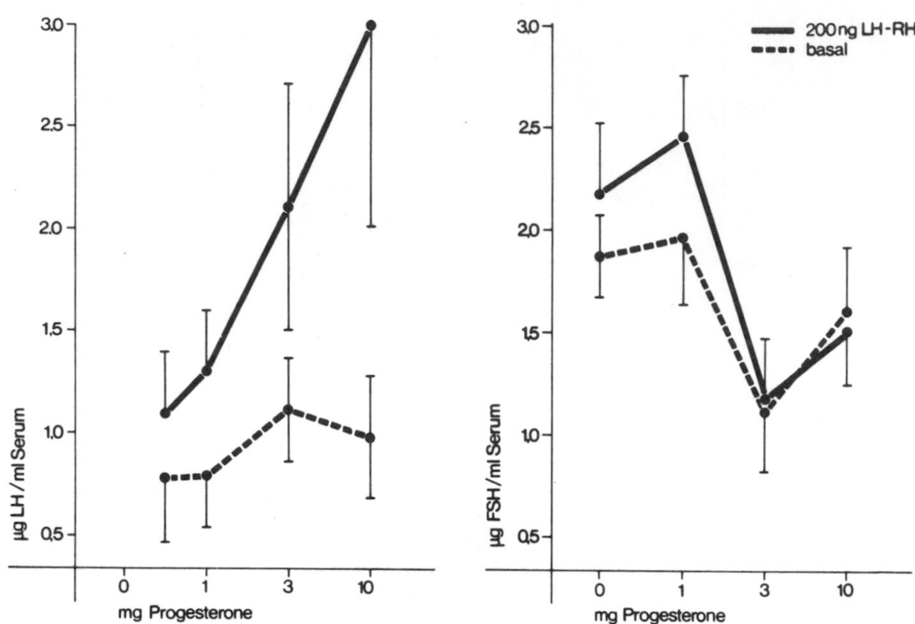

FIG. 7. Basal and LH-RH-stimulated LH and FSH release in female rats treated with progesterone 7 days after ovariectomy.

Identical displacement curves were again found when ^{3}H-E_2 was used as tracer and either unlabelled estrone (E_1) or estriol (E_3) were used as standards (Fig.2): relative affinity constants of 2×10^{-8} M were estimated. P and T did not compete for estrogen-binding sites in the hypothalamic cytosol samples.

Binding of tracer at zero concentration of standard was 10-times greater with pituitary cytosol samples than with those derived from hypothalamic tissue. The sensitivity of radioligand-receptor assays with pituitary cytosol samples was found to be between 1 and 2×10^{-10} M for E_2 and EE_2 (Fig.3). Essentially identical displacement curves were recorded when ^{3}H-E_2 and ^{3}H-EE_2 were used as tracers and when the same unlabelled hormones were used as standards in homologous and heterologous systems (Fig.3). Relative affinity constants of 1×10^{-9} M were estimated for these systems. Again, identical displacement curves were obtained when ^{3}H-E_2 was used as tracer and E_1 and E_3 were used as standards. Relative affinity constants of 7×10^{-9} M were estimated for these interactions (Fig.4). In addition, P and T at concentrations up to 2×10^{-5} M did not compete for binding sites at the estrogen receptor.

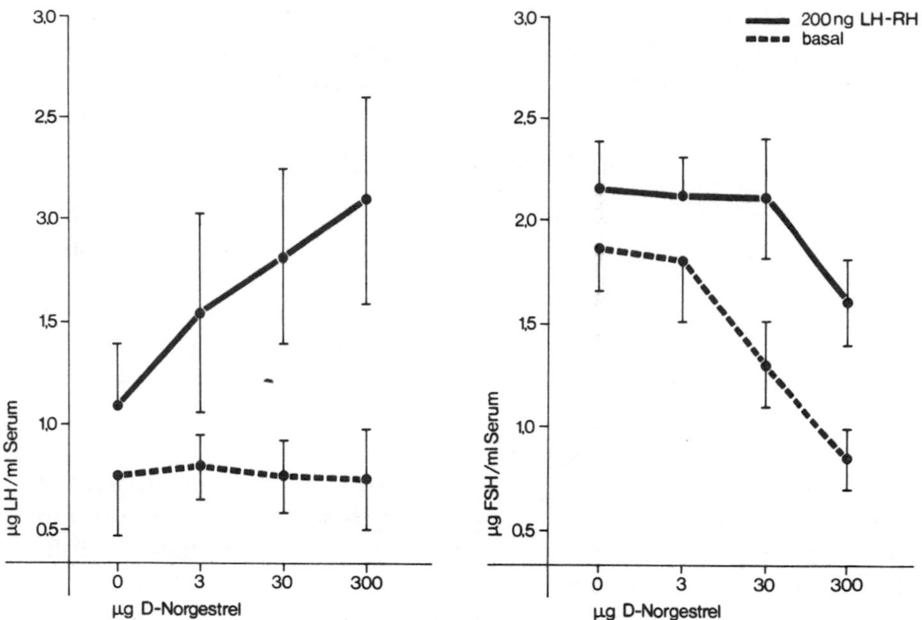

FIG.8. Basal and LH-RH-stimulated LH and FSH release in female rats treated with D-Norgestrel 7 days after ovariectomy.

Similar sedimentation patterns were registered for pituitary cytosol samples that were labelled with ^{3}H-E$_2$, ^{3}H-E$_3$ or ^{3}H-EE$_2$, and a protein moiety sedimenting in the 8 S region was recorded for the estrogens (Figs 5 and 6). No radioactive peak was found in the presence of a 1000 -fold excess of unlabelled material. Similar results were recorded for E$_1$ (data not shown). In contrast, no binding of P, T and 17,21-dimethyl-19-nor-4,9-pregnadiene-3,20-dione-6,7 (R 5020) by cytosol samples was found upon gradient analysis.

The in-vivo administration of LH-RH to castrated female rats resulted in a small, but significant, rise of both LH and FSH serum levels (Figs 7 and 8). Administration of P did not alter basal LH serum levels significantly, but provoked an increase of LH-RH-stimulated LH levels. On the other hand, a suppression of FSH serum levels was noted (Fig.7). Administration of D-Nor provoked an increase in LH-RH-stimulated LH levels, whereas basal LH levels remained unaffected (Fig.8). Again, both basal as well as LH-RH-stimulated FSH levels were suppressed by the progestogen.

DISCUSSION

Current trends in the development of new oral contraceptives have resulted in the reduction of steroid doses [21,22]. In addition, new steroids with greater biological activity have been synthesized. The biological potencies of these synthetic steroids have to be evaluated before they can be used in oral contraceptives. A major drawback of previously used biological test methods was that none of them took into account the central action of the material to be tested. Therefore, an in-vitro radioligand-receptor assay procedure for estrogens and an in-vivo model for progestogens were worked out. The assay procedure here is based on an earlier observation [23] of a 17β-estradiol receptor in the cytosol of the rat pituitary and hypothalamus. The ontogeny of estrogen-binding sites was described recently [13,14] and the biological role of the cytosol receptor was evaluated by studying its nuclear translocation [15]. The assay procedure, which can be performed on either pituitary or hypothalamic cytosol samples, provides a means of determining the structural requirement for binding to the estrogen receptor. The relative affinity of the estrogen may be calculated from the displacement curves at 50% binding (Figs 1–4). The assay performed on hypothalamic cytosol samples (Figs 1,2) was found to differentiate best between the biological activities of the steroids tested, though other factors contributing to the biological activity have to be considered. For example, the biological half-life is increased by the addition of an ethinyl group at position C-17α [24]. This is due to a decreased metabolism of this substituted estrogen. The discrepancy between the somewhat lower affinity of EE_2 than of 17β-estradiol for the hypothalamic estrogen receptor and its greater biological activity may be explained on these grounds. Another possible explanation could lie in differences in the cellular uptake of the steroids. The similar affinities of the two estrogens for pituitary receptor may be considered on the same basis. In addition, a difference was noted between the relative affinities of E_1 and E_3 in our system and in figures reported [25] for the two estrogens in a uterine cytosol system. These discrepancies may be explained by differences in uterotrophic activity and potency of central action. The relatively high binding activity of estrone compared with its activity in vivo may be explained partially by the relatively high metabolic clearence rate of the steroid [26]. Furthermore, intranuclear binding of 17β-estradiol and estrone was reported in female ovine pituitaries after incubation with estrone sulphate [27]. The assay procedure described may also be useful in evaluating the action of estrogens and anti-estrogens acting at the hypothalamic pituitary level.

Sedimentation patterns (Figs 5, 6) found for cytosol samples labelled with the estrogens used in this study are in agreement with data published by us previously [13] and with the results of the studies on the radioligand-receptor assay.

Another approach to evaluating the central action of steroids was used for testing the biological potency of progestogens (Figs 7, 8). The biological activity of P and D-Nor, based on the ability to modulate the gonadotrophin release stimulated by LH-RH, correlates well with data derived from the Clauberg test [24].

It was interesting to note that we could not find a radioactive peak upon gradient analysis of pituitary cytosol samples labelled with ^{3}H-P and ^{3}H-R 5020 in our system. But, a different modulation by the progestogens of the provoked LH and FSH release was noteworthy (Figs 7 and 8).

When considered as a whole, the findings reported in the present paper suggest that the radioligand-receptor assay for estrogens and the in-vivo model for evaluating the central action of progestogens may be valuable tools for testing new steroids to be used in oral contraceptives.

ACKNOWLEDGEMENTS

The authors would like to extend their thanks to C.Ehrig and L. Gschwantler for their technical assistance and to Mrs. E. Friedel for her help with the manuscript. The gift of materials for the radioimmunoassay of rLH and rFSH from the National Institute of Arthritis, Metabolism and Digestive Diseases, Rat Pituitary Hormone Distribution Program and from Dr. A.F. Parlow is gratefully acknowledged.

REFERENCES

[1] ARIMURA, A., SCHALLY, A.V., Endocrinology **87** (1970) 653.
[2] HILLIARD, J., SCHALLY, A.V., SAWYER, C.H., Endocrinology **88** (1971) 730.
[3] ARIMURA, A., SCHALLY, A.V., Proc. Soc. Exp. Biol. Med. **136** (1971) 290.
[4] DEBELJUK, L., ARIMURA, A., SCHALLY, A.V., Proc. Soc. Exp. Biol. Med. **139** (1972) 774.
[5] REEVES, J.J., ARIMURA, A., SCHALLY, A.V., Biol. Reprod. **4** (1971) 88.
[6] THOMAS, K., CARDON, M., DONNEZ, J., FERIN, J., Contraception **7** (1973) 289.
[7] SPONA, J., LUGER, O., FEBS Letters **32** (1973) 49.
[8] SPONA, J., LUGER, O., FEBS Letters **32** (1973) 52.
[9] SPONA, J., Endocrinol. Exp. **8** (1974) 19.
[10] SCHALLY, A.V., REDDING, T.W., ARIMURA, A., Endocrinology **93** (1973) 893.
[11] SPONA, J., "Hypothalamic hormone receptors", Basic Application and Clinical Use of Hypothalamic Hormones, Excerpta Medica International Congress Series No.374 (1976) 87.
[12] SPONA, J., Endocrinol. Exp. **9** (1975) 167.
[13] SPONA, J., BIEGLMAYER, Ch., ADAMIKER, D., JETTMAR, W., FEBS Letters **76** (1977) 306.
[14] SPONA, J., BIEGLMAYER, Ch., ADAMIKER, D., JETTMAR, W., (in preparation).
[15] BIEGLMAYER, Ch., PÖCKL, E., SPONA, J., ADAMIKER, D., JETTMAR, W., FEBS Letters (in press).
[16] MARTIN, R.G., AMES, B.N., J. Biol. Chem. **236** (1961) 1372.
[17] SPONA, J., Z. Immun.-Forsch. **143** (1972) 192.

[18] GITSCH, E., SCHNEIDER, W.H.F., SPONA, J., "Der Radioimmunoassay", Radioisotope in Geburtshilfe und Gynäkologie (GITSCH, E., Ed.), Walter de Gruyter, Berlin, New York (1977) 373.
[19] YALOW, R.S., BERSON, S.A., "Labelling of proteins – problems and practices", Radioactive Pharmaceutical, AEC, Symposium Series 6 (1966) 265.
[20] SPONA, J., "Rapid assay for luteinizing hormone and evaluation of data by new computer program", Radioimmunoassay and Related Procedures in Medicine (Proc. Symp. Istanbul, 1973) 1, IAEA, Vienna (1974) 123.
[21] SPONA, J., SCHNEIDER, W.H.F., Acta Obstet. Gynecol. Scand., Suppl. **54** (1976) 45.
[22] SCHNEIDER, W.H.F., SPONA, J., MATT, K., Contraception **9** (1974) 81.
[23] DAVIES, I.J., SIU, J., NAFTOLIN, F., RYAN, K.J., "Cytoplasmic binding of steroids in brain tissues and pituitary", Advances in the Biosciences (RASPE, G., Ed.), Pergamon Press, New York 15 (1975) 89.
[24] BROTHERTON, J., Sex Hormone Pharmacology, Academic Press, London, New York (1976).
[25] KORENMANN, S.G., Steroids **13** (1969) 163.
[26] NICOL, T., VERNON–ROBERTS, B., QUANTOCK, D.C., J. Endocrinol. **25** (1966) 119.
[27] PAYNE, A.H., LAWRENCE, C.C., FOSTER, D.L., JAFFE, R.B., J. Biol. Chem. **236** (1971) 1043.

DISCUSSION

H. BREUER: Your results are of great interest as regards the interaction of hormones at the hypophyseal-hypothalamic level. J. Axelrod has recently published (Science, September 1977) figures on the concentration of the 2-hydroxylated metabolite of 17α-ethinyl-17β-estradiol in hypothalamic tissue. He found fairly high values, which indicate that an interaction takes place between catechol estrogens and catecholamines. Do you have reliable figures for the concentrations of estradiol-17β and 17α-ethinyl-17β-estradiol in the different brain regions?

J. SPONA: The purpose of the present experiments was to investigate the interactions in vitro, and so we did not look at estrogen concentrations in various brain regions. Neither did we correct for any metabolism of estrogens in our studies, since the experiments were performed at 4°C and degradation should therefore be quite slow. Work is in progress, however, to study such effects in more detail.

O.A. JÄNNE: Do you think that estrogen receptors in the hypophysis and the hypothalamus have different ligand specificities?

J. SPONA: Our data suggest that there is ligand specificity. The cytosol estrogen receptor exhibits different affinities in binding the various estrogens.

DETERMINATION OF ESTRADIOL, ESTRONE AND PROGESTERONE IN SERUM AND HUMAN ENDOMETRIUM IN CORRELATION WITH THE CONTENT OF STEROID RECEPTORS AND 17β-HYDROXYSTEROID DEHYDROGENASE ACTIVITY DURING THE MENSTRUAL CYCLE

M. SCHMIDT-GOLLWITZER, J. EILETZ, J. PACHALY
Frauenklinik und Poliklinik Charlottenburg,
Berlin (West)

K. POLLOW
Institut für Molekularbiologie und Biochemie,
Freie Universität Berlin,
Berlin (West)

Abstract

DETERMINATION OF ESTRADIOL, ESTRONE AND PROGESTERONE IN SERUM AND HUMAN ENDOMETRIUM IN CORRELATION WITH THE CONTENT OF STEROID RECEPTORS AND 17β-HYDROXYSTEROID DEHYDROGENASE ACTIVITY DURING THE MENSTRUAL CYCLE.

A study has been carried out to compare the influence of estradiol, estrone and progesterone on the estradiol and progesterone receptor levels and 17β-hydroxysteroid dehydrogenase (17β-HSD) activity in human endometrium. The steroid hormone concentrations were measured simultaneously in both serum and endometrial tissue. The estradiol receptor levels were highest during the early proliferative phase and were inversely correlated to the endometrial tissue and serum concentrations of estradiol and progesterone. The highest progesterone binding capacity was found in endometrial cytosol during the late proliferative phase (midcycle) of the menstrual cycle. The midcycle peak of the progesterone receptor level correlated well with the first peak of the serum and tissue concentrations of estradiol. During the luteal phase, in contrast to the proliferative phase, the progesterone receptor level decreased whereas serum progesterone concentrations were high. Estrone concentrations were higher in secretory than proliferative endometrium and were correlated to the increase of progesterone receptor content and 17β-HSD activity during the early secretory phase. The 17β-HSD activity was approximately 10-fold higher during the early secretory than during the proliferative phase. The progesterone receptor level was highly correlated to the specific 17β-HSD activity of the microsomal fraction, whereas a significant inverse correlation between the enzyme activity and the estradiol receptor level was observed.

INTRODUCTION

It has been shown that the levels of the cytoplasmic estradiol and progesterone binding components [1 – 5] and the 17β-hydroxysteroid dehydrogenase

(17β-HSD) [6 – 10] are under steroidal control. Estrogen treatment increases the progesterone receptor concentration by promoting the synthesis of uterine progesterone receptors, whereas progesterone seems to be a negative effector of its own receptor. Progesterone that antagonizes estrogen stimulation of uterine growth inhibits estrogen action by interfering with the replenishment of cytoplasmic receptor molecules, thereby reducing the number of receptor-estrogen complexes that are translocated and retained by uterine nuclei [5]. The correspondence between the 17β-HSD activity and the serum concentrations of progesterone during the menstrual cycle suggest the possibility that this hormone has an inductive effect upon the endometrial enzyme [6 – 10].

This paper summarizes the authors' recent studies on the correlation between serum and human endometrial tissue levels of various steroid hormones and the concentration of binding sites of cytoplasmic estrogen and progesterone receptors as well as microsomal 17β-HSD activity. The aim of the present study was to determine directly whether estrogens or progestagens are responsible for the changes in receptor levels and enzymatic activity in human endometrium during the menstrual cycle.

MATERIAL AND METHODS

Endometrial tissue

Normal human endometrium (120 cases) from normally menstruating patients was obtained in the course of hysterectomy or diagnostic curettage for myomata uteri and prolapsus uteri. Immediately after hysterectomy the endometrium was scraped from the uterine cavity. Samples were examined histologically. For the receptor assay, 17β-HSD and steroid measurements, the specimens were chilled in ice-cold buffer composed of 50mM Tris/HCl, pH7.0, 1.25 mM EDTA, 12 mM mercaptoethanol and 20% glycerol (TEM-glycerol buffer). Further processing of the samples was initiated within the next 30 min. Blood samples were withdrawn simultaneously with the biopsies or the hysterectomy. The menstrual age of the endometrium was based on a 28-day cycle according to the method of Noyes et al. [11].

Preparation of cytosol and microsomal fraction

Tissue processing and experiments were done at 4°C. The tissue was washed several times in ice-cold TEM-glycerol buffer, weighed and homogenized in 4 volumes (wt/vol.) of the same buffer by five strokes with a Potter-Elvehjem-type homogenizer. The homogenate was centrifuged for 15 min at 850 × g to remove the nuclear fraction. The supernatant was centrifuged at 12 000 × g for 15 min. After removing the floating fat the supernatant was carefully decanted and centrifuged in a Spinco L2-65B ultracentrifuge (Beckman Instruments) using a Ti 50 rotor at 105 000 × g for 90 min. The final supernatant was designated "cytosol". Microsomes were obtained from the resulting pellet after washing twice in TEM-glycerol buffer. Total cytosol was divided according to the tissue content in aliquots for the different methods.

Determination of progesterone and estradiol binding

Cytosols were diluted with TEM-glycerol buffer to a final protein concentration of approximately 1 mg/ml. For progesterone binding measurement the equilibrium dialysis was performed according to the method described in detail by Davies [12]. The diluted cytosols were incubated at 4°C for 16 h, with shaking, in the presence of increasing concentrations of H^3-R 5020 (0.2 – 2nM).

For the determination of estradiol binding the diluted cytosols were incubated at 4°C for 16 h with ^{3}H-estradiol over a 30-fold concentration range (0.5 – 15nM). Binding was then measured using the charcoal adsorption technique. Tubes containing μM amounts of unlabelled estradiol were used to correct for non-specific binding. The number of binding sites and the association constant were determined from a Scatchard plot of the data [13].

17β-HSD activity measurement

For the oxidation reaction the standard reaction mixtures (total volume 4.1 ml) contained 0.01M Tris/HCl buffer, pH7.4, 0.1 μCi (4–14C)-estradiol-17β (0.47 μg) plus 10μM of unlabelled steroids (dissolved in 0.1 ml of propyleneglycol, 2.4% vol./vol.), 500 μM NAD and microsomal preparations. The incubation temperature was 37°C. Reactions were started by addition of coenzymes and terminated (after 30 min of incubation) by addition of 5 ml of ether/chloroform (3:1 vol./vol.). The extracts of the reaction mixtures (3 × 5 ml ether/chloroform) were pooled and evaporated under nitrogen and dissolved in 0.5 ml of benzene. An aliquot (50 μl) was removed for liquid scintillation counting (Berthold BF 5000 liquid scintillation counter, Wildbad, FRG) in order to estimate the total amount of radioactive steroids present in the extract. The benzene extracts were evaporated under nitrogen and the dry residues were transferred with 0.2 ml of chloroform/methanol (1:1 vol.vol.) to thin-layer plates (silica gel, 0.25 mm, Woelm, Eschwege, FRG). Thin-layer chromatography and identification of reaction products were performed as described previously [14 – 17].

Protein assay

Protein concentration was measured by the method of Lowry et al. [18] using bovine serum albumin as standard.

Extraction of steroids

Tritiated internal standards (approximately 1000 counts/min) were added to every cytosol containing 5 – 200 mg of tissue and kept for 30 min in an ice-bath. After equilibration, 3 vol. of diethyl ether (Merck, Darmstadt, FRG) was added to the cytosol samples. The contents were mixed for 15 s. The diethyl ether was decanted and evaporated under nitrogen at 40°C. The residue was dissolved in 1 ml of 0.1% gelatine PBS buffer, pH7.0, and aliquots were taken for determination of recovery and radioimmunoassay of steroids.

Radioimmunoassays

The radioimmunoassays for estradiol-17β, estrone and progesterone were performed without chromatography by using specific antisera. Estradiol-17β was determined with an anti-estradiol-6-BSA-serum donated generously by Dr. G.D. Niswender, Colorado State University [19]. Estrone was measured by an anti-estrone-6(CMO)BSA-serum obtained commercially from Steranti Research Ltd, St. Albans, UK. Progesterone was determined by specific radioimmunoassay using an 11-OH-progesterone-BSA-antiserum [20].

In brief, aliquots of the extracted serum or cytosol specimen were incubated for 16 h with 100 μl of antiserum in appropriate dilution and 100 μl of tritiated steroid (approx. 5 000 counts/min of estradiol-1,4,6,7-3H, estrone-2,4,6,7-3H and progesterone-1,2,6,7-3H purchased from Amersham Buchler, Braunschweig, FRG. Bound and free fractions were separated using 1 ml of dextran-coated charcoal. The bound fraction was transferred to a liquid scintillation cocktail and counted in an automatic scintillation counter (Nuclear Chicago, Isocap 300). Statistical analysis of the raw radioimmunoassay data was done by a computer program described by Schmidt-Gollwitzer and Pachaly [21].

The recovery of the three steroids under investigation was assessed by adding known amounts of tritiated or untritiated steroids to the endometrial samples before homogenization and to the cytosol samples. Mean percentage recoveries for all hormones were between 70% and 80% for endometrial specimens and over 95% for serum samples. Blank values in all assays were negligible, if present. The cross-reactivities have been calculated in the conventional manner [22]. In the three assay systems the cross-reactivities of the relevant steroids (estradiol, estrone, estriol, progesterone, 17-hydroxyprogesterone, testosterone, androstenedione and cortisol) were below 0.5%. The detection level at 95% probability was 5, 12 and 15 pg for estradiol-17β, estrone and progesterone, respectively. The coefficient of variation within and between assays was below 12% for all hormones.

Text continued on page 266

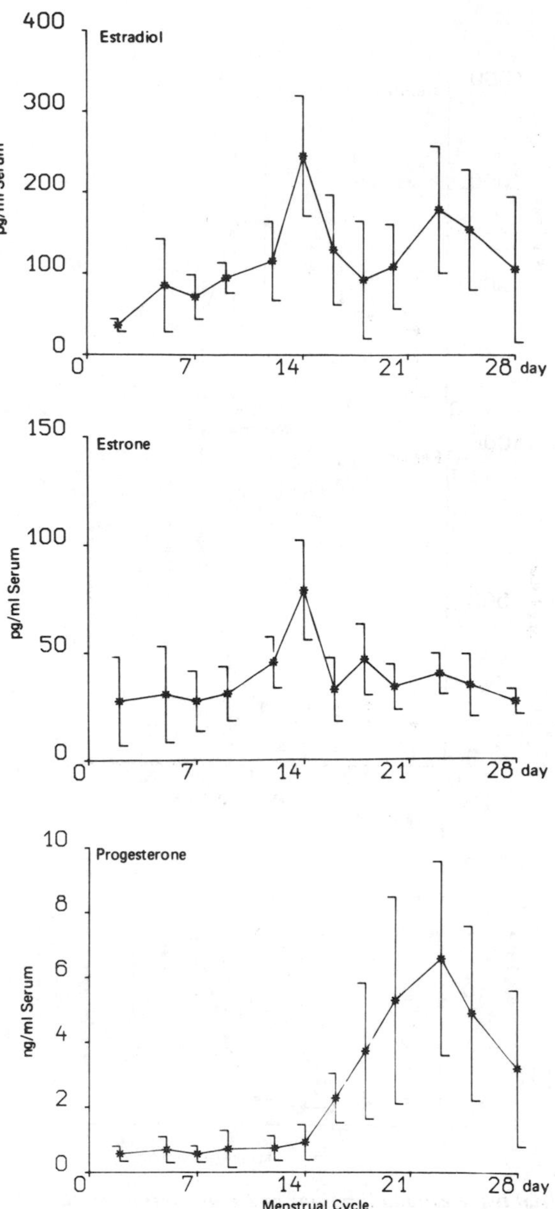

FIG.1. Serum estradiol, estrone and progesterone levels of 120 women between 20 and 48 years of age, in relation to the day of the menstrual cycle. Each point represents the mean ± SD.

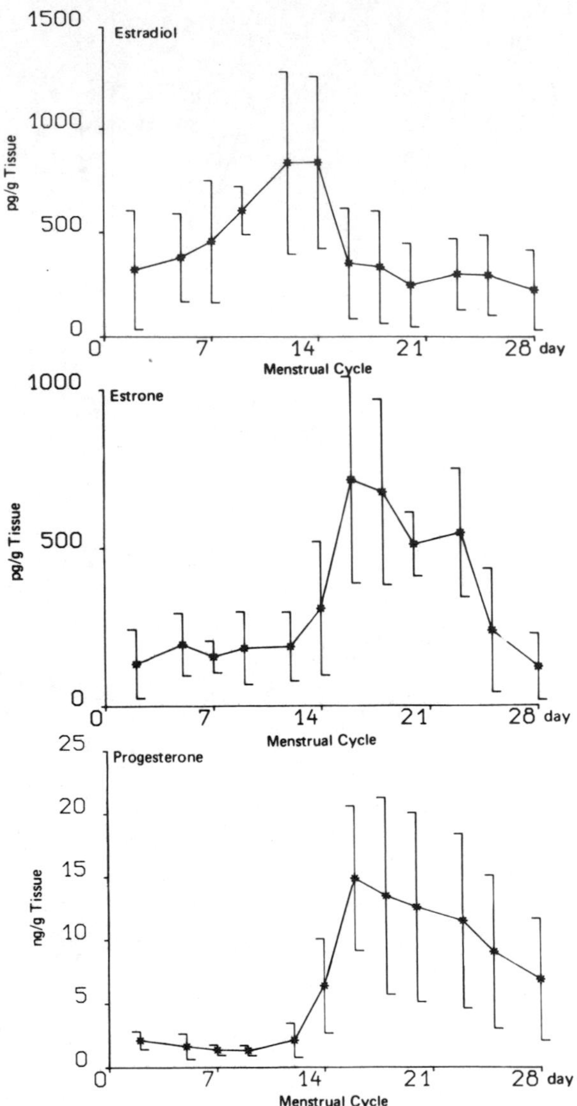

FIG.2. Endometrial tissue estradiol, estrone and progesterone levels in 120 women in relation to the day of the menstrual cycle. Each point represents the mean ± SD.

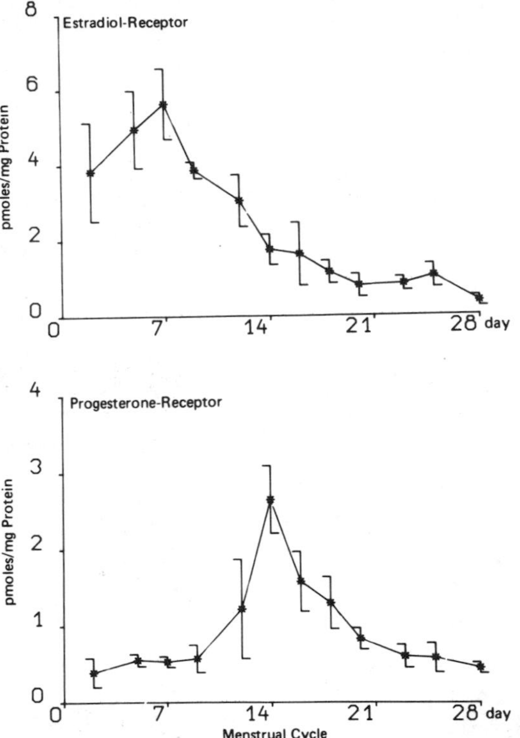

FIG.3. Concentration of specific estradiol and progesterone binding sites of normal human endometrium in relation to the day of the menstrual cycle. Each point represents the mean ± SD.

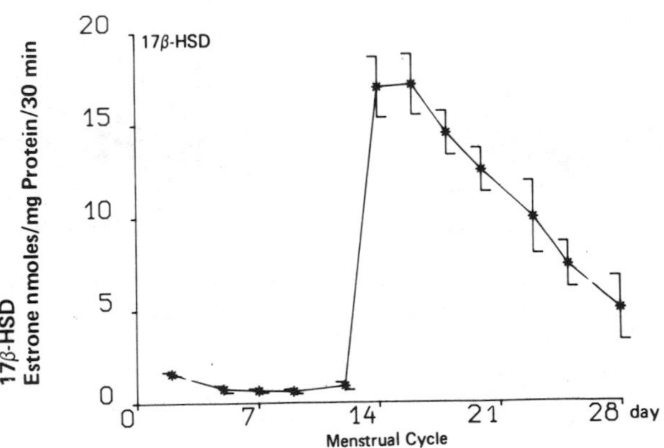

FIG.4. Dependence of specific 17β-HSD activity in microsomes of normal human endometrium on the phase of the menstrual cycle. Each point represents the mean ± SD.

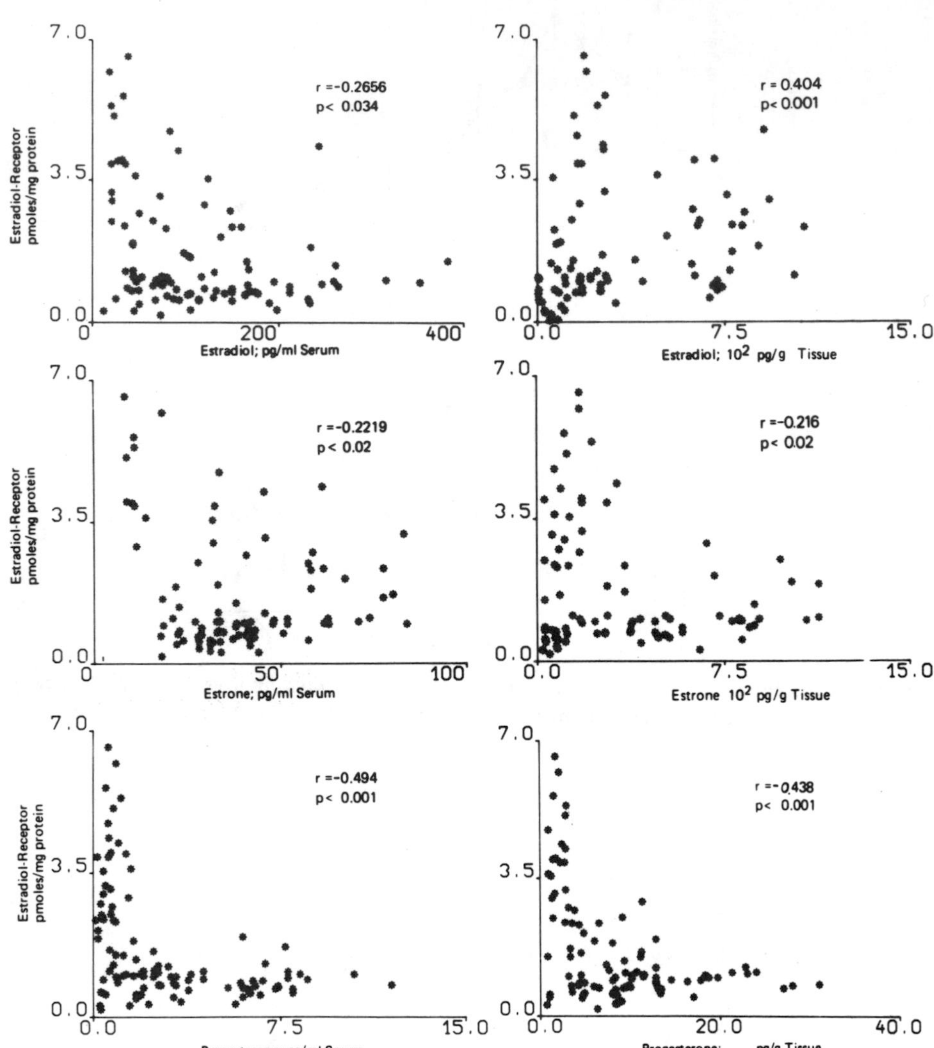

FIG.5. Correlation of the specific estradiol-binding capacity of endometrial cytosol with serum and tissues levels of estradiol, estrone and progesterone.

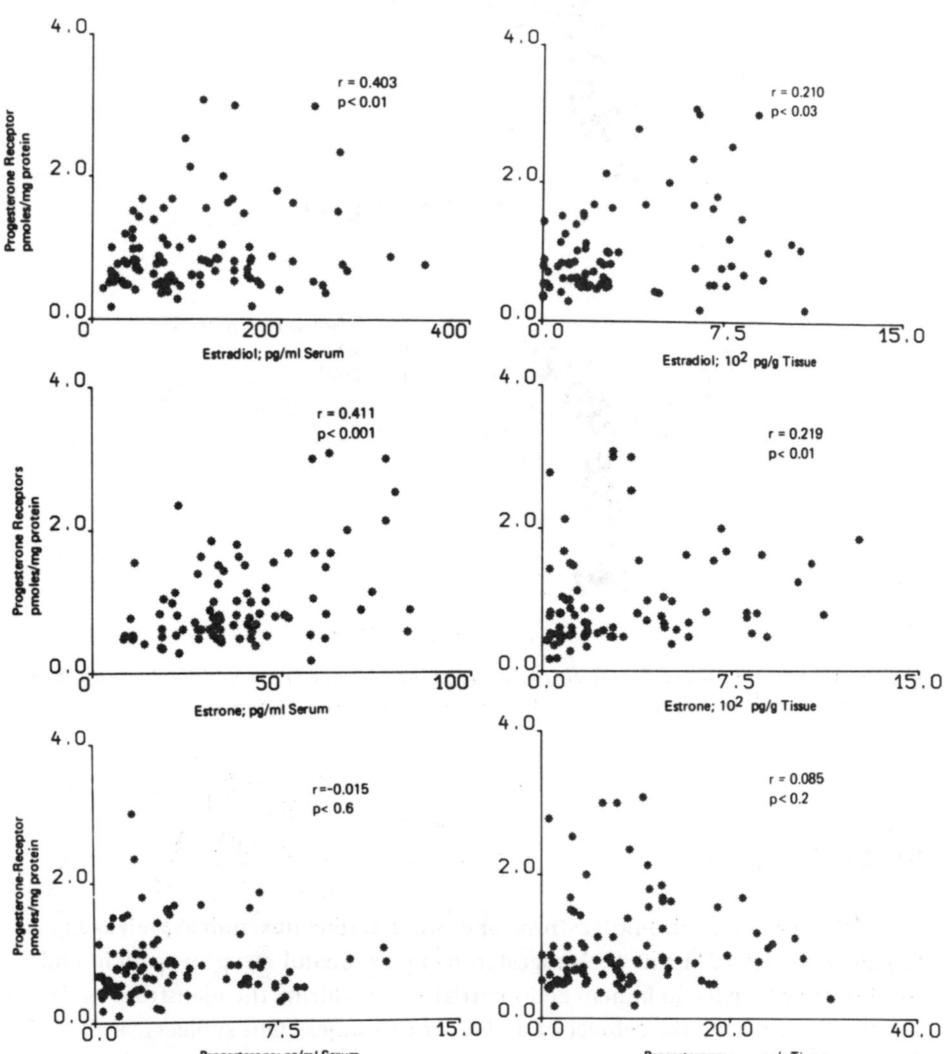

FIG.6. Correlation of the specific progesterone binding capacity of endometrial cytosol with serum and tissue levels of estradiol, estrone and progesterone.

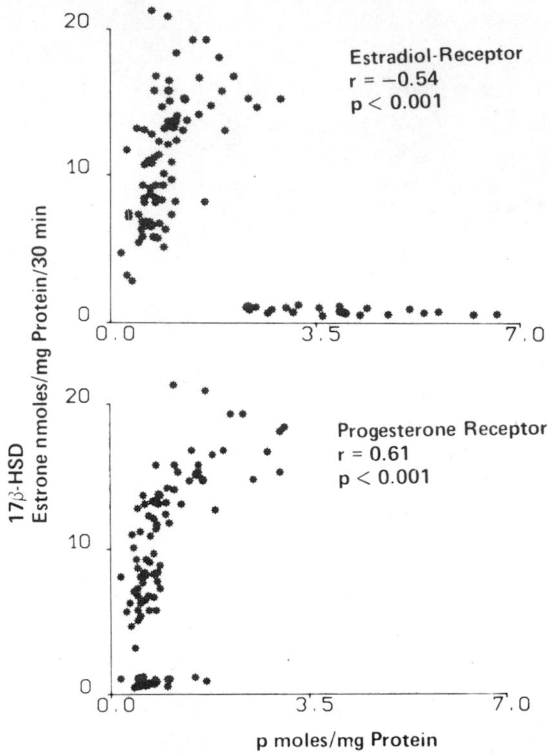

FIG. 7. Correlation of specific 17β-HSD activity in microsomes of normal endometrium with the specific estradiol and progesterone cytoplasmic receptor concentration.

RESULTS

The values for estradiol, estrone and progesterone in serum as well as in human endometrial tissue, the progesterone and estradiol receptor content and the 17β-HSD activity in human endometrial tissues during the menstrual cycle in women have been the subject of a number of studies. Our subjects, aged between 20 and 48 years, were selected with a history of regular cycles characterized by a biphasic basal body-temperature curve. The serum values for estradiol, estrone and progesterone, shown in Fig. 1, were not different from those described by others for women in this age group [23 – 27].

In Fig. 2, endometrial tissue concentrations of estradiol, estrone and progesterone in the different phases of the menstrual cycle are depicted. The overall picture of endometrial hormone concentrations shows similarities to the serum levels of these steroids. The progesterone tissue concentration parallels the serum levels of progesterone, whereas the estradiol and estrone tissue levels were partly different from their serum pattern. The mean estradiol concentration in endometrium culminate in a peak of 840 pg/g tissue during midcycle but dropped steeply after ovulation without rising in the luteal phase. In contrast to the serum levels, the estrone concentration in endometrial tissue reached its highest level during the secretory phase.

Figure 3 shows that estradiol and progesterone receptor levels in normal endometrial tissue are directly dependent on the stage of the menstrual cycle. The level of the ^{3}H-R 5020 binding sites (progesterone receptor) was low in the early proliferative phase but increased towards the 14th day of the menstrual cycle, having its highest value around the time of ovulation, and declined sharply during the secretory phase. The estradiol receptor level was highest during the early proliferative phase. The specific 17β-HSD activities of microsomal fractions of normal human endometrium are plotted against the day of the menstrual cycle in Fig.4. It was interesting to observe that the specific activity of the 17β-HSD in microsomes was approximately 10-fold higher during the early secretory than during the proliferative phase.

In Figs 5 and 6, progesterone and estradiol cytoplasmic receptor levels are correlated with serum and endometrial tissue concentrations of progesterone, estradiol and estrone. There seems to be correlation between the cytosol progesterone receptor level and the serum and tissue concentration of estrone and estradiol, pointing to a possible positive control by estrogen on the progesterone receptor level. In addition, no significant correlation was found between the progesterone receptor concentration and the serum or tissue levels of progesterone.

In Fig.7 the specific microsomal 17β-HSD activity is plotted against the cytosol estradiol and progesterone binding capacity. It was interesting to observe that the cytosol progesterone receptor level was highly correlated to the specific 17β-HSD activity and that there was a significant inverse correlation between the cytosolic estradiol receptor level and the enzyme activity.

DISCUSSION

In this study estradiol and progesterone receptor levels in human endometrium cytosol were simultaneously measured in the different phases of the menstrual cycle. At the same time, the specific 17β-HSD activity of the microsomal fraction as well as progesterone, estradiol and estrone concentrations in serum and endometrial tissue were determined. There was evidence for cyclic changes in the estradiol and progesterone receptor concentrations in human endometrium: highest receptor binding of estradiol occurred in specimens taken during the early proliferative phase, whereas the highest specific progesterone binding was observed at midcycle. Similar results have been reported by other workers [28 – 32]. The observed variations in apparent receptor site concentration can be explained by occupation of receptor sites by endogenous steroid hormones, as documented by an inverse correlation between serum estrogen concentration and measured receptor binding activity.

Serum hormone levels showed the well-known changes during the menstrual cycle [23 – 27]. Endometrial steroid concentrations demonstrated also cyclic profiles during menstrual cycle. This agrees with the findings of other groups [27, 33 – 36]. Simultaneous measurements of serum and tissue hormone concentrations and endometrium receptor binding capacity showed an inverse correlation between the estradiol receptor level and the serum concentration of estradiol. However, the rapid decrease of serum estradiol after ovulation is not followed by an inversely correlated increase of estradiol receptor levels. It is interesting to note that the estradiol concentration in the endometrial cell conforms only partly to the serum pattern: in endometrial tissue the isolated peak of estradiol in the preovulatory period of the menstrual cycle could be found, but not the high plateau during the secretory phase. In contrast, the tissue levels of estrone parallel the serum levels but the increase in estrone concentration found in the luteal phase was higher in endometrial tissue than in serum. Since estrone and estradiol have similar affinities to the highly specific estrogen receptor binding sites, it is possible that high estrone levels decrease estrogen binding capacity in the same manner as estradiol.

Furthermore, the results in this study demonstrate that the midcycle peak of the progesterone receptor concentration correlated well with the first peak of the serum and tissue concentration of estradiol. During the first half of the menstrual cycle the amount of progesterone bound by endometrial supernatant correlated well with the progesterone concentration in serum and endometrial tissue, whereas during the main part of the luteal phase the binding capacity seemed to be inversely correlated with serum progesterone concentrations. The tissue progesterone levels correlate to the progesterone receptor content during midcycle but not thereafter. These data clearly demonstrate that the level of the progesterone receptor is under steroidal control. Estrogens increase the progesterone receptor concentration. These findings clearly agree with the results of earlier experiments using animal models. These studies showed that estradiol induces the synthesis of the progesterone receptors in the mammalian uterus. The same may be true for the increase of the cytoplasmic progesterone receptor during the secretory phase of the menstrual cycle.

In addition, it was observed that progesterone increases the inactivation rate of its own receptor [1 – 5]. We could not confirm these results for the second half of the menstrual cycle. Whether or not the low estradiol receptor level during the luteal phase is influenced by high serum and tissue concentrations of progesterone remains to be clarified, but the results show that there is a significant inverse correlation between both parameters ($p < 0.001$).

Some studies showed that progesterone interferes with the replenishment of the cytoplasmic estrogen receptor and this reduction is correlated with a reduced sensitivity of the uterus to estrogen. These findings are in good agreement with clinical and experimental observations that progesterone is able to antagonize and/or modify the action of estrogen and that estrogen pretreatment enhances tissue sensitivity to progesterone.

The observed changes in the specific 17β-HSD activity of the microsomal fractions in the course of the menstrual cycle should be discussed in connection with the findings for the steroid hormone receptors. There is a close correlation between the progesterone receptor level and the specific 17β-HSD activity in the endometrial cell. This finding is consistent with in-vitro and in-vivo results obtained by Tseng and Gurpide [6, 7] who pointed out that progesterone is the agent responsible for the 10-fold increase in endometrial 17β-HSD activity observed during the luteal phase in menstruating women. In addition, Pollow et al. [8, 9] could show that in well-differentiated endometrial carcinoma, which possesses a relatively high concentration of progesterone receptors, there is a steep increase of the 17β-HSD activity after gestagen treatment in vivo, just as there is in the normal endometrial cell after ovulation.

We conclude that the 17β-HSD activity is induced by the progesterone receptor mechanism, while the latter in turn is enhanced by estradiol concentration (by way of the receptor mechanism?). Since a high intracellular activity of the 17β-HSD during the luteal phase leads to a rapid decrease in the intracellular concentration of estradiol, the progesterone receptor concentration also decreases. While the intracellular concentration of estradiol is lowest during the secretory phase, the estrone concentration is highest. At the moment the physiological significance of these observations is unclear, but it can be expected from superfusion experiments [37, 38] that estrone is a metabolite that competes poorly with estradiol for binding to nuclear receptors and diffuses out of the cells more easily than estradiol. On the basis of the above hypothesis the measurement of the 17β-HSD activity could be a simple and rapid method to determine the intactness of the above-named chain of the reactions.

REFERENCES

[1] FEIL, P.D., GLASSER, S.R., TOFT, D.O., O'MALLEY, B.W., Endocrinology **91** (1972) 738.

[2] MILGROM, E., ATGER, M., PERROT, M., BAULIEU, E.-E., Endocrinology **90** (1972) 1071.

[3] O'MALLEY, B.W., Endocrinology **94** (1974) 1041.

[4] KONTULA, K., J. Steroid Biochem. **6** (1975) 1555.

[5] HSUEH, A.J.W., PECK, E.J., CLARK, J.H., Endocrinology **98** (1976) 438.

[6] TSENG, L., GURPIDE, E., Endocrinology **94** (1974) 419.

[7] TSENG, L., GURPIDE, E., Endocrinology **97** (1975) 825.
[8] POLLOW, K., LÜBBERT, H., BOQUOI, E., KREUZER, G., JESKE, R., POLLOW, B., Acta Endocrinol. **79** (1975) 134.
[9] POLLOW, K., BOQUOI, B., LÜBBERT, H., POLLOW, K., J. Endocrinol. **67** (1975) 131.
[10] BUIRCHELL, B.J., HÄHNEL, R., J. Steroid Biochem. **6** (1975) 1489.
[11] NOYES, R.W., HERTIG, A.T., ROCK, J., Fert. Steril. **1** (1950) 3.
[12] DAVIES, I.J., In: Molecular Techniques and Approaches in Developmental Biology (CHRISPEELS, M.J., Ed.), J. Wiley and Sons (1973) pp.39–54.
[13] SCATCHARD, G., Ann. Acad. Sci. **51** (1949) 660.
[14] POLLOW, K., LÜBBERT, H., POLLOW, B., J. Steroid Biochem. **7** (1976) 45.
[15] POLLOW, K., LÜBBERT, H., JESKE, R., POLLOW, B., Acta Endocrinol. **79** (1975) 146.
[16] POLLOW, K., LÜBBERT, H., POLLOW, B., Acta Endocrinol. **80** (1975) 355.
[17] POLLOW, K., LÜBBERT, H., POLLOW, B., J. Steroid Biochem. **7** (1976) 315.
[18] LOWRY, O.H., ROSEBROUGH, N.J., FARR, A.L., RANDALL, R.J., J. Biol. Chem. **193** (1951) 265.
[19] ENGLAND, B.G., NISWENDER, G.D., MIDGLEY, A.M., Jr., J. Clin. Endocrinol. Metab. **38** (1974) 42.
[20] HOFFMANN, B., KYREIN, H.J., ENDER, M.L., Horm. Res. **4** (1973) 302.
[21] SCHMIDT-GOLLWITZER, M., PACHALY, J., Radioimmunoassay Paket. Computer program, Freie Universität, Berlin (1974).
[22] ABRAHAM, G.E.J., J. Clin. Endocrinol. Metab. **28** (1969) 866.
[23] BAIRD, D.T., GUEVARA, A., J. Clin. Endocrinol. Metab. **29** (1969) 149.
[24] ROSS, G.T., CARGILLE, C.M., LIPSETT, M.B., RAYFORD, P.L., MARSHALL, J.R., STROTT, C.A., RODBARD, D., Recent Progr. Hormone Res. **26** (1970) 1.
[25] VANDE WIELE, R.L., BOGUMIL, J., DYRENFURTH, J., FERIN, M., JEWELEWICZ,R., WARREN, M., RIZKALLAH, T., MIKHAIL, G., Recent Progr. Hormone Res. **26** (1970) 63.
[26] SHERMAN, B.M., KORENMAN, S.G., J. Clin. Invest. **55** (1975) 699.
[27] GUERRERO, R., LANDGREN, B.-M., MONTIEL, R., CEKAN, Z., DICZFALUSY, E., Contraception **11** (1975) 169.
[28] RAO, B.R., WIEST, W.G., ALLEN, W.M., Endocrinology **95** (1974) 1275.
[29] KONTULA, K., JAENNE, O., LUUKKAINEN, T., VIHKO, R., Biochim. Biophys. Acta **328** (1973) 148.
[30] ILLINGWORTH, D.V., WOOD, G.P., FLICKINGER, G.I., MIKHAIL, G., J. Clin. Endocrinol. Metab. **40** (1975) 1001.
[31] CROCKER, S.G., MILTON, P.J.D., KING, R.J.B., J. Endocrinol. **62** (1974) 145.
[32] BAYARD, F., DAMILANO, S., ROBEL, P., BAULIEU, E.-E., C.R. Hebd. Acad. Sci. **281** (1975) 1341.
[33] GRUNDSELL, H., NILSSON, J., NORDQVIST, S., Lancet **i** (1973) 888.
[34] BATRA, S., BENGTSSON, L.P., J. Steroid Biochem. **7** (1976) 599.
[35] BAYARD, F., LOUVET, J.P., MONROZIES, M., BOULARD, A., PONTONNIER, G., J. Clin. Endocrinol. Metab. **41** (1975) 1322.
[36] BATRA, S., GRUNDSELL, H., SJÖBORG, N.-O., Contraception **16** (1977) 217.
[37] TSENG, L., GURPIDE, E., L. Steroid Biochem. **5** (1974) 273.
[38] TSENG, L., GURPIDE, E., Am. J. Obstet. Gynecol. **114** (1972) 1002.

DISCUSSION

O.A. JÄNNE: Do you have any information on nuclear receptor levels during the menstrual cycle?

M. SCHMIDT-GOLLWITZER: During the menstrual cycle the nuclear estradiol receptor exhibits a pattern similar to that of the cytoplasmic receptor.

SPECIFIC BILE ACID RADIOIMMUNOASSAYS FOR SEPARATE DETERMINATIONS OF UNCONJUGATED CHOLIC ACID, CONJUGATED CHOLIC ACID AND CONJUGATED DEOXYCHOLIC ACID IN SERUM AND THEIR CLINICAL APPLICATION*

S. MATERN, W. GEROK
Medizinische Universitätsklinik,
Freiburg im Breisgau,
Federal Republic of Germany

Abstract

SPECIFIC BILE ACID RADIOIMMUNOASSAYS FOR SEPARATE DETERMINATIONS OF UNCONJUGATED CHOLIC ACID, CONJUGATED CHOLIC ACID AND CONJUGATED DEOXYCHOLIC ACID IN SERUM AND THEIR CLINICAL APPLICATION.

Specific radioimmunoassays have been developed for separate determinations of unconjugated cholic acid, conjugated cholic acid and conjugated deoxycholic acid in serum. Before carrying out the radioimmunoassay, the serum bile acids were extracted with Amberlite XAD-2. Unconjugated cholic acid was separated from glyco- and taurocholic acids by thin-layer chromatography. At 50% displacement of bound labelled glyco-[^{3}H]-cholic acid, using antiserum obtained after immunization with cholic acid-bovine serum albumin-conjugate, the cross-reactivity of taurocholic acid was 100%, cholic acid 80%, glycochenodeoxycholic acid 10%, chenodeoxycholic acid 7%, conjugated deoxycholic acid 3% and conjugated lithocholic acid $< 1\%$. Conjugated cholic acid and conjugated deoxycholic acid were determined by radioimmunoassays already described. Unconjugated cholic acid was determined by a solid-phase radioimmunoassay uisng the cholic acid antibody chemically bound to Sepharose. The displacement curve of [^{3}H]-cholic acid in the solid-phase radioimmunoassay was linear on a logit-log plot from 5 to 200 pmol of unlabelled cholic acid. The coefficient of variation between samples was 5%. The clinical application of these bile acid radioimmunoassays is shown by an "oral cholate tolerance test", which is a sensitive indicator of liver function, and by an "oral cholylglycine tolerance test" which is a useful test for bile acid absorption.

INTRODUCTION

Techniques for measuring bile acids in serum are of great importance for the study of liver and intestinal functions [1–4]. Although there is a radioimmunoassay for almost every steroid of biological significance, it was only recently that Simmonds et al. [5] introduced a radioimmunochemical method for measuring a bile acid in serum. Since then, radioimmunoassays for conjugated cholic

* This work was supported by the Deutsche Forschungsgemeinschaft (Grant No.Ma 567/3).

acid [6–10] and conjugated deoxycholic acid [11, 12] in serum have also been described. The present paper describes the separate determinations of unconjugated (free) cholic acid, conjugated cholic acid and conjugated deoxycholic acid by specific radioimmunoassays. Clinical applications of these bile acid radioimmunoassays are shown by an "oral cholate tolerance test", which is a sensitive indicator of liver function, and by an "oral cholylglycine tolerance test" which is a useful test for bile acid malabsorption.

RADIOIMMUNOASSAYS FOR SEPARATE DETERMINATIONS OF UNCONJUGATED CHOLIC ACID, CONJUGATED CHOLIC ACID AND CONJUGATED DEOXYCHOLIC ACID IN SERUM

Antigens were prepared by coupling the carboxyl group of the side chain of either cholic acid or deoxycholic acid to amino groups of bovine serum albumin by a mixed anhydride reaction, as described by Erlanger et al. [13]. Both the cholic acid-bovine serum albumin-conjugate and the deoxycholic acid-bovine serum

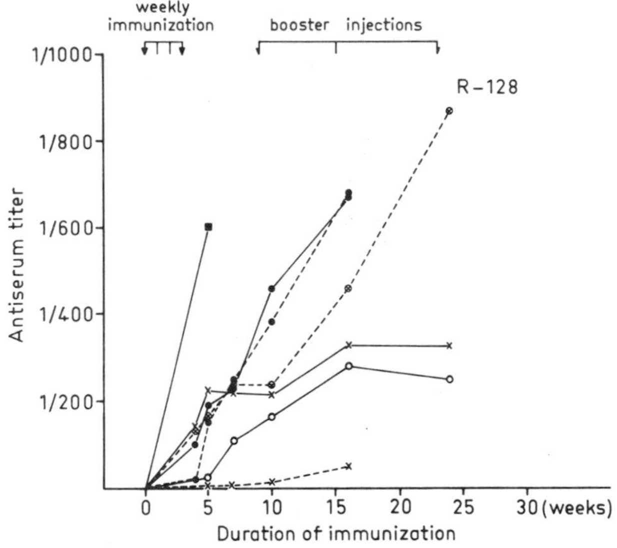

FIG.1. Development of antiserum titres of seven rabbits after weekly multiple site, intradermal immunization with 1 mg of cholic acid-bovine serum albumin-conjugate emulsified with 1 ml of Freund's complete adjuvant-saline (1 : 1, vol./vol.) and after booster injections with 100 μg of conjugate. Titres were determined as described previously [7]. *(End points of curves show when antisera were harvested from the* V. cava inferior *in urethane narcosis and when animals were killed. Antiserum of rabbit R-128 was used to develop the cholic acid radioimmunoassay.)*

TABLE I. CROSS-REACTION OF VARIOUS BILE ACIDS WITH ANTISERUM R-128 OBTAINED AFTER IMMUNIZATION OF RABBITS WITH CHOLIC ACID-BOVINE SERUM ALBUMIN-CONJUGATE (see Fig.1).

Bile acid	% Cross-reaction
Taurocholic	100
Glycocholic	100
Cholic	80
Glycochenodeoxycholic	10
Chenodeoxycholic	7
Taurodeoxycholic	3
Glycodeoxycholic	3
Deoxycholic	< 1
Taurolithocholic	< 1
Glycolithocholic	< 1
Lithocholic	< 1

albumin-conjugate contained 12 mol of bile acid per mol of albumin [14, 15] determined by gas-liquid chromatography [16, 17]. Specific antiserum to deoxycholic acid was obtained after injections of the deoxycholic acid-albumin-conjugate into rabbits using the previously described immunization procedure [18]. The development of the antiserum titres of seven rabbits immunized with cholic acid-bovine serum albumin-conjugate is shown in Fig.1. Investigation of the specificity of the antiserum R-128 (Fig.1) by adding other common bile acids to a solution containing labelled glyco-[^{3}H]-cholic acid and antiserum showed (see Table I) that it was necessary to separate conjugated cholic acid (glyco- and taurocholic acids) from unconjugated cholic acid for the separate radioimmunochemical determination of these bile acids in serum.

The simultaneous determination of unconjugated cholic acid, conjugated cholic acid and conjugated deoxycholic acid in the same serum sample by separate radioimmunoassays was performed as shown in Fig.2. After extraction of serum bile acids with Amberlite XAD-2 [19] and separation of unconjugated cholic acid from conjugated cholic acid (glyco- and taurocholic acids) by thin-layer chromatography [20], conjugated cholic acid and conjugated deoxycholic acid were determined by the previously described radioimmunoassays [7, 11, 12]. The separated unconjugated cholic acid (see Fig.2) was determined by a solid-phase radioimmunoassay (manuscript in preparation).

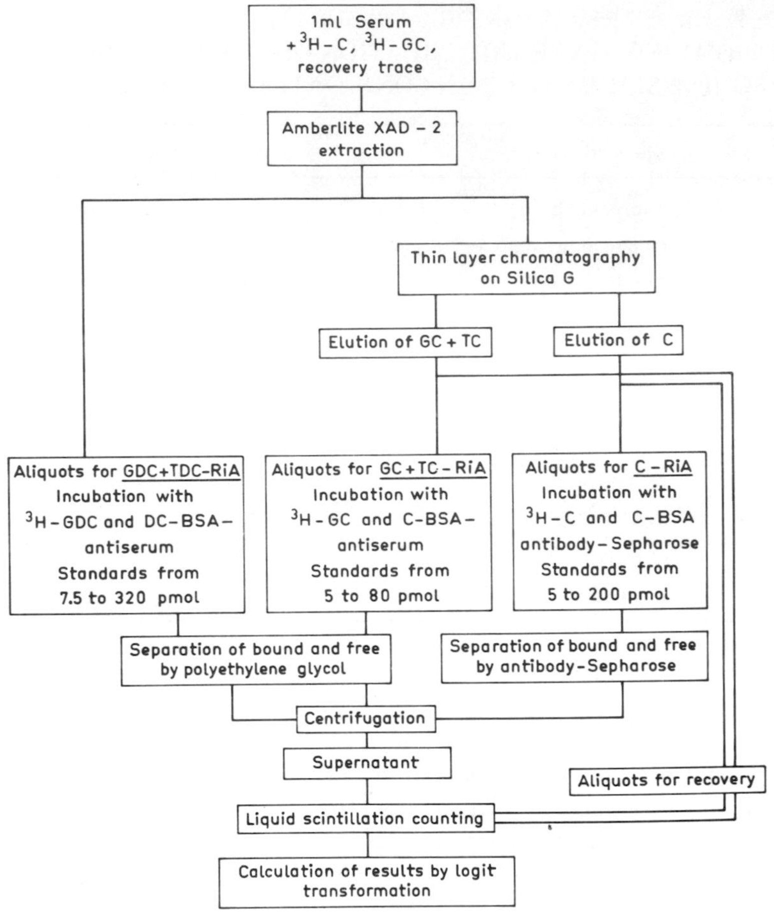

FIG.2. Scheme of simultaneous radioimmunoassays for unconjugated cholic acid (C), conjugated cholic acid (GC, TC) and conjugated deoxycholic acid (GDC, TDC) in serum.

SOLID-PHASE RADIOIMMUNOASSAY OF UNCONJUGATED CHOLIC ACID IN SERUM

Three millilitres of the antiserum R-128 (Table I) were purified from the low molecular material by gel-filtration on Sephadex-G-25 medium; 6 ml of the eluted fraction containing the serum protein were coupled to CNBr-activated Sepharose 4-B (9 g) and, after washing, the cholic acid antibody-Sepharose was made up to a volume of 90 ml with phosphate buffer (0.01M KH_2PO_4/K_2HPO_4, 1M NaCl, 3mM NaN_3, pH7.4) to give a stock solution, as described by van den Berg et al.[8].

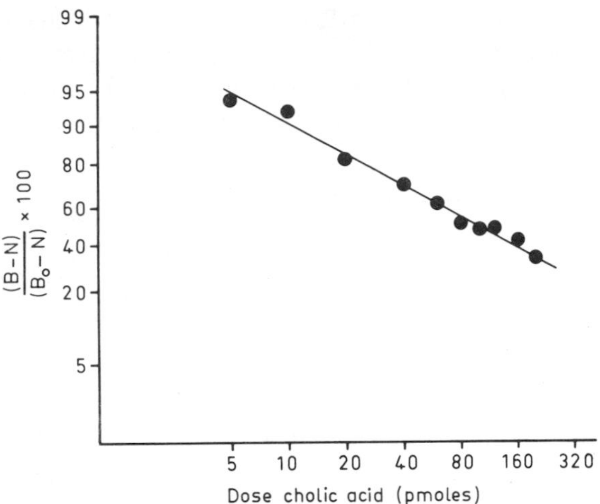

FIG.3. Standard curve in logit transformation of the solid-phase radioimmunoassay for unconjugated cholic acid. Ordinate B/B_0, on logit scale (B, antibody-bound labelled [^3H]-cholic acid in counts/min; B_0, antibody-bound labelled [^3H]-cholic acid in counts/min at zero dose of unlabelled cholic acid; N, non-specific bound labelled [^3H]-cholic acid in counts/min). The 'N' and the 'B_0' were determined with serum from a non-immunized rabbit, purified by gel-filtration on Sephadex-G-25 and coupled to Sepharose. The abscissa is the logarithm of the dose of cholic acid.

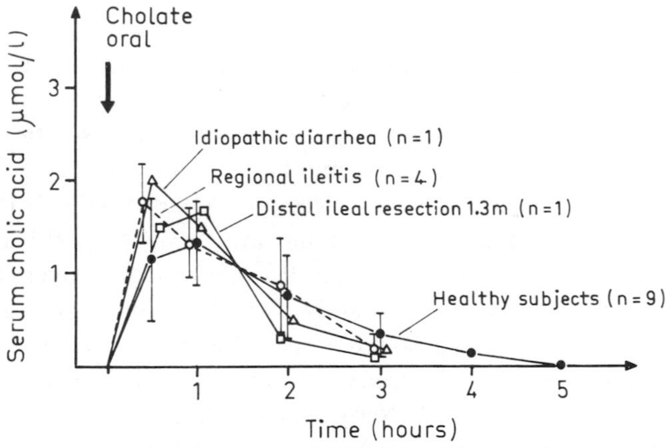

FIG.4. Effect of oral cholate administration – 0.5 g or 7 mg/kg body weight – on serum cholic acid levels in fasting healthy subjects and in fasting patients with regional ileitis (Crohn's disease), distal ileal resection (1.3 m) and idiopathic diarrhœa. Ordinate: the serum cholic acid values are expressed as the mean (± SE) of the measured values minus the corresponding fasting values of free and conjugated cholic acids in serum.

TABLE II. INTEGRATED AREA (MEAN ±SE) UNDER THE CURVES FOR SERUM CHOLIC ACID CONCENTRATIONS VERSUS TIME IN HEALTHY SUBJECTS (SEE FIG.4) AND IN PATIENTS WITH DIFFERENT LIVER DISEASES BETWEEN 0 AND 2 HOURS OF THE "ORAL CHOLATE TOLERANCE TEST"

Group[a]	Integrated area $\int_0^2 C(t)\,dt^b\,[\mu M \times h]$
Healthy subjects (9)	1.9 ± 0.5
Fatty liver/fatty liver hepatitis (5)	2.4 ± 0.2 ($p > 0.05$)
Cirrhosis without portal hypertension (10)	2.5 ± 1.3 ($p > 0.05$)
Granulomatous hepatitis (3)	4.1 ± 2.4 ($p < 0.05$)
Cirrhosis with portal hypertension (17)	12.3 ± 7.5 ($p < 0.001$)

[a] Figures in parentheses represent No. of subjects.

[b] The observed serum cholic acid values minus the fasting cholic acid value (C) after oral cholate administration were plotted against the time (t), and the area under the cholic acid concentrations-vs.-time curve was integrated between 0 and 2 hours.

In the immunoassay procedure, the standard curve included 10 dose levels between 5 and 200 pmol of sodium cholate dissolved in saline, containing 4 g/l bovine serum albumin and 3mM NaN_3 (cholic acid standard solution). The reaction mixture comprised: 3000 counts/min of [^{3}H]-cholic acid (specific activity 5.6 Ci/mmol; NEN Chemicals, Boston, Mass., USA) dissolved in 0.1 ml of saline containing 0.01 mg of bovine serum albumin and 3mM NaN_3; 0.1 ml of the unlabelled cholic acid standard solution or 0.1 ml of the thin-layer chromatographically separated serum sample dissolved in saline containing 4 g/l bovine serum albumin and 3mM NaN_3; and 0.5 ml of the cholic acid antibody-Sepharose solution (1 : 3 dilution of the cholic acid antibody-Sepharose stock solution diluted with 0.01M phosphate buffer, 1M NaCl, 3mM NaN_3, pH7.4). Incubation and separation of antibody-bound and antibody-free antigen was performed as described by van den Berg et al. [8]. The sample values were extrapolated from a straight-line standard curve which was linear between 5 and 200 pmol of unlabelled cholic acid (see Fig.3). The coefficient of variation between samples was 5%.

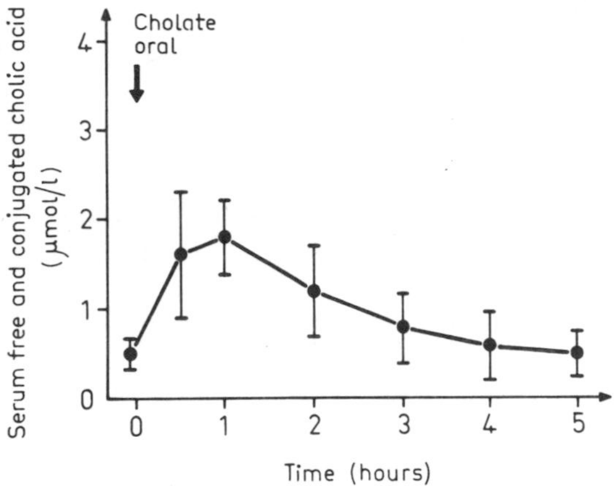

FIG.5. Effect of oral cholate administration – 0.5 g or 7 mg/kg body weight – on free and conjugated cholic acid levels (mean ± SE) in serum of nine healthy fasting subjects. (The fasting value was not subtracted.)

ORAL CHOLATE TOLERANCE TEST

Oral administration of 0.5 g of cholate or about 7 mg of cholate per kg body weight to nine fasting healthy volunteers caused an elevation of peripheral serum cholic acid levels (Fig.4) which represents incomplete hepatic clearance of the bile acid absorbed from the intestine. Intestinal diseases do not disturb the intestinal absorption of the administered unconjugated cholate, as patients with regional ileitis (Crohn's disease), distal ileal resection (1.3 m) or idiopathic diarrhoea did not show significantly less elevation of the peripheral serum cholic acid concentrations after oral cholate administration than that shown by the healthy subjects (Fig.4). This can be explained by the absorption of the unconjugated cholic acid in the whole small intestine. Furthermore, since in healthy subjects and in patients with hepatobiliary diseases and hepato-renal syndrome, the urinary excretion of intraveneously injected labelled cholic acid-24-[^{14}C] was less than 5% during 24 hours after the injection [21], the degree of elevation of peripheral serum cholic acid levels after oral cholate administration is also independent of renal function and depends on the hepatic clearance of the intestinal absorbed bile acid. Therefore, the degree of elevation of peripheral cholic acid levels in serum after oral cholate administration reflects the hepatic extraction of intestinal absorbed bile acid, which depends on liver function and shunting from portal to systemic circulation. Thus, for healthy subjects and for patients with liver disease, the area under the cholic acid concentration versus

TABLE III. COMPARISON BETWEEN THE NUMBER OF PATIENTS WITH ELEVATED FASTING SERUM CONJUGATED CHOLIC ACID CONCENTRATIONS (> 1.0 μmol/l) AND THE NUMBER OF PATIENTS WITH ELEVATED SERUM FREE AND CONJUGATED CHOLIC ACID LEVELS AFTER ORAL CHOLATE ADMINISTRATION (> 2.8 μmol/l) IN DIFFERENT LIVER DISEASE (For values in healthy subjects, see Fig.5).

Diagnosis	Total number of patients	Number of patients with elevated free and conjugated cholic acid levels in serum				
		Fasting (> 1.0 μmol/1)	After cholate administration (> 2.8 μmol/l)			
			1/2h	1h	2h	3h
Fatty liver/fatty liver hepatitis	5	2	4	0	0	0
Granulomatous hepatitis	3	0	2	0	0	0
Cirrhosis without portal hypertension	10	3	4	1	2	1
Cirrhosis with portal hypertension	17	15	17	0	0	0
Extrahepatic cholestasis	4	4	4	0	0	0

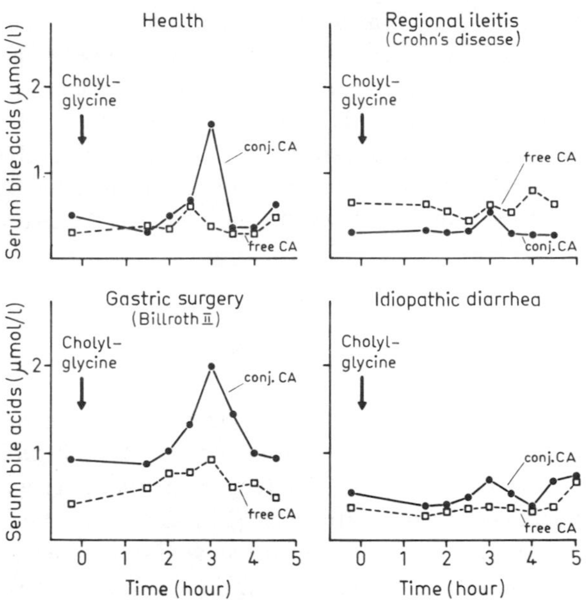

FIG.6. Effect of oral cholylglycine administration – 0.5 g or about 7 mg/kg body weight – on serum conjugated cholic acid (conj. CA) and unconjugated cholic acid (free CA) levels in a healthy subject, a patient with gastric resection (Billroth II), a patient with extensive regional ileitis (Crohn's disease) and a patient with idiopathic diarrhoea.

time curve of the "oral cholate tolerance test", which was integrated between 0 and 2 hours after oral cholate administration

$$\left(\int_0^2 C(t)\,dt\right),$$

increases with increasing severity of the liver injury (see Table II). This reflects an increased disturbance of the hepatic fractional extraction of cholic acid from portal blood and shunting from portal to systemic circulation.

As the measurement of serum bile acids in fasting subjects has been claimed to be a more sensitive indicator of disease activity than conventional tests of liver function [22], we investigated whether the determination of free and conjugated cholic acids in serum after oral cholate administration is an even more sensitive test of liver function than is the concentration of conjugated cholic acid in serum of fasting subjects. In nine fasting healthy volunteers the conjugated cholic acid concentrations in the serum did not exceed 1.0 μmol/l before cholate administration, and the free and conjugated cholic acid levels (without subtraction of the value for conjugated cholic acid in serum during fasting) did not exceed

2.8 μmol/l within 5 hours after oral cholate administration of about 7 mg cholate/kg body weight (Fig.5). A comparison of the number of patients with elevated fasting conjugated cholic acid concentrations in serum (> 1.0 μmol/l) and the number of the patients with elevated free and conjugated cholic acid levels within 3 hours of oral cholate administration (> 2.8 μmol/l) in different liver diseases shows (see Table III) that the "oral cholate tolerance test" is a more sensitive indicator of liver function than the bile acid levels in serum of fasting subjects.

ORAL CHOLYLGLYCINE TOLERANCE TEST

Conjugated cholic acid (for example cholylglycine) is mainly absorbed in the distal ileum by an active transport mechanism and only a small part is deconjugated to give free cholic acid and a small part 7α-dehydroxylated to give conjugated or free deoxycholic acid per enterohepatic cycle [23]. Since in patients with normal liver function the major factor determining peripheral serum bile acid concentrations is the rate of intestinal bile acid absorption [24], the determination of the kinetics of conjugated cholic acid, free cholic acid and conjugated deoxycholic acid in serum after oral cholylglycine administration might be useful clinically for characterization of intestinal function in diarrhoeal states. Therefore an "oral cholylglycine tolerance test" was performed, that is the determination of the kinetics of free cholic acid, conjugated cholic acid and conjugated deoxycholic acid in serum before and after oral administration of 0.5 g of cholylglycine or about 7 mg of cholylglycine/kg body weight to fasting subjects.

As exemplified in Fig.6, the patient with extensive regional ileitis (Crohn's disease) and the patient with idiopathic diarrhoea showed, in contrast to the healthy subject and the patient with gastric resection (Billroth II), no elevation of peripheral serum conjugated cholic acid levels after oral cholylglycine administration, reflecting a disturbed intestinal absorption of the conjugated bile acid. Thus, the "oral cholylglycine tolerance test" might be a useful test for bile acid malabsorption.

REFERENCES

[1] SANDBERG, D.H., SJÖVALL, J., SJÖVALL, K., TURNER, D.A., J. Lipid Res. **6** (1965) 182.

[2] MAKINO, I., NAKAGAWA, S., MASHIMO, K., Gastroenterology **56** (1969) 1033.

[3] KAPLOWITZ, N., KOK, E., JAVITT, N.B., J. Am. Med. Assoc. **225** (1973) 292.

[4] HOFMANN, A.F., SIMMONDS, W.J., KORMAN, M.G., LaRUSSO, N. F., HOFFMAN, N.E., "Radioimmunoassay of bile acids", Advances in Bile Acid Research (MATERN, S., HACKENSCHMIDT, J., BACK, P., GEROK, W., Eds), F.K. Schattauer Verlag, Stuttgart-New York (1975) 95.

[5] SIMMONDS, W.J., KORMAN, M.G., GO, V.L.W., HOFMANN, A.F., Gastroenterology **65** (1973) 705.
[6] MURPHY, G.M., EDKINS, S.M., WILLIAMS, J.W., GATTY, D., Clin. Chim. Acta **54** (1974) 81.
[7] MATERN, S., KRIEGER, R., GEROK, W., Clin. Chim. Acta **72** (1976) 39.
[8] VAN DEN BERG, J.W.O., VAN BLANKENSTEIN, M., BOSMAN-JACOBS, E.P., FRENKEL, M., HÖRCHNER, P., OOST-HARWIG, O.I., WILSON, J.H.P., Clin. Chim. Acta **73** (1976) 277.
[9] MIHAS, A.A., SPENNEY, J.G., HIRSCHOWITZ, B.I., GIBSON, R.G., Clin. Chim. Acta **76** (1977) 389.
[10] DEMERS, L.M., HEPNER, G.; Clin. Chem. **22** 5 (1976) 602.
[11] MATERN, S., HAAG, M., HANS, Ch., GEROK, W., Bile Acid Metabolism in Health and Disease (PAUMGARTNER, G., STIEHL, A., Eds), MTP Press Ltd., Lancaster (1977) 253.
[12] MATERN, S., KRIEGER, R., HANS, C., GEROK, W., Scand. J. Gastroent. **12** (in press).
[13] ERLANGER, B.F., BOREK, F., BEISER, S.M., LIEBERMAN, S., J. Biol. Chem. **228** (1957) 713.
[14] MATERN, S., LIOMIN, E., BUSCHER, H., OEHLERT, W., GEROK, W., Digestion **12** (1975) 331.
[15] MATERN, S., SCHMIDT, C., BUSCHER, H., OEHLERT, W., GEROK, W., Verh. Dtsch. Ges. Inn. Med. **81** (1975) 1308.
[16] CRONHOLM, T., ERIKSSON, H., MATERN, S., SJÖVALL, J., Eur. J. Biochem. **53** (1975) 405.
[17] MATERN, S., SJÖVALL, J., POMARE, E.W., HEATON, K.W., LOW-BEER, T.S., Med. Biol. **53** (1975) 107.
[18] BOCK, K.W., MATERN, S., Eur. J. Biochem. **38** (1973) 20.
[19] MAKINO, I., SJÖVALL, J., Analyt. Letters **5** (1972) 341.
[20] BRUUSGAARD, A., Clin. Chim. Acta **28** (1970) 495.
[21] ALSTRÖM, T., NORMAN, A., Acta Med. Scand. **191** (1972) 521.
[22] KORMAN, M.G., HOFMANN, A.F., SUMMERSKILL, W.H.L., New Engl. J. Med. **290** (1974) 1399.
[23] HEPNER, G.W., HOFMANN, A.F., THOMAS, P.J., J. Clin. Invest. **51** (1972) 1889.
[24] LaRUSSO, N.F., KORMAN, M.G., HOFFMAN, N.E., HOFMANN, A.F., New Engl. J. Med. **291** (1974) 689.

DISCUSSION

R. VIHKO: Did you perform cholic acid tolerance tests by intravenous administration of the bile salt? In this way the potential error of abnormalities in absorption of cholic acid given orally could be avoided.

S. MATERN: We did not, because we found that intestinal diseases did not disturb the outcome of tests in which the cholic acid was administered orally.

RADIOIMMUNOASSAY OF PRIMARY AND SECONDARY BILE ACIDS IN SERUM WITH SPECIFIC ANTISERA AND ^{125}I-LABELLED LIGANDS

O.A. JÄNNE, O.K. MÄENTAUSTA
University of Oulu,
Oulu, Finland

Abstract

RADIOIMMUNOASSAY OF PRIMARY AND SECONDARY BILE ACIDS IN SERUM WITH SPECIFIC ANTISERA AND ^{125}I-LABELLED LIGANDS.

The authors have developed methods for radioimmunological determination of two primary (cholic acid and chenodeoxycholic acid) and two secondary (deoxycholic acid and lithocholic acid) bile acid conjugates from human serum. The antibodies against BSA conjugates of the different bile salts were raised in rabbits. ^{125}I-iodohistaminyl-bile acid conjugates were prepared with a Chloramine-T labelling technique, purified by thin-layer chromatography and subsequently used as tracers in the RIA. The method for radioimmunoassay of serum bile acids was briefly as follows: (i) precipitation of serum (0.1 ml) with 9 vols of absolute ethanol; (ii) evaporation of duplicate 0.1–0.2 ml aliquots from ethanol to dryness; (iii) redissolving of the residue in 0.01M phosphate buffer, pH 7.4, and incubation of the samples in the presence of an appropriate antiserum and ^{125}I-iodohistaminyl bile acid (ca. 25 000 counts/min per tube) at + 4°C for 14–18 h; (iv) precipitation of bound radioactivity with polyethylene glycol (final concentration 12.5%), and (v) counting of the precipitate with a gamma-counter. The sensitivity of the present methodology permits determination of all the four bile salts from 0.1 ml of serum. The recoveries of cholylglycine and chenodeoxy-cholylglycine added to serum were excellent and no blank values were noticed in assays of bile acid-free sera. Serum cholic acid conjugate levels in normal female and male serum (n = 47) were 0.51 ± 0.09 μmol/1, while chenodeoxycholic acid conjugate concentrations were 0.78 ± 0.59 μmol/l. Greatly elevated levels of these two primary bile salts were determined in sera from patients suffering from intrahepatic cholestasis during pregnancy (3.8–78.4 μmol/l for cholic acid conjugates and 0.96–40.9 μmol/l for chenodeoxycholic acid conjugates).

1. INTRODUCTION

Reports from a number of laboratories have indicated the usefulness of serum bile acid estimations in the early detection of disturbed liver function [1–5]. In the past, techniques utilized for measurement of serum bile salts have been rather insensitive, cumbersome and tedious, thus preventing a large-scale application of these determinations to clinical chemistry. The introduction in 1973 of a radioimmunoassay (RIA) for conjugates of cholic acid in human serum [1] has rendered bile salt estimations much simpler and more easily applicable to routine clinical chemical work. In almost all contemporary RIA techniques for serum bile acid measurements, however, only tritium-labelled ligands have been employed [1, 5–9] which necessitates liquid scintillation counting. To further simplify serum bile salt determinations we have developed techniques for labelling bile acids with $Na^{125}I$ and for purifying the radiolabelled products, and have subsequently used individual ^{125}I-radiolabelled bile acids as tracers in the radioimmunoassay for primary and secondary bile acid conjugates from human serum.

2. MATERIALS AND METHODS

2.1. Chemicals

Non-radioactive bile salts were purchased from Steraloids, Inc., Wilton, NH, USA, 1-ethyl-3-(dimethylaminopropyl)-carbodiimide-HC1 (EDC) from Fluka AG, Bucks, Switzerland, $Na^{125}I$ (SA 11–17 Ci/μg) from the Radiochemical Centre, Amersham, UK and various tritium-labelled bile acids from New England Nuclear, Boston, Mass., USA. When not otherwise indicated, other chemicals were from Merck AG, Darmstadt, the Federal Republic of Germany, and were of the highest purity grade available.

2.2. Preparation of immunogens

Various bile acid conjugates were joined to fatty acid-free BSA [10] by the carbodiimide reaction as follows: 5 mg of EDC were first mixed with 5 mg of BSA in 1 ml of water, after which 5 mg of the individual bile acid (in 0.2 ml pyridine) were added. To monitor the efficiency of the coupling reaction, each reaction mixture also contained the corresponding ^{3}H-labelled bile acid conjugate (ca. 3×10^{6} counts/min in 0.05 ml ethanol). The pH of the reaction was kept at 5.4 with the aid of 1M HCl. The reaction was allowed to proceed for 72 h at room temperature. After dialysis of the product against distilled water, the ^{3}H-content of the bile acid-BSA complex was measured, and the conjugates were subsequently used for immunization of rabbits. Under the above conditions, 20–35% of the bile salts were conjugated to BSA and the following molar bile salt/BSA ratios in the immunogens were obtained: cholylglycine (CG)/BSA 25/1; chenodeoxycholylglycine (CDCG)/BSA 28/1; deoxycholylglycine (DCG)/BSA 24/1, and lithocholylglycine (LCG)/BSA 44/1.

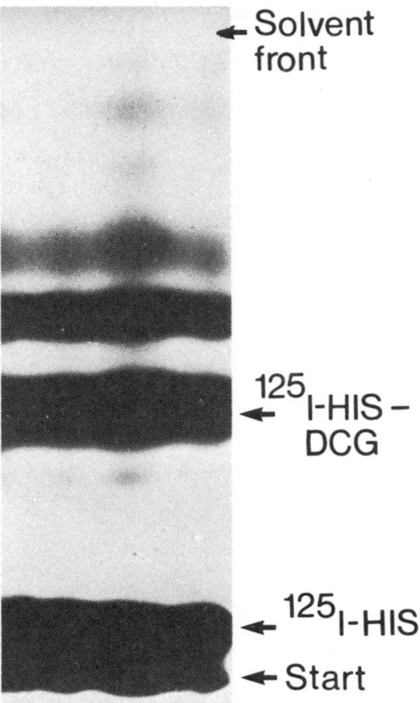

FIG.1. Autoradiograph of the thin-layer chromatography plate employed for the purification of ^{125}I-iodohistaminyl-deoxycholyl glycine (^{125}I-HIS-DCG) from other reaction products (^{125}I-HIS = ^{125}I-iodohistamine). The solvent system employed was n-butanol: acetic acid: water (85:10:5, by vol.).

2.3. Immunizations

Rabbits were injected intradermally at multiple sites with 0.5–1.0 mg of the immunogen emulsified with Freund's complete adjuvant. The immunogens were first given at one-week intervals for one month and then at one-month intervals. Serum was harvested 7–10 days after each booster injection, and stored at -20°C until use.

2.4. Preparation of ^{125}I-labelled bile acid conjugates

Synthesis of bile acid-histamine complexes: 3.3 μmol of histamine-HCl and 5.2 μmol of EDC were first dissolved in 0.2 ml of water, after which 2.0 μmol of glycine-conjugated bile acid in 0.04 ml pyridine were added to the solution, which was adjusted to pH 5.4 with 1M HCl. The reaction was allowed to continue for 72 h at room temperature. This mixture was used directly in the radioiodination and no attempt to separate free histamine from histaminyl-bile acid was made.

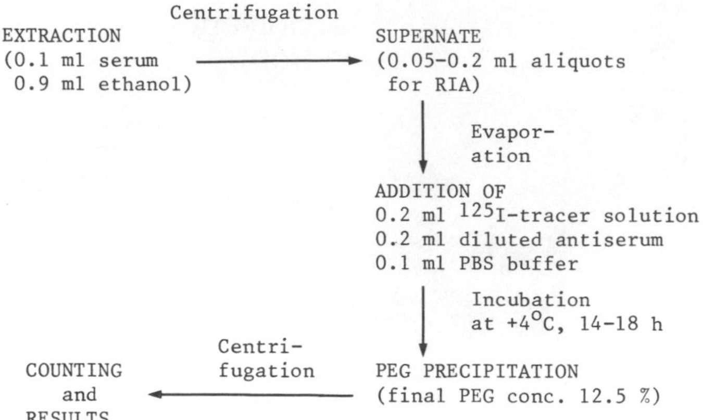

FIG.2. Flow diagram of the method for determination of serum CG, CDCG, DCG and LCG.

Radioiodination of histaminyl-bile acids: Approximately 100 nmol of bile acid-histamine complex was radioiodinated with the Chloramine-T technique principally as described by Nars and Hunter [11], employing 1 mCi of $Na^{125}I$ and 0.1M phosphate buffer, pH 7.4. The reaction time was 60 s. After addition of 150 μg of sodium metabisulphite (in 0.01 ml phosphate buffer), the reaction mixture was diluted with 0.5 ml of phosphate buffer, and the radiolabelled bile acid conjugates extracted with 1 ml of n-butanol.

Purification of the labelled ligands: The extracted bile acids in n-butanol were applied onto a silica gel (F 254) thin-layer chromatography plate and run in a solvent system n-butanol:acetic acid:water (85:10:5, by vol.). Radioiodinated bile acids were located with the aid of radioautography, scraped off the plate and eluted from the silicic acid with 2 ml of methanol, in which they were stored at +4°C. In the above solvent system, ^{125}I-iodohistaminyl-bile acids had the following R_f values: HIS-CG 0.19; HIS-CDCG 0.59; HIS-DCG 0.34 and HIS-LCG 0.48. The R_f for free ^{125}I-iodohistamine was 0.09. An example of the autoradiogram from the purification of ^{125}I-iodohistaminyl-DCG is shown in Fig. 1.

2.5. Radioimmunoassay conditions for serum bile acid measurement

A flow sheet of the RIA method is shown in Fig. 2. Bile acids were extracted from the serum by adding 9 vols of absolute ethanol to serum (usually 0.9 ml ethanol per 0.1 ml serum). The resulting mixture was vortexed for 15 s and then centrifuged at 1500 × g for 10 min. Two portions (0.1 and 0.2 ml) from each

TABLE I. SPECIFICITY OF THE ANTISERA AGAINST BSA-CONJUGATES OF CHOLYLGLYCINE (CG), CHENODEOXYCHOLYLGLYCINE (CDCG), DEOXYCHOLYLGLYCINE (DCG) AND LITHOCHOLYLGLYCINE (LCG)

Antigen	Antiserum against			
	CG	CDCG	DCG	LCG
Cholic acid	100	0.1	0.2	–
Cholylglycine	100	0.8	0.1	–
Cholyltaurine	100	0.4	1.3	–
Chenodeoxycholic acid	1.5	100	–	1.2
Chenodeoxycholylglycine	4.2	100	0.5	1.2
Chenodeoxycholyltaurine	1.3	50	1.1	1.2
Deoxycholic acid	0.9	–	30	–
Deoxycholylglycine	1.2	–	100	3.4
Deoxycholyltaurine	3.7	–	50	1.7
Lithocholic acid	0.1	0.6	30	100
Lithocholylglycine	1.4	8.0	100	100
Lithocholyltaurine	0.3	1.5	100	100

– = Less than 0.1% displacement of the corresponding ^{125}I-iodohistaminyl-bile acid.

supernatant in duplicate were transferred into disposable glass tubes and evaporated to dryness. The dry residue was dissolved in 0.1 ml of 0.01M phosphate-buffered saline (PBS), pH 7.4. After addition of the appropriate ^{125}I-iodohistaminyl-bile acid tracer (ca. 25 000 counts/min per tube in 0.2 ml PBS containing 0.2% human gamma globulin) and diluted antiserum (in 0.2 ml of PBS-gamma globulin buffer) the samples were incubated for 14–18 h at +4°C. Precipitation of the bound antigen was achieved by polyethylene glycol (Carbowax 6000) at a final concentration of 12.5%. After centrifuging for 45 min at +4°C at 2000 × g, the supernatants were aspirated and the radioactivity of the tubes counted in a gamma-counter (LKB-Wallac 1280 Ultro gamma). Each series of assays also contained a standard curve with 0 to 200 pmol/tube of the corresponding bile acid. The standards were processed in a manner identical with that of serum samples. The working dilutions of the antisera used for the determination of individual bile salts were as follows: CG 1 : 20 000; CDCG 1 : 10 000; DCG 1 : 10 000 and LCG 1 : 6 000.

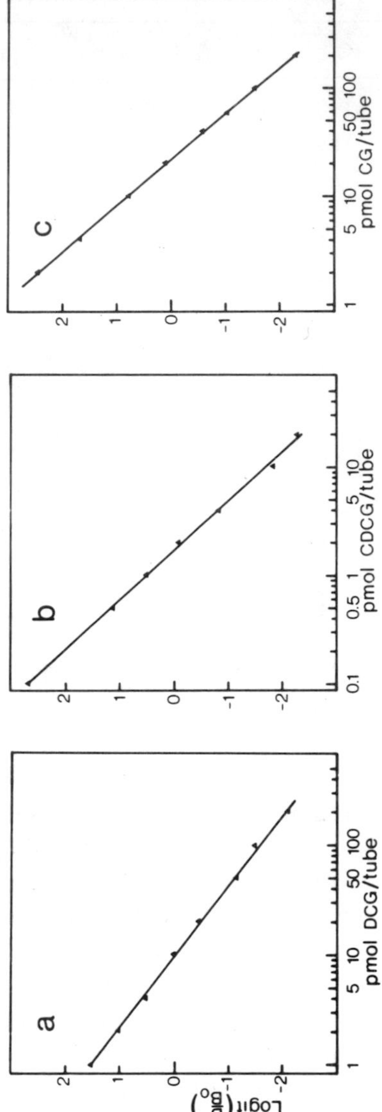

FIG.3. Standard curves for the radioimmunoassay of deoxycholylglycine (DCG, 3a), chenodeoxycholylglycine (CDCG, 3b) and cholylglycine (CG, 3c).

3. RESULTS

3.1. Specificity of the antisera

Table I illustrates the specificity of the antisera raised in rabbits against the two primary (CG and CDCG) and two secondary (DCG and LCG) bile acid conjugates. As seen in the table, the individual antisera were fairly group specific, i.e. they only cross-reacted with a given grimary or secondary bile acid and its conjugates.

3.2. Characteristics of the RIA procedure

Figure 3 shows standard curves for the assays of DCG, CDCG and CG. With the present methodology, normally circulating serum bile acid concentrations were easily measurable from a 0.1-ml serum sample, since the linear ranges of the standard curves were from 1 to 50 pmol for DCG (3a), from 0.5 to 20 pmol for CDCG (3b) and from 2 to 100 pmol for CG (3c). When CG and CDCG were added to serum at various concentrations (10–100 pmol), their recoveries were very good, being 94–113%. The blank values, studied by taking samples from bile acid-free serum through the entire procedure were always negligible. The intra-assay variation coefficients were 3.4% for CG-RIA and 3.2% for CDCG-RIA, while inter-assay variation coefficients were 11.2% and 10.0%, respectively. The assays were routinely performed at +4°C for 14–18 h, although an incubation for 2 h at +37°C yielded similar results.

3.3. Serum bile acid levels

Cholylglycine (CG) and chenodeoxycholylglycine (CDCG) values measured by the present RIAs from serum samples from normal females and males were as follows: 0.51 ± 0.09 μmol/l for CG and 0.78 ± 0.59 μmol/l for CDCG (n = 47). The corresponding values for women during early pregnancy were 0.24 ± 0.02 μmol/l for CG and 0.46 ± 0.15 μmol/l for CDCG (n = 15), while the values measured at late pregnancy were 0.65 ± 0.03 μmol/l for CG and 0.37 ± 0.01 μmol/l for CDCG (n = 7). Bile acid levels were greatly elevated in sera collected from patients suffering from intrahepatic cholestasis during pregnancy, being 22.5 (3.8–78.4) μmol/l for CG and 8.5 (0.96–40.9) μmol/l for CDCG. Since the antisera used in the present RIAs cross-reacted with a given bile acid and its conjugates, the values depicted above represent total serum cholic acid and chenodeoxycholic acid concentrations rather than the glycine conjugate levels only.

4. DISCUSSION

In the present investigation, we have prepared ^{125}I-iodohistaminyl-bile acid conjugates and used them as tracers in the RIA for two primary and two secondary bile acids in human serum. The antisera used were rather group specific and cross-reacted only with one bile acid and its glycine and taurine conjugates, with the exception that the deoxycholic acid antiserum also recognized some monohydroxy bile acids (Table I). The sensitivity of the methods allows a very convenient measurement of bile acid conjugates from normal and phathological sera, since only 0.1 ml of serum is needed for the assay of all the four bile salts. A simple ethanol extraction was used for serum before RIA, since the binding of bile acids to serum proteins was found to cause spurious results in the final RIA: serial dilutions of serum did not give identical values, but higher concentrations were measured from more diluted samples. The same has also been reported by Murphy et al. [6].

The values for serum CG and CDCG in normal female and male serum were in good agreement with those reported by others using either RIA or gas-liquid chromatography [1, 5–8]. Our RIA results were also compared with values measured by gas-liquid chromatography in the case of about 40 serum samples, and a close agreement between the values was found (Mäentausta, Laatikainen and Jänne, to be published).

In harmony with reports by Sjövall and Sjövall [12] and Laatikainen and Hesso [4], all the patients with intrahepatic cholestasis of pregnancy showed elevated concentrations of serum cholic acid and chenodeoxycholic acid conjugates, the former being clearly more elevated. This further supports the consensus of opinion expressed in recent publications from several laboratories [1–5] which has emphasized the usefulness of serum bile salt estimations in early detection of disturbed liver function. The RIA method presented in this work is simple and convenient to handle and offers, therefore, a potential tool for the large-scale monitoring of liver function by serum bile acid estimations.

REFERENCES

[1] SIMMONDS, W.J., KORMAN, M.G., GO, V.L.W., HOFMANN, A.F., Gastroenterology **65** (1973) 705.

[2] KORMAN, M.G., HOFMANN, A.F., SUMMERSKILL, W.H.J., New Engl. J. Med. **290** (1974) 1399.

[3] KOPLOWITZ, N., KOK, M.S., JAVITT, N.B., J. Am. Med. Assoc. **225** (1973) 292.

[4] LAATIKAINEN, T., HESSO, A., Clin. Chim. Acta **64** (1975) 63.

[5] DEMERS, L.M., HEPNER, G., Clin. Chem. **22** (1976) 602.

[6] MURPHY, G.M., EDKINS, S.M., WILLIAMS, J.W., CATTY, D., Clin. Chim. Acta **54** (1974) 81.

[7] MATERN, S., KRIEGER, R., GEROK, W., Clin. Chim. Acta **72** (1976) 39.
[8] MIHAS, A.A., SPENNEY, J.G., HIRSCHOWITZ, B.I., GIBSON, R.G., Clin. Chim. Acta **76** (1977) 389.
[9] SPENNEY, J.G., JOHNSON, B.J., HIRSCHOWITZ, B.I., MIHAS, A.A., GIBSON, R., Gastroenterology **72** (1977) 305.
[10] CHEN, R.F., J. Biol. Chem. **242** (1967) 173.
[11] NARS, P.W., HUNTER, W.M., J. Endocrinol. **57** (1973) xlvii.
[12] SJÖVALL, K., SJÖVALL, J., Clin. Chim. Acta **13** (1966) 207.

DISCUSSION

S. MATERN: I have a question concerning the specificity of the bile acid antisera, especially the specificity of the antiserum against lithocholyl conjugates. Did the latter antiserum also cross-react with sulphated lithocholyl conjugates?

O.A. JÄNNE: We have not yet tested the cross-reactivity of sulphated lithocholic acid derivatives in the lithocholic acid RIA.

THE RADIOIMMUNOASSAY OF CLOMIPRAMINE (ANAFRANIL-GEIGY)
A tricyclic antidepressant

G.F. READ, D. RIAD-FAHMY
Tenovus Institute for Cancer Research,
Welsh National School of Medicine,
Cardiff, United Kingdom

Abstract

THE RADIOIMMUNOASSAY OF CLOMIPRAMINE (ANAFRANIL-GEIGY): A TRICYCLIC ANTIDEPRESSANT.

A radioimmunoassay has been developed for the tricyclic antidepressant, clomipramine (Anafranil-Geigy) which allows accurate determination of plasma levels without a pre-assay purification step. This is achieved by generation of specific antisera using an antigen produced by conjugation of clomipramine to bovine serum albumin via the 10, 11 bridge positions. As expected, cross-reaction of the pharmacologically active major metabolite, desmethylclomipramine was $< 5\%$ and that of didesmethylclomipramine $< 1\%$. Specificity was confirmed by comparing titres achieved in the routine assay with those observed in an assay incorporating a pre-assay thin-layer chromatographic purification step. Pharmacokinetic data were in agreement with double radioisotope derivative assays and also with previously reported assays using GC or GC/MS techniques. The sensitivity is superior to any previous assay known to us for this class of compound. The specificity and precision, coupled with the high sample turnover (greater than 300 samples a week per technician), make the assay ideal for supervision of patient compliance and routine assay of samples generated in large clinical trials.

Clomipramine, a lipophilic, tricyclic drug (Fig.1), is widely used in the treatment of depression. Considerable interest exists in the correlation between therapeutic response and circulating clomipramine concentrations, since marked differences in plasma levels have been reported for patients on the same drug regimen. Although many methods exist for measuring tricyclic drugs, only those based on gas chromatography/mass spectrometry (GC/MS) [1] or double radioisotope derivative (DRID) techniques [2] have the required sensitivity, specificity and accuracy. A major drawback of both methods, however, is their relatively low sample throughput capability and, in addition, GC/MS requires a large capital investment. A radioimmunoassay (RIA), however, combines specificity, sensitivity and accuracy with the ability to handle large numbers of samples. Such an assay has been established.

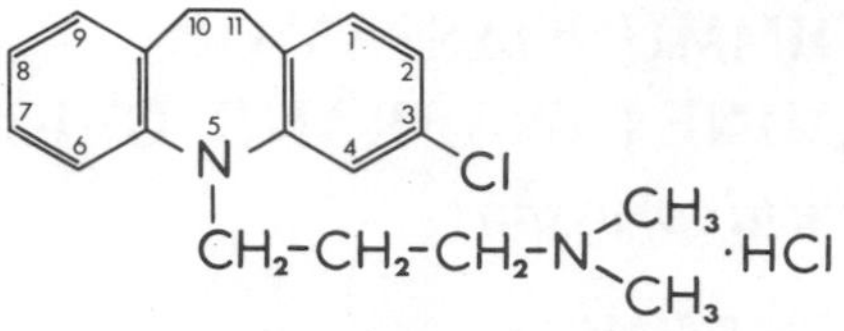

ANAFRANIL (CLOMIPRAMINE)
3-chloro-5-(3-dimethylaminopropyl)-10,
11-dihydro-5H-dibenz [b,f] azepine
hydrochloride

FIG.1. Clomipramine, showing the numbering system.

An antiserum of high specificity obviates the need for chromatography and is mandatory for high sample throughput. This requires a rational choice of antigen. Previous studies on the RIA of tricyclic drugs have produced antisera of relatively poor specificity because of a non-optimal choice of antigen. Nortriptyline antisera prepared by coupling through the terminal amino group of the side chain had a cross-reaction of 153% with the related compound, amitriptyline [3]. Antisera raised against imipramine coupled by the diazo reaction to an antigenic protein, have 100% cross-reaction with all side-chain metabolites [4]. Detailed studies on clomipramine metabolism are lacking, but information is available for the closely related non-chlorinated compound, imipramine. Such studies indicate that 10,11-hydroxy compounds are not likely to be major metabolites. This compound was therefore synthesized and coupled to bovine serum albumin by conventional techniques, and an immunization programme was started in four rabbits. The antiserum having the highest titre with the radioligand [10,11-$^3H_2$]-clomipramine, specific activity 39 Ci/mmole, was therefore chosen for specificity studies. Cross-reactions are shown in Table I. The cross-reactions of drugs often given concomitantly with Anafranil, namely Librium, Valium and Mogadon, are negligible. The cross-reaction of desmethylclomipramine, a major metabolite known to have antidepressant properties, is, as predicted, low and that of didesmethylclomipramine is negligible. The cross-reactions of other sterically similar tricyclic drugs, imipramine and amitriptyline, are significant but are not co-administered with Anafranil, and therefore cause no interference.

A ten-point standard curve was set up covering the range of 0–200 pg and the coefficient of variation at each point in twenty replicate assays was in no case greater than 4.0%. The sensitivity of the curve was less than 10 pg, corresponding to a plasma level of less than 0.2 ng/ml. This is significantly lower than other published methods and is adequate for assaying all samples currently envisaged. Samples from patients receiving placebo only did not differ from zero.

TABLE I. CROSS-REACTIONS OF ANTI-ANAFRANIL SERUM R_3b_3

Compound	Cross-reaction (%)	Compound	Cross-reaction (%)
Clomipramine	100	Amitriptyline	7.0
Desmethyl-clomipramine	4.1	Nortriptyline	0.55
Didesmethyl-clomipramine	0.74	Chlorpromazine	13.0
Imipramine	20	Chlordiazepoxide	<0.002
Desmethyl-imipramine	0.55	Carbamazepine	<0.002
Prothiaden	19	Nitrazepam	<0.002
Maprotiline	0.34	Diazepam	<0.002

The extraction procedure is based on standard methods. Plasma aliquots, in duplicate, were made alkaline with ammonia/saline, then extracted with redistilled petroleum ether. After extraction, samples were deep-frozen for one hour: this allowed the organic phase to be decanted and minimized carry-over of base into the petroleum ether. Extracts and standards were dried down together under nitrogen, and then taken up and incubated with antiserum at 30°C. [^{3}H]-Radioligand was added before a second incubation at 30°C for one hour. Free and bound steroid were then separated by dextran-coated charcoal and aliquots of supernatant taken for scintillation counting.

The efficiency of the extraction procedure was checked by monitoring the recovery of [^{3}H]-clomipramine, pre-incubated overnight in plasma containing 10 and 250 pg/assay tube. Recoveries were 96 ± 2.1%, n = 11; and 95.5 ± 2.2%, n = 12, respectively. A further check on the assay was performed by the serial-dilution procedure. A sample known to assay at high titre was diluted with varying volumes of a blank plasma. On plotting the apparent titre against the volume of high-titre plasma taken, a correlation r = 0.994 was observed.

In the absence of detailed metabolic studies on the fate of clomipramine in man, it was necessary to rule out the possibility of some unforeseen metabolite contributing to the apparent titre. This was checked by investigating the effect of a pre-assay thin-layer chromatographic step. The system chosen had been shown to separate clomipramine from its bridge and ring metabolites, and from its desmethyl derivatives. Samples were taken from a patient who had been on high dose Anafranil (150 mg/day) for at least 14 days who would be expected to show maximum metabolism of the drug. In no case did the difference between titres, achieved with and without the TLC purification step, exceed the calculated inter-assay variance.

The clinical value of the assay was evaluated by assaying samples from several clinical trials, set up to correlate clinical response and drug levels in plasma. The high throughput of the assay was invaluable in these studies, which generated large numbers of samples, since it allowed processing of 300 samples per week. This study showed that plasma levels determined by RIA were in accordance with previously published data [5]. In another series, samples previously assayed by the DRID technique were re-assayed by RIA and an acceptable correlation was achieved (r = 0.898, n = 60).

In conclusion, a RIA for Anafranil has been set up having adequate specificity, sensitivity and precision, which gives results in good agreement with other assay techniques whilst allowing significantly more samples to be assayed. The strategy of antigen formation is of wide application in the area of psychotropic drugs and it is likely to contribute significantly to current knowledge of the relation between plasma levels and therapeutic efficacy of this important class of compounds.

REFERENCES

[1] DUBOIS, J.P., Clin. Chem. **22** (1976) 892.
[2] CARNIS, G., GODBILLON, J., METAYER, J.P., Clin. Chem. **22** (1976) 817.
[3] AHERNE, G.W., PIALL, E.M., MARKS, V., Br. J. Clin. Pharmac. **3** (1976) 561.
[4] SPECTOR, S., SPECTOR, N.L., ALMEIDA, M.P., Psychopharmacol. Comm. **1** (1975) 421.
[5] JONES, R.B., LUSCOMBE, D., Proc. of the B.P.S. (1976) 430.

DISCUSSION

G. BOZLER: Is there any reason for not treating the standards in the same way as samples?

G.F. READ: We have good evidence for the stability of standards in ethanol and find the use of plasma standards to be wasteful in plasma. The latter is not economical unless we can thereby develop a direct assay. We have also shown that addition of ammonia/saline to the standards does not cause any significant alteration in the standard curve.

M. TORTEN: Do you have any data on the affinity of your antibodies? If you have, how do they relate to the site of conjugation?

G.F. READ: We have not performed any Scatchard plots with our antisera, so I am afraid I do not have these data.

IAEA-SM-220/63

THE SPECIFIC RADIOIMMUNOASSAY IN PHARMACOKINETICS

Its potency, requirements and development for routine use as illustrated by an assay for Pirenzepin

G. BOZLER
Dr. Karl Thomae GmbH,
Biberach,
Federal Republic of Germany

Abstract

THE SPECIFIC RADIOIMMUNOASSAY IN PHARMACOKINETICS: ITS POTENCY, REQUIREMENTS AND DEVELOPMENT FOR ROUTINE USE AS ILLUSTRATED BY AN ASSAY FOR PIRENZEPIN.

Requirements for using RIA in pharmacokinetics are specified. An assay system developed for Pirenzepin was used to illustrate the general strategy in striving mainly for specificity, sensitivity and reliability. The type of error in the final data is considered. It is a widespread assumption that weak cross-reactions with metabolites result in a 'relative' error and, therefore, have no relevance to the determination of the parent drug. In contrast to this assumption, it was shown that such weak cross-reactivity in biological samples gives rise to an 'absolute' error which is independent of concentration and analogous to that caused by a 'blank' value in chemical analysis.

1. RADIOIMMUNOASSAY IN DRUG MONITORING

To establish the pharmacokinetic profile of a new drug it is inevitable that the level of the effective compound has to be monitored with a specific and sensitive routine assay. The assay should be capable of routinely detecting nanogram, or even more often, picogram amounts of a single compound of low molecular weight in small samples (preferably 0.1 ml or less) of biological fluids. For the determination of one plasma-level curve in one person after the administration of a particular substance, it is usual that as many as 30 samples (each in triplicate) are required. It is only in the preclinical stage of an investigation that some 3 000 samples (~ 10 000 determinations) have to be handled. For example, when the plasma and urine of 10 to 12 healthy volunteers are monitored after a drug has been administered by 4 or 5 different routes.

TABLE I. CONDITIONS TO SATISFY THE REQUIREMENTS FOR RIA OF PIRENZEPIN

Requirement	mainly for:	Some conditions
Antibody		
(1) High affinity for one compound	Sensitivity,	Proper haptens
(2) Weak cross-reactivity for closely related biotransformation products	specificity	More than one hapten
Tracer		
(3) High specific activity	Sensitivity	^{3}H-labelled
(4) High degree of similiarity to the compound to be determined	Accuracy	parent compound as tracer
(5) Stability, shelf-life	Costs, reliability	
Assay procedure		
(6) Same general procedure for all drugs	Costs, suitability for automation	
(7) Minimal sample preparation	Reliability	Specific antibody
(8) Fast incubation		
(9) Easy separation of bound and free antigen	Reproducibility,	$(NH_4)_2SO_4$
(10) Proper choice of phase for counting	suitability for automation	Suitable cocktail
Evaluation		
(11) Calibration	Reliability,	A suitable curve-fitting procedure [7]
(12) Data transfer counter/calculator	automation,	Automated data transfer
(13) Protocol	documentation	Advanced calculator
(14) Evaluation of type of errors	Pharmacokinetic analysis	

RIA seems to be especially suited for this type of investigation if certain requirements for the assay system are satisfied. It is advisable to have similar assay systems for different drugs. Some conditions to meet these requirements are listed in Table I for the RIA of Pirenzepin.

Firstly, a specific antibody has to be developed taking into account the biotransformation of the active compound to very similar products. In the case of Pirenzepin (MO), two metabolites, M1 and M2, are present in biological samples.

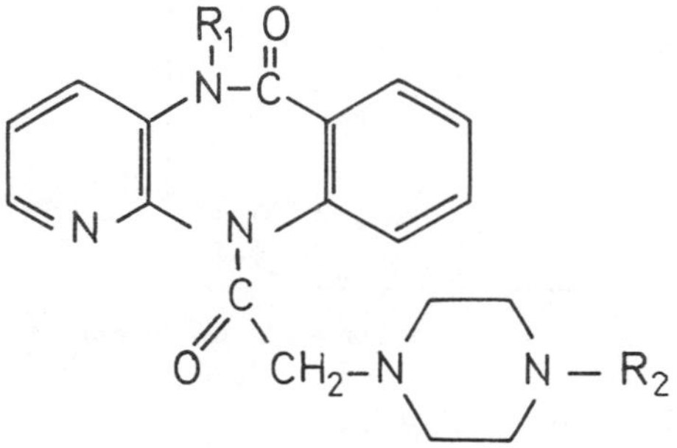

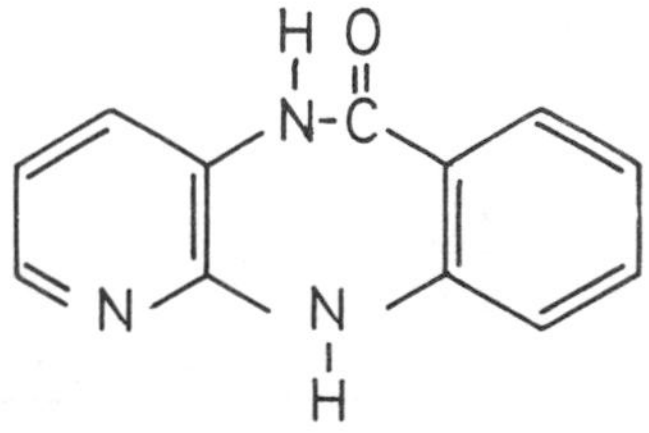

M2

MO:	$R_1 \triangleq H$	$R_2 \triangleq CH_3$
M1:	$R_1 \triangleq H$	$R_2 \triangleq H$
A1:	$R_1 \triangleq H$	$R_2 \triangleq CO(CH_2)_2COOH$
A2:	$R_2 \triangleq CH_3$	$R_1 \triangleq (CH_2)_2COOH$

To convert the compound into an immunogenic form it is linked covalently to a macromolecular carrier. Usually, simple derivatization of the compound is not sufficient to fix it in a proper topographical position on the carrier. Several analogues have to be synthesized[1] with ligands suitably located for coupling [1]. It was expected that antibodies raised against analogue A1 as hapten would specifically detect the intact tricyclus, whereas those against A2 would have more specificity for the methyl piperazine moiety. The latter was expected to be more suitable with respect to the metabolites already known.

Secondly, one major requirement for sensitivity is the availability of a suitable tracer compound. The label should be in a chemically stable position and should result in a tracer of high specific activity with a molecular structure

---

[1] The synthesis of the compounds by Dr. G. Schmidt is gratefully acknowledged.

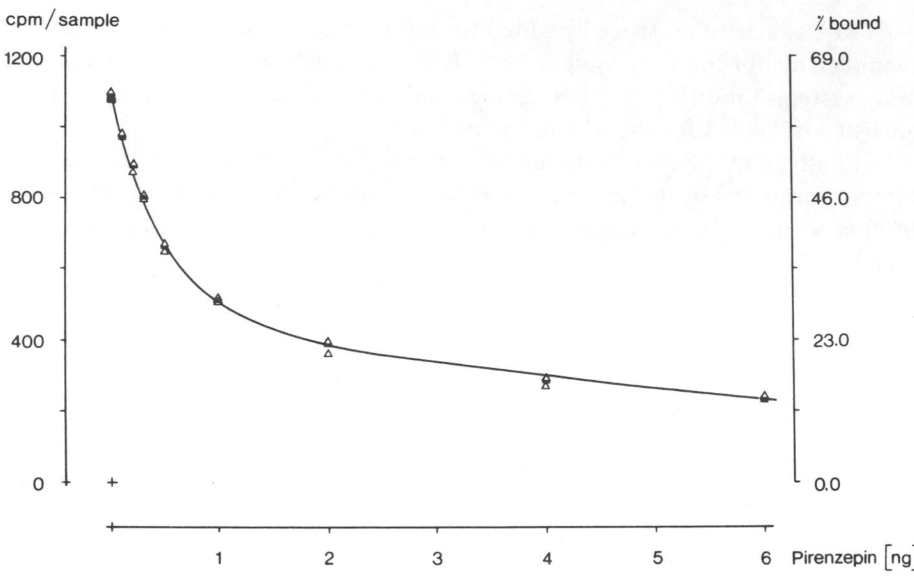

FIG.1. Typical calibration curve (assay A2) for Pirenzepin.

identical to that of the effective compound [2]. With small molecules like drugs, a ^{3}H-labelled compound would therefore be the one of choice. But still another analogue of the parent compound is necessary for the preparation of the tracer. ^{3}H-Pirenzepin (11.61 Ci/mmol) was synthesized from an analogue with a halogen substituent in the benzene moiety by a catalytic exchange reaction.

As selectivity and sensitivity are primarily established by antiserum (raised against hapten A1 and A2 in rabbits) and tracer, the reliability – that means accuracy, precision and reproducibility – is optimized by the assay procedure. The proper choice of haptens is the best strategy for avoiding laborious sample preparation [1]. In the case of Pirenzepin, the sample (plasma, urine, or saliva properly diluted with the same fluid) can be added directly to the antiserum (final concentration 1:3 000 to 1:10 000) and tracer (86 pg/0.1 ml) in buffer and incubated at 25°C for 4 h to reach equilibrium. To separate the antibody-antigen complex from free antigen, adsorption of the antigen to dextrane-coated charcoal is not advisable because of the hydrophilic nature of Pirenzepin [3]. Precipitation of the protein with $(NH_4)_2SO_4$ proved to be a useful method, especially with drugs [2]. In our laboratory we have been able to confirm these findings with all drugs so far tested (see, for example, Refs [4] and [5]).

TABLE II. INTRA-ASSAY AND INTER-ASSAY VARIATION FOR ASSAY A2 USING POOLED PLASMA CONTAINING PIRENZEPIN AND METABOLITES AT VARIOUS DILUTIONS AND A CONTROL PLASMA

No. of determinations in triplicate	Dilution	Concn of MO (pg/0.1 ml)	Coefficient of variation
Intra-assay			
5	1 + 3	570	4.6%
4	1 + 1	988	3.6%
14	1 + 3	562	4.5%
1	1 + 1	1022	–
1	1 + 0	2023	–
Inter-assay			
3	1 + 3	536	6.3%

Because of the high salt content of the supernatant it is difficult to measure the radioactivity in scintillation fluids. Instead, the precipitate may be counted after it has been rinsed, centrifuged and dissolved in H_2O. However, these additional steps are not well suited for automatic procedures. Therefore, an attempt was made to measure an aliquot of the supernatant. After mixing the aliquot with 3 volumes of MeOH and adding a scintillation mix (RIASOLVE®, W. Zinsser, Frankfurt, FRG), the clear phase above the precipitated salt contained all the activity and could be counted without any difficulty. No correction for quench is necessary because of the uniform quality of the samples.

Most of the assay is performed using automatic devices. Full automation is possible and a prototype of the respective RIAMAT [6] is already working. By using other antibodies and tracers the system is readily changed for assaying different drugs. Calibration curves were obtained by plotting the % bound against the amounts of standard added and fitting the data points to a triexponential function [7] (Fig. 1). Iterative non-linear regression analysis was performed with a desk-top calculator. Data input by punch tape prevents errors in transfer. This kind of fit has the advantage that equal weight is given to each point of the calibration curve, including the initial value without antigen added. The concentrations are automatically calculated, and the data are documented by tables and plots and recorded on magnetic discs.

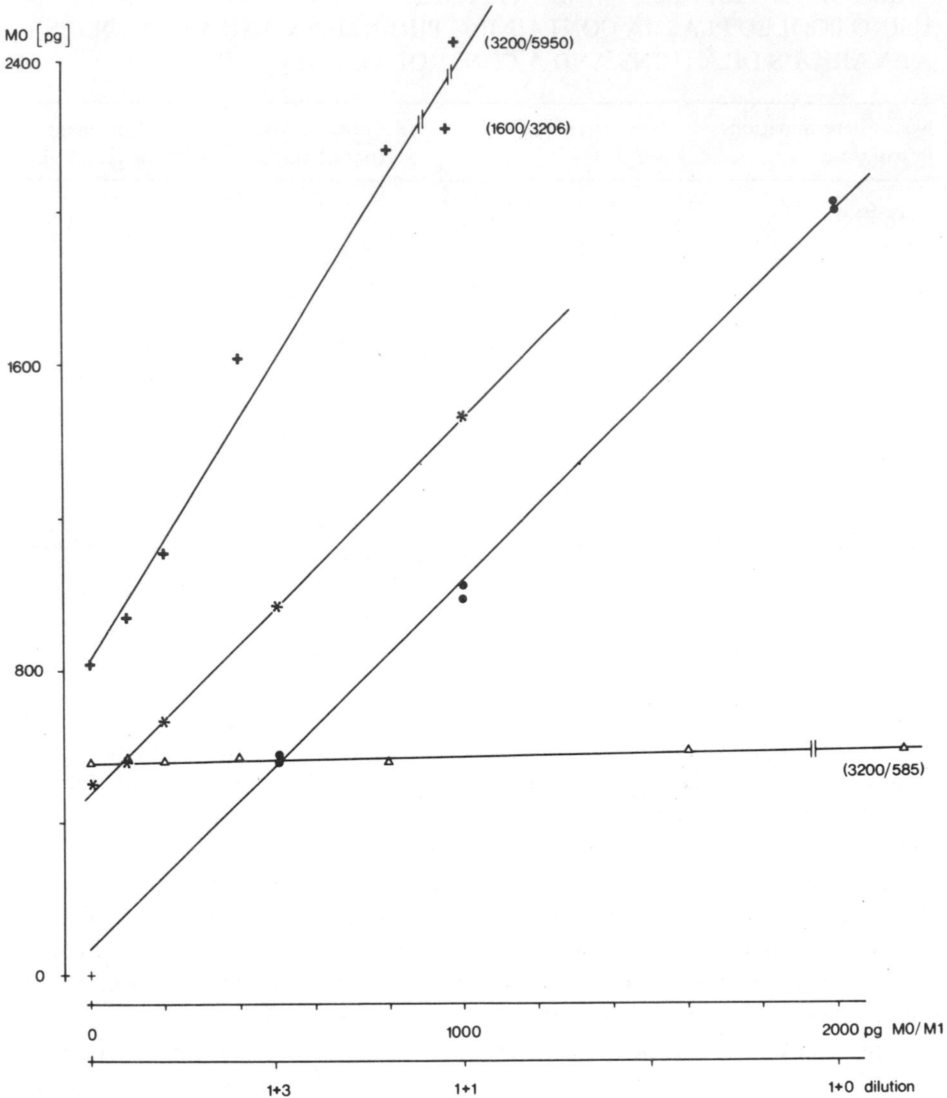

FIG.2. Evaluation of recovery of amounts of MO added to pooled plasma (mean of triplicates, – regression line) with antibody A2.*
Evaluation of cross-reactivity with M1 added to pooled plasma (Δ mean of triplicates) with antibody A2.
Evaluation of cross-reactivity with M1 added to pooled plasma (+ mean of triplicates, – regression line) with antibody A1.
Evaluation of response to pooled plasma at different dilutions (● mean of several determinations in one assay, – regression line).

2. SPECIFICATIONS OF THE RIA FOR PIRENZEPIN

All specifications are given for the assay with antibodies raised against hapten A2 using 0.1-ml samples, unless otherwise specified.

2.1. Limit of detection

With the routine use of six determinations of the initial value (no antigen added), 3 SD were subtracted from the mean. This value corresponds to 24 pg MO/sample (or less) in the calibration curve. Alternatively, determinations (6-fold each) of the initial value and of the samples spiked with 25 pg of Pirenzepin were compared statistically using the t-test which yielded a significant difference at the 1% level. Since the routine assay with a limit of detection of 25 pg/sample was sufficient for pharmacokinetic studies, no further attempt was made to increase the sensitivity.

2.2. Precision

Intra-assay precision was determined using human plasma with an unknown concentration of Pirenzepin (pooled plasma obtained from various subjects who had received Pirenzepin orally). Inter-assay precision was determined using the same plasma (diluted 1 + 3) in three different assays (see Table II).

2.3. Accuracy

Since there is no equally sensitive method for determining Pirenzepin, accuracy was tested by recovery of amounts added to pooled plasma diluted 1 + 3. Recovery for 100 to 1000 pg/sample was 98% ± 2.0% (slope of regression line ± SD, $r^2 = 0.998$). The concentration of Pirenzepin in the pooled plasma was found to be 480 ± 10.4 pg/0.1 ml (intercept ± SD). The linearity of the response was further checked against the various dilutions of pooled plasma shown in Table II. From the slope of the regression line ($r^2 = 0.998$), the Pirenzepin concentration (plasma 1 + 3) was 486 ± 13 pg/0.1 ml, the blank being (intercept ± SD) 61 ± 30 pg/0.1 ml (Fig. 2).

2.4. Cross-reactions

With antibodies against hapten A2, cross-reactivity of M1 and M2 was checked with and without unlabelled Pirenzepin at various concentrations of the metabolites. For M2, no measurable displacement of tracer was observed up to 6 ng/sample under either condition. Cross-reactivity with M1 was slight and concentration-dependent when no Pirenzepin was present (20% to 8% in the

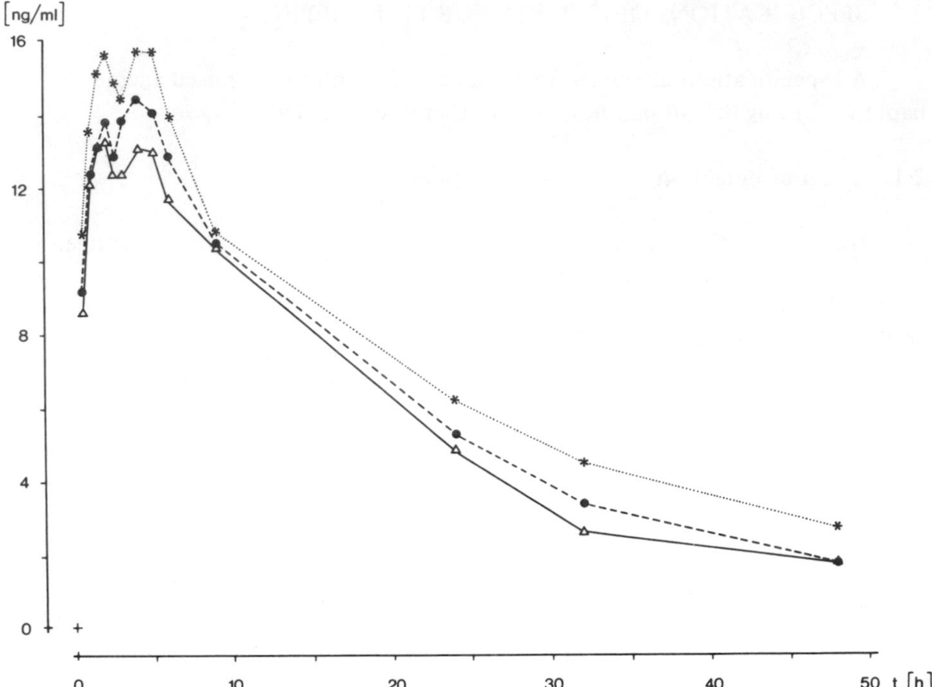

FIG.3. Plasma levels of Pirenzepin in one volunteer after oral administration of a 25-mg tablet.
* *total radioactivity (in ng equivalents/ml)*
● *Pirenzepin + M1 (RIA with antibodies A1)*
Δ *Pirenzepin (RIA with antibodies A2).*

range of 0.25 to 1 ng/sample). Addition of various concentrations of M1 to pooled plasma (1 + 3 as in Table II) containing Pirenzepin and metabolites yielded no cross-reaction (range 0.1 to 3.2 ng M1 sample) since, by analysis of variance, no significant difference between samples could be verified. The Pirenzepin concentration was determined as 569 pg/sample (CV = 2.1%) or as 579 pg/sample (CV = 5.1%) in a replicate of the whole assay. With antibodies against hapten A1, cross-reactivity with M1 was over 100% when no Pirenzepin was added. Recovery from pooled plasma yielded 158% ± 3.8% cross-reaction ($r^2 = 0.990$) and 827 ± 53 pg/sample of Pirenzepin including metabolites.

3. DISCUSSION

For pharmacokinetic analysis it is important to have an idea about the magnitude and type of error in the final data [8]. There are two general types of error which require different treatment in kinetic analysis. Either a constant uncertainty (e.g. a blank) contributes to each individual data point regardless of the concentration measured (absolute error), or the error is concentration dependent, so that one can give a percentage range of error (e.g. coefficient of variation) for all concentrations. Usually, RIA data are considered to be predominantly subject to the latter type of error because of the small dynamic range of the calibration curve and the necessity of choosing properly diluted samples. However, this generalization is not supported in our case.

The main problem in the RIA for drugs is the cross-reactivity of the antibodies with metabolites. With Pirenzepin, there is evidence that in one assay system there is a heterogenous population of antibodies of different specificity and avidity. As a consequence, even a small cross-reaction can contribute significantly to the error. At least two assay systems are required to exclude gross errors due to the main metabolites. With one assay (A2) for Pirenzepin, one can monitor almost exclusively the parent compound, whereas with the second assay (A1) for selected samples, one can prove that the biotransformation product does not interfere significantly. With Pirenzepin it was shown that the concentration of metabolite M1 in biosamples is less than half that of the parent compound. For most persons and at all sampling times, M1 is present in only very small amounts ($< 15\%$ of Pirenzepin, see Fig. 3). This was confirmed also by TLC of ^{14}C-labelled Pirenzepin administered to volunteers [9]. On the other hand, it is possible that very small amounts of M1 cross-react quite extensively with a small percentage of the antibody population (A2). This can be seen by comparing the data from pooled plasma at various dilutions (Table II); to the same plasma either more Pirenzepin (Section 2.3) or more M1 (Section 2.4) has been added. Obviously a 'blank' due to M1 present in biological samples may simulate a concentration of MO of about 50–100 pg/sample, which might be decreased by changing the Pirenzepin-to-antibody ratio, but is not changed at all by further addition of M1. For this reason it is impractical to strive to decrease the limit of detection in biological samples, even though this is easily possible for pure samples of Pirenzepin. An interesting possibility is the addition of sufficient amounts of M1 to standards and samples to block this small portion of antibodies and enhance specificity for Pirenzepin. This strategy might be of general use also for other assays, where this problem is more pronounced than in our case. Here, the 'blank' is within the inter-assay variation, if only the part of the calibration curve from 0.8 ng/0.1 ml to 5 ng/0.1 ml is used.

In conclusion, the validity of the general strategy for assaying drugs with RIA was illustrated by an example showing that sensitivity, reliability and routine performance of such a system suits the needs of the pharmacokineticist. But this is true only if all phases of the assay are well planned and controlled with regard to the special tasks in question.

REFERENCES

[1] LEVINE L., Pharmacol. Rev. **25** (1973) 293.
[2] BUTLER, V.P., BEISER, S.M., Adv. Immunology **17** (1973) 255.
[3] EBERLEIN, W., SCHMIDT, G., REUTER, A., KUTTER, E., Z. Arzneimittelforsch. (Drug Res.) **27** (1977) 356.
[4] KOPITAR, Z., ZIMMER, A., Z. Arzneimittelforsch. (Drug Res.) **26** 7a (1976) 1450.
[5] KOPITAR, Z., KOMPA, H.E., Z. Arzneimittelforsch. (Drug Res.) **25** 10 (1975) 1469.
[6] KAUBISCH, N., et al., (in preparation).
[7] TEMBO, A.V., SCHORK, M.A., WAGNER, J.G., Steroids **28** (1976) 387.
[8] BOZLER, G., et al., Z. Arzneimittelforsch. (Drug Res.) **27** 4a (1977) 897.
[9] HAMMER, R., et al., Therapiewoche **27** 9 (1977) 1575.

DISCUSSION

M. TORTEN: Do you have any data on the affinity of your antibodies? If you have, how do they relate to the site of conjugation?

G. BOZLER: We don't have these data. We regard the assay simply as an analytical tool, and since we do not routinely evaluate the data by Scatchard plots, no further information is available at this time.

M. JOUSTRA: Did I correctly understand that you do not extract your plasma samples before assay?

G. BOZLER: This is correct. We do not perform any extraction whatsoever. We only dilute the biological specimens and standards strictly in the same manner.

M. JOUSTRA: Did you not experience any interference from the serum protein binding of your analyte? Being a tricyclic substance, it should be bound to albumin to a fair extent.

G. BOZLER: The binding of this compound in plasma is very low (10–15%) in the range of therapeutic concentrations, and this is in accordance with the hydrophilic nature of the compound (see Ref. [3] in the paper), as opposed to other tricyclic agents. But even in the case of compounds with higher binding to albumin, often no extraction is necessary if you treat samples in the same way as standards, if you dilute biological specimens with inert material (e.g. globulins etc.) and if you use a proper evaluation method.

IAEA-SM-220/35

THE RADIOIMMUNOASSAY OF BIOLOGICALLY ACTIVE COMPOUNDS IN PAROTID FLUID AND PLASMA

R.F. WALKER, G.F. READ, D. RIAD-FAHMY
Tenovus Institute for Cancer Research,
Welsh National School of Medicine,
Cardiff, United Kingdom

Abstract

THE RADIOIMMUNOASSAY OF BIOLOGICALLY ACTIVE COMPOUNDS IN PAROTID FLUID AND PLASMA.

Parotid fluid collection is a simple stress-free procedure. The potential value of parotid fluid estimations of clomipramine, a tricyclic antidepressant, d-norgestrel, a synthetic contraceptive steroid and cortisol have been evaluated for assessment of clinical status and patient compliance. These compounds circulate bound largely to plasma proteins. Their concentration in parotid fluid, which reflects the non-protein bound fraction, is low but assay sensitivity (10, 1 and 30 pg/tube respectively) is adequate. Excellent agreement ($r > 0.9$) was observed when parotid fluid samples were assayed with and without chromatographic purification. Clomipramine levels following oral dosage (150 mg) rose steadily to a maximum in plasma but showed wide fluctuations in parotid fluid. Clomipramine therapy can only be assessed by plasma assays, but patient compliance may be checked by parotid fluid concentrations. Following an oral dose of d-norgestrel (0.3 mg), parotid fluid levels rose steadily to a maximum but plasma response was biphasic making correlation impossible. The sensitivity and high throughput of the d-norgestrel methodology suggests its use in evaluating patient compliance in large-scale fertility control programmes. Changes in circulating cortisol concentrations were rapidly and accurately reflected in parotid fluid in normal volunteers. Parotid fluid cortisol showed a marked diurnal rhythm, suppression to low levels after dexamethasone, and elevation following Synacthen. Low levels after Synacthen stimulation in a patient with secondary adrenal atrophy and constant high levels in Cushingoid patients indicate that parotid fluid cortisol levels could be used for accurate adrenocortical evaluation. The value in rapid screening procedures is stressed since the assay can be performed directly on only 10 μl of parotid fluid.

Parotid fluid, collected by a non-invasive technique, facilitates sample collection in clinical situations where skilled personnel are not readily available. The concentration of most biologically active compounds in parotid fluid reflects the non-protein bound concentration of the compound in plasma [1]. This is of clinical significance since it is now generally accepted that the biological activity of a compound parallels the 'free' or non-protein bound concentrations. However, parotid fluid concentrations of compounds which circulate mainly bound to plasma proteins are so low that accurate, routine determinations are only possible using sensitive, specific radioimmunoassay techniques.

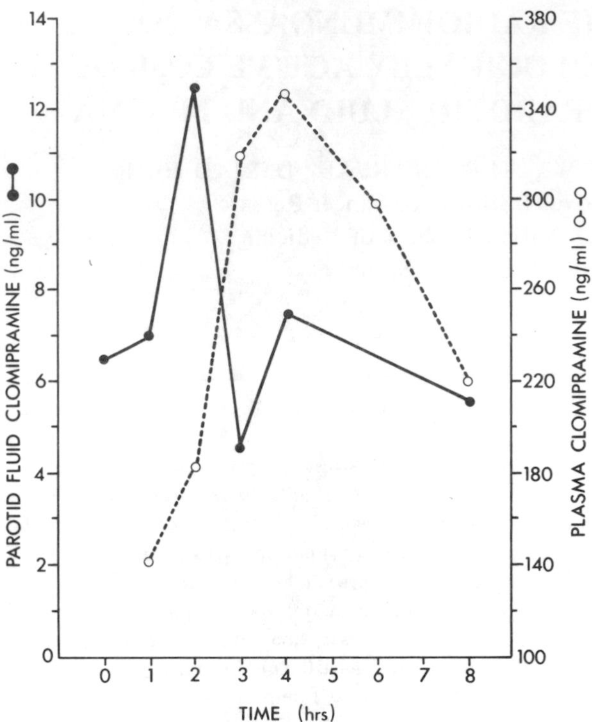

FIG.1. Plasma and parotid fluid levels after administration of clomipramine (150 mg).

Comparative data are presented on the problems concerned with assaying three biologically active compounds, clomipramine, d-norgestrel and cortisol in both parotid fluid and plasma. Parotid fluid was collected using a Curby cup and, since available evidence suggests that salivary excretion of biologically active compounds is independent of flow rate [2], collection rate was maximized by stimulation with a citric-acid syrup. Blood was collected in lithium heparin tubes, and the plasma separated by centrifugation. Plasma and parotid fluid samples were stored at -20°C until assayed.

Clomipramine, a tricyclic, lipophilic drug widely used in the treatment of depression, was determined in parotid fluid by a radioimmunoassay procedure developed in the Tenovus Institute for clomipramine in plasma [3]. The assay required only slight modification to give adequate sensitivity (10 pg/tube) [4] and was shown to be specific since parotid fluid samples assayed with and without thin-layer chromatographic pre-assay purification showed excellent correlation ($r = 0.99$). Hospital patients, known to be in a steady state and to have taken a 150-mg oral dose, had clomipramine levels in plasma which increased steadily to

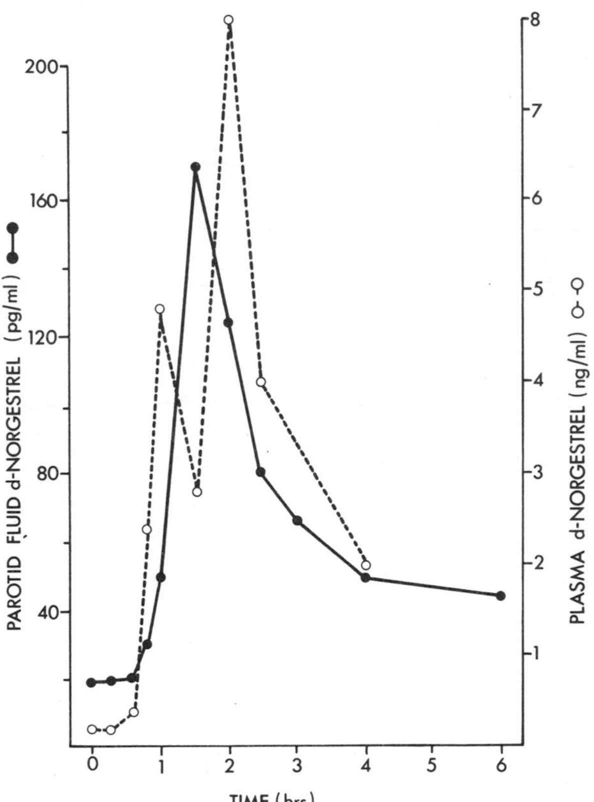

FIG.2. Plasma and parotid fluid levels after administration of d-norgestrel (0.3 mg).

a maximum 2–4 h after administration. In parotid fluid, however, the response was multiphasic (Fig.1). The lack of correlation between plasma and parotid fluid levels probably arose because transfer of a basic drug like clomipramine from plasma (pH 7.4) to saliva (pH 5.5 – 7.5) is dependent on salivary pH, known to be influenced by various external stimuli [5]. It is therefore believed that plasma levels are mandatory for monitoring dose-response but that patient compliance, a very pressing problem in general practice, could well be monitored by parotid fluid, clomipramine concentrations.

d-Norgestrel is a synthetic contraceptive steroid largely bound in plasma to a specific binding protein similar to α_1-acid glycoprotein [6]. It was determined in parotid fluid by a radioimmunoassay procedure based on techniques established in the Institute for the determination of this steroid in human milk and plasma [7].

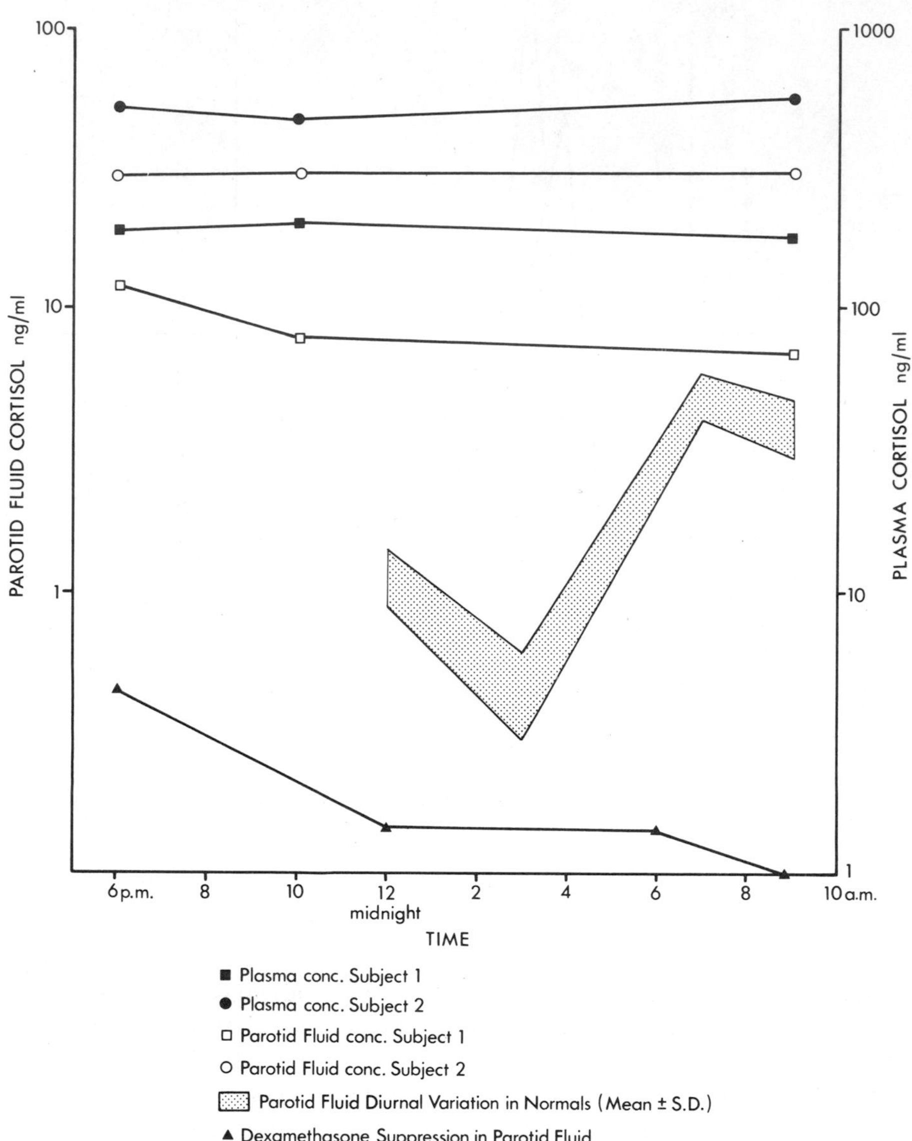

FIG.3. Diurnal variation of parotid fluid cortisol in four normals; diurnal variation in plasma and parotid fluid cortisol in two subjects (Cushingoid) and parotid fluid cortisol suppression by dexamethasone.

The use of an ^{125}I-radioligand increased assay throughput and reduced running costs. Following a single oral dose of d-norgestrel (0.3 mg), parotid fluid levels never exceeded 2% of the total plasma concentration. This result is in accordance with the plasma binding studies of Uniyal and Laumas [6], indicating that circulating d-norgestrel is almost completely protein bound. In all subjects [5] the response was biphasic in plasma but uniphasic in parotid fluid (Fig.2). The correlation between parotid fluid and total plasma d-norgestrel levels was consequently poor. The reason for the biphasic plasma response is obscure, but has been noted by other workers [8]. This anomalous plasma response makes it impossible to equate parotid fluid levels with plasma-free steroid in a simple pharmacodynamic model. The ease of sample collection and high throughput of the assay suggests the use of parotid fluid for evaluating patient compliance in large-scale fertility control programmes where medical personnel are not readily available.

Cortisol determinations are widely used in assessing adrenocortical function. Since plasma sampling is associated with stress which may mask response, and urinary studies are complicated by collection difficulties, determination of parotid fluid cortisol levels could become the method of choice in assessing adrenal function. Parotid fluid cortisol, efficiently extracted (>95%) by dichloroethane was determined by a radioimmunoassay procedure similar to that developed at the Tenovus Institute for plasma cortisol [9]. This assay had a sensitivity of 30 pg/tube, and is highly specific since agreement in titres ($r = 0.98$) between parotid fluid samples assayed with and without thin-layer chromatography purification was excellent.

Matched parotid fluid and plasma samples were obtained from normal volunteers [7] for investigation of diurnal rhythms, short-term Synacthen stimulation and dexamethasone suppression tests. A well-defined diurnal rhythm was observed in the parotid fluid of healthy volunteers. This was in marked contrast to the consistently high parotid fluid levels seen in two Cushingoid patients (Fig.3).

In normal subjects, cortisol levels reached peak values in both parotid fluid and plasma 60 min after intramuscular injection of Synacthen (25 μg) and returned to baseline levels after 5.5 h (Fig.4). The increase in parotid fluid levels (8-fold) was greater than that of plasma (3-fold). A patient with secondary adrenal atrophy had plasma and parotid fluid cortisol levels approximating to those seen in dexamethasone-treated normal volunteers. Synacthen stimulation caused no change in either parotid fluid or circulating cortisol concentrations (Fig.4).

The influence of elevated transcortin levels in parotid fluid cortisol was investigated in three healthy volunteers who had been taking an estrogen-containing contraceptive for at least three months (Fig.4). Cortisol titres in parotid fluid were normal and the response to Synacthen stimulation was within the normal range, although the time taken to achieve maximal response was doubled. Baseline

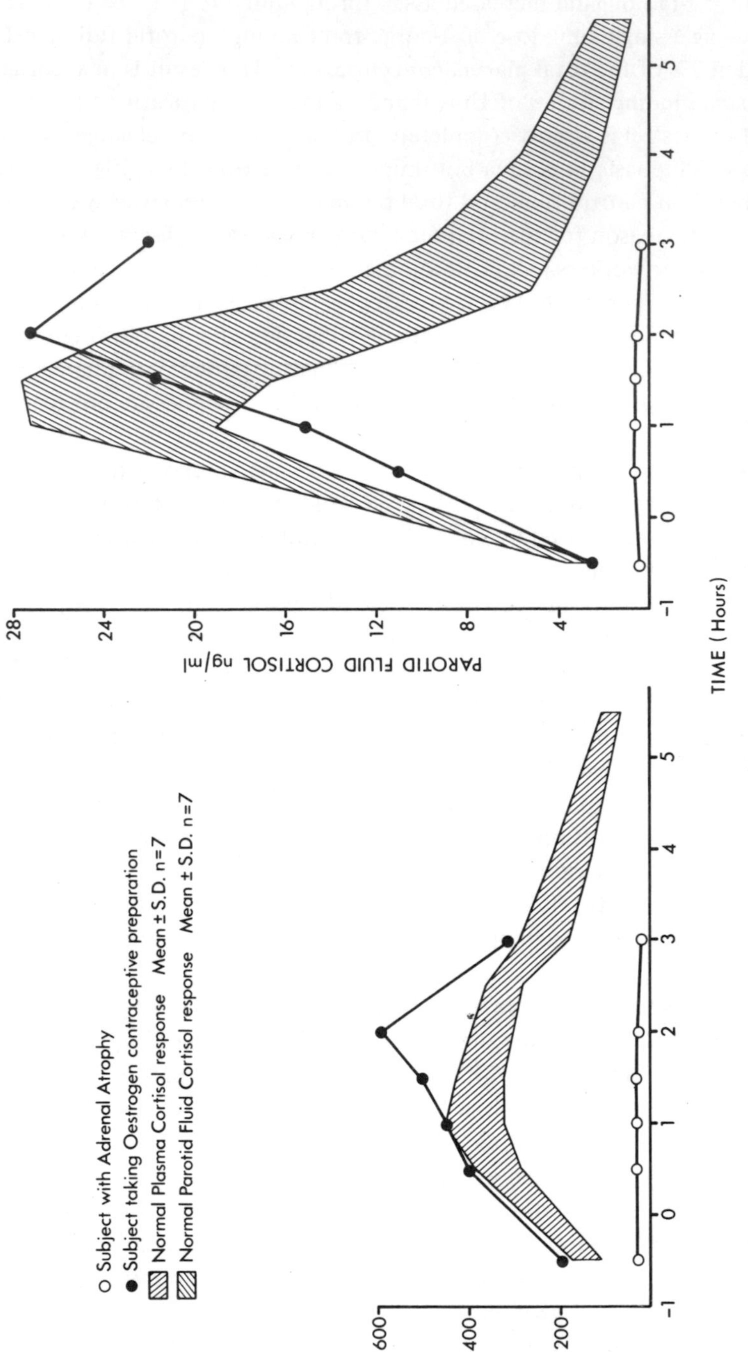

FIG.4. Parotid fluid and plasma cortisol levels in a patient with secondary adrenal atrophy and a woman taking an estrogen-containing contraceptive pill after stimulation with 250 μg of Synacthen (i.m.).

plasma levels however were elevated and on stimulation the response was considerably greater than normal. The disparate results in parotid fluid and plasma of these subjects are presumably due to an increase in circulating transcortin induced by the pill [10].

Only slight modification of the assay procedure was required for parotid fluid cortisol determination in patients taking Metyrapone, an 11β-hydroxlyase enzyme inhibitor. Metyrapone, used as a test of adrenal function or for treatment of Cushingoid patients, blocks the synthesis of cortisol from 11-deoxycortisol, thus causing elevated circulating levels of 11-deoxycortisol. As a result of cross-reaction (10%) with the antiserum used, elevated 11-deoxycortisol levels would cause erroneous results. Interference of this steroid in the assay can easily be eliminated by prior extraction of parotid fluid with petroleum ether : benzene (65 : 35) which extracts 80% of 11-deoxycortisol with no significant loss of cortisol.

Parotid fluid is reported to contain no corticosteroid-binding protein [2]. It would therefore appear to be an ideal biological fluid for the direct determination of cortisol. The correlation in cortisol titres in parotid fluid assayed directly and following dichloroethane extraction was excellent ($r = 0.99$). Serial dilution of a high titre sample of parotid fluid assayed by both procedures also gave results in good agreement ($r = 0.99$). It is therefore apparent that cortisol determinations in parotid fluid, which can be done directly on as little as 10 μl of sample, are of considerable value not only as a screening procedure but for accurate assessment of adrenocortical function.

REFERENCES

[1] HORNING, M.G., et al., Clin. Chem. **23** 2 (1977) 157.
[2] KATZ, H.F., SHANNON, I.L., J. Clin. Invest. **48** (1969) 848.
[3] READ, G.F., FAHMY, D.R., WALKER, R.F., "Biological aspects of Anafranil" (Proc. Conf. Gibraltar, 1977), Postgraduate Medical Journal (in press).
[4] KAISER, H., SPECKER, M., Z. Anal. Chem. **149** (1956) 46.
[5] JENKINS, G.N., The Physiology of the Mouth, 3rd Edn, Blackwell Scientific Publications.
[6] UNIYAL, J.P., LAUMAS, K.R., Biochim. Biophys. Acta **427** (1976) 218.
[7] THOMAS, M.T., et al., Steorids (submitted for publication).
[8] ELSTEIN, M., et al., Fertility and sterility **27** 8 (1976) 892.
[9] FAHMY, D.R., READ, G.F., HILLIER, S.G., Steroids **26** (1975) 267.
[10] DOE, R.P., FERNANDEZ, R., SEAL, H.S., J. Clin. Endocrinol. Metab. **24** (1964) 1029.

DISCUSSION

G. BOZLER: This paper has nicely shown the use of saliva as sampling site. I should like to point out that this may be a useful method even when plasma concentrations and concentrations in parotid fluids do not correlate. There are papers in the pharmacokinetic literature showing correlation of concentrations in peripheral compartments with saliva concentrations. Thus, valid information may be obtainable from the latter although only indirectly after kinetic analysis.

Session VIII, Part 1

APPLICATIONS

Assays for thyroid-related hormones

Chairman

C.A. TAFURT
Colombia

Invited review paper

PATHOPHYSIOLOGICAL ASPECTS OF RECENT ADVANCES IN CURRENT THYROID FUNCTION TESTING

R.-D. HESCH
Medizinische Hochschule Hannover,
Hanover,
Federal Republic of Germany

Abstract

PATHOPHYSIOLOGICAL ASPECTS OF RECENT ADVANCES IN CURRENT THYROID FUNCTION TESTING.

The paper first discusses thyroid function and thyroid "status", which is determined by thyroid gland function in secreting T_4, and peripheral bio-transformation of T_4. The accuracy of a current in-vitro diagnostic strategy ensures high reliability in clinical routine. More recent test procedures for iodothyronines and immunological phenomena need further evaluation. Later, the bio-transformation of T_4 to bioactive and regulatory iodothyronines is discussed with respect to its possible clinical implications. Finally, the significance of TBG in the interpretation of T_4 and T_3 concentrations is determined and more attention is directed to its functional heterogeneity.

The current strategy for testing thyroid function depends very much on the nature of the individual case. This review therefore considers in more detail those aspects that have become more important as a result of recent progress in thyroid hormone pathophysiology, namely:

(1) The current status of thyroid function testing.
(2) The function of the thyroid gland, the importance of TSH and thyroid stimulating immunoglobulins.
(3) The transformation of T_4 to iodothyronines.
(4) The importance of TBG.

1. Current status of testing thyroid function

Our most important clinical interest is to define "thyroid status" in an individual, but this is complicated by the problems of classification and nomenclature. The classification of the American Thyroid Association is based primarily on thyroid gland function and is presented in the abridged classification

TABLE I. CLINICAL VALUE OF CURRENT TEST PROCEDURES TO TEST THYROID FUNCTION, THYROID "STATUS", THYROID STIMULATING ANTIBODIES, PITUITARY THYROID FUNCTION AND THYROID HORMONE BINDING

	Euthyroidism	Euthyroid goitre	Euthyroid Endocr. ophth.	Thyrotoxicosis	Hypothyroidism (primary)
T_4	Age-related "euthyroid ranges"; correct diagnosis in 95% of an unselected population	n to ↓ ("euthyroid range")	n	↑ in 80% n in 20%	n in 20% ↓ in 80%
T_3		n to ↑ correct diagnosis in 100%	n	↑ in 95% n in 5%	↑ in 20% n in 20% ↓ in 60%
TBG	Age-related variation	n	n	n(?)	n(?)
TRH test	Positive by definition with rare exceptions	Neg. in 20% Pos. in 80%	Neg. in 70% Pos. in 20% Exag. in 10%	Neg. in 100%	Exaggerated with high basal TSH in 100%
Ig-autoantibodies Microsomal antibodies	Usually negative with exceptions		Pos. in about 20%	Pos. in 20–50%	Pos. in 30%
HTS, MTS, TSI, HTACS MIF-test	Increased frequency in apparently healthy first-degree relatives of patients with Graves' disease and Hashimotos thyroiditis		Pos. (depending on methods used) in 20–50%	Pos. (depending on methods used) 60–100%	Pos. (depending on methods used) in ~ 50%
^{131}I-suppression test	Positive with rare exceptions	Positive (Neg. in some cases with neg. TRH test)	Neg. in 70% Pos. in 30%	Neg. in 100%	Not done

HTACS: human thyroid adenyl cyclase stimulator. HTS: human thyroid stimulator. MIF-test: migration inhibition factor test. MTS: mouse thyroid stimulator. TSI: thyroid-stimulating immunoglobulins.

TABLE II. LABORATORY AND SCINTIGRAPHIC CHARACTERIZATION OF AUTONOMOUS THYROID NODULES

	Autonomous Thyroid Nodule	
	Iodine exposed	controls
T_4 ↑	60%	20 %
T_3 ↑	67%	56 %
TRH-test neg	100%	92,5%
clinically hyperthyroid	41%	34 %

	Scintigraphic Diagnosis		
	compensated	transition	decompensated
T_4n, T_3n	50%	49%	29%
T_4n, T_3↑	43%	36%	42%
T_4↑, T_3↑	7%	15%	29%
n	(28)	(39)	(52)

as (1) euthyroidism, (2) hyperthyroidism and (3) hypothyroidism. Although goitre and ophthalmopathy do occur in all conditions of normal and disturbed thyroid gland function, I will consider them separately. Also, for didactic reasons, I shall discuss extrathyroidal variables separately. The nonthyroidal fate of thyroid hormones, i.e. their binding to specific plasma proteins and the biotransformation of T_4, seem to determine the "thyroid status" of an individual to a yet unexpected extent. Thus, the "thyroid status" of an individual will ultimately be determined by both the thyroid gland function and the biochemical events induced by transformation of the main thyroid gland hormone, thyroxine (T_4). So we should no longer talk about "thyroid function tests" but rather about "thyroid status tests". Since I believe that direct tests of thyroid gland function by means of radioisotopic methods should be restricted to special diagnostic evaluations, I will now discuss the diagnostic value of the currently available in-vitro methods. The radioimmunochemical determination of T_4, T_3 and TSH and the indirect tests of thyroid hormone binding have enabled us to distinguish thyroid status in euthyroid subjects and in those with disturbed thyroid function with an accuracy of more than 95%.

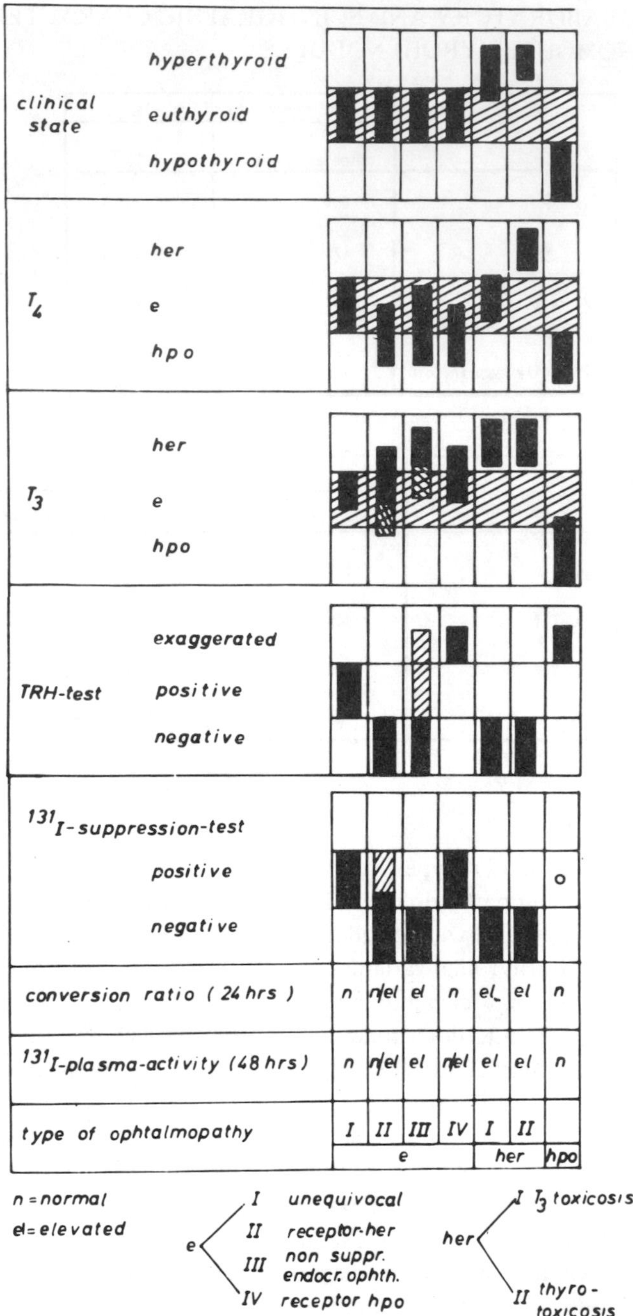

FIG.1. Staging of the types of endocrine exophthalmos by means of laboratory data and data from the TRH test and the ^{131}I-suppression test [4]. When data for immunopathogenesis are considered [12], a more complex classification is obtained which may be related to that in the figure.

T_3 \ T_4	low	normal	elevated
low	15	2	–
normal	17	13	1
elevated	1	–	5

T_3 \ TRH-test	exagg.	positive	negative
low	7	2	5
normal	17	4	7
elevated	1	11	–

T_4 \ TRH-test	exagg.	positive	negative
low	15	3	12
normal	–	1	14
elevated	–	–	7

FIG.2. Data from thyrotoxic patients under antithyroid drug therapy. The combination of T_4/T_3, T_3/TRH test and T_4/TRH test allowed several conclusions:

(1) Normal T_3 is most frequently combined with low and normal values of T_4.

(2) A T_3 value between 1.0 and 2.0 is the most reliable parameter in euthyroid patients under therapy irrespective of the T_4 concentration of the result of the TRH test.

The determination of thyroid hormones and TSH is beset at the outset by technical problems. A recent interlaboratory comparison of the "Sektion Schilddrüse" of the German Society of Endocrinology has demonstrated that the inter-assay coefficient of variation for T_3 was between 4 and 43% and for T_4 between 4.5 and 30% due to technical insufficiency [1]. In another similar study initiated by the European Thyroid Association, the variance was 26–44% for T_3 and 23% for T_4 [2]. Apart from technical misclassification, insufficient inhibition of TBG binding by TBG blockers was responsible for the wide variation and the disappointing results. The same survey for TSH was even more disappointing, exhibiting an interlaboratory precision of 128% and recovery rates ranging from 50 to 926%. Some of these problems could be solved in the meantime for the T_3, the T_4 and the TSH assays by using appropriate TSH-free plasma for standards and delayed addition of the tracer [3]. Thus, governmental or other surveys by permanent interlaboratory control, as exemplarily realized in the Supraregional Assay Service in the UK, must optimize quality control of the in-vitro procedures. Under appropriate conditions [4], thyroid status may be correctly diagnosed as follows: At a constant concentration of binding proteins, T_4 reflects a static measure of thyroid gland secretion, T_3 represents the overall function of peripheral biotransformation of T_4 to T_3 and the TRH test indicates how pituitary T_4 and T_3 tissue concentrations would regulate the responsiveness of the thyrotrophes to TRH. From this we may derive a current strategy to differentiate between different forms of thyroid status; we can define diffuse and nodular thyroid diseases and those related to immunological phenomena associated with thyroid diseases by means of scintigraphic examinations and pure in-vitro diagnostic procedures (Table I). The description of such a strategy for euthyroid status, for euthyroid goitre and for the different forms of hyperthyroidism is now probably generally accepted. The primary diagnosis of thyrotoxicosis with or without

TABLE III. POSSIBLE DEFINITIONS AND CLASSIFICATION OF HYPOTHYROIDISM [6]

1. Hypothyroidism is not an "all or none" phenomenon but a "graded" one.
2. The frontier between euthyroidism and hypothyroidism is not defined (definable?).
3. Attempts to clarify the "grey zone" between hypo- and euthyroidism lead to concepts of:

latent	hypothyroidism
preclinical	"
compensated	"
subclinical	"
mild	"
borderline	"
early	"
incipient	"
premyxoedema	"

Preclinical hypothyroidism:

1. Clinically asymptomatic phase of hypothyroidism, showing normal results with conventional serum parameters, but an increased TSH-response to TRH (see Hall (1972) and Pickardt et al. (1972) in Ref.[6]).
2. Clinically euthyroid patients with asymptomatic thyroiditis; risk factor with increased prevalence of myocardial infarction, obesity, diabetes and hypertension (see Bastenie et al. (1971) in Ref.[6]).

Subclinical hypothyroidism:

Asymptomatic state in which a reduction of thyroid activity has been compensated by an increased TSH output to maintain a euthyroid state (see Evered and Hall (1973) in Ref. [6]).

Latent hypothyroidism:

1. Synonymously used with "preclinical" hypothyroidism (see Pickardt et al. (1972) in Ref. [6]).
2. Synonymously used with "premyxoedema" and "preclinical" hypothyroidism (see Bastenie et al. (1971) in Ref. [6]).
3. Pre-stage to premyxoedema (see Fowler et al. (1970) in Ref. [6]).

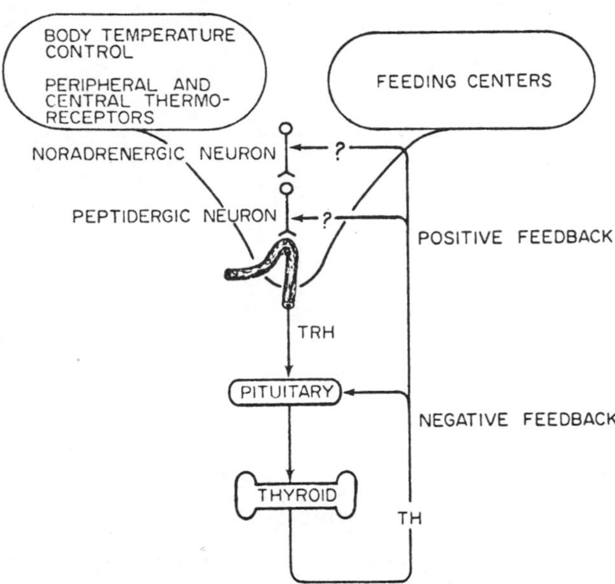

FIG.3. Hypothalamic-pituitary-thyroid system for control of thyroid activity. It is proposed that T_4, after conversion to T_3 in the pituitary and in the hypothalamus, exerts a positive feedback effect on TRH secretion and that the set point of control is determined by the interaction between positive stimulatory effects of T_3 on TRH secretion and inhibitory effects on the thyrotrope [8]. It is hypothesized that iodothyronines with neurotransmitter information locally converted from T_4 in the hypothalamic regions control the noradrenergic neuron [7].

endocrine exophthalmos and with or without goitre can be clearly differentiated and may be better subdivided later by immunological tests. Autonomous thyroid nodules can easily be characterized by scintigraphy and by laboratory data (Table II). Euthyroid endocrine exophthalmos is a syndrome associated with many forms of thyroid diseases and it may even be without a clear relationship to such a manifestation, in which case we need as many laboratory, biochemical and immunological tests as possible for its classification (Table I and Fig.1). It is obvious that the multiple and partly confusing combinations of results need great clinical experience for correct treatment and indeed an important difference of opinion exists on this point. The same is true for surveys of thyrotoxic patients under treatment. Laboratory tests are less helpful and all combinations may be found (Fig.2 from Ref.[4]). Experienced clinical examination is very important. So far, the most reliable parameter during and after any antithyroid therapy (antithyroid drug $\pm T_4$ replacement, radioiodine, surgery) is, in fact, T_3 which, independent of T_4, should not exceed 1.5 – 2.0 ng/ml and should never be below 1.0 ng/ml. None of these tests has any value in predicting healing or relapse of

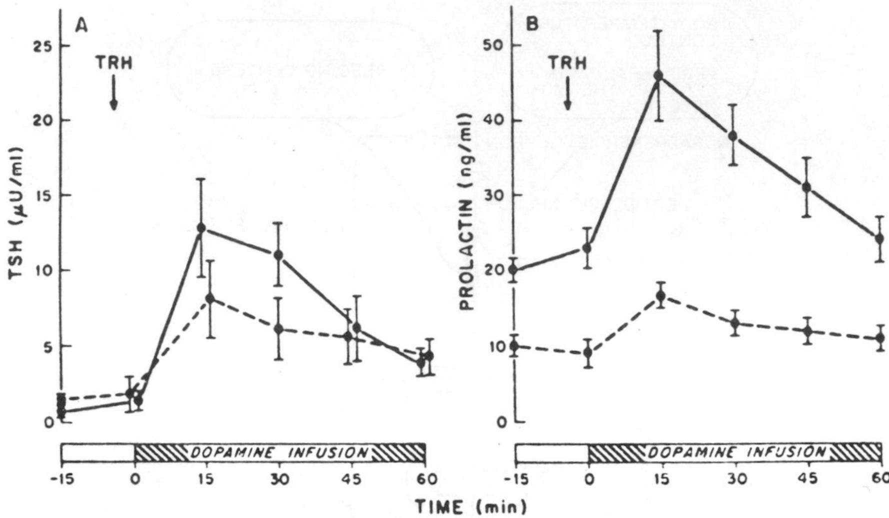

FIG.4. Effect of T_3 administration on the dopamine-mediated inhibition of TRH-stimulated TSH (A) and prolactin secretion (B) [9].

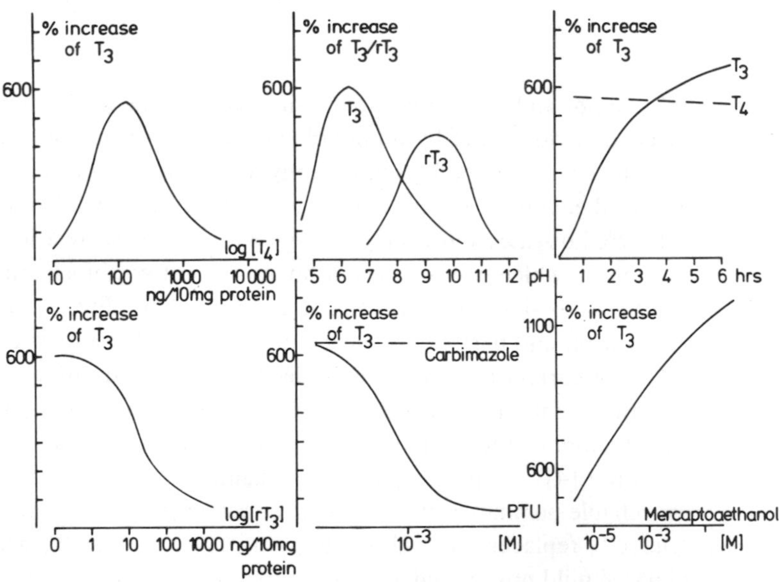

FIG.5. Cascade-enzymatic bio-transformation of T_4 [7].

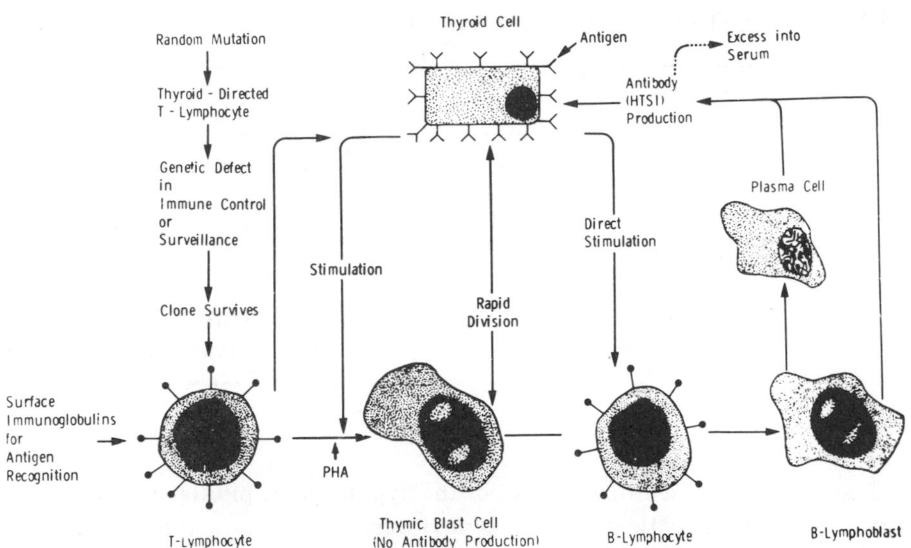

FIG.6. Schematic representation of immune-surveillance of the thyroid gland [13].

the disease, but it is possible that the determination of thyroid stimulating IgG may help in the near future [5]. Another problem is how to define graded deviations from euthyroid status. This is best exemplified, for example, by the characterization of hypothyroidism which was recently described by Krüskemper [6]. The whole semantic problems are portrayed by three of his statements regarding hypothyroidism (Table III). Laboratory data are therefore difficult to interpret (Table I). But the same is true for hyperthyroidism, especially with respect to the occurrence of 20% negative TRH tests as a phenomenon which we observed for example in euthyroid goitre. Another discrepancy not yet explained is the incidence of a positive TRH test and a negative ^{131}I-suppression test, and vice versa, which was observed in numerous patients after successful treatment of thyrotoxicosis [7].

2. Function of the thyroid gland: importance of TSH and thyroid stimulating immunoglobulins

The phylogeny of the thyroid suggests that under physiological conditions the function of this gland is to extract optimal amounts of iodide and to transform it to T_4. As only trace amounts (about 10^{-5}%) of iodide occur in the geosphere, an ingenious mechanism for active iodide transport, accumulation, conservation, organification and secretion of T_4 is necessary. Thyroid T_4 production is

TABLE IV. TESTS FOR THYROID AUTOIMMUNITY

Tests for humoral immunity
Thyroid stimulating immunoglobulins
Circulating anti-Tg and anti-microsomal antibodies
Circulating anti-Tg-immunocomplexes
Anti-thyroxine and anti-triiodothyronine antibodies
Tests for cellular immunity
Determination of migration inhibitor factor (MIF)
Determination of lymphocyte determinants in culture

under the extremely sensitive control of the hypothalamic pituitary system (Fig.3 from Ref. [8]). However, this is phylogenetically a more primitive adaptative mechanism to the low environmental iodide concentration. This ancestral mechanism does not seem adequate to cope with the conditions of iodide deficiency of our modern civilisation. Recent data on the interaction of iodothyronine at the hypothalamic level, like the T_3-modulated effects of TRH and dopamine on pituitary hormone secretion in man (Fig.4 from Ref.[9]), suggest that in higher vertebrates biotransformed iodothyronines (Fig.5 from Ref.[7]) may exert highly specific neuroendocrine actions; probably a more important feedback control than that of iodide extraction. Another important observation is the sympathetic control of the thyroid gland function [10]. Except by the TRH test, we cannot yet determine parameters that allow the activities of other important feedback regulators in normal thyroid gland function to be measured.

A genetic predisposition to euthyroid goitre and Graves' disease is suggested by the occurrence of both diseases in first-degree relatives [11]. There has been a search for a genetic link between the HLA system and thyrotoxicosis [12], but the evidence is not convincing. Our present understanding of genetic disposition to disturbed immune surveillance and lymphocyte control is certainly better. Genetically predisposed desuppression of normally suppressed T-lymphocytes responsible for the control of thyroid surface antigen results in two reactions: the production of immunoglobulins directed towards the TSH receptor membrane protein and the proliferation of B-lymphocytes and K-lymphocytes which directly destroy the thyrocyte (Fig.6 from Ref.[13]). There are several methods for determining the immune reactions (Table IV).

2.1. Immunoglobulins that bind to the TSH receptor and/or have a stimulatory effect on it are detectable by several methods, each detecting a different moiety of the immunoglobulin by using different target effects. Hence, one cannot expect absolute correlation between results of different tests. This is

Postulated interrelationship LATS, LATS-P, HTS, and TSI

Serum	1	2	3	4
KaH	+ + + +	+ + + +	+ + +	+
KaM	–	+ +	+	–
LATS	–	+ +	+	–
LATS-S	+ +	+ +	+ +	+
HTS	+ +	+ +	+	–
TSI	+ +	+ +	+ +	+

FIG.7. Nomenclature of thyroid stimulating antibodies [41]. KaH and KaM represent the average affinity of IgG in representative sera (1–4) for the human and mouse thyroid antigens respectively. Strength of affinity increases from zero (–) to maximal (+ + + +). Results of assays for LATS, LATS-P, HTS and TSI are similarly represented as negative (–) to strongly positive (+ +).

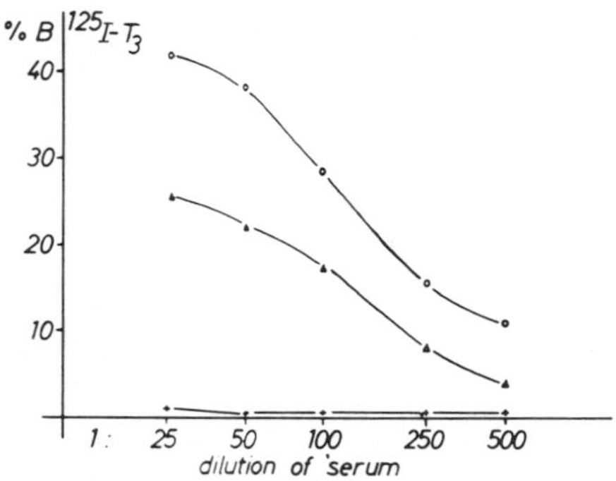

○ before treatment with radioiodine, clinically hyperthyroid, total T_3 = 6.6 ng/ml
△ 6 months after treatment with radioiodine, clinically slightly hypothyroid, total T_3 = 3.3 ng/ml
+ Antibody negative control, normal serum, total T_3 = 1.1 ng/ml.

FIG.8. Demonstration of antibodies against T_3 which may interfere with radioimmunochemical determination of the hormone [17].

the major problem in interpreting the results of these tests. Since IgGs have been found in the relatives of euthyroid persons with normal suppressible thyroid function or in absolutely euthyroid ophthalmopathy, caution must be exercised in misinterpreting the results. Blocking antibodies and receptor refractoriness against some IgG populations must be considered (Fig.7).

2.2. The high incidence of antithyroid antibodies in the relatives of persons with Graves' disease points to the importance of cell-mediated autoimmunity. Tests to determine anti-Tg antibodies and antimicrosomal antibodies are readily available.

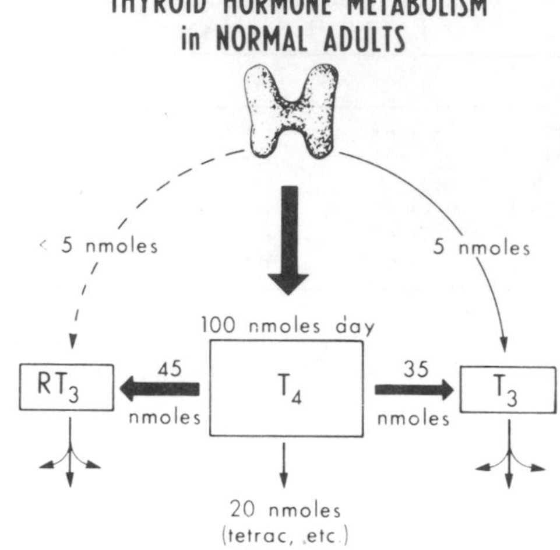

FIG.9. Schematic representation of T_4 pathways [27].

2.3. A more complex way of testing for Tg-anti-Tg-immunocomplexes in patients with ophthalmopathy is by radiometric measurements [14]. These complexes may in fact be inhibitory to stimulating IgG when deposited at the thyroid cell surface. More interestingly, they may migrate via the lymph-vessels from the thyroid to the orbita. It has been recently suggested that these immuno-complexes, when bound to the orbital muscle tissue, may be of etiologic importance in the precipitation of endocrine exophthalmos [15]. This is one of the most fascinating hypotheses regarding a possible relationship between thyroid and ocular disease.

2.4. Observations of others [16] and our group [17] (Fig.8) suggest that in a few cases with disturbed thyroid function there are anti-thyroid-hormone-antibodies. The pathophysiological significance of these antibodies is unclear, but they may give rise to false thyroid hormone measurements and can easily be determined when there is a discrepancy between the clinical state and the hormone determinations and/or a divergence between the T_3 and T_4 determinations.

2.5. The determination of cell-mediated immunity by the MIF test [18, 19], i.e. by the inhibition of leucocyte or lymphocyte migration, has been considered to be a reliable indicator of autoimmunity in thyroid diseases. In fact, all hyper-thyroid patients in the series studied by Munro and coworkers [18] exhibited a positive test; a high incidence of positive tests was also shown in euthyroid endocrine exophthalmos. The test procedure is complicated so the results are few, but they would have an enormous clinical importance if they enabled one to

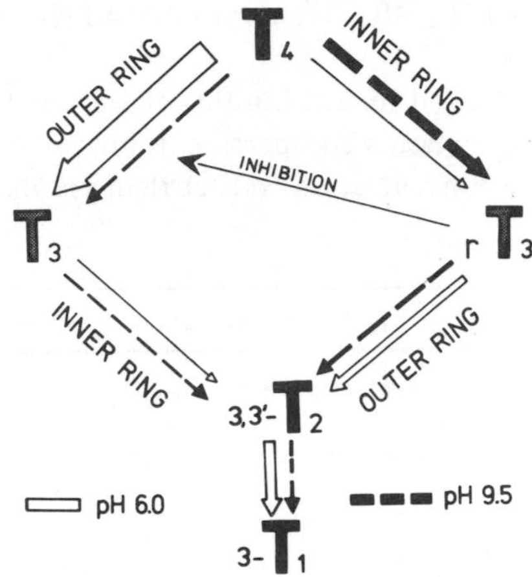

FIG.10. pH-dependence of major pathways of T_4 bio-transformation [42].

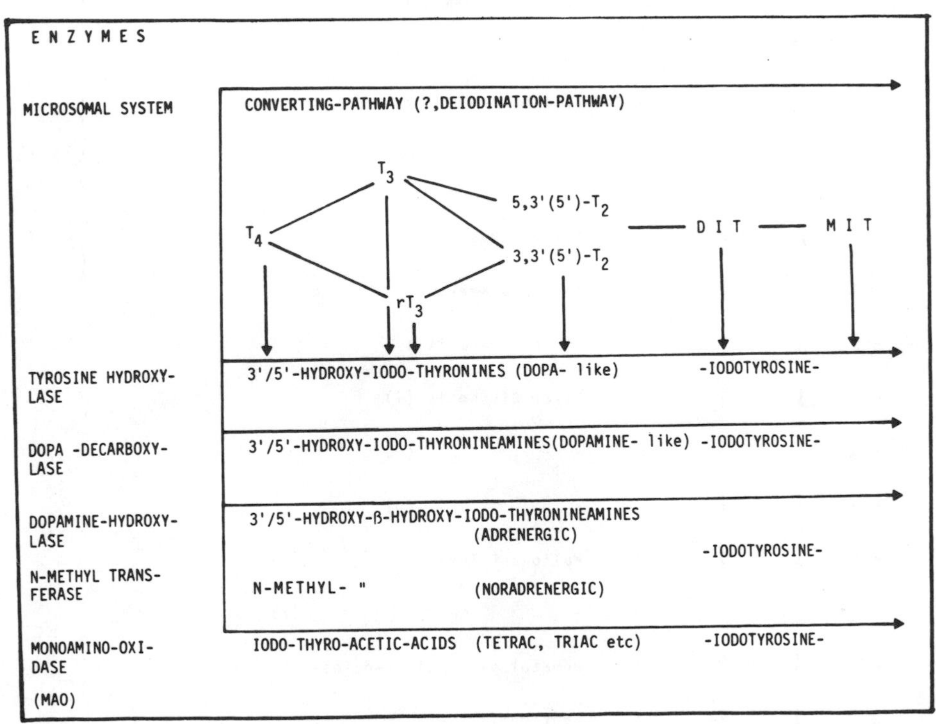

FIG.11. Cascade-enzyme system for bio-transformation of T_4.

TABLE V. PATTERN OF T_4 BIO-TRANSFORMATION IN DIVERSE CLINICAL CONDITIONS

Since all iodothyronines have different binding characteristics and different metabolic clearances in the plasma compartment, binding characteristics (TBG) and tissue iodothyronine concentrations rather than plasma values will determine thyroid "status"

T_4	T_3	rT_3	rT_2	T_4 Biotransformation in diverse clinical conditions
↓	↓	↑	↑	Normal Human Neonates
↑	↑	n	n	Adolescence
n	n	n	n	Adult (middle age)
(↓)	↓	(↓)	?	Adult (old age)
↓	↑	n	?	Hypothyroidism (1)
↓	n↓	(↓)	?	- (2)
↓	↓	↓	↓	- (3)
↑	↑	↑	↑	Hyperthyroidism (1)
n	↑	n	?	- (2)
↓	n	↑	?	-(iodide induced) (3)
n	↓	↑	?	Dexamethasone Therapy
n	↓	↑	?	Caloric Restriction
n(↓)	↓	↑	?	Anorexia Nervosa
n(↑)	↓	↑	n	Chronic Hepatitis
n	↓	↑	n	Liver Cirrhosis (1)
n ↓	↓	n	n	- (2)
n ↓	↓	↓	n ↓	- (3)
n(↑)	↓	↑	?	Malignant Tumor (1)
↓	↓	n	?	- (2)
n	↓	↑	?	Hematologic Malignancies
n	↓	↑	?	Septicemia

test for the occurrence of endocrine exophthalmos during treatment of thyrotoxicosis with a view to immunosuppressive therapy, as has been stated by Mahieu and Winand [19]. However, for unknown reasons, this statement has never been reinforced by a double-blind study [20, discussion].

3. Transformation of T_4 to iodothyronines

The important observation of the conversion of T_4 to T_3 by Braverman and coworkers [21] was the beginning of a new area of research in thyroid hormone metabolism. This new area was initiated by the original communication of Pitt-Rivers and colleagues [22] on the conversion of T_4 to T_3 in 1955. Later, Pittman's group [23] and Surks and coworkers [24] added important contributions to our knowledge of the extent of this process which has since been regarded as the main pathway of T_3 formation. Further work by Chopra [25] on the formation of rT_3 and rT_2 from T_4 gave new insight into possible pathways of T_4 metabolism in vivo. These studies have been supplemented by our in-vitro investigations since 1973 [26]. The whole field was recently reviewed by Cavalieri and Rapoport [27] and by us [28]. It may be summarized by the schematic representation in Fig.9.

From these data it is evident that 80% of T_4 is metabolized through a deiodinating pathway and 20% by a non-deiodinative pathway. We call the whole complex of reactions the "bio-transformation" of T_4 since the conversion process is not a simple one. We have followed these reactions by in-vitro methods and found that rT_3 is the most active naturally occurring inhibitor of the T_4 to T_3 deiodination. This regulation is extremely sensitive to pH. This is important because rT_3 has been reported not to be calorigenic [29, 30], though only recently Fishman and coworkers [31] found that rT_3 appears to be approximately as potent as T_3 in increasing hepatic activity of T_3-aminotransferase, an important enzyme catalysing the transamination of iodothyronine, i.e. it functions in a degradative capacity. This supports, in an unexpected way, our current model of a pH- and substrate-dependent bio-transformation of T_3 (Fig.10). Under physiological conditions the metabolic need for bioactive hormone will regulate the different steps and, with respect to the deiodination pathway of T_4, we have schematically proposed a whole cascade of enzymatic processes which regulate the metabolic fate of T_4 and the biological expression of iodothyronines (Fig.11). It is evident that different organs may respond differently to the T_4 supply, depending upon their enzymatic equipment, and this may determine the organ-selective effects of iodothyronines so well known from clinical observations [32].

To restate the facts more subtly, one could say that T_4 intoxication and T_4 deficiency are the primary thyroid diseases whilst transformation of T_3 modulates the character of the diseases. Under physiological conditions, however, the function of the thyroid in extracting iodine is relatively rudimentary compared with

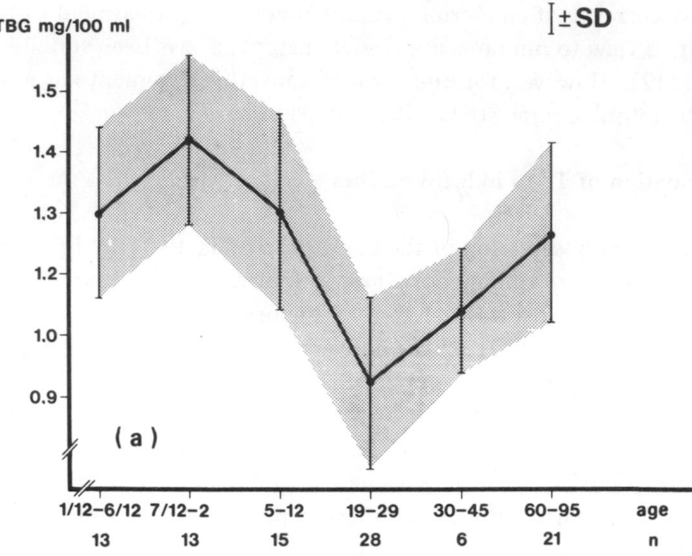
TBG mg/100 ml
± SD
1.5
1.4
1.3
1.2
1.0
0.9
(a)
1/12–6/12 7/12–2 5–12 19–29 30–45 60–95 age
13 13 15 28 6 21 n

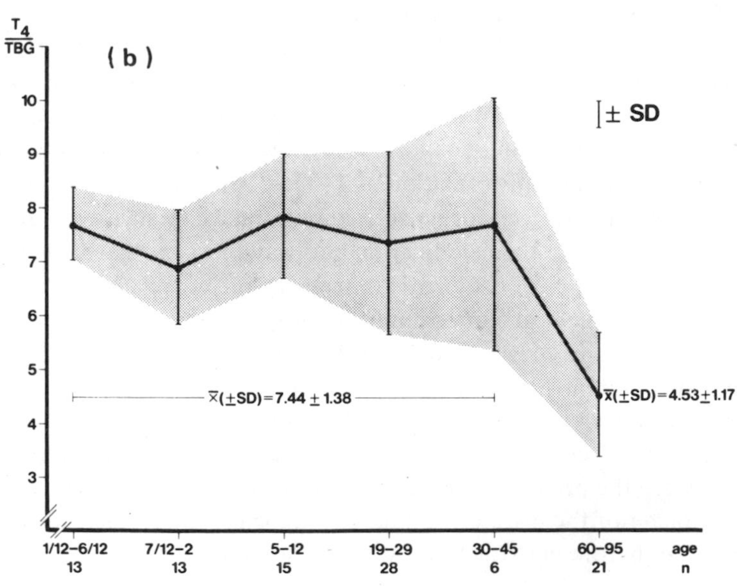
T4/TBG
(b)
10
9
8
7
6
5
4
3
± SD
x̄(±SD)=7.44 ± 1.38
x̄(±SD)=4.53±1.17
1/12–6/12 7/12–2 5–12 19–29 30–45 60–95 age
13 13 15 28 6 21 n

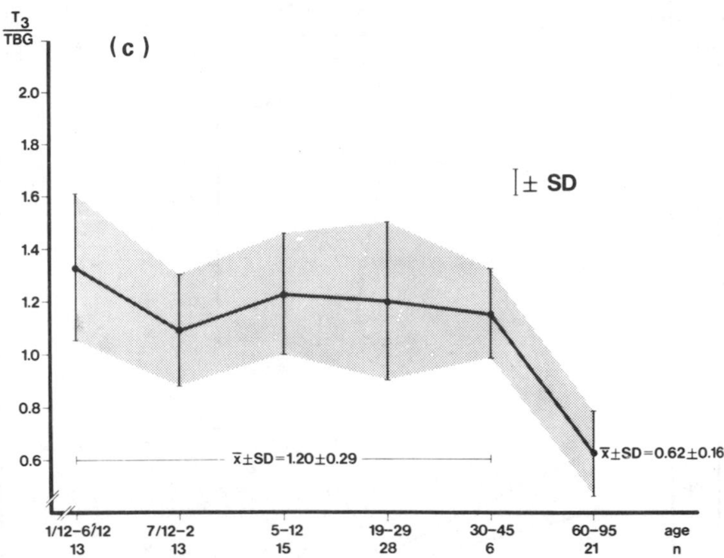

FIG.12(a). Age-related variation of TBG concentration.
(b,c). Smoothing of age-dependent variations of T_4 and T_3 by forming T_4/TBG and T_3/TBG ratios. A divergence in the pattern of T_4 and T_3 versus TBG ratios is only apparent in old age [39].

the processes of bio-transformation of T_4 which are even more important in relation to extrathyroidal disturbances of these processes. Further testing of "thyroid status" must endeavour to complete our knowledge by evaluating the bioactivity of plasma iodothyronines in a purely descriptive way. However, they are beginning to be seen as of limited clinical value (Table V). Recent work by Morreale de Escobar [33] has demonstrated that intracellular T_3 derived from T_4 is not rapidly and completely exchangeable with extracellular compartments. That means that even if we knew the plasma kinetics we would not know the local mitochondrial effects summarized recently by Sterling and Bull [34], nor the nuclear events proposed by Oppenheimer [35] and Samuels and colleagues [36] which ultimately determine the bio-expression of T_4 bio-transforming reactions.

4. Importance of TBG

Bound hormone fractions represent the main extrathyroidal pool for iodothyronines, above all T_4. The current belief is that bound T_4 represents a reservoir for rapid exchange of free T_4 between plasma and intracellular compartments. It is however conceivable that some of the TBG-T_4 complex undergoes active transmembranous transport, as recently hypothesized in Refs [37] and [38].

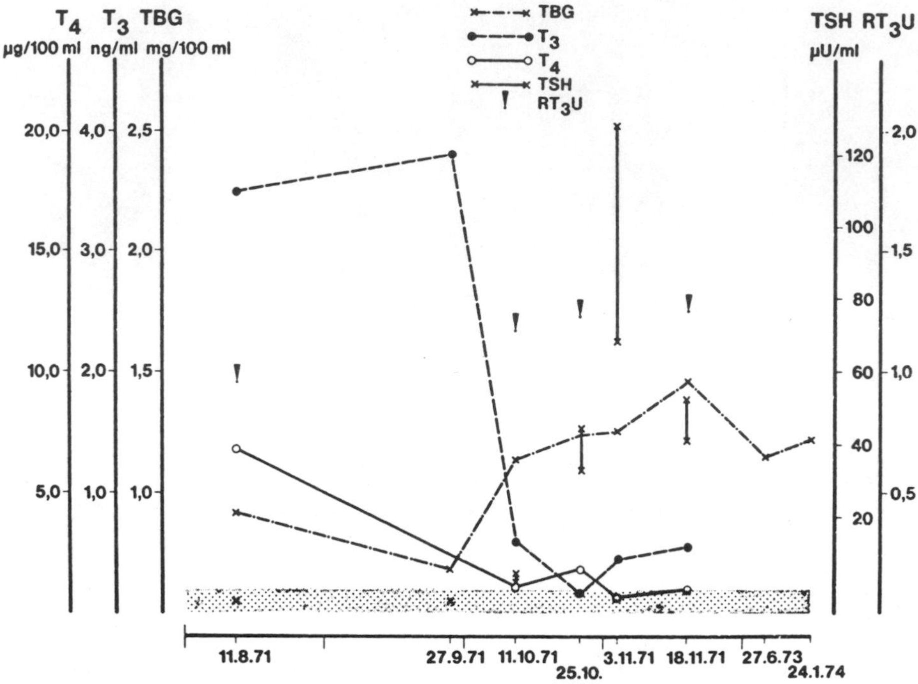

FIG.13. Results of T_4, T_3, TBG and the TRH tests in thyrotoxic patients under antithyroid drug therapy. From the typical example in the figure it is evident that TBG increases when the TRH test becomes positive and vice versa, suggesting the functional importance of TBG for the bio-availability of thyroid hormones.

TABLE VI. EVIDENCE FOR FUNCTIONAL HETEROGENEITY OF TBG

Two different species of TBG molecules, only one binding T_3
Age-related variations in TBG concentration with euthyroidism
Change of affinity in thyrotoxicosis and hypothyroidism
Exogenous T_4 and T_3 application alters binding kinetics of TBG
Increase of TBG concentration coincident with positive TRH test during treatment of thyrotoxicosis
Resynthesis of hormone-devoid TBG in patients after plasmapheresis for thyrotoxicosis

As TBG has a more static function as a purely binding protein it seems to be involved in the regulation of bio-available T_4 for intracellular transformation. Protein concentration of TBG and its functional alterations of binding characteristics would hence modify the bio-availability of iodothyronines. The concentration of TBG varies with age (Fig.12) and the usually wide range of bound concentrations for T_4 and T_3 is restricted by hormone/TBG ratios. This finding is especially relevant for neonatal screening of hypothyroidism since TBG, and hence T_4 (and T_3) concentrations, depend very much on neonatal liver function [39]. This seems to open a new possibility of better discrimination of differing thyroid status with regard to hormone concentrations in cases with borderline clinical signs of disturbed thyroid gland function and peripheral transformation. Recent evidence indicates that the bio-availability of T_4 may depend on the functional heterogeneity of TBG (Fig.13 from Ref.[32]).

From these findings we would like to emphasize that more attention should be directed to the enormous importance of TBG as a peripheral mediator of thyroid gland function. Since the determination of TBG concentration is now generally possible, more clinical data need to be accumulated and our scientific interest should focus on the determination of functional alterations in the TBG molecule (Table VI).

SUMMARY

I have tried to review the current status of thyroid function testing with test procedures which are already available for clinical use. Furthermore, I have discussed the pathophysiological background of possible new ways to understand and test disturbed thyroid function and thyroid hormone metabolism. Our main interest with respect to the thyroid gland concerns the thyroid stimulating immunoglobulins and the whole area of immune reactions. The peripheral fate of the main product of thyroid gland function, namely the bio-transformation of T_4, will probably open a new means of understanding different and organ-specific effects of iodothyronines. Another main interest would be the further investigation of the physiological and pathophysiological importance of thyroid binding proteins.

REFERENCES

[1] HORN, K., MARSCHNER, I., SCRIBA, P.C., J. Clin. Chem. Clin. Biochem. **14** (1976) 353.

[2] GORDON, A., GROSS, J., Acta Endocrinol. **83** (1976) 539.

[3] MARSCHNER, I., ERHARDT, F.W., SCRIBA, P.C., J. Clin. Chem. Clin. Biochem. **14** (1976) 345.

[4] HESCH, R.-D., Schilddrüse 1973 (SCHLEUSENER, H., WEINHEIMER, B., Eds), G. Thieme Verlag, Stuttgart (1975) 120.
[5] HALL, R., Rational Diagnosis of Thyroid Disease. A Current Concept (Proc. Bernstein Workshop, 1976) (HÖFER, R., Ed.), H. Egermann Verlag, Vienna (1977) 43.
[6] KRÜSKEMPER, H.L., ibid. p.143.
[7] HESCH, R.-D., MÜHLEN, A. von zur, HÖFFKEN, B., KÖDDING, R., SIMON, R., ibid. p.121.
[8] REICHLIN, S., MARTIN, J.B., MITNICK, M.A., BOSHANS, R.L., GRIMM, Y., BOLLINGER, J., CORDON, J., MALACARA, J., Rec. Progr. Horm. Res. **28** (1972) 229.
[9] BURROW, G.N., MAY, P.N., SPAULDING, S.W., DONABEDIAN, R.K., J. Clin. Endocrinol. Metab. **45** (1977) 65.
[10] MELANDER, A., Endocrinology, Excerpta Medica, Amsterdam – Oxford, Vol. 1 (1977) 221.
[11] SKILLERN, P., Mayo Clinic Proc. **47** (1972) 848.
[12] CHOPRA, I.J., SOLOMON, D.H., CHOPRA, U., YOSHIHARA, E., TERASAKI, P.I., SMITH, F., J. Clin. Endocrinol. Metab. **45** (1977) 45.
[13] VOLPE, R., Rational Diagnosis of Thyroid Disease. A Current Concept (Proc. Bernstein Workshop, 1976) (HÖFER, R., Ed.), H. Egermann Verlag, Vienna (1977) 46.
[14] IAKEDA, A., KRISS, J.P., J. Clin. Endocrinol. Metab. **44** (1977) 46.
[15] MULLIN, B.R., LEVINSON, R.R., FRIEDMAN, A., HENSEN, D.E., WINAND, R.J., KOHN, L.D., Endocrinology **100** (1977) 351.
[16] STAEHELIN, V., VALLOTON, M.B., BURGER, A., J. Clin. Endocrinol. Metab. **41** (1975) 699.
[17] HEHRMANN, R., HÖFFKEN, B., MÜHLEN, A. von zur, CREUTZIG, H., THIELE, J., HESCH, R.–D., Horm. Metab. Res. **9** (1977) 326.
[18] MUNRO, R.E., LAMKI, L., ROW, V.V., VOLPE, R., J. Clin. Endocrinol. Metab. **37** (1973) 286.
[19] MAHIEU, P., WINAND, R.J., J. Clin. Endocrinol. Metab. **34** (1972) 1090.
[20] WINAND, R., KOHN, L.D., Rational Diagnosis of Thyroid Disease. A Current Concept (Proc. Bernstein Workshop, 1976) (HÖFER, R., Ed.), H. Egermann Verlag, Vienna (1977) 93.
[21] BRAVERMAN, L.E., INGBAR, S.H., STERLING, K., J. Clin. Invest. **49** (1970) 855.
[22] PITT-RIVERS, R., STANBURY, J.B., RAPP, B., J. Clin. Endocrinol. Metab. **15** (1955) 616.
[23] PITTMAN, C.S., CHAMBERS, J.B., READ, W.N., J. Clin. Invest. **50** (1971) 1187.
[24] SURKS, M.I., SCHADLOW, A.R., STOCK, J., OPPENHEIMER, J.N., J. Clin. Invest. **52** (1973) 805.
[25] CHOPRA, I.J., J. Clin. Invest. **58** (1976) 32.
[26] HESCH, R.–D., BRUNNER, G., SÖLING, D., Clin. Chim. Acta **59** (1975) 209.
[27] CAVALIERI, R.R., RAPOPORT, B.R., Ann. Rev. Med. **28** (1977) 57.
[28] HÖFFKEN, B., HESCH, R.–D., Dtsch. Med. Wschr. **102** (in press).
[29] LARSON, F.C., ALBRIGHT, E.C., J. Clin. Invest. **40** (1961) 1132.
[30] PITTMAN, L.S., PITTMAN, J.A., Handb. Physiol. **3** (1974) 233.
[31] FISHMAN, N., HUANG, Y.P., TERGIS, D.C., RIVLIN, R.S., Endocrinology **100** (1977) 1055.
[32] HÖFFKEN, B., KÖDDING, R., HEHRMANN, R., MÜHLEN, A. von zur, HESCH, R.–D., Biochim. Biophys. Acta (in press).
[33] MORREALE de ESCOBAR, G., Regulation of Thyroid Function, F.K. Schattauer, Stuttgart (1976) 109.
[34] STERLING, K., BULL, N.Y., Acad. Med. **53** (1977) 260.

[35] OPPENHEIMER, J.H., N. Engl. J. Med. **292** (1975) 1063.
[36] SAMUELS, A.A., TSAI, J.S., CASANOVA, J., STANLEY, F., J. Clin. Invest. **54** (1974) 853.
[37] COOPER, E., BURKE, C.W., Personal communication.
[38] SACK, J., FISHER, D.A., Perinatal Thyroid Physiology and Disease (FISHER, D.A., BURROW, G.N., Eds.), New York (1975) 49.
[39] HESCH, R.–D., GATZ, J., JÜPPNER, H., STUBBE, P., Horm. Metab. Res. **9** (1977) 141.
[40] CAMUS, M.M., STERLING, K., HESCH, R.–D., ERMANS, A.M., Excerpta Medica, International Congress Series **86** (1975) 361.
[41] McKENZIE, J.M., ZAKARIJA, M., J. Clin. Endocrinol. Metab. **42** (1976) 7787.
[42] HÖFFKEN, B., KÖHRLE, J., KÖDDING, R., HESCH, R.–D., Annual Meeting European Thyroid Association, Lyon, 1977 (Abstract).

DISCUSSION

D.K. HAZRA: What, in your opinion, is the significance of isolated T_4 elevation in the presence of a normal T_3?

R.-D. HESCH: You may refer to "T_4 euthyroidism" or to elevated T_4 values with low T_3 in thyrotoxic patients. In my own experience I have only observed "T_4 euthyroidism" in old age and elevated T_4 values with low T_3 in thyrotoxic patients suffering from other extrathyroidal diseases such as pneumonia or cancer. They could also be observed in thyrotoxic cases with anti-T_3-antibodies.

D.K. HAZRA: Alterations in T_4/T_3 conversion after acute myocardial infarction have been associated with a poor prognosis. Is there any evidence to suggest that such alterations may be worth treating?

R.-D. HESCH: We observed a decrease in T_3 values during acute myocardial infarction, which we reported last year. Investigations carried out at the Physiological Institute of the University of Warsaw have shown extreme T_3 toxicosis in the infarct region of the myocardium, indicating a definite local disruption of T_4/T_3 metabolism. It is conceivable that drugs may be used in future to treat such local T_3 accumulation.

G. PINEDA: When you speak of the TRH test, do you mean measurement of both TSH and T_3 response to TRH, or only TSH?

We find from our experience that the T_3 response is basic in defining the thyroidal status.

R.-D. HESCH: We perform the TRH test by measuring only TSH, just before and 30 min after injecting 200 μg of TRH. Under these conditions you will not observe a change in T_3. We showed several years ago that when we infused TRH continuously over several hours, T_3 increased. But this is not of diagnostic importance and I do not think that T_3 measurement is of clinical relevance.

D. RODBARD: Is it possible that the antibodies in human sera which react with thyroxine or tri-iodothyronine are really anti-thyroglobulin antibodies? It seems unlikely that T_4 or T_3 would be immunogenic, in view of their size and immunological tolerance.

Secondly, is the relative importance of the deiodinating and non-deiodinating pathways influenced by iodine deficiency or excess?

R.-D. HESCH: They are certainly not anti-thyroglobulin antibodies. We checked that possibility. Other proteins may be involved, but certainly not thyroglobulin.

As to your second question, we did not investigate the point, and neither do I know of any such investigation reported in the literature.

S.A. SIDDIQUI: Referring to the assessment of thyroid status, you suggest that a whole battery of laboratory investigations – eight or nine, in fact – should be carried out. It would be uneconomical, in my opinion, to carry out all of them for each patient. Would it not be more practical and economical to perform after the clinical examination a selected combination of laboratory investigations, followed by a provocative test to confirm the outcome?

R.-D. HESCH: You have raised a very important point, namely whether there may be a general procedure for the assessment of thyroid status. In my view there are so many variable circumstances that I would not impose such a procedure. For example, in an out-patient clinic much depends on where the patients come from and whether a recall is easy or not. The next deciding factor is whether you want to exclude or to prove a deviation from euthyroidism. In our Department we routinely perform, in the former case, a T_4 and T_3 determination by RIA and, in the latter, a TRH test. In all cases of goitre a scan is performed immediately with ^{99m}Tc. In cases of endocrine exophthalmos, we perform as many tests as possible. (For more details I would refer you to Rational Diagnosis of Thyroid Disease: A Current Concept (HÖFER, R., Ed.), Verlag H. Egermann, Vienna, 1977.)

THYROXINE AND THYROTROPHIN RADIOIMMUNOASSAYS USING DRIED BLOOD SAMPLES ON FILTER PAPER FOR SCREENING OF NEONATAL HYPOTHYROIDISM*

C. BECKERS, C. CORNETTE
Centre de médecine nucléaire,
Ecole de médecine

B. FRANÇOIS
Centre de dépistage des anomalies
métaboliques néonatales

A. BOUCKAERT, M. LECHAT
Unité d'épidémiologie,

Université de Louvain,
Brussels, Belgium

Abstract

THYROXINE AND THYROTROPHIN RADIOIMMUNOASSAYS USING DRIED BLOOD SAMPLES ON FILTER PAPER FOR SCREENING OF NEONATAL HYPOTHYROIDISM.

A routine and automated methodology for thyroxine (T_4) and thyrotrophin (TSH) radioimmunoassay (RIA) using dried blood samples on filter paper is described. Five-mm-diameter 'dots' were prepared. One dot eluate, corresponding to 4 μl of plasma, was used for the T4 RIA while two were necessary for the TSH RIA. Reference dot eluates were included in each assay for quality control. In a preliminary study on 1903 newborns, samples were generally obtained between the 5th and 7th day. The mean dot T_4 concentration was 7.38 ± 2.5 μg/dl. The mean dot TSH concentration was 11.83 ± 9.1 μU/ml, the equation of the regression line between dot TSH (y) and serum TSH (x) being $y = 10.29 + 0.623x$.

INTRODUCTION

The importance of early treatment of congenital hypothyroidism is a well-recognized fact. However, the diagnosis is often subtle because it is difficult to be certain on clinical grounds only. Also, the diagnosis is often delayed which has catastrophic consequences for the patient. To face this difficult problem, pilot screening programs were started a few years ago in Quebec, Pittsburgh and

* Partially supported by the Fonds de la Recherche Scientifique Médicale, Belgium (grant No. 20.393).

Toronto [1–4]. Since then, the determinations of blood thyroxine (T_4) and of blood thyrotrophin (TSH) have appeared as tools of considerable interest for the early detection of congenital hypothyroidism.

The aim of this paper is to describe the experience we have gained in this field by using a sensitive T_4 radioimmunoassay (T_4 RIA) that is complemented by the radioimmunological determination of TSH, both assays being performed on minute amounts of serum obtained from dried blood samples on filter paper. When used for the screening of neonatal hypothyroidism, the methodology can be extended to other applications, especially to solve various thyroid problems in countries where samples have sometimes to be sent from remote places.

MATERIAL AND METHODS

Subjects under study and collection of blood samples

The present report deals with a total of 1903 newborns surveyed between November 1976 and January 1977 for T_4. In 90% of the cases, TSH was also determined. Blood samples were obtained from newborns in the University Clinics and other related hospitals spread throughout Belgium that are connected with our Central Laboratory. The group included 52% males and 48% females. It was requested that, ideally, the specimens should be taken on the 5th day after birth, but this request could be fulfilled in 28% of the cases only, 77% of the samples being obtained between the 5th and 7th day.

Blood samples were adsorbed on Schleisser and Schull No.2992 filter paper, a material already routinely used for phenylketonuria screening. A standard paper punch was used to obtain 5-mm-diameter 'dots' of standards and unknowns. Control experiments indicated that a 5-mm-diameter paper dot corresponds to a mean of 8.5 μl of whole blood. Taking into account the coefficient of extraction by elution of one dot (overnight incubation in clean polystyrene tubes at 4°C with 0.3 ml barbital buffer, pH8.6, ionic strength 0.075 and containing 1% normal rabbit serum) and a mean haematocrit value of 55%, it can be calculated that the eluate from each dot corresponds to an average of 3.8 μl of serum [2, 4].

Thyroxine radioimmunoassay (T_4 RIA)

The methodology previously reported for T_4 RIA was used with appropriate dilutions of the T_4 antibody to obtain a maximal sensitivity in the low range of serum T_4 concentrations [5, 6]. Routinely, one dot per subject was used for the T_4 RIA. T_4-specific rabbit antiserum was used at a final dilution of 1:20 000. High specific activity ^{125}I-T_4 tracer (200 μCi/μg) was obtained from The Radiochemical Centre (Amersham, UK). The results were expressed in μg T_4/dl serum

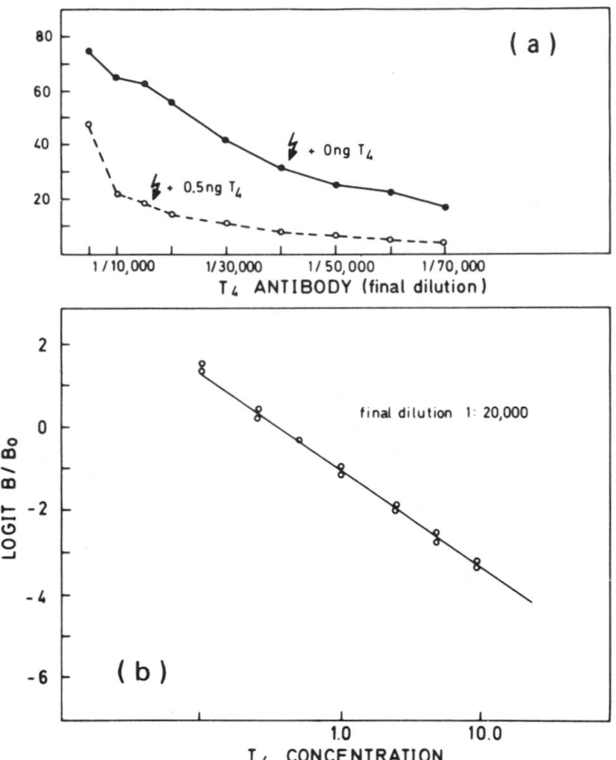

FIG.1. (a) Titration curve of anti-T_4 antibodies with and without addition of cold T_4 (0.5 ng/tube). (b) Typical calibration curve for thyroxine by radioimmunoassay.

by running, with each assay, 30 different dots used as references for quality control. The T_4 content of these dots had also been directly determined several times by competitive protein-binding analysis of samples obtained by venipuncture at the same time as the sample was obtained for preparing the dot of dried blood (see Results).

Thyrotrophin radioimmunoassay (TSH RIA)

Our double-antibody radioimmunoassay [7, 8] was adapted to achieve maximal sensitivity in the low range of TSH concentrations to satisfy the goals of the screening program. ^{125}I-hTSH was obtained from the Institut National des Radioéléments (I.R.E., Belgium) at a specific activity of 100 μCi/μg. Specific anti-human TSH antibodies were purchased from Serono Laborat. (Italy) and used at a final dilution of 1:500 000. TSH research standard 68/38, obtained

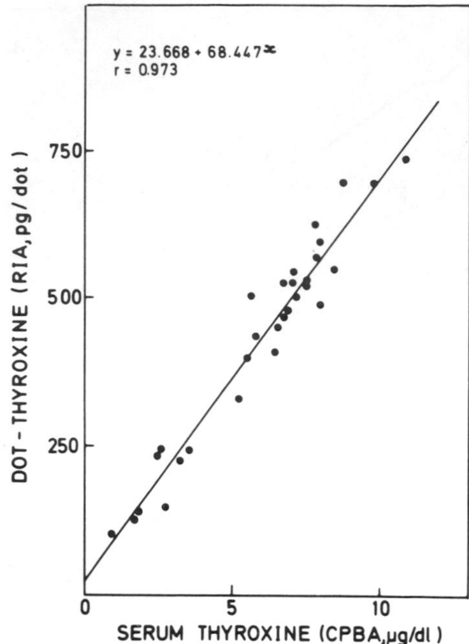

FIG. 2. Correlation between the T_4 value (pg/dot) obtained by RIA by the dot method and the serum T_4 concentration (µg/dl) obtained by competitive protein-binding analysis.

from the Medical Research Council (UK), was routinely used for the calibration curve. After correcting for the elution factor, the results were expressed in µU/ml. Each assay included dot eluates for which a concomitant serum sample obtained by venipuncture had been previously assayed for TSH by our routine TSH RIA [7, 8] (see Results).

General methodology

When the filter papers were not obtained from our hospital, they were received by mail and kept at 4°C until being processed within the next few days. Under these conditions of preservation, the per cent elution remained unchanged for several weeks.

The general methodology for T_4 and TSH radioimmunoassays was adapted to full automatization on a Micromedic pipetting station (Micromedic System, USA). A well-type gamma-scintillation counter equipped with a spectrometer was connected to a teletype and a punched system so that the data could be processed

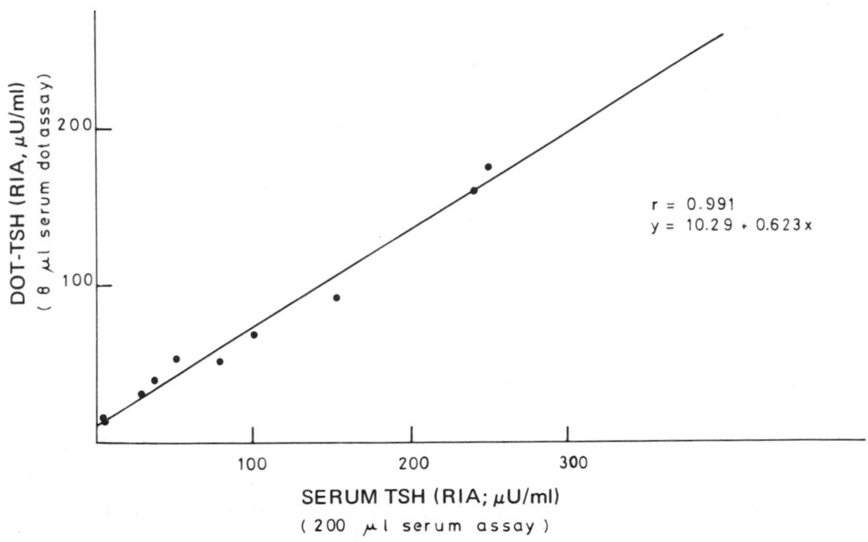

FIG.3. Correlation between the TSH value (μU/ml) obtained by the RIA by the dot method and the serum TSH concentration (μU/ml) obtained by radioimmunoassay.

directly through a Wang 600 calculator and the calibration curve, the main parameters for quality control and the results of the hormonal determinations obtained immediately.

Except where otherwise stated, all the data are given as the mean ± one standard deviation.

RESULTS

T_4 radioimmunoassay (T_4 RIA)

A typical dilution curve of our T_4 antibody is presented in Fig.1. Although we had the possibility to use the T_4 antibody at a dilution higher than 1:20 000, this titre was selected to obtain the maximal sensitivity in the lower concentration range of T_4.

A typical calibration curve is also given in Fig.1. In 11 quality-control experiments, the determination of T_4 in 29 different samples measured in parallel by the dot method and the classical competitive protein-binding technique on serum gave a correlation coefficient of 0.930 ± 0.034 SEM (Fig.2).

The mean serum T_4 concentration for the whole group was 7.38 ± 2.5 μg/dl.
In the 1767 cases (93%) in which the sex of the newborn was known, the mean T_4 concentration in 903 males was found to be 7.14 ± 2.37 μg/dl and in 864 females it was found to be 7.55 ± 2.47 μg/dl ($p < 0.05$).

TSH radioimmunoassay (TSH RIA)

As previously mentioned, the TSH RIA was adapted to be very sensitive in the low range of serum TSH concentrations. The correlation coefficient between the TSH values measured on dots and sera was 0.991 (Fig.3).

The dot TSH RIA was adapted not only to detect minute amounts of TSH in the eluates from two dots (about 8 μl of serum) but also to cover the useful range of TSH concentrations for the neonatal hypothyroidism screening. As a result of the methodology adopted, the TSH values from the dot eluates (y) were systematically higher than the ones obtained directly from the serum of the same patient (x) ($y = 10.29 + 0.623x$) (Fig.3). This difference was considered to be of little importance since the purpose of the methodology was to be able to detect, with the highest degree of certainty, any case of hypothyroidism. In 1700 subjects, the mean dot TSH was 11.83 ± 9.1 μU/ml. No significant difference in TSH was observed after the 3rd day after birth.

DISCUSSION

The exceptional possibilities of radioimmunology allow a unique application to mass screening of neonatal hypothyroidism, the incidence of which lies around 1/8000 births (if not higher when partial defects are considered). The RIA of T_4 and TSH can – under appropriate conditions – be fully automated which, in turn, allows a better quality control of the assays and therefore a better screening quality.

Endless discussions could be envisaged as to which assay, the T_4 or the TSH, is the superior for screening. Indeed, the pediatrician needs both values for a screening procedure that is 100% foolproof. The T_4 assay is probably the more fundamental approach, but it could be misleading in cases of ectopic thyroid gland (partial hypothyroidism) or in subjects with low thyroxine-binding globulin (TBG), a situation which may have a higher incidence than generally expected [9]. The T_4 RIA is also cheaper than the TSH RIA which is a more delicate technique with regard to TSH labelling, storage of the tracer and the methodology itself. On the other hand, TSH determination would probably recognize mild cases of hypothyroidism more easily though it is of no help in the diagnosis of infants with hypothyroidism secondary to TSH deficiency.

The T_4 and TSH values of the dot eluates correlate well with those of serum, indicating the good reliability of the dot assay. In our experience, T_4 and TSH in dried blood spots on filter paper remain stable, thus allowing the specimens to be easily mailed. Keeping the dots at room temperature does not alter the results at least one month, although it is recommended that the filter papers be kept at 4°C if possible.

As illustrated in Figs 2 and 3, the sensitivities of the T_4 RIA and TSH RIA satisfy the prerequisites of a good quality screening test for neonatal hypothyroidism, even in mild cases of thyroid dysfunction. It should be recalled here that in the 21 cases with proven congenital hypothyroidism that were detected by the dot screening method, the T_4 values were less than 7 μg/dl and the TSH levels higher than 50 μU/ml [9]

The dot TSH RIA gives a higher value than that obtained directly on the serum of the same sample (see equation of the regression line in Fig.3), but this is probably an indirect consequence of the effort to maximize the sensitivity of the dot TSH RIA which was finally done on the equivalent of about 8 μl of serum. It should indeed be pointed out here that the detection of neonatal hypothyroidism is only one facet of a screening program for metabolic diseases. A compromise had thus to be adopted in order to save enough dots for other assays (phenylketonuria, etc.).

ACKNOWLEDGEMENTS

The skilful technical assistance of Mrs C. Veulemans-Grevy, Miss M.A. Lecroart and Mr J.M. Alley is gratefully acknowledged.

REFERENCES

[1] DUSSAULT, J.H., COULOMBE, P., LABERGE, C., LETARTE, J., GUYDA, H., KHOURY, K., Preliminary report on a mass screening for neonatal hypothyroidism, Pediatrics **96** (1975) 670.

[2] WALFISH, P.G., Evaluation of three thyroid function screening tests for detecting neonatal hypothyroidism, Lancet **i** (1976) 1208.

[3] DUSSAULT, J.H., COULOMBE, P., LABERGE, C., in Perinatal Thyroid Physiology and Disease (FISHER, D.A., BURROW, G.N., Eds), New York (1975) 221.

[4] LARSEN, P.R., BROSKIN, K., Thyroxine (T_4) immunoassay using filter paper blood samples for screening of neonates for hypothyroidism, Pediatr. Res. **9** (1975) 604.

[5] BECKERS, C., CORNETTE, C., THALASSO, M., Serum thyroxine radioimmunoassay, Horm. Metab. Res. **4** (1972) 406.

[6] BECKERS, C., CORNETTE, C., THALASSO, M., Evaluation of serum thyroxine by radioimmunoassay, J. Nucl. Med. **14** (1973) 317.

[7] BECKERS, C., CORNETTE, C., Dosage radio-immunologique de la thyréostimuline en pathologie thyroïdienne, Ann. Andocrinol. **30** (1969) 291.

[8] BECKERS, C., MASKENS, A., CORNETTE, C., Thyrotropin response to synthetic thyrotropin-releasing hormone in normal subjects and in patients with nontoxic goiter, Europ. J. Clin. Invest. **2** (1972) 220.

[9] Recommendations for screening programs for congenital hypothyroidism (Newborn Committee of the American Thyroid Association), Canad. Med. Assoc. J. **116** (1977) 631.

IAEA-SM-220/71

LE DOSAGE RADIOIMMUNOLOGIQUE DE LA THYREOSTIMULINE HYPOPHYSAIRE A PARTIR D'UN ECHANTILLON DE SANG CAPILLAIRE RECUEILLI SUR PAPIER FILTRE

Intérêt dans le dépistage de l'hypothyroïdie néonatale

J. INGRAND, M.A. DUGUE, A.M. MAMARBACHI
Laboratoire de radioimmunologie,
Hôpital Cochin,
Paris, France

P. BOURDOUX, F. DELANGE
Service des radioisotopes,
Hôpital St-Pierre,
Bruxelles, Belgique

Abstract–Résumé

RADIOIMMUNOASSAY OF THYROID-STIMULATING HORMONE (TSH) USING A CAPILLARY BLOOD-SAMPLE COLLECTED ON FILTER PAPER: VALUE OF THE METHOD FOR DETECTING NEONATAL HYPOTHYROIDISM.

Hypothyroidism is the thyroid disturbance most commonly encountered in paediatrics. Its average frequency is estimated at around one case per 6000 births. It is an exceptionally serious disease in newborn infants as it is accompanied by imperfect brain development leading to cerebral atrophy, degenerescence of the cortical neurons, defective myelinization and, most often, in children, irreversible psychomotor retardation. It should be possible to avoid this complication provided that a substitutive therapy using thyroid hormone is initiated very rapidly. For this it is necessary that the hypothyroidism be detected during the first few days of life since the chances of the therapy being successful decline very quickly. Save in a few exceptional cases, early detection cannot be based on clinical signs alone. The laboratory can play a decisive part by bringing to light either a defect in the production of thyroid hormone or a high blood level of TSH. The paper presents a description of the micromethod used together with a detailed analysis of certain important technical points, a study of the quality of the results obtained and a general discussion of the strategy for detecting neonatal hypothyroidism.

LE DOSAGE RADIOIMMUNOLOGIQUE DE LA THYREOSTIMULINE HYPOPHYSAIRE A PARTIR D'UN ECHANTILLON DE SANG CAPILLAIRE RECUEILLI SUR PAPIER FILTRE: INTERET DANS LE DEPISTAGE DE L'HYPOTHYROIDIE NEONATALE.

L'hypothyroïdie est l'affection thyroïdienne la plus fréquente en pédiatrie; sa fréquence moyenne est estimée à environ 1 cas pour 6000 naissances. Il s'agit d'une maladie exceptionnellement grave chez le nouveau-né car elle s'accompagne d'un développement imparfait du cerveau entraînant atrophie cérébrale, dégénérescence des neurones corticaux et défaut de myélinisation, et, le plus souvent, chez l'enfant, un retard psychomoteur irréversible.

Cette complication doit pouvoir être évitée dans la mesure où un traitement substitutif à base d'hormones thyroïdiennes est instauré très rapidement. Pour cela, il faut dépister l'hypothyroïdie dès les premiers jours de la vie car les chances de succès de la thérapeutique s'amenuisent très rapidement. A quelques exceptions près, le dépistage précoce ne peut s'appuyer sur les seuls signes cliniques; en fait, le laboratoire peut jouer un rôle déterminant en mettant en évidence ou bien un déficit de production des hormones thyroïdiennes, ou bien un taux sanguin élevé de TSH. Le mémoire comprend la description de la microméthode utilisée, avec l'analyse détaillée de certains points techniques importants, l'examen de la qualité des résultats obtenus, ainsi qu'une discussion générale sur la stratégie de dépistage de l'hypothyroïdie néonatale.

L'hypothyroïdie est l'affection thyroïdienne la plus fréquente en pédiatrie; sa fréquence moyenne est estimée à environ 1 cas pour 6000 naissances [1–5]. Il s'agit d'une maladie exceptionnellement grave chez le nouveau-né car elle s'accompagne d'un développement imparfait du cerveau, entraînant atrophie cérébrale, dégénérescence des neurones corticaux et défaut de myélinisation [6–11] et, le plus souvent, chez l'enfant, un retard psychomoteur irréversible.

Cette complication doit pouvoir être évitée dans la mesure où un traitement substitutif à base d'hormones thyroïdiennes est instauré très rapidement [12–14]. Pour cela, il faut dépister l'hypothyroïdie dès les premiers jours de la vie car les chances de succès de la thérapeutique s'amenuisent très rapidement.

A quelques exceptions près [15–16], le dépistage précoce ne peut s'appuyer sur les seuls signes cliniques; en fait, le laboratoire peut jouer un rôle déterminant en mettant en évidence:
- ou bien un déficit de production des hormones thyroïdiennes [17–20],
- ou bien un taux sanguin élevé de TSH, qui reflète le plus souvent un hypofonctionnement de la glande thyroïde [4, 21–22].

Dans cet exposé, nous nous proposons dans un premier temps de décrire la méthode utilisée (dosage de TSH dans le sang total prélevé le cinquième jour) en insistant sur un certain nombre d'aspects techniques, pour analyser ensuite la qualité des résultats obtenus. Nous terminons par une discussion générale sur la stratégie de dépistage de l'hypothyroïdie néonatale.

1. MATERIEL ET METHODES

1.1. Recueil du sang

Le sang est prélevé vers le cinquième jour après la naissance par piqûre du talon au vaccinostyle et dépôt sur une feuille de papier filtre Schleicher-Shull 2992 (fig.1). Après séchage en position verticale, à la température ordinaire, le prélèvement est conservé à + 4°C jusqu'au moment de l'analyse. Les caractéristiques du papier utilisé jouent un très grand rôle au niveau des performances analytiques; elles ont fait l'objet d'un certain nombre d'études.

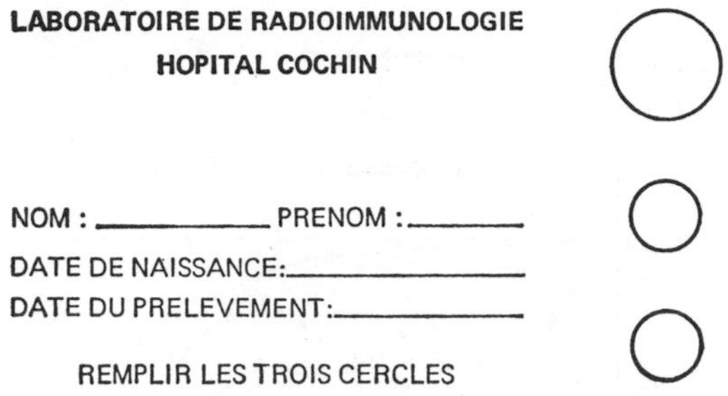
LABORATOIRE DE RADIOIMMUNOLOGIE
HOPITAL COCHIN

NOM : __________ PRENOM : ______
DATE DE NAISSANCE: ____________
DATE DU PRELEVEMENT: __________

REMPLIR LES TROIS CERCLES

FIG.1. Fiche de papier filtre utilisée pour le recueil du sang total.

TABLEAU I. VARIANTES DU PROTOCOLE EXPERIMENTAL UTILISABLES POUR LE DOSAGE DE TSH A PARTIR D'UNE PASTILLE DE PAPIER FILTRE
Volumes et instructions

	A	B
Echantillon ou standard	20 μl (1 pastille 8 mm)	6 μl 1 pastille de 4,2 mm (ou 2 de 3 mm)
Suspension d'anticorps (Sephadex®)	400 μl	50 μl
	Laisser une nuit à température du laboratoire	
TSH marquée	100 μl	100 μl
	Laisser une nuit sous agitation	
NaCl 0,9%	3 ml	2 ml
	Centrifuger à 1500 × g pendant 5 minutes Répéter le lavage; compter le culot	

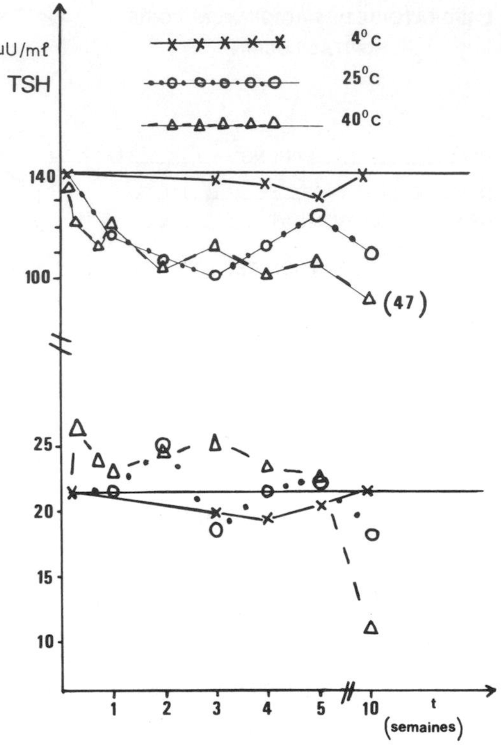

FIG.2. Etude de l'influence de la température sur la conservation des échantillons.

1.2. Dosage radioimmunologique de la TSH sanguine

Le dosage de la TSH est réalisé[1] après élution de l'hormone à partir de pastilles découpées à l'emporte-pièce dans la tache de sang total. Le protocole expérimental comporte différentes variantes (tableau I), selon le volume de sang analysé; l'élution est effectuée pendant 18 heures à l'aide d'une suspension de Sephadex[1] renfermant l'anticorps, en l'absence d'hormone marquée. Après ce délai, le traceur est ajouté et on termine l'incubation sous agitation pendant une nuit supplémentaire.

La séparation de la fraction B comporte plusieurs centrifugations et lavages; la courbe d'étalonnage est habituellement construite en ordonnée à partir des valeurs B/B_1 et en abscisse à partir des concentrations d'un standard secondaire de TSH (1 à 200 µU/ml) (calibré par rapport au standard MRC 68–38).

---

[1] Réactifs fournis par Pharmacia (TM), Uppsala.

TABLEAU II. CARACTERISTIQUES DU PAPIER FILTRE UTILISE

Masse surfacique	180 g/m^2
Durée nécessaire à l'élution	t $\geqslant$ 1 heure
Mode d'étalement	dépôt d'une grosse goutte de sang *en 1 fois*

N.B.: Il est contre-indiqué d'effectuer des dépôts en couches superposées. Exemple:

Concentration du sang (μU de TSH par ml)	Concentration mesurée à partir des étalements	
	a: 1 $\times$ 150 μl	b: 3 $\times$ 50 μl
12,5	12,5	18,5
25	25	39

TABLEAU III. COEFFICIENT D'EXTRACTION DE LA TSH A PARTIR DU PAPIER FILTRE; INFLUENCE DU DIAMETRE DES PASTILLES

Diamètre (mm)	Coefficient
8	x_1 (env. 60%)
6	$x_2 = x_1 \times 1,1$
4	$x_3 = x_1 \times 1,4$

La gamme étalon est préparée à partir de sangs supplémentés en TSH, déposés sur papier filtre et traités dans les mêmes conditions que les sangs à analyser (deux tubes par échantillon).

2. RESULTATS ET COMMENTAIRES

2.1. Etude des conditions de conservation des échantillons

Les études de stabilité de la TSH sur le papier effectuées à différentes températures (+ 4, + 25 et + 40°C) (fig.2) montrent que la conservation est possible pendant au moins 14 semaines à 4°C, une semaine à 25°C et un jour à 40°C.

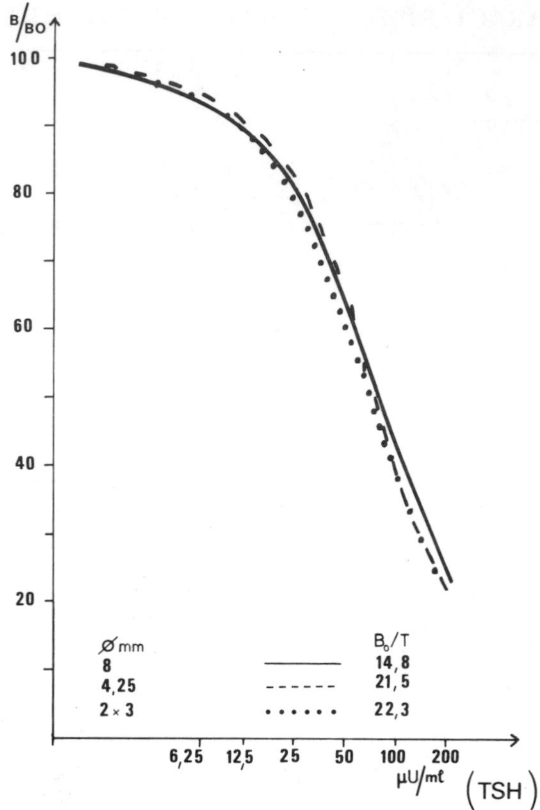

FIG.3. Courbes d'étalonnage obtenues par élution des pastilles de papier filtre.

2.2. Etude des caractéristiques du papier filtre

Le tableau II indique qu'une durée de contact du tampon de une heure avec le disque de papier est suffisante pour obtenir une extraction convenable de la TSH; il révèle également l'importance du mode d'étalement, dont la reproductibilité devra faire l'objet d'une surveillance attentive.

Le coefficient d'extraction de la TSH à partir du papier filtre augmente lorsque le diamètre du disque diminue (tableau III); la pente de la courbe reproduisant la variation de B/B_1 en fonction de la quantité de TSH n'est pas sensiblement modifiée lorsque le volume de sang analysé passe de 20 à 6 microlitres (fig.3).

TABLEAU IV. ANALYSE DE LA QUALITE DES RESULTATS

Taux de recouvrement (exactitude)	100% (95–105%)	
Sensibilité (seuil minimal détectable) (μU/ml de sang)	7 (5,4–9,3)	
Précision (reproductibilité)		
	Concentration (μU/ml)	
	16	100
C.V.% Intraessai	11,9	6,4
C.V.% Interessai	6,6	4,4
Spécificité (taux % de réactivité croisée)		
LH: 0,1; FSH: 0,01; HCG: 0,002		

2.3. Qualité des analyses effectuées

Le tableau IV rassemble les données objectives concernant la qualité des analyses. La technique utilisée est reproductible et permet d'atteindre un seuil de détection voisin de 7 μU/ml de sang, ce qui correspond à environ 13 μU/ml dans le sérum pour un hématocrite de 45%.

2.4. Résultats obtenus (tableau V)

– Equipe parisienne (2499 analyses en double au 10 octobre 1977): les valeurs obtenues ont été séparées en plusieurs plages de concentration: inférieures au seuil de détection ($<$ 6,25), subliminales (6,25–13), en zone de doute (13–25) et en zone d'alerte ($>$ 25).

– Equipe bruxelloise (4446 analyses en double au 30 décembre 1976): les valeurs frontières sont ici 10 et 20 μU/ml.

3. DISCUSSION GENERALE

Les caractéristiques de la méthode utilisée pour le dosage radioimmunologique de la TSH dans un éluat de sang séché sont très satisfaisantes au plan analytique.

TABLEAU V. REPARTITION DES RESULTATS EN FONCTION DE LA CONCENTRATION

Hôpital St-Pierre (Bruxelles) n = 4446 (1974-07-01 – 1976-12-30)		Hôpital Cochin (Paris) n = 2499 (1977-02-15 – 1977-10-10)	
< 10 μU/ml	98,6%	< 6 μU/ml	74,3%
10 – 19 μU/ml	0,8%	6 – 13 μU/ml	23,6%
> 20 μU/ml	0,6%	13 – 25 μU/ml	2 %
		> 25 μU/ml	0,1%

Une ligne stratégique cohérente devrait conduire à considérer comme normaux les résultats égaux ou inférieurs à 13 μU/ml; elle devrait inciter à répéter l'analyse sur le même prélèvement en cas de valeurs comprises entre 13 et 25 μU/ml pour tenir compte d'un éventuel et imperceptible défaut d'étalement du sang lors du prélèvement en salle. Tout résultat de cette zone, après confirmation, serait classé en zone d'alerte et déclencherait, au même titre que les résultats déjà classés dans cette zone, les mesures suivantes:

– confirmation par le laboratoire du taux élevé sur un deuxième prélèvement (élimination d'une hypothyroïdie transitoire, due à un traitement de la mère ou associée à des troubles de la période néonatale) [23];
– prise en charge par l'équipe de pédiatrie (bilan clinique, scintigraphie thyroïdienne, dosages de T_4, T_3 et TSH sur plasma; traitement).

Revenons maintenant sur les raisons qui nous ont guidés dans le choix du liquide biologique, du temps de prélèvement et de l'hormone analysée pour le dépistage biologique de l'hypothyroïdie congénitale.

Le recueil du sang total (prélevé par piqûre au talon) doit, à notre sens, être préféré à celui du sang du cordon pour des raisons essentiellement pratiques (identification, stockage et transfert au laboratoire).

Le choix du cinquième jour après la naissance tient compte de la fin du séjour de la mère à la clinique et de la pratique d'un autre dépistage, le test de Guthrie (détection de la phénylcétonurie); il est compatible avec le niveau de fonctionnement atteint par la glande thyroïde (fig.4) [24–29].

Le choix de l'hormone, par contre, pose a priori un certain nombre de problèmes.

Le dosage de la thyroxine offre l'avantage d'alerter aussi bien sur les concentrations basses que sur les concentrations élevées et de ne pas se limiter au dépistage de l'hypothyroïdie primaire. Il présente par contre l'inconvénient

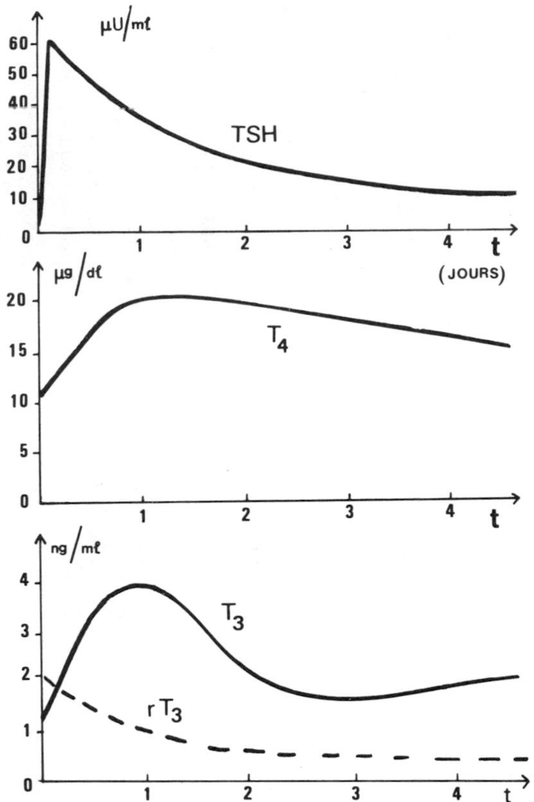

FIG.4. Evolution des concentrations hormonales plasmatiques (TSH, T_3, T_4, r T_3) pendant les 5 jours qui suivent la naissance [24–29].

d'obliger les pédiatres à reconvoquer un nombre important de nouveau-nés; ce taux de rappel important (0,9 à 4,4% selon les auteurs) est dû essentiellement à la difficulté du tri statistique des valeurs basses; par ailleurs, il n'est pas à l'abri des faux négatifs, comme l'a montré Delange à l'occasion d'un cas d'ectopie thyroïdienne et de plusieurs cas de dysfonctionnement analysés à la suite d'une amniographie (tableau VI).

Le dosage, au cinquième jour de la vie, de la thyroxine libre, ou celui des autres hormones thyroïdiennes (T_3, r T_3), ne paraît pas convenir au dépistage envisagé.

En fait, les tenants de la détection de l'hypothyroïdie néonatale à l'aide du dosage de TSH disposent d'atouts importants: sensibilité du dosage, reproductibilité, démarcation nette entre valeurs normales et pathologiques, taux de rappel réduit (0,1% environ).

TABLEAU VI. RESULTATS DES EXAMENS DE CONTROLE EFFECTUES SUR DIX CAS ANORMAUX **(expérience bruxelloise)**

Patient (âge en jours)	TSH (μ U/ml) 1	TSH (μ U/ml) 2	T_4 (μg/dl)	T_3 (ng/ml)	Remarques[a]
1 (9)	27	14,7	14,8	–	AFG (T: 13e – 36e jour)
2 (16)	50	> 250	3,2	–	AFG (T: 23e – 39e jour)
3 (17)	50	51	2,4	2,90	AFG (T: 17e – 54e jour)
4 (17)	> 50	> 50	0	1,16	AFG (T: 22e – 38e jour)
5 (16)	> 50	> 50	3,3	1,97	AFG (T: 21e – 35e jour)
6 (21)	> 50	50	8,7	2,10	Thyr. linguale (T: 32e jour)
7 (15)	13	14	14,5	3,55	N à 1 mois
8 (17)	50	10,5	14,2	3,95	N à 2 mois 3/4
9 (15)	40	47	17,7	2,00	Scinti.: thyroïde haute; T_4, T_3: N; TSH: élevée jusqu'à 3 mois
10 (12)	34	23,5	2,7	–	Scinti.: N; T_4, T_3: N; TSH: N au 25e jour

[a] AFG: amniofœtographie; T: traitement suivi du ....

L'objection concernant la non-mise en évidence d'une hypothyroïdie secondaire (par insuffisance hypothalamo-hypophysaire) ne peut être réfutée, mais doit être analysée en tenant compte d'une part de la fréquence extrêmement réduite de cette affection et d'autre part d'une évolution clinique qui, différente, pourrait orienter le diagnostic.

Quoi qu'il en soit, puisqu'il existe des possibilités de faux négatifs avec l'une ou l'autre méthode, le protocole le plus rigoureux sur le plan conceptuel consiste en un dosage, effectué sur le même échantillon, de la T_4 et de la TSH [30, 31]. Ce protocole alourdit sensiblement la tâche du laboratoire chargé du dépistage de masse.

Si, pour des raisons essentiellement économiques, les organismes de tutelle étaient contraints de se contenter d'un seul type d'analyse, notre préférence irait au dosage systématique de la TSH, en raison de la sensibilité et de la précision d'une méthode dont les résultats faussement positifs, quant au myxoedème congénital, traduisent en fait très fréquemment l'existence d'une hypothyroïdie néonatale induite (souvent iatrogène), dont il importera de vérifier le caractère transitoire.

REMERCIEMENTS

Le travail effectué à l'Hôpital St-Pierre, à Bruxelles, a été réalisé à l'aide d'une subvention du Fonds de la recherche scientifique médicale (FRSM) et d'un contrat du Ministère de la politique scientifique (Belgique) dans le cadre de l'Association Euratom-Université de Bruxelles-Université de Pise.

Les auteurs remercient Mme Branders et Mlle Vinard pour leur collaboration technique.

REFERENCES

[1] KLEIN, A.H., AGUSTIN, A.V., FOLEY, T.P., Lancet **2** (1974) 77.

[2] DUSSAULT, J.H., LETARTE, J., GUYDA, H., LABERGE, C., J. Pediatr. **89** (1976) 541.

[3] FISHER, D.A., J. Pediatr. **86** (1975) 822.

[4] WALFISH, P.G., Lancet **1** (1976) 1208.

[5] DE JONGE, G.A., Lancet **1** (1976) 143.

[6] LEGRAND, J., C.R. Hebd. Acad. Sci. **261** (1965) 544.

[7] EAYRS, J.H., «Thyroid and central nervous development», *In* Scientific Basis of Medicine, Athlone Press, London (1966) 317.

[8] BALASZ, R., *In* Human Development and the Thyroid Gland, Adv. Exp. Med. Biol. **30** (1972) 385.

[9] ROSMAN, N.P., MALONE, M.J., HELFENSTEIN, M., FRAFT, E., Neurology **22** (1972) 99.

[10] BRAZEL, J.O., BOYD, D.B., *In* Perinatal Thyroid Physiology and Disease (Fisher, D.A., Burrow, G.N., Eds), Raven Press, New York (1975) 59.
[11] GALI, P., Biomedicine **22** (1975) 62.
[12] RAITI, S., NEWNS, G.H., Arch. Dis. Child. **46** (1971) 692.
[13] KLEIN, A., MELTZER, S., KENNY, F., J. Pediatr. **81** (1972) 912.
[14] MacFAUL, R., GRANT, D.B., Arch. Dis. Child. **52** (1977) 87.
[15] NEIMAN, N., *In* Journées Fr. Péd., Flammarion, Paris (1972) 159.
[16] SMITH, D.W., KLEIN, A.H., HENDERSON, J.R., MYRIANTHOPOULOS, N.C., J. Pediatr. **87** (1975) 958.
[17] DUSSAULT, J.H., LABERGE, C., Union Méd. Canad. **102** (1973) 2062.
[18] WALFISH, P.G., *In* Perinatal Thyroid Physiology and Disease (Fischer, D.A., Burrow, G.N., Eds), Raven Press, New York (1975) 239.
[19] DUTAU, G., AUGIER, D., BAYARD, F., ROCHICCIOLI, P., Arch. Fr. Pédiatr. **32** (1975) 957.
[20] LAFRANCHI, S., MURPHEY, W., BUIST, M., LARSEN, P., FOLEY, T., Pediatr. Res. **2** (1977) 427.
[21] KLEIN, A.H., FOLEY, T.P., LARSEN, P.R., AGUSTIN, A.V., HOFWOOD, N.J., J. Pediatr. **89** (1976) 545.
[22] DELANGE, F., CAMUS, M., WINKLER, M., DODION, J., ERMANS, A.M., Arch. Dis. Child. **52** (1977) 89.
[23] RODESCH, F., CAMUS, M., ERMANS, A.M., DODION, J., DELANGE, F., Am. J. Obstet. Gynecol. **126** (1976) 723.
[24] FISHER, D.A., ODELL, W.D., J. Clin. Invest. **48** (1969) 1670.
[25] CZERNICHOW, P., GREENBERG, A.H., TYSON, J., BLIZZARD, R.M., Pediatr. Res. **5** (1971) 53.
[26] MONTALVO, J.M., WAHNER, H.W., MAYBERRY, W.E., LUN, R.K., Pediatr. Res. **7** (1973) 706.
[27] DAVIES, R.H., LAWTON, K., WARING, D., Arch. Dis. Child. **49** (1974) 410.
[28] ERENBERG, A., DALE, L., PHELPS, D.L., LAM, R., FISHER, D.A., Pediatrics **53** (1974) 211.
[29] SIMILA, S., KOIVISTO, M., RANTA, T., LEPPALUOTO, J., REINILA, M., HAAPALAHTI, J., Arch. Dis. Child. **50** (1975) 565.
[30] BUIST, N.R., MURPHEY, W.F., BRANDON, G.R., FOLEY, T.P., Lancet **2** (1975) 872.
[31] DUSSAULT, J.H., PARLOW, A., LETARTE, J., GUYDA, H., LABERGE, C., J. Pediatr. **89** (1976) 550.

DISCUSSION

R.-D. HESCH: Do you really think that the four patients whom you mentioned during the presentation and who exhibited a T_4 value above 14 μg% and a T_3 value higher than 2.0 n/ml are, in spite of elevated TSH, cases of neonatal hypothyroidism? What about the TBG?

I think that, for statistical reasons, it may be dangerous to include such cases when you give data on the incidence of neonatal hypothyroidism.

J. INGRAND: Those cases were not intended for inclusion in a table of epidemiological statistics for congenital myxoedema. The purpose was to show that very often TSH assay only can indicate a "tendency" for hypothyroidism or transient hypothyroidism during a period when hormone deficiency can have grave consequences for the future.

In fact, paediatricians often encounter iatrogenic hypothyroidism, the frequency of which is much higher than that of congenital myxoedema. One advantage of TSH assay is that it enables us to follow the recovery of the thyroid function *even under treatment,* whether or not the treatment is intentional.

Regarding TBG, the analysis was not made regularly.

S.A. SIDDIQUI: A short question on the technique of application of blood spots and cutting of dots: According to a recent report, the TSH concentration is greater at the periphery of the spot than at the centre. If this is correct, could it explain the slightly decreased recovery in your experiments?

J. INGRAND: You have raised an important point, that of homogeneity of spots. This is a practical problem (sampling in bed during maternity) which it does not seem possible entirely to overcome. In about 98% of cases, however, the values of duplicates (obtained from the same spot) were found to be almost identical. In some cases the possibility of higher TSH concentration at the periphery should be borne in mind. In any case, before requesting a second sampling the assay should be repeated where limiting values (13–25 μU/ml) are involved in order to avoid any unjustified recall.

As for the variations in the recovery rate from one series to another, we would point out that the proposed technique does not require calculation of an extraction coefficient because the standard curve is achieved in each series with the help of dots cut in spots from blood containing known TSH concentrations (6.25–200 μU/ml).

A. HADZILOUKA-MANTAKA: Do you treat new-born babies with borderline levels of TSH and T_4?

The rôle of thyroxine in the action of growth hormone is well known and so low levels of thyroid hormones must affect neonatal growth. What, in your opinion, should be the dose?

P. BOURDOUX: We perform a full check-up on the patients with borderline values. If necessary, they are treated with L-T_4 or L-T_3 (5–10 ng/day in 2 to 4 doses). Treatment with T_3 seems to be better in this case because it enables us to see if there is a rise of endogenous T_4.

What is important is not to have a large number of screened babies but screening of good quality. This is why we do both T_4 and TSH screening on capillary blood samples and on serum; it is only for practical reasons that TSH screening has been presented here.

J. INGRAND: I should like to add that the problems of the hypothyroid child (lingual thyroid) would not have been detected by T_4 assay alone (8.7 μg per 100 ml). Also, the problems of treatment strategy were left aside intentionally in the paper, for we considered that the methodological aspects should have priority and that it was for another forum to discuss the important question of treatment.

CONTROL OF TREATMENT OF DIFFERENTIATED THYROID CARCINOMA BY MEASUREMENT OF THYROGLOBULIN IN SERUM

J. HAGEMANN, C. SCHNEIDER
Universitätskrankenhaus,
Eppendorf, Hamburg,
Federal Republic of Germany

Abstract

CONTROL OF TREATMENT OF DIFFERENTIATED THYROID CARCINOMA BY MEASUREMENT OF THYROGLOBULIN IN SERUM.

The presence of thyroglobulin in serum of patients with differentiated thyroid carcinoma was studied by a specific radioimmunoassay. Seventy-three patients with thyroid carcinomata were examined, 16 of whom had pulmonary or skeletal metastase, 11 local metastases, and the others no metastases. Patients with generalized metastases had very high serum thyroglobulin concentrations while those with local metastases had slightly elevated or normal concentrations. Those with remaining thyroid tissue had mainly normal thyroglobulin levels and patients with neither metastases nor remaining thyroid tissue had undetectable serum thyroglobulin. In seven patients with metastases it was possible to observe the development of serum thyroglobulin after ^{131}I treatment. In all cases the serum thyroglobulin concentration paralleled the development of the clinical status. Elevated serum thyroglobulin was also found in benign thyroid diseases such as hyperthyroidism and endemic goitre. Measurement of thyroglobulin in serum is therefore of little value in differentiating between benign and malignant thyroid diseases, but it is a good method for the follow-up control of patients with differentiated thyroid carcinomata. Because normal thyroglobulin levels do not exclude local metastases, additional examinations are necessary if normal thyroglobulin levels are found. When thyroglobulin is undetectable, metastases can be excluded and the measurement of thyroglobulin in serum can replace all other methods in the follow-up control.

In 1967 Roitt and Torrigiani [1] described a radioimmunoassay for measuring thyroglobulin (Tg) in human serum. They found elevated Tg levels in nearly all thyroid disorders. Elevated Tg levels in patients with differentiated thyroid carcinoma were observed by van Herle and Uller [2] in 1975. They also found high Tg levels in six patients with metastases of thyroid carcinomata after thyroidectomy, whereas patients without metastases had normal Tg levels. Our study was made to further improve the significance of serum thyroglobulin in the follow-up control of thyroid carcinoma.

Subjects

We examined 73 patients with thyroid carcinomata: 30 had papillary carcinomata, 24 follicular, 2 undifferentiated and 1 a medullary carcinoma.

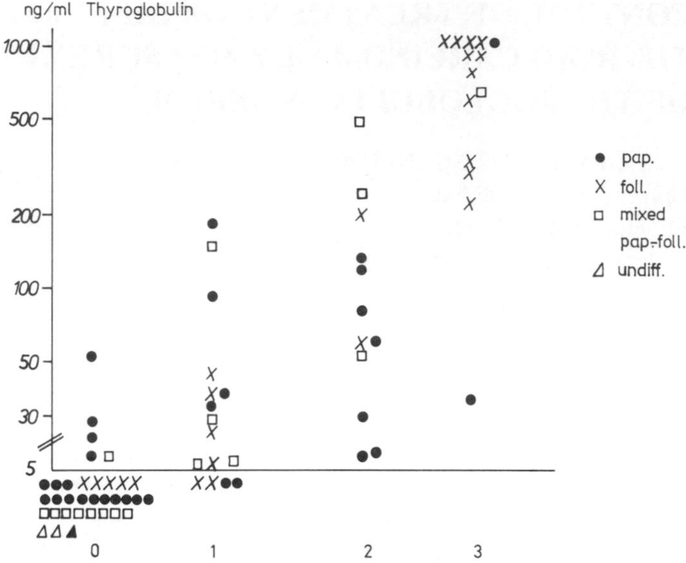

FIG.1. Serum thyroglobulin concentration in patients with metastases of thyroid cancer. 0 = no remaining thyroid tissue, no metastases; 1 = remaining thyroid tissue, no metastases; 2 = local metastases; 3 = general metastases. ● = papillary carcinoma, X = follicular carcinoma, □ = mixed papillary-follicular carcinoma, Δ = undifferentiated carcinoma.

Seventy-one patients had undergone total thyroidectomies and 2 had undergone hemithyroidectomies. All of them had had one or more ^{131}I treatments. At the time of our blood test all patients underwent a regular check-up. This check-up included: whole-body scintigraphy with ^{131}I, roentgenological examinations and clinical examinations including laboratory tests. The patients were divided into four groups according to the following criteria: Group 0 – patients without any detectable thyroid tissue and without metastases. Group 1 – patients with remaining thyroid tissue but without metastases. Group 2 – patients with only local metastases (it is unimportant in this context whether these patients have thyroid tissue or not). Group 3 – patients with general metastases, usually pulmonary or skeletal. The division into these groups was made by one of the authors without knowledge of the serum Tg concentration.

Thyroglobulin assay

The Tg assay was done on plasma using, with some modifications, the radioimmunoassay procedure described by Roitt and Torrigiani [1]: human Tg was obtained from a goitre by homogenization in 0.25M sucrose followed by elution once from Sephadex G-200 and twice from Bio-Gel A 1.5 m [3]. This preparation was shown to be homogeneous by rechromatography on Bio-Gel A 1.5 m and by sodium dodecyl sulphate chromatography (SDS). It was used as the standard in the assay and for preparation of the tracer. The tracer was prepared according to the method of Greenwood and Hunter. Antibodies to Tg were produced in rabbits. Dilutions of the standards were made in Tg-free serum. After pre-incubation of antibody and serum for 48 h the tracer was added and an incubation of 24 h followed. Double-antibody precipitation was used to separate the bound and free Tg. The standard curve and the serum dilution curve of a patient without antithyroglobulin auto-antibodies were parallel, whereas the serum dilution curve of a patient with high anti-Tg antibody titre was not parallel. The least detectable concentration was 5 ng/ml using a serum volume of 100 μl. The intra-assay coefficient of variation was 9.8%; the inter-assay coefficient of variation was 12.1%. Subjects with positive anti-Tg antibodies were excluded from all analyses.

Results

Of the 31 patients in group 0, 26 had undetectable Tg in serum, 4 nearly undetectable and 1 was in the normal range. In group 1, the serum Tg concentration ranged from undetectable in 4 out of 16 patients to 180 ng/ml. The 12 patients in group 2 had serum Tg levels of 10 to 490 ng/ml. Patients in group 2 had significantly higher concentrations than those in group 1. The average Tg level was 10 times higher in the 16 patients of group 3, the values ranging from 220 to 1600 ng/ml. All patients with metastases had measureable serum Tg concentrations (Fig.1).

In one patient there was a clinical suspicion of local metastases but no detectable Tg in the serum. After surgical removal of the suspicious nodule a diagnosis of myositis ossificans without any suspect of cancer was made on the basis of histological examination. In one patient with pulmonary metastases of a medullar carcinoma the serum Tg was undetectable. One patient with pulmonary metastases of a follicular carcinoma, but without iodinophilia of the metastases, had a serum Tg concentration of 800 ng/ml. Patients with follicular thyroid carcinomata had significantly higher serum Tg levels than those with papillary or mixed papillary follicular carcinomata, reflecting the fact that from the 16 patients with general metastases 14 had follicular carcinomata.

In four patients with regional metastases and three with general metastases we were able to observe the development of the serum Tg concentration after treatment with ^{131}I. In one patient with a follicular carcinoma there was a worsening in spite of treatment. The serum Tg level in this patient rose from 60 ng/ml to 200 ng/ml. All other patients showed an improved state of health.

TABLE I. CLINICAL STATUS AND SERUM THYROGLOBULIN LEVELS IN THE COURSE OF TREATMENT OF THYROID CANCER

All patients had total thyroidectomy and ^{131}I treatment

Initials, age, histology	Date	Clinical status	Thyroglobulin level (ng/ml) (Normal range 69.2 ± 37.2)
K.G., 37y	9/76	rem. thyr. tiss., reg. ln. met.	80
pap.	3/77	no rem. thyr. tiss., no met.	<5
F.K., 59y	7/76	rem. thyr. tiss., pulm. met.	500
foll.	11/76	rem. thyr. tiss., no met.	26
I.S., 25y	1/77	rem. thyr. tiss., reg. ln. met.	244
pap.-foll.	4/77	rem. thyr. tiss., reg. ln. met. reduced	55
S.B., 27y	6/76	rem. thyr. tiss., reg. ln. met.	30
pap.	8/76	small thyr. res., no met.	10
E.R., 65y	7/76	small thyr. res., small met.	60
foll.	3/77	met. larger, ^{131}I uptake increased	200
R.T., 45y	5/76	reg. ln. met., pulm. met.	>1000
pap.	10/76	reg. ln. met., no pulm. met.	122
	5/77	no rem. thyr. tiss., no met.	900
W.K., 58y	10/76	pulm. met.	>1000
foll.	1/77	improvement of pulm. met.	329
	4/77	further improvement of pulm. met.	200

rem. thyr. tiss. = remaining thyroid tissue
reg. ln. met. = regional lymph node metastases
pulm. met. = pulmonary metastases
pap. = papillary
foll. = follicular

In four patients the local or pulmonary metastases vanished, in two others the metastases shrank markedly in extent and number. In all patients with clinical improvement the serum Tg concentration decreased parallel with the degree of the improvement (Table I).

Discussion

Differentiated carcinomata of the thyroid and their metastases are able to accumulate and store iodine. This ability is based on the synthesis of thyroglobulin. The immunological identity of Tg from normal thyroid tissue and from metastases is shown in our radioimmunoassay by the parallelism of the Tg standard curve and the serum dilution curves of patients with metastases of a differentiated thyroid carcinoma. This is in accordance with Valenta and colleagues [4] who showed that Tg from metastases is physico-chemically identical with normal Tg, except for a lower iodine content of the tumour thyroglobulin. van Herle [2] furnished proof that patients with differentiated thyroid carcinomata had elevated serum Tg levels. Unfortunately, elevated serum Tg levels are observed in a lot of thyroid diseases such as hyperthyroidism, thyroiditis and endemic goitre, as shown by other investigators and our own examinations [5–7]. Therefore, the determination of serum Tg is of low significance in the diagnosis of thyroid cancer. This has been proven by Schneider and colleagues [8] who examined 904 persons after childhood neck irradiation and concluded, as we do, that the Tg assay is without value in distinguishing benign from malignant thyroid diseases.

We have found other conditions after total thyroidectomy because of thyroid cancer. In such cases, elevated serum Tg clearly proves the presence of metastases. We found elevated Tg levels in patients with general metastases and in some patients with local metastases. Similarly, elevated Tg levels were also seen by van Herle [2] in six patients with metastases, whereas his patients without metastases had normal serum Tg levels. We do not know whether his six patients had local or general metastases. We saw normal Tg levels in patients with remaining thyroid tissue without metastases as well as in patients with local metastases. Normal Tg levels therefore do not exclude local metastases but do exclude general metastases. A proven exclusion of metastases is only possible if serum Tg is undetectable. We had cases of undetectable serum Tg in patients without metastases mostly after total thyroidectomy and elimination of the remaining thyroid tissue by means of ^{131}I.

Our results suggest that a long follow-up control of patients with differentiated thyroid carcinomata by measuring the serum Tg concentration is possible only if, beforehand, the serum Tg is made undetectable by surgery and radiotherapy.

REFERENCES

[1] ROITT, I.M., TORRIGIANI, G., Endocrinology **81** (1967) 421.

[2] HERLE, A.J. van, ULLER, R.P., J. Clin. Invest **56** (1975).

[3] PEAKE, R.L., WILLIS, D.B., ASIMAKIS, G.K., Jr., DEISS, W.P., Jr., J. Lab. Clin. Med. **84** (1974) 907.

[4] VALENTA, L., LISSINSKI, S., ROQUE, M., ROLLAND, M., Thyroid Cancer (HEDINGER, C.E., Ed.), Springer Verlag New York Inc., New York **12** (1969) 234.

[5] TORRIGIANI, G., DONIACH, D., ROITT, I.M., J. Clin. Endocrinol. Metab. **29** (1969) 305.

[6] HERLE, A.J. van, ULLER, R.P., MATTHEWS, N.L., BROWN, J., J. Clin. Invest. **52** (1973) 1320.

[7] HAGEMANN, J., SCHNEIDER, C., ENGELS, J., Acta Endocrinol. **84** Suppl. 208 (1977), (Abstract).

[8] SCHNEIDER, A.B., FAVUS, M.J., STACHURA, M.E., ARNOLD, J.E., RYO, U.Y., PINSKY, S., COLMAN, M., ARNOLD, M.J., FROHMAN, L.A., Ann. Int. Med. **86** (1977) 29.

DISCUSSION

P. BOURDOUX: Is your Tg labelled with ^{125}I?

According to van Herle, ^{125}I-labelled Tg is not stable and is a very poor immunoreactive material. What is your opinion?

J. HAGEMANN: We use ^{125}I-labelled Tg. This preparation remains stable for four weeks. There are no special problems with labelled Tg that do not exist with other labelled proteins. It is important to store the tracer in several vials and use a new vial for each assay in order to prevent damage by repeated thawing.

A. MALKIN: What proportion of your patients had anti-thyroglobulin antibodies? Did such patients show any differences on histologic examination of their thyroids, as compared to the patients without anti-thyroglobulin antibodies? Also, were there any other differences in the manifestations of their disease?

J. HAGEMANN: We made our determinations by the Wellcome test. Patients with an anti-thyroglobulin antibody titre of up to 1/40 were defined as normal, and under these circumstances we had to exclude about 10% of the patients. As far as we know, these patients did not differ from the others.

NEW CONCEPTS FOR THE ASSAY OF UNBOUND THYROXINE (FT_4) AND THYROXINE BINDING GLOBULIN (TBG)

G. ODSTRCHEL, W. HERTL, F.B. WARD,
K. TRAVIS, R.E. LINDNER, R.D. MASON
Corning Glass Works,
Sullivan Science Park,
Corning, New York,
United States of America

Abstract

NEW CONCEPTS FOR THE ASSAY OF UNBOUND THYROXINE (FT_4) AND THYROXINE BINDING GLOBULIN (TBG).

Two new concepts for the assay of thyroid-related substances are presented. One assay (FT_4) is based on a kinetic measurement of T_4 as it desorbs from binder proteins onto solid-phase T_4 antibody. This reaction can be described by a second-order rate equation: $r = k\,[IMA]\,[FT_4]$. The assay is rapid (2 h) and gives good agreement (correlation coefficient = 0.92) with the results of equilibrium dialysis and gives a normal range of 0.9–2.3 ng/dl. This assay uses a small sample size (25 μl) and is unaffected by drugs such as aspirin and dilantin. Pregnant and estrogen-treated women gave normal FT_4 values. A new method for the measurement of functionally active TBG is also presented. In this case, the labelled T_4 is partitioned between bovine serum albumin and the patient's samples. The complex is then removed from solution by solid-phase anti-TBG. A curve reminiscent of an immunoradiometric assay is obtained. The assay has a sensitivity of 4 μg/ml and is unaffected by aspirin, dilantin or the patient's T_4 concentrations. Correlation with "rocket" electrophoresis gives good agreement (correlation coefficient = 0.90). The normal range is 20 ± 7 μg/ml, with pregnant women giving values greater than 30 μg/ml. Five hereditarily deficient patients gave a value equivalent to zero TBG concentration.

Unbound or "free" thyroxine (FT_4) changes with varying total T_4 (TT_4) and the concentration of specific protein binder molecules. This parameter, when measured, is particularly useful in those physiological conditions where there are measurable changes in these protein levels (e.g. pregnancy, estrogen therapy). In these situations, T_4 and binder concentrations will increase but the FT_4 will remain relatively constant. Although FT_4 has long been recognized as an important parameter to measure, the assay for FT_4 is difficult and complex [1]. The only common direct measurement of FT_4 in the past has been accomplished by use of equilibrium dialysis [2]. This method is time consuming with many technical problems (e.g. poor counting statistics, need for an accurate T_4 value).

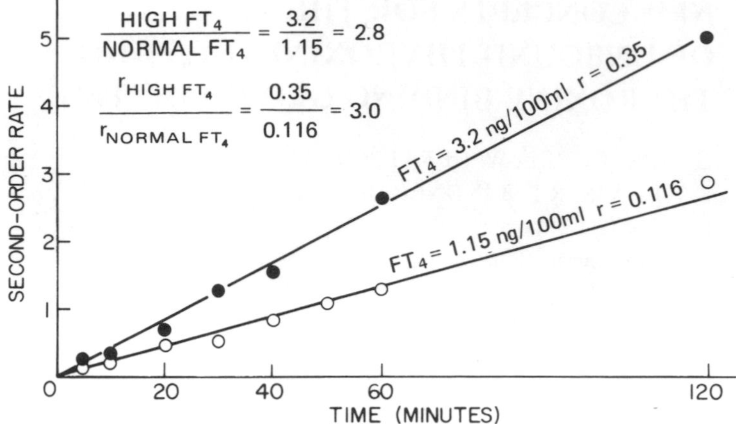

FIG.1. The assay, treated as an apparent second-order reaction, of two patient samples, one containing a normal level (1.15 ng/dl) and the other a high level (3.2 ng/dl) of FT_4, as determined by equilibrium dialysis.

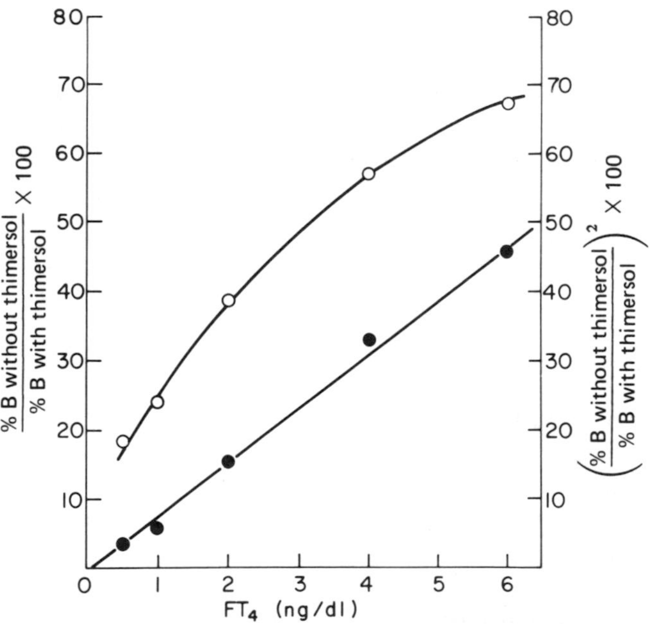

FIG.2. The two procedures used for reduction of data in the kinetic FT_4 assay.

TABLE I. FT_4 VALUES OBTAINED WITH THE KINETIC ASSAY ARE SHOWN TO BE INDEPENDENT OF DILUTION OR SAMPLE SIZE

Sample size	FT_4 (ng/dl) A	FT_4 (ng/dl) B	Dilution	FT_4 (ng/dl) A	FT_4 (ng/dl) B
10	1.40	3.00	Undiluted	1.40	3.10
25	1.40	3.10	1:2	1.35	2.90
50	1.35	3.10	1:3	1.35	3.00
100	1.40	2.95	1:4	–	3.00

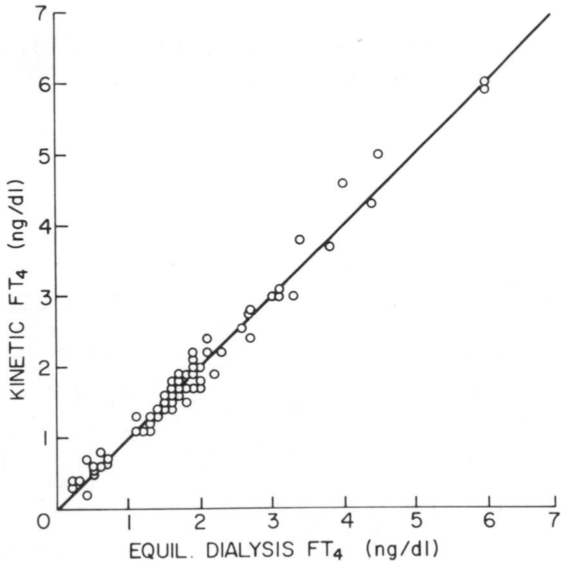

FIG. 3. The linear correlation of 93 patient samples analysed by kinetic analysis with the same samples analysed by equilibrium dialysis.

To circumvent these problems, laboratories have resorted to a number of indices which are computed from total T_4 data and the measurement of available thyroxine binding globulin (TBG) binding sites using labelled T_3 uptake of a patient's serum sample relative to a pool of normal serum [3]. Clearly, a need for a faster and more direct measurement for FT_4 is indicated.

A detailed study of the kinetics and thermodynamics of the interaction of T_4 binding to it's specific immobilized antibodies (IMA) demonstrated that the

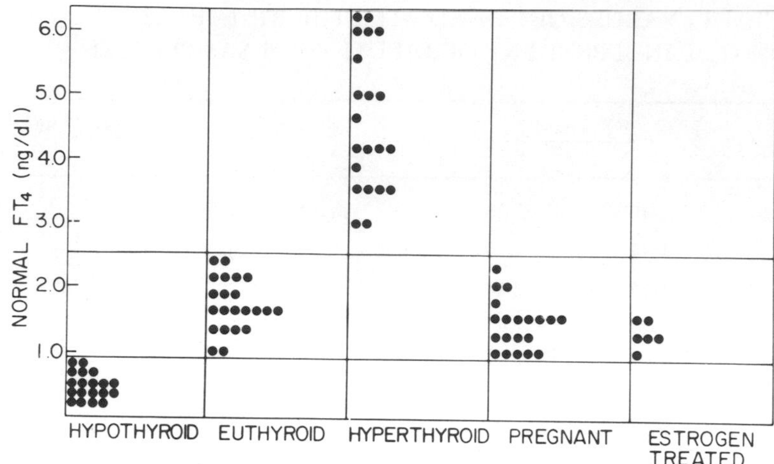

FIG.4. Status agreement between FT_4 values obtained by the kinetic FT_4 assay and current acceptable ranges of FT_4 using diagnosed patient samples.

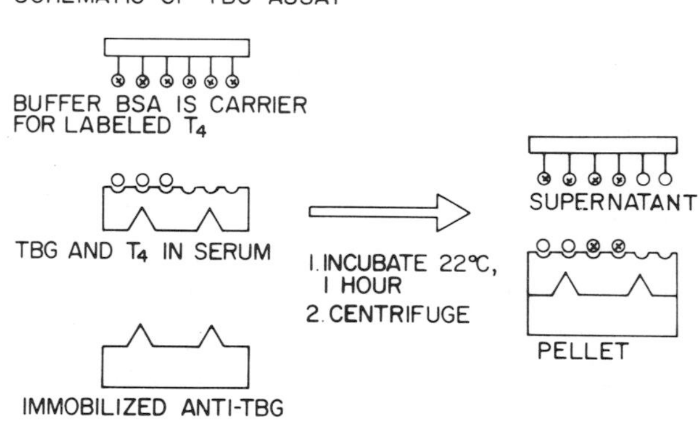

FIG.5. Mechanism of the ligand partitioning assay for TBG shown schematically.

rate at which T_4 desorbs from its respective binder proteins onto the IMA was proportional to the FT_4 in the presence of constant antibody.

$$r = k\,[IMA]\,[FT_4] \tag{1}$$

The kinetic data obtained could be treated with an apparent second-order rate equation, as demonstrated in Fig.1. These data indicated that by the use of kinetic analysis of each patient sample one could obtain an FT_4 assay. Obviously the time and labour necessary to do each test under these conditions would be

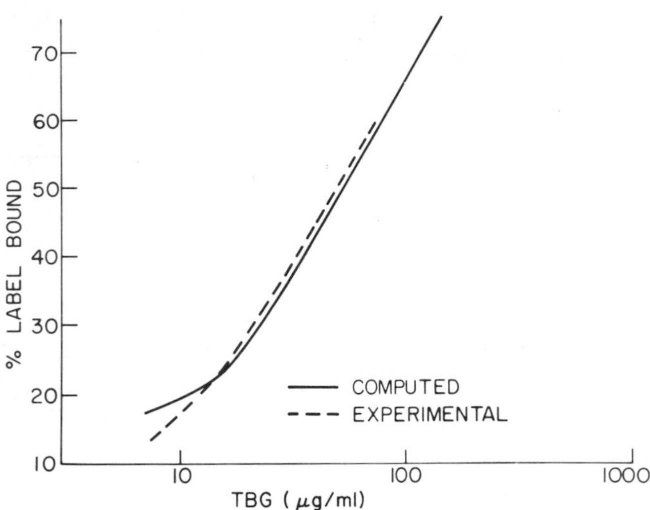

FIG.6. Comparison of a computer-simulated curve (– – –) with an experimental curve (———) obtained in the TBG assay.

prohibitive with a large number of samples. However, the data necessary for a rapid assay can be gathered by a two-tube measurement in which the end point of the reaction, expressed in % bound, can be obtained in the presence of sufficient thimersol to completely release the T_4 from binder molecules. A second tube without thimersol is run in the assay for the same controlled incubation time as the previous tube. The extent of binding is visualized with labelled T_4 which is allowed to pre-equilibrate with the sample for 20–30 min followed by a 30-min kinetic response initiated by the addition of IMA to each tube. The reaction is terminated by centrifuging at 1 100 X g for 5 min, decanting, blotting and counting the radioactivity bound to the IMA. The rate of reaction can be estimated in terms of the expression:

$$\frac{\%\text{ B without thimersol}}{\%\text{ B with thimersol}} \times 100$$

A plot of this type as a function of FT_4 concentration approximates a parabola, as shown in Fig.2. This curve can be conveniently linearized (Fig.2) in terms of the expression:

$$\left(\frac{\%\text{ B without thimersol}}{\%\text{ B with thimersol}}\right)^2 \times 100$$

TABLE II. RECOVERY OF TBG CONCENTRATIONS USING MIXTURES AND DILUTIONS OF KNOWN ANALYSED CONTROL SERA

In the mixtures, they represent equal volumes of each control serum

Controls	Expected	Found	% Recovery
A	25	24.8	99
B	18	18	100
C	15	14	94
(A+B)	21	20.6	98
(B+C)	16.5	16.1	97
D	43.2	46	106
E	25.6	27	105
F	18	18	100
G	7.2	7.5	104

These standard curves are linear over the range of 0.2–6.0 ng/dl with a sensitivity of 0.2 ng/dl FT_4. As predicted thermodynamically, Table I shows that the concentration of FT_4 is independent of the sample volume and the dilution of the sample.

Correlation with equilibrium dialysis (93 samples) was excellent (Fig.3) and gave a correlation coefficient of 0.92 with a slope of 0.96. Status correlation with diagnosed patient samples was excellent, as shown in Fig.4. This assay in our laboratories showed a normal range of 0.9–2.3 ng/dl with no interference by therapeutic levels of known releasing agents such as aspirin and dilantin. The assay is rapid, requiring a total assay time of less than 2 h for 96 tubes which is a significant advance in the measurement of FT_4 when compared with current methodology.

In recent years there has been an increasing interest in the measurement of TBG. This interest has been stimulated by the identification of an increasing number of people whose serum levels of TBG are either hereditarily too high or too low [4]. This interest has also been fuelled by the reports of increased TBG in liver disease [5]. A number of assays has been proposed in which either competitive binding procedures or rocket electrophoresis is used [4–6]. These procedures are based on an immunological identification which may or may not be representative of the functional level of TBG. In addition, there has been much controversy over what are considered to be the normal levels of TBG. These reported values range from a mean of 11 μg/ml to 48 μg/ml.

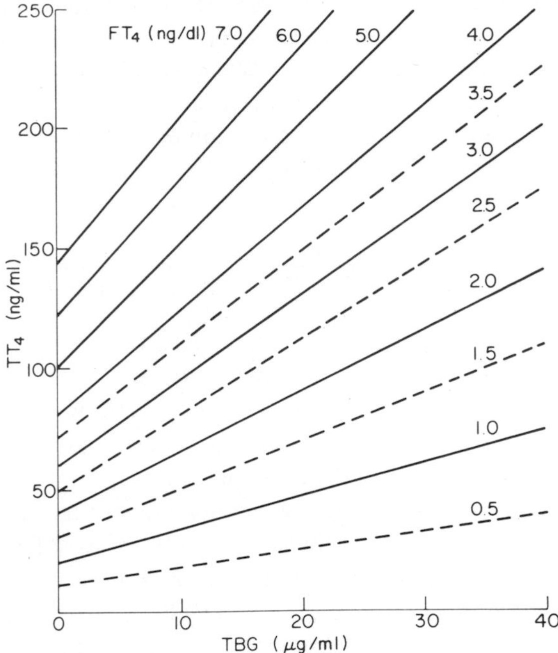

FIG. 7. A linearized version of Eq.(2) which can be used to calculate FT_4 from known values of TT_4 and TBG.

A computer model using binding constants taken from the literature has allowed us to predict that, in dilute solutions, one could partition labelled T_4 between the TBG in the serum and a known fixed concentration of bovine serum albumin. The fraction of T_4 bound to the TBG is then a direct function of the TBG concentration. This mechanism is shown in Fig.5. The separation of the labelled TBG-T_4* complex could then be accomplished by the addition of excess specific immobilized anti-TBG. Figure 6 shows a comparison of the expected curve obtained by computer modelling and the experimental curve obtained in this assay system. The assay is conveniently run using 25 μl of a sample prediluted 1:40 with water or saline. The diluted sample, labelled T_4 and excess antibody are added to the assay tubes consecutively to give a final serum dilution of 1:1 000 and are then incubated for 1 h at room temperature, centrifuged at 1 100 × g, decanted and counted. The total assay time is about 90 min with a curve having a range of 4–72 μg/ml of TBG. Standards are conveniently prepared from analysed serum added in increasing volumes to water and standardized against purified TBG. The assay is unaffected by aspirin, dilantin or endogenous T_4. Dilution recovery experiments using this assay are shown in Table II. In this assay procedure, normal TBG values were 20 μg/ml ± 7 and those of pregnant women were higher than 30 μg/ml. Five samples from patients identified as being hereditarily deficient in TBG gave assay results that could not be distinguished from zero, thus confirming the diagnosis. When compared with samples measured by rocket electrophoresis, a correlation coefficient of 0.90 was obtained.

An equation demonstrating the distribution of T_4 to its respective binder proteins, TBG, albumin (ALB) and thyroxine binding pre-albumin (TBPA), was derived:

$$FT_4 = \frac{[TT_4]}{K_1\,([TBG] - [TBG\text{-}T_4]) + K_2\,[ALB] + K_3\,[TBPA]} \qquad (2)$$

From the solution of this equation a calculated FT_4 value can be obtained from known values of TT_4 and TBG (Fig.7). Correlation of free T_4 values obtained with this expression gave a correlation coefficient of 0.90 with either equilibrium dialysis or the previously described kinetic FT_4 assay and provides a convenient internal cross-check for FT_4 and TBG assay procedures.

In summary, we have presented new methodologies for the assay of FT_4 and TBG. The FT_4 or kinetic assay, in addition to measuring FT_4, provides a technology that can be extended to measure the unbound concentrations of many substances in serum (e.g. T_3, cortisol). The ligand partitioning assay for TBG can also be applied to a functional measurement of other binder molecules when a specific antiserum and radioligand are available for the system to be assayed.

REFERENCES

[1] STERLING, K., HEGEDUS, A., Measurement of free thyroxine concentrations in human serum, J. Clin. Invest. **41** (1962) 1031.

[2] OPPENHEIMER, J.H., SQUEF, R., SURKS, M.I., HAUER, H., Binding of thyroxine by serum proteins evaluated by equilibrium dialysis and electrophoretic techniques, J. Clin. Invest. **24** (1964) 486.

[3] HOWORTH, P.J.N., MADOGAN, N.F., Clinical application of serum total thyroxine estimation, resin uptake and free thyroxine index, Lancet **i** (1969) 224.

[4] LEVY, R.P., MARSHALL, J.S., VELAYO, N.L., Radioimmunoassay of human TBG, J. Clin. Endocrinol. **32** (1971) 372.

[5] HESCH, R.D., GATZ, J., McINTOSH, C.H.S., JANZYN, J., HERRMANN, R., Radioimmunoassay of TBG in human plasma, Clin. Chim. Acta **70** (1976) 33.

[6] BRADWELL, A.R., BURNETT, D., RAMSDEN, D.B., BURR, W.A., PRINCE, H.P., HOFFENBERG, R., Preparation of a monospecific antiserum to TBG for its quantitation by rocket immunoelectrophoresis, Clin. Chim. Acta **71** (1976) 501.

DISCUSSION

D. RODBARD: First of all I would like to congratulate you on having solved at least two major problems. The kinetics of separation of bound and free have been investigated to some extent by us[1], but we were concerned with the measurement of B/T or B/F rather than with the free fraction as such. My colleagues[2] at the National Institutes of Health have used a similar approach, following the kinetics of dialysis, for the measurement of testosterone-estradiol binding globulin (TeBG or SHBG) and/or free testosterone. Hence your approach is broadly applicable, as you have noted.

Use of a nomogram relating total thyroxine, free thyroxine and TBG levels is analogous to the use of a nomogram for total calcium, free calcium and albumin concentration. Such nomograms should be used with extreme caution; for instance, with the advent of the "free-calcium electrode" methods, it became apparent that the nomograms and related computational methods were extremely unreliable.

G. ODSTRCHEL: As regards the mathematics of preparing the nomograms, I would just point out that to obtain a 10% change in free T_4 we evidently require doubling or halving of the albumin.

I agree that we must be cautious about this kind of simplistic approach. However, it provides a convenient cross-check.

T.C. SMEATON: Have you tried any different forms of solid support for antibodies in your free T_4 assay other than glass particles – cellulose or Sepharose, for example? Are the glass particles readily available yet?

G. ODSTRCHEL: We haven't tried other solid supports because the glass particles are excellent for the assay and have all the properties we need. Besides, it is the glass-making company which is financing the work! These particles are not yet available.

I should like to point out in connection with the glass that it is important to have spheres with 1-μm pores, and this for two reasons. The pore size should be such as would give good suspendibility in solution so as to avoid constant vortexing and also good surface area to ensure optimal loading. All this involves a lot of preparation, so that starting from 500 lb of glass we obtain about 900 g of porous glass.

D. RODBARD: Is the antibody located on the surface of the glass bead or interspersed throughout the matrix?

G. ODSTRCHEL: The antibody is dispersed throughout the matrix but little is known relative to the functionality of pore-dispersed versus surface-attached antibody. We feel that for small molecules all antibodies are involved because antigen binding capacity for a solid particle is a direct function of surface area which is a function of porosity.

---

[1] RODBARD, D., CATT, K.J., Mathematical theory of radioligand assays: the kinetics of separation of bound from free, J. Steroid Biochem. **3** (1972) 255.

[2] VIGERSKY, R.L., LIPSETT, M.B., LORIAUX, D.L., J. Clin. Endocrinol. Metab. (in press).

D. RODBARD: Would a coating of glass surrounding the antibody result in a diffusion chamber which would help to separate the free thyroxine from the serum proteins and thus improve performance?

G. ODSTRCHEL: The present beads could possibly be used in such a manner, as their structure when viewed by electron microscopy is sponge-like. Attachment of antibody to either exposed or internal surfaces is a random phenomenon. Our studies indicate a rapid reaction with little or no diffusion control with or without porous particles. Larger particle-size beads would appear to be more useful for an application such as you suggest. On the other hand, the suspension properties of the particle-size beads is very good and they require centrifugation to sediment.

D. RODBARD: Could the antibody-coated beads be used as a microdialysis bag turned inside out?

G. ODSTRCHEL: Such a system could be constructed, but would be technically difficult. Controlled porous glass can be made in a variety of geometries and thus could serve as a micro-dialysis chamber.

A. MALKIN: While I agree with Dr. Rodbard on the need to exercise caution in using nomograms to derive data, I suggest that we should also be cautious in using a calcium electrode as a standard for measuring free calcium.

IAEA-SM-220/54

DEVELOPMENT OF A TWO-SITE RADIOIMMUNOASSAY FOR ANTITHYROGLOBULIN ANTIBODIES USING ^{125}I-THYROGLOBULIN*

J.P. LEONARD, F. TAYMANS, C. BECKERS
Centre de médecine nucléaire,
Ecole de médecine,
Université de Louvain,
Brussels, Belgium

Abstract

DEVELOPMENT OF A TWO-SITE RADIOIMMUNOASSAY FOR ANTITHYROGLOBULIN ANTIBODIES USING ^{125}I-THYROGLOBULIN.

A two-site radioassay for human antithyroglobulin auto-antibodies has been developed using human thyroglobulin (Tg) labelled with ^{125}I. The technique is based on (1) the use of polystyrene tubes coated with Tg, (2) the binding of the antibodies to the solid-phase Tg, and (3) the reaction of the labelled Tg with the insolubilized antibodies. The factors affecting the assay that were evaluated included: (a) the effect of temperature, Tg concentration and coating time on the adsorption of Tg, (b) the stability and storage of the solid-phase Tg, (c) the variations in temperature, reaction times and incubation volumes, (d) the effect of the serum proteins, and (e) the influence of the variations in concentration and specific activity of the labelled Tg. Increasing sensitivity resulted from a prolonged incubation at low temperature, the addition of serum proteins and the use of an appropriate specific activity of ^{125}I-Tg. Non-specific radioactive uptake normally averaged 1% or less of the total radioactivity added. The use of Tg-coated tubes makes the technique rapid and simple to operate. The ability of the coated tubes to be stored and the relative insensitivity of the test to fluctuations in the quality of the tracer represent additional advantages in the routine application of the method.

INTRODUCTION

The presence of antithyroglobulin antibodies has been demonstrated in the serum of patients suffering from various thyroid diseases, especially in the serum of those suffering from Hashimoto's thyroiditis [1].

Among the various techniques proposed to detect these antibodies in the blood, radioimmunoassay offers the advantages of its specificity and high sensitivity [2–4]. The aim of this paper is to describe a two-site radioassay [5,6] using thyroglobulin-coated tubes. The uptake of antithyroglobulin antibody to the solid phase is measured by subsequent reaction with thyroglobulin labelled with ^{125}I.

* This work has been partly supported by the Fonds de la Recherche Scientifique Médicale, Belgium (grant No. 20.393).

MATERIAL AND METHODS

Human thyroglobulin (Tg) from thyroid glands removed by surgery was prepared by salting-out with ammonium sulphate and purified by column chromatography on Sepharose 6B (Pharmacia, Sweden) equilibrated and eluted with 0.02M phosphate buffer, pH 7.4, containing 0.1M KCl [7]. The top of the protein peak corresponding to Tg was used for labelling with ^{125}I by the lactoperoxidase method [8].

The antithyroglobulin auto-antibodies were purified by adsorption chromatography. The purified Tg was bound to the CNBr activated Sepharose 4B (Pharmacia, Sweden). The gamma-globulin fraction from a human serum with a high titre of anti-Tg antibodies was incubated with the immuno-adsorbant for 24 h at room temperature. The gel was poured into a column and washed with 0.01M phosphate buffer, pH 7, containing 0.5M NaCl. The anti-Tg antibodies were eluted with 0.5M NaCl – 0.01N HCl.

Two-site assay procedure

Five-millilitre polystyrene tubes were coated with human thyroglobulin (0.3 ml) which had been diluted at 1 μg/ml in KCl-phosphate buffer. After 3 h at room temperature, the tubes were washed 3 times with 0.01M phosphate buffer, pH 7, containing 0.15M NaCl (PBS) and once with PBS containing 0.5% bovine serum albumin. 0.3 ml of unknown serum or purified anti-Tg solution was added and incubated for 18 h at 24°C. Then, the content of the tubes was aspirated and the tubes were washed 3 times with PBS. ^{125}I-Ig in 5% serum was added in a volume of 0.3 ml and incubated for 6 h at 37°C. The unbound ^{125}I-Tg was discarded by aspiration and the tubes were washed 3 times with 0.15M NaCl. The tubes were finally counted in an automatic well scintillation counter.

RESULTS

The effects of various parameters on optimal two-site assay conditions were examined by determining the relative activity, i.e. the per cent increase of the activity bound to the antibodies over the bound activity in the presence of normal serum (non-specific binding or zero concentration of the antibodies).

Conditions for coating

The tubes were coated at room temperature with a series of Tg solutions (100 pg/ml – 10 mg/ml) in the KCl-phosphate buffer for periods ranging from 0.5 h to 24 h. The adsorption of Tg on the tubes rose rapidly during the first

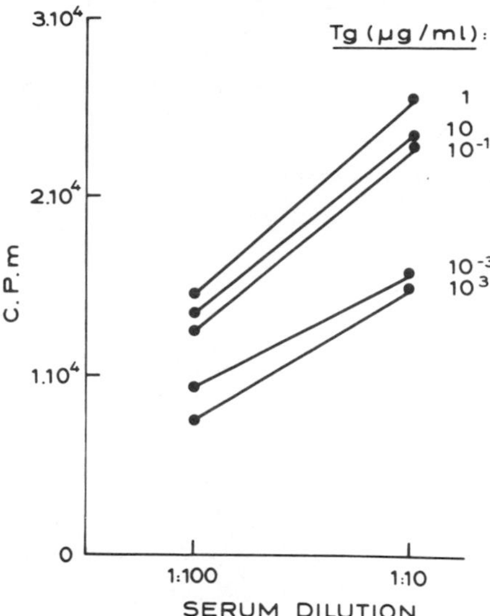

FIG.1. Effect of the concentration of Tg, used in the coating, on the subsequent binding of anti-Tg antibodies by the Tg-coated tubes.

hours, then increased more slowly after the 3rd hour. However, when the Tg concentration was high, the maximum binding of Tg was rapidly reached. The adsorption at 4°C was not much different to that at 37°C.

The subsequent fixation of the antibody reached a maximum for a concentration of Tg of 1 μg/ml and decreased when the Tg concentrations were either higher or lower (Fig.1). Moreover, the maximum binding was already obtained with a coating time of 2 h for a Tg concentration of 1 μg/ml. Increasing the duration of coating did not cause any further increase in the subsequent antibody binding.

To examine the stability of the solid-phase Tg, tubes were coated with ^{125}I-Tg tracer. Freshly prepared tubes and dried tubes stored at 4°C for one week were incubated for 24 h after the addition of an excess of cold Tg or serum proteins. Less than 5% of the ^{125}I-Tg fixed on the tubes was displaced from the walls.

Effect of time and temperature on incubation of antibodies and ^{125}I-Tg

The antibodies and the ^{125}I-Tg were incubated for up to 72 h at 4°C, room temperature and 37°C, the other incubation being maintained at room temperature for 24 h.

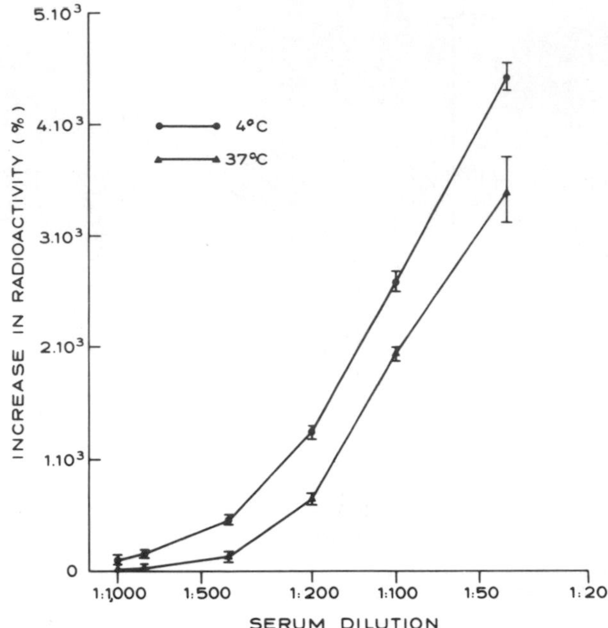

FIG.2. Various dilution curves of a serum showing the effect of different periods and temperatures of incubation on serum and ^{125}I-Tg : ● — ● 3 days at 4°C; ▲ — ▲ 24 h at 37°C. Vertical lines indicate ± SEM.

The binding of the antibody to the solid-phase Tg was accelerated at the higher temperatures and reached its maximum around the 24th hour at room temperature and 37°C, and on the 3rd day at 4°C.

The kinetics of the heteroantibodies, obtained in rabbits injected with human Tg, was almost identical to those of the autoantibodies.

The non-specific binding did not vary proportionally to the bound activity in the presence of antibodies. It was found that the relative activity was the highest when the antibodies were incubated at 24°C. During the incubation of ^{125}I-Tg, the relative activity decreased over the first 24 h of incubation at 37°C but continued to rise at 4°C up to 3 days. The improvement in sensitivity was obvious when both incubations were performed for 3 days at 4°C rather than for 24 h at 37°C (Fig.2).

Effect of serum proteins

The effect of the serum proteins in the incubation medium was investigated. The purified anti-Tg antibodies were incubated in human or rabbit serum, and in serum diluted to 1 : 5 or 1 : 20 with PBS. A reduction of the binding was

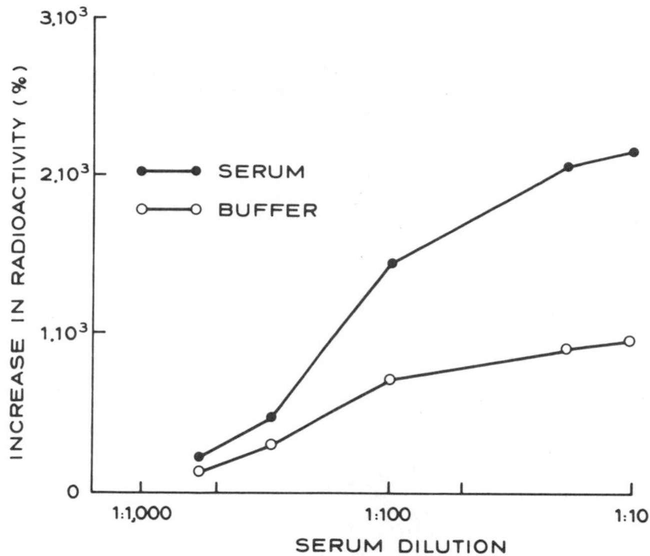

FIG.3. Dose-response curves obtained with ^{125}*I-Tg solutions in 2% albumin (○—○) and 5% serum (●—●).*

observed with undiluted serum. There was no striking difference between the curves obtained with serum diluted 1 : 5 and serum diluted 1 : 20. However, an inhibition of the non-specific binding was observed simultaneously, so that the relative activity was finally slightly enhanced in the presence of serum.

When ^{125}I-Tg was incubated in buffer containing either 2% serum albumin or 5%, 10% and 20% serum, there was a reduction of the activity bound in the presence of serum. However, the measured activity compared with the non-specific binding was significantly higher than when the incubation was performed in buffer containing serum albumin (Fig.3). The dose-response curves obtained by varying the concentrations in serum from 5% to 20% were most comparable.

Variations of the specific activity of the ^{125}I-Tg

The dose-response curves were examined by varying the specific activity of ^{125}I-Tg from 0.1 mCi/mg to more than 20 mCi/mg. Increasing the specific activity considerably enhanced the bound radioactivity but caused only a little improvement in sensitivity (Fig.4). A plateau was progressively reached, no further increase in tracer binding being achieved when a higher specific activity was used; the sensitivity of the assay was even decreasing.

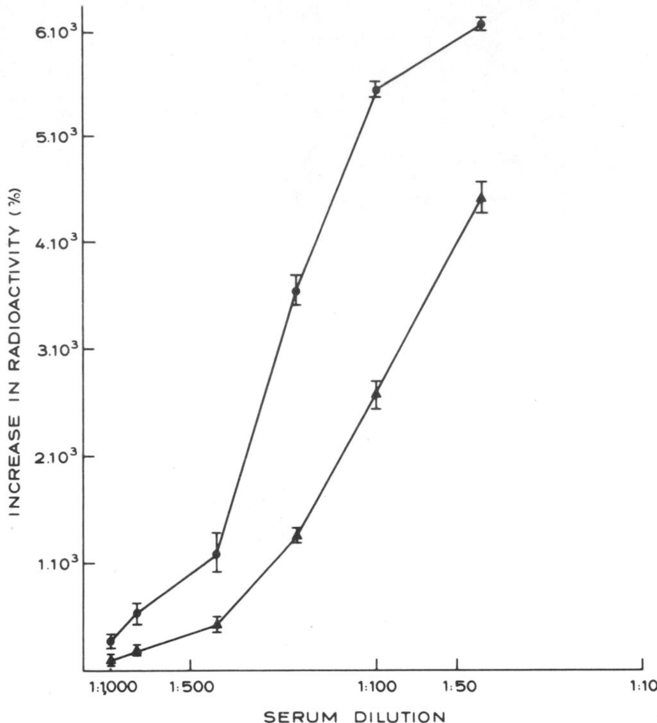

FIG.4. Effect of varying the specific activity of the labelled Tg : ●—● 4.05 mCi/mg; ▲—▲ 0.5 mCi/mg. Vertical lines indicate ± SEM.

Variations of the concentration of ^{125}I-Tg and of the reaction volume

No improvement in the sensitivity was obtained when the ^{125}I-Tg concentration was increased from 10 000 to 500 000 cpm per tube. When coating and incubation volumes from 0.2 ml to 2 ml were compared, no substantial modification of the results was observed.

Storage of the reagents

No modification of the sensitivity of the dose-response curve occurred when the assay was performed with coated tubes kept at 4°C for 40 days or with freshly prepared tubes.

The contamination of the solution of ^{125}I-Tg by iodide or denatured Tg had relatively little effect on the sensitivity of the assay, even when the per cent of

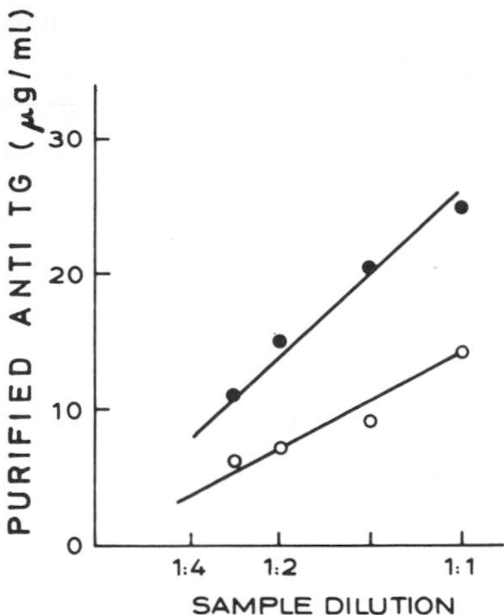

FIG.5. Serial dilution of sera showing a proportional reduction in the measured anti-Tg concentrations.

immunoreactive Tg was as low as 20% of the total radioactivity. Satisfactory results could still be obtained with Tg labelled for several months, without any significant increase of the non-specific binding.

Evaluation of the assay

The non-specific binding was low, ranging between 0.2% and 2% of the total activity. Individual values from 12 normal sera and from 10 replicate analyses of a normal serum were all distributed within ± 3 standard deviations of the mean. The bound radioactivity which was higher than 5 standard deviations from the normal control mean had been selected as the minimal detectable level of antibodies. A 100 times increase of the radioactivity of the tube could be observed with a high level of antibodies. At high concentration, a paradoxal drop of the bound activity was sometimes observed.

The within-assay variation was assessed by performing triplicate measurements of successive dilutions of a serum rich in antibodies; the coefficient of variation throughout the dilution curve averaged 6% and was virtually constant, even with low concentration of antibodies. Six sera characterized by low levels of antibodies were measured on two successive occasions, using two different batches of labelled Tg. The standard deviation (SD) was calculated according to Snedecor [9]: $SD = \sqrt{\Sigma d^2/2N}$ where d is the difference between two successive measurements and N is the number of pairs. Under these conditions, the coefficient of variation was 26.5%, the antibodies being repeatedly detected in all the sera. Serial dilution of sera containing antibodies showed a proportional reduction of the measured concentrations of purified anti-Tg (Fig.5).

The radioimmunoassay was compared with the tanned red cell haemagglutination test (TRCH). Of 220 sera examined simultaneously with both methods, 25 were positive by radioassay and 15 by the haemagglutination test. Only one patient's serum, positive in TRCH, was negative in the radioassay. The positive sera preincubated with an excess of cold Tg showed levels of radioactivity similar to the non-specific binding.

DISCUSSION

This two-site radioassay represents a simple and sensitive measurement of the antithyroglobulin antibodies. The main advantage of our method is that it avoids most of the difficulties encountered with other radioassays of anti-thyroglobulin [2–4]. Indeed, in the double-antibody radioimmunoassay using ^{125}I-Tg, it is essential to purify the tracer before each assay in order to avoid any significant contamination of the specific precipitate by some degraded ^{125}I-Tg [3,4]. In the presence of a normal serum, the blank is higher than in the two-site radioassay. Finally, the presence of Tg in an unknown serum may decrease the specific activity of the tracer and therefore the sensitivity of the test. Other methods in solid phase based on the use of anti-Tg antibodies labelled with radioiodine require delicate preliminary steps of purification and labelling of the antibody [2, 10].

The two-site radioassay reported here is characterized by a very low non-specific binding of the tracer, a fact which improves the detection of low levels of antibodies. As indicated by the present experiments, the optimal conditions for the test much depend on the quantity of Tg adsorbed on the tubes, the temperature and the duration of the incubations. The sensitivity of the test may be improved by prolonged incubations at 4°C and by the use of a buffer containing serum and of labelled Tg of adequately high specific activity. It should however be stressed that, under these conditions, the gain in sensitivity is finally relatively low and, indeed, the method appears to be relatively independent of the specific activity of the tracer and its purity.

The use of Tg as a tracer represents a remarkable advantage since the protein can be easily purified. Moreover, in our method, the labelled Tg does not need repeated purifications before each assay.

Aside from its extreme simplicity of execution, this two-site radioimmunoassay presents the advantage of the long shelf-life of the reagents. The coated tubes may be prepared a long time in advance and the ^{125}I-Tg remains utilizable for weeks after the labelling procedure.

REFERENCES

[1] ROITT, I.M., DONIACH, D., Br. Med. Bull. **16** (1960) 152.
[2] MORI, T., FISHER, J., KRISS, J.P., J. Clin. Endocrinol. Metab. **31** (1970) 119.

[3] SALABE, G.B., FONTANA, S., ANDREOLI, M., Hormones **3** (1972) 1.
[4] PEAKE, R.L., WILISS, D.B., ASIMAKIS, Jr., G., DEISS, Jr., W.P., J. Lab. Clin. Med. **84** (1974) 907.
[5] CATT, K., TRAEGER, G.W., Science **158** (1967) 1570.
[6] MILES, L.E.M., BIEBER, C.P., ENG, L.F., LIPSCHITZ, D.A., Radioimmunoassay and Related Procedures in Medicine (Proc. Symp. Istanbul, 1973) **1**, IAEA, Vienna (1974) 149.
[7] SALVATORE, G., SALVATORE, M., CAHNMANN, H.J., ROBBINS, J., J. Biol. Chem. **239** (1964) 3267.
[8] THORELL, J.I., JOHANSSON, B.G. Biochim. Biophys. Acta **251** (1971) 363.
[9] SNEDECOR, G.W., Biometrics **8** (1952) 85.
[10] TAKEDA, Y., KRISS, J.P., J. Clin. Endocrinol. Metab. **44** (1977) 46.

DISCUSSION

D.K. HAZRA: We can confirm the excellent stability of labelled antibody. In our case, the labelled anti-IgG used in glycoprotein assay showed reproducible results without further repurification for as long as six months. We feel this long stability is very important in that it permits distribution of a centrally produced labelled antibody and improves assay reproducibility.

D. RODBARD: Your dose-response curve for a "two-site" immunoradiometric assay (IRMA) appears to be smooth and symmetrical. In such cases one can use the four-parameter logistic model to describe the curve empirically (Rodbard, D. and Feldman, Y., Immunochemistry (in press)). Moreover, your data clearly show that the standard deviation of the response is directly proportional to the response. We have found similar results in the two-site IRMAs of ferritin and glial fibrillary acidic protein (GFAP)(Ref.[3] of paper SM-220/58), and indeed this can be shown to be a general rule for two-site IRMAs. This is in contrast to most labelled antigen RIAs, where the standard deviation of the response is proportional to the square root of the response, i.e. the response variable behaves as a Poisson variable, with variance of response proportional to the response. Your data very nicely illustrate this point.

D.K. HAZRA: Doesn't the "hook" effect cause difficulty in feeding the infinite dose variable required for four-parameter curve-fitting, as suggested by Dr. Rodbard?

J.P. LEONARD: The "hook" effect to which you are referring can perhaps be avoided by increasing the number of washings after each stage and then by raising the concentration of the radioactive tracer in the final stage.

D. RODBARD: In the presence of a "hook" effect (due to incomplete washing or heterogeneity of the first, solid-phase antiserum), it is often necessary to abandon the "four-parameter logistic" model (which applies in those assays approaching the "ideal" case) and to utilize other, empirical methods to describe the dose-response curve for two-site IRMA. Polynomials, exponentials, splines or related functions may be used in such cases.

A. MALKIN: Using the more sensitive techniques which you described, have you been able to detect an increased incidence of antithyroglobulin antibodies in so-called normal individuals?

J.P. LEONARD: We did not do a full screening of normal subjects. However, it is very difficult to define the term 'normal'. There are normal subjects who have chronic thyroiditis but do not know it themselves. We have not carried out a systematic comparison of the two methods.

Session VIII, Part 2 and Session IX

APPLICATIONS

Assays for peptides

Chairmen

C.A. TAFURT
Colombia

J. HAMMERSTEIN
Federal Republic of Germany

A RADIOIMMUNOASSAY OF PLASMA CORTICOTROPHIN*

L. HUMMER
Rigshospitalet,
Copenhagen, Denmark

Abstract

A RADIOIMMUNOASSAY OF PLASMA CORTICOTROPHIN.

An assay has been established, based on high-affinity antibodies against the N-terminal part of the ACTH molecule, with a detection limit of 2 pg ACTH when assaying 200 μl of unextracted plasma and allowing a total incubation time of 3 days. The antibody has been obtained by immunizing guinea-pigs with synthetic human 1–24 ACTH coupled to bovine serum albumin. The selected antibody has an equilibrium constant of 4×10^{11} litres/mole in a final dilution of 1/320 000. The antiserum reacts with synthetic human 1–39 ACTH as well as with synthetic human 1–24 ACTH; the hormonally inactive synthetic human 11–24 ACTH fragment and the α- and β-melanocyte-stimulating hormones do not cross-react in the assay. The inter-assay coefficient of variation of replicate estimates was 11–13%. The reproducibility of the standard curve was evaluated by calculating the amount of ACTH corresponding to 5% of the $(B/T)_0$ value, 1.2 ± 0.4 pg ACTH/tube ± SD and 50% of the $(B/T)_0$ value, 15.7 ± 2.6 pg ACTH/tube ± SD. Validation of the assay was obtained by assaying samples from patients with verified adrenal disorders, and the accuracy was supported by ACTH determinations in tests where metyrapon had been administered intravenously. Stimulation of ACTH production by insulin-induced hypoglycaemia was found as well. Special attention was always paid to the conditions under which the blood was sampled. A reference interval of 10–76 ng/l was found (115 normal subjects).

INTRODUCTION

More than ten years ago the production of antibodies to ACTH was described [1] and subsequently a radioimmunoassay technique for the determination of ACTH was introduced [2–5]. However, few reports have been published on the clinical use of ACTH measurements [6–10]. The main difficulties in establishing an ACTH assay are: the production of antibodies [11], the labelling of the ACTH and the rapid degradation of the labelled molecule, conditions which all have an influence on the reliability of the results of the assay. Because of the very low concentrations of ACTH in plasma of normal subjects, it is necessary to obtain an antibody with a very high avidity to ACTH in order to circumvent an ACTH extraction before assay. Further, an antibody directed to the N-terminal part of the ACTH molecule can be expected to give assay results in better agreement with results obtained by bioassay [12].

---

* This study was supported by grants from the Danish Medical Research Council.

An assay has been established, based on high-affinity antibody raised against the N-terminal part of the ACTH molecule, with a detection limit of 2 pg ACTH, when assaying 200 μl of unextracted plasma and allowing a total incubation time of 3 days.

The accuracy of the assay has been evaluated by indirect stimulation of the ACTH level by lowering the cortisol level with metyrapon and by direct stimulation of the ACTH production by hypoglycaemia.

MATERIALS

Immunization

Ten guinea-pigs were immunized with synthetic human 1–24 ACTH (Synacthen, short-acting, Organon, Netherlands) coupled to bovine serum albumin from Behringwerke, Marburg. The conjugate was mixed with complete Freund's adjuvant, Difco, USA.

Assay

Synthetic human 1–39 ACTH supplied by CIBA was used for labelling with ^{125}I (IMS 30, The Radiochemical Centre, Amersham, UK).
Different standards were used in the assay:

Synthetic human 1–39 ACTH (CIBA).
Synthetic human 1–24 ACTH (CIBA).
Fragments of synthetic human 11–24 ACTH (CIBA).
Synthetic α-MSH (CIBA).
Synthetic β-MSH (CIBA).
α-human corticotrophin 75/555, Medical Research Council, London.

Hormone-free plasma was obtained from normal persons, who had taken 1 mg of dexamethasone four times over a period of 24 hours before blood sampling [11].

All blood samples were taken into heparinized plastic tubes (10 IU/ml blood) and centrifuged immediately at 4°C. The plasma was removed from the blood with a plastic pipette. All samples were immediately frozen and stored at −20°C until assayed.

METHODS

Synthetic human 1–24 ACTH was coupled to BSA by means of 1-ethyl-3 (3-dimethyl-aminopropyl) carbodiimide, (ethyl-CDI) [13]. For 10 animals, a

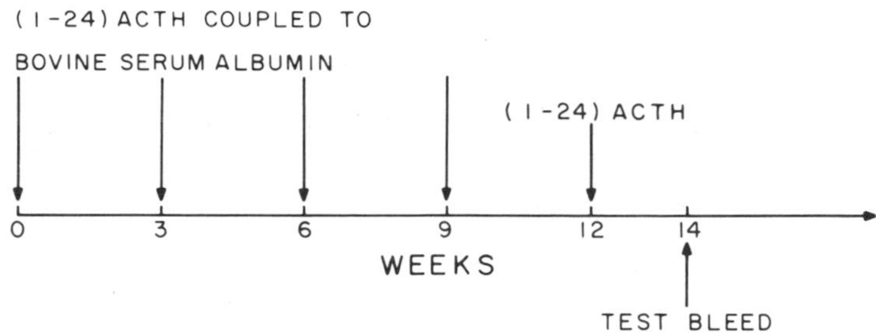

FIG.1. Immunization schedule for 10 guinea-pigs immunized with 1–24 ACTH.

reaction product of 10 mg ACTH, 200 mg BSA, and 100 mg ethyl-CDI was prepared in 3 ml. The dialysate was mixed with double the volume of complete Freund's adjuvant to make a stable water-in-oil emulsion [14]. Two aliquots of 0.5 ml of this emulsion were injected subcutaneously in the back of the guinea-pigs. Booster injections were administered at 3-week intervals, blood was collected by cardiac puncture for assessment of antibody production (Fig.1). Several of the animals produced antibodies against ACTH. The serum presented in this paper is from the first bleed and is coded No.3. A dilution curve of this antiserum is shown in Fig.2.

Labelling procedure

^{125}I-labelled ACTH is prepared by the Cloramine-T method [11]. 1 μg of synthetic human 1–39 ACTH in 5 μl of 0.01M phosphate buffer, pH 7.4, and 25 μg of Chloramine-T in 10 μl of 0.24M phosphate buffer, pH 7.4, are added to 10 μl of ^{125}I, 500 μCi.

As stated by Virasoso et al. [16], a rapid labelling procedure is of great importance. Therefore, the addition of the ACTH and the Chloramine-T is performed by using a polyethylene tube (1 mm diameter) connected to a Hamilton syringe. In the tube, 5 μl of ACTH, 20 μl of air, and 10 μl of Chloramine-T are sucked up successively. The outlet of the tube is then placed in the bottom of the V-vial containing ^{125}I-solution and, by pressing the piston into the syringe, all the reactants are rapidly added to the reaction mixture and stirred by the air bubbles at the same time. With a 5-μl pipette containing 200 μg of metabisulphite, the labelling reaction is ended. The complete labelling procedure is performed within 10 s. An aliquot of the iodination mixture is removed for electrophoresis and the labelled hormone is purified by adsorption

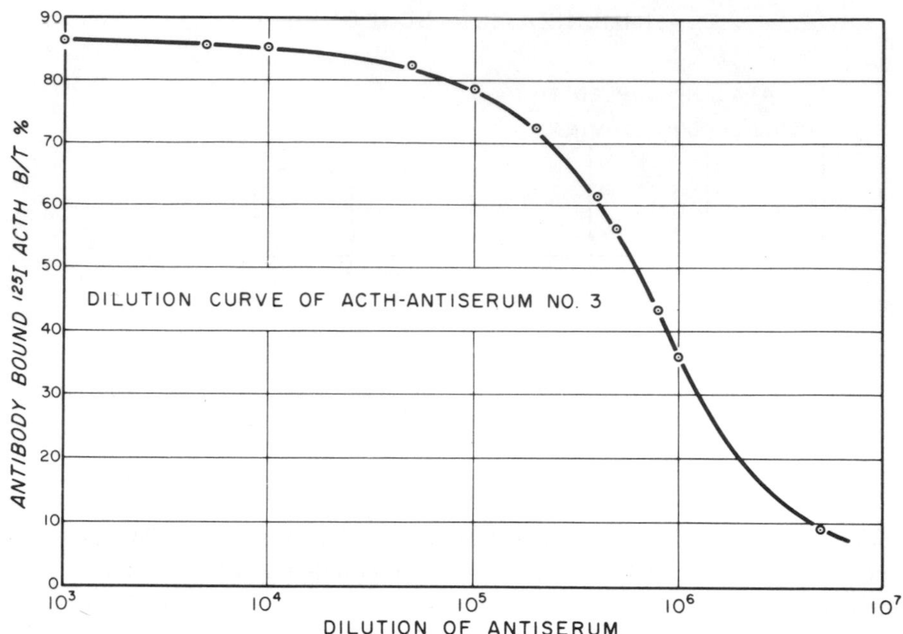

FIG.2. Antiserum dilution curve using sera from animal No.3 incubated with 50 pg of ^{125}*I-(1−39)-ACTH for 3 days.*

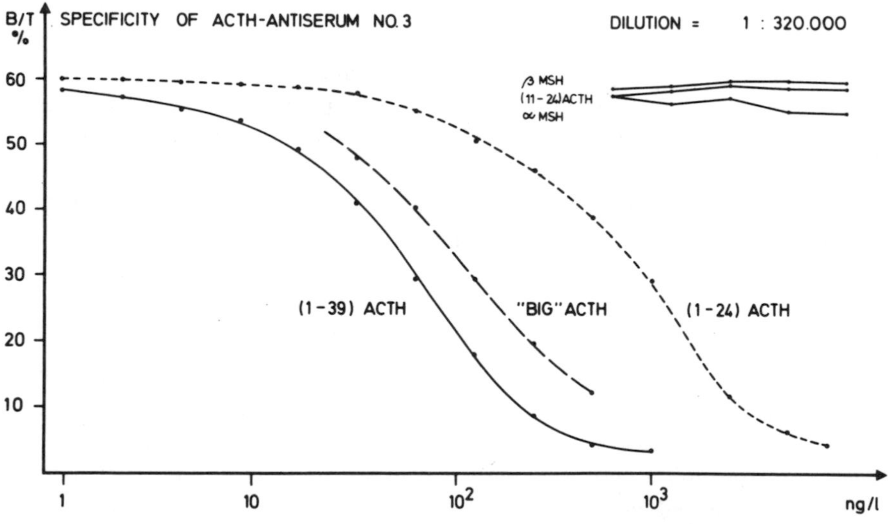

FIG.3. Testing of the cross-reactivity of different fragments of ACTH in the ACTH assay.

on microfine precipitated silica granules (QUSO 32) according to Berson and Yalow [4]. ACTH is eluted with 2 ml of a 1% acetic acid-40% acetone-water mixture. The QUSO-eluate is checked by electrophoresis, and the eluate shows only one peak and is completely free from "damage-products" and free iodide. Because of the very short shelf-life of the labelled ACTH, only freshly labelled ACTH (iodinated the same day) is added to the incubation mixtures.

Assay procedure

Incubation mixtures of 2.2 ml are prepared in disposable polystyrol tubes, 70 mm × 11 mm. All steps in the assay procedure are performed at 4°C. An amount of 0.2 ml of plasma sample or standard, prepared in ACTH-free plasma, are added to 2 ml of ACTH-antibody diluted 1:320 000 (final dilution) by 0.02 ml of diemal buffer, pH 8.16, containing 0.4% mercaptoethanol, 400 KIE Trasylol/ml and 1% BSA. Tubes are capped and incubated at 4°C until the next day.

The following day the labelling procedure is performed and the QUSO-eluate diluted in the above-mentioned buffer. Approximately 3000 cpm/200 μl are added to each test-tube and mixed on a Vortex mixer. After another 20 hours of incubation at 4°C, the antibody-bound and the free ACTH are separated by addition of 200 μl of activated charcoal suspension containing 3% Norite A and 0.75% Dextran T-80 in 0.02 m of diemal buffer, pH 8.6. The tubes are incubated for 15 min and then centrifuged at 4°C for 15 min at 2000 rpm. The supernatant is discarded and the charcoal residue is counted in a gamma scintillation counter. The labelled ACTH bound to antibody is calculated in percentage of the total activity in the incubation mixture and correction for non-specific binding in the individual sample is made. Figure 3 shows a standard curve prepared by means of ACTH-free plasma.

Standard

The standard is human 1–39 ACTH Code No.73/555 MRC. In our hands this standard seems to have a perfect stability and a very low variability of contents between the individual micro-ampoules.

RESULTS

Characterization of the antiserum

The specificity of the antiserum used in the assay was evaluated by testing the cross-reactivity of certain ACTH fragments in the assay. Figure 3 shows that the hormonally inactive 11–24 ACTH as well as the α-melanocyte-stimulating hormone and β-melanocyte-stimulating hormone did not cross-react at the

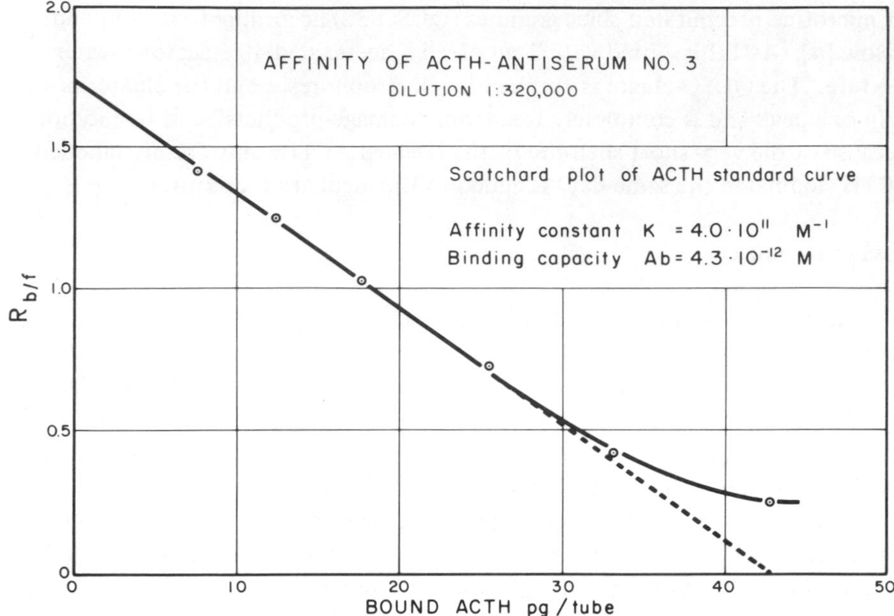

FIG.4. A Scatchard plot calculated from a standard curve for ACTH (3rd International Standard) diluted in ACTH-free plasma.

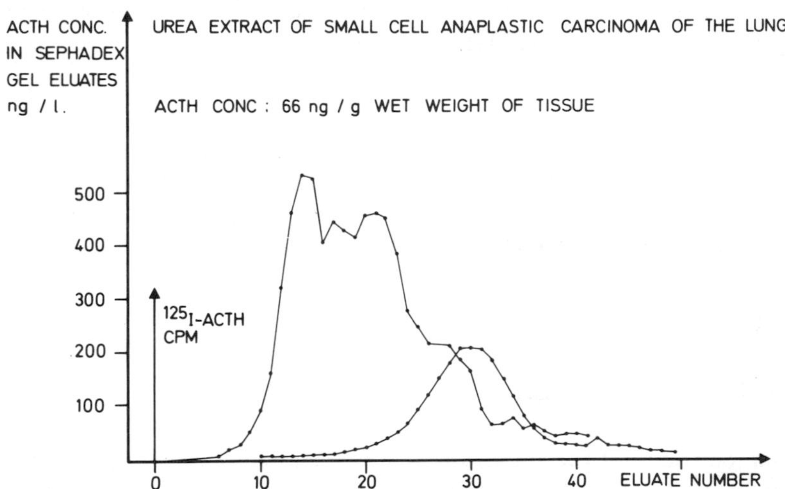

FIG.5. Distribution of immunoreactive ACTH in the eluates from Sephadex G-50 gel-filtration of an urea extract of a small cell anaplastic carcinoma of the lung.

TABLE I. REPRODUCIBILITY OF ACTH STANDARD CURVE

Lowering of initial binding $(B/T)_0$	5%	50%
pg ACTH/tube ± SD	1.2 ± 0.4	15.7 ± 2.6

TABLE II. RECOVERY EXPERIMENT OF ACTH

Plasma sample (ng/l)	Added ACTH (ng/l)	Measured ACTH (ng/l)	Recovery (ng/l)	Recovery (%)
65	10	73	8	80
65	20	83	18	90
65	40	103	38	95
65	60	120	55	92
65	80	135	70	88

concentrations tested. The antiserum reacts with the intact hormone 1–39 ACTH and with the 1–24 ACTH fragment which retains the full biological activity on a molecular basis.

Figure 3 shows a dilution curve of plasma from a patient with an extremely high concentration of ACTH due to ectopic ACTH production (Code No.74/555 MRC, a gift from Dr. Lesley H. Rees, St. Bartholomew's Hospital, London).

From a Scatchard plot [17], the equilibrium constant was calculated to be 4.0×10^{11} M^{-1} and the concentration of antibody binding sites to be 4.3×10^{-12} M at the dilution of the antibody used in the assay (Fig.4).

From a patient (plasma ACTH 2530 ng/l) with a small cell anaplastic carcinoma of the lung, a urea extract was made from the tumour removed at necropsy. The extract was prepared according to the method described by Gewirtz and Yalow [21] and subjected to gel-filtration at 4°C on a Sephadex G-50 fine column 1 cm × 50 cm. The ACTH concentrations in the eluates were determinated. From the elution pattern, Fig.5, it can be seen that 90% of the ACTH content of the tumour is a component with ACTH immunoreactivity and a molecular weight higher than the ACTH-tracer eluted around fraction number 30.

Sensitivity

The sensitivity, defined as the smallest amount of unlabelled hormone that can be distinguished from no hormone, is calculated as 6.0 ng/l (Standard 73/555), i.e. 1.2 pg/test-tube.

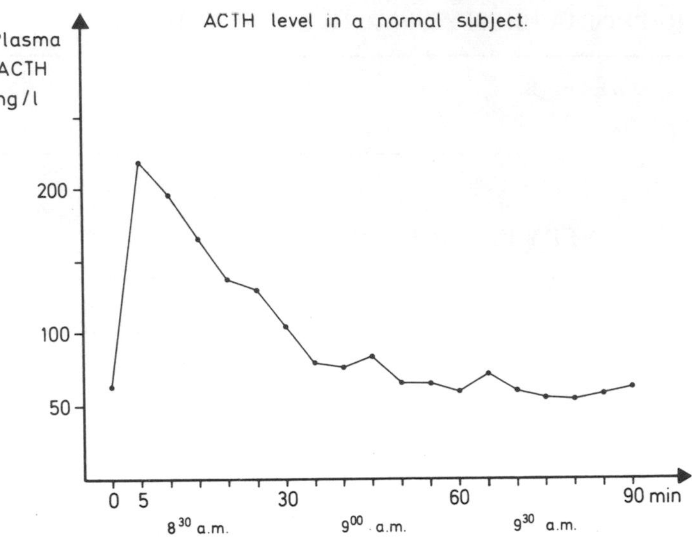

FIG. 6. Plasma ACTH concentration in a normal subject measured at 5-min intervals.

Precision and reproducibility

Two plasma samples were determined in duplicate in 15 different assays. One had an average content of 42 ng/l, and the other contained 134 ng/l. The inter-assay coefficients of variation of duplicate determinations based on a weekly set-up during one year were 11% and 13% respectively. The reproducibility of the standard curve was evaluated by calculating the amount of ACTH corresponding to 5% and to 50% lowering of the $(B/T)_0$ value, as a mean evaluation index of sensitivity and of average slope, respectively.

Table I shows the indices calculated from 26 dose-response curves run over a period of one year.

Recovery

Recovery of exogenous ACTH added to plasma samples ranged from 80–95%, as shown in Table II.

Reference interval

It is shown [18] that ACTH, like cortisol, is secreted episodically in periods of very short duration. Measured at 5-min intervals from 1.00 to 9.00 a.m. there were 18 episodes of ACTH secretion. The half-life of ACTH is stated to

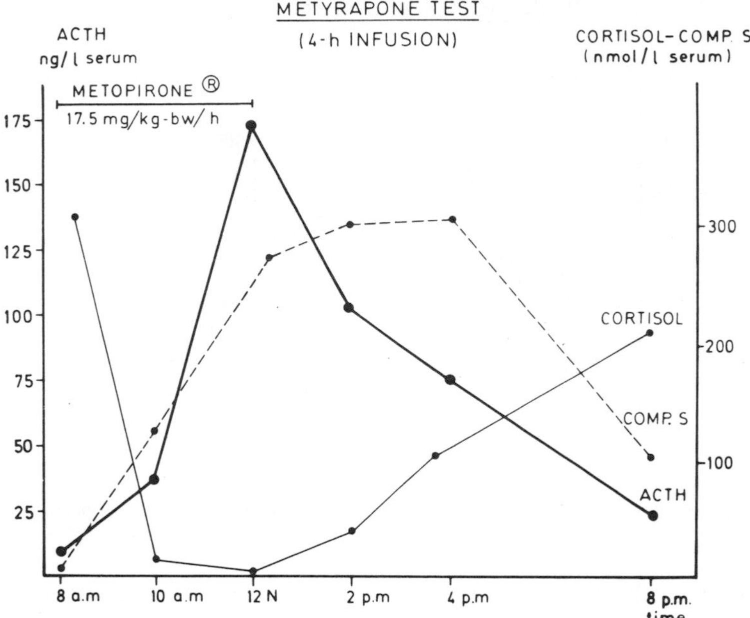

FIG. 7. Metyrapon-infusion test performed in a normal person.

range from 4 to 15 min. These facts make it very difficult to determine a reference interval for ACTH concentration in plasma. In addition, acute stress due to anxiety or pain may result in an increase in ACTH concentration more than 4 times the basic level (see Fig.6). As a result of this observation, blood sampling for ACTH determination is performed by taking two samples with an interval of 5 min. If the results from these two samples differ by more than 50% of the mean value, another blood sample has to be drawn.

Morning concentrations of ACTH in plasma

A total of 115 fasting healthy volunteers, 60 females and 55 males, aged 20–94 years, had blood samples drawn between 7.30 a.m. and 8.30 a.m. The 95% range observed was 10–76 ng/l.

ACTH response to metyrapone stimulation

Metyrapone was administered intravenously in doses of 17.4 mg of Metopiron (CIBA) per kg body weight per hour, between 8 a.m. and noon. The blocking

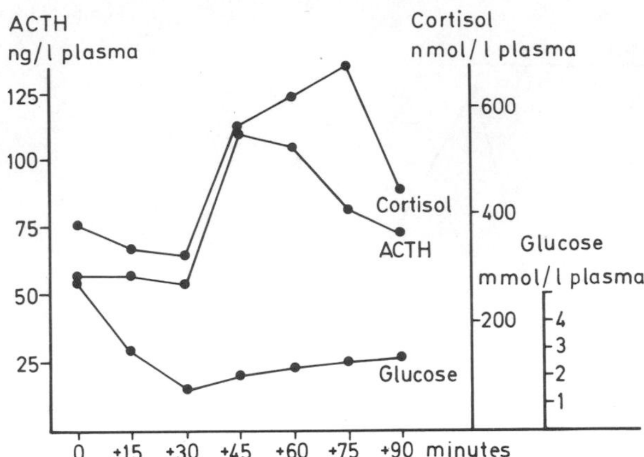

FIG.8. Insulin-induced hypoglycaemia test performed in a normal person.

effect was checked by determining the decrease in cortisol level and the increase in 11-deoxycortisol (Comp. S) level in plasma according to the double-isotope-derivative technique [23]. The results of such a test are graphically illustrated in Fig.7.

ACTH-response to insulin-induced hypoglycaemia

On the day of examination the subjects were fasting and the hypoglycaemia test was started by giving crystalline insulin intravenously. Blood for determination of cortisol, glucose, and ACTH was drawn through an intravenous needle just before the insulin injection and 15, 30, 45, 60, 75 and 90 min after the injection. The test was considered adequate only if the blood sugar fell to at least 2 mmol/l and the patient sweated [20]. The results of such a test are shown in Fig.8.

The validation of the ACTH assay has been obtained by assaying samples from patients with verified adrenal disorders.

1. Two patients with cortisol-producing adrenal adenomas: 5–7 ng/l.
2. Six patients with Cushing's syndrome without pituitary tumor: 20–83 ng/l.
3. Six patients with ACTH-dependent Cushing's syndrome due to ectopic ACTH production: 98–273 ng/l.
   One patient with a small cell anaplastic carcinoma of the lung: 2350 ng/l. The ACTH concentration in the carcinoma was 66 ng/g wet weight.
4. Ten patients with pituitary ACTH-dependent Cushing's syndrome subjected to total adrenalectomy: 260 – > 1000 ng/l (post-operatively).
5. Two patients with Nelson's syndrome: > 1000 ng/l.
6. One patient with Addison's disease: 730 ng/l.

CONCLUSION

The present radioimmunoassay is well established in our laboratory. ACTH can be measured directly in 200 μl of plasma, and the antibody binding site is the N-terminal part of the ACTH molecule. Special attention has to be paid to the blood-sampling procedure in order to obtain results reflecting the basal ACTH concentration in the plasma of the patient.

The application of the ACTH radioimmunoassay in adrenal pathology seems helpful in differentiating different forms of Cushing's syndrome. If the disease is caused by an adrenal adenoma, very low ACTH values are obtained, implying that the feed-back mechanism in the patient is intact as the elevated cortisol level is suppressing the ACTH secretion.

Patients with adrenal hyperplasia without pituitary tumour show ACTH levels in the reference interval. Distinctly elevated ACTH values are seen if the Cushing's syndrome is caused by ectopic ACTH production. In patients with Cushing's disease in maintenance therapy after bilateral adrenalectomy, the ACTH levels are increased in most of the patients.

Lastly, the ACTH responses to insulin-induced hypoglycaemia and to metyrapon seem promising for information about the pituitary function in cases of pituitary pathology.

ACKNOWLEDGEMENTS

The author is grateful to the Department of Endocrine Surgery and the Department of Neurosurgery, Division of Neuroendocrinology, Rigshospitalet, for providing the plasma samples, and to the Department of Pathology, Frederiksberg Hospital, Copenhagen, for the tissue from the pulmonary carcinoma. The technical assistance of Ilse Aalund and Tove Sibbernsen is much appreciated. The author would also like to express her gratitude to Drs P.A. Desaulles and W. Rittel, CIBA, Basle for the most valuable gift of the ACTH fragments and the ACTH for labelling. The ACTH standards were kindly supplied by the Medical Research Council, London.

REFERENCES

[1] FELBER, J.P., Experientia **19** (1963) 227.
[2] DEMURA, H., WEST, C.D., NUGENT, C.A., NAKAGAWA, K., TYLER, F.H., J. Clin. Endocrinol. Metab. **26** (1966) 1297.
[3] LANDON, J., GREENWOOD, F.C., Lancet **i** (1968) 273.
[4] BERSON, S.A., YALOW, R.S., J. Clin. Invest. **47** (1968) 2725.
[5] GALSKOV, Aa., Radioimmunochemical Corticotropin Determination (Thesis), Copenhagen, Forum (1972).

[6] BESSER, G.M., LANDON, J., Brit. Med. J. **iv** (1968) 552.
[7] ORTH, D.N., ISLAND, D.P., NICHOLSON, W.E., ABE, K., WOODHAM, J.P., "ACTH radioimmunoassay: interpretation, comparison with bioassay and clinical application", Radioisotopes in Medicine: In vitro Studies (HAYES, R.L., GOSWITZ, F.A., MURPHY, B.E.P., Eds), USAEC, Div. Tech. Inf., Oak Ridge, Tenn. (1968) 251.
[8] BESSER, G.M., CULLEN, D.R., IRVINE, W.J., RATCLIFFE, J.G., LANDON, J., Br. Med. J. **1** (1971) 374.
[9] CROUGHS, R.J.M., TOPS, C.F., de JONG, F.H., J. Endocrinol. **59** (1973) 439.
[10] GENAZZANI, A.R., FRAIOLI, F., CONTI, C., FIORETTI, P., J. Nucl. Biol. Med. **18** (1974) 67.
[11] PROESCHEL, M.F., COURVALIN, J.C., DONNADIEU, M., BINOUX, M., GIRAUD, F., Acta Endocrinol. **75** (1974) 461.
[12] ORTH, D.N., NICHOLSON, W.E., MITCHELL, W.M., ISLAND, D.P., LIDDLE, G.W., J. Clin. Invest. **52** (1973) 1756.
[13] McGUIRE, J., McGILL, R., LEEMAN, W., GOODFRIEND, T., J. Clin. Invest. **44** (1965) 1672.
[14] HURN, B.A.L., LANDON, J., "Antisera for radioimmunoassay", Radioimmunoassay methods (HUNTER, W.M., KIRKHAM, K.E., Eds), Churchill Livingstone, Edinburgh and London (1971) 121.
[15] GREENWOOD, F.C., HUNTER, W.M., Nature (London) **194** (1962) 495.
[16] VIRASORO, E., COPINSCHI, G., BRUNO, O.D., "Degradation of labelled hormone in radioimmunoassay of ACTH", Radioimmunoassay and Related Procedures in Medicine (Proc. Symp. Istanbul, 1973) **1**, IAEA, Vienna (1974) 323.
[17] SCATCHARD, G., Ann. N.Y. Acad. Sci. **51** (1949) 660.
[18] GALLAGHER, T.F., YOSHIDA, K., ROFFWARG, H.D., FUKUSHIMA, D.K., WEITZMANN, E.D., MELLMAN, L., J. Clin. Endocrinol. Metab. **36** (1973) 1058.
[19] BLICHERT-TOFT, M., HUMMER, L., J. Gerontol. **31** (1976) 539.
[20] LANDON, J., GREENWOOD, F.C., STAMP, T.C.B., WYNN, V., J. Clin. Invest. **45** (1966) 437.
[21] GEWIRTZ, G., YALOW, R.S., J. Clin. Invest. **53** (1974) 1022.
[22] RAUX, M.C., BINOUX, M., LUTON, J.P., GOURMELEN, M., GIRAUD, F., J. Clin. Endocrinol. Metab. **40** (1975) 186.
[23] BUUS, O., Excerpta Medica, International Congress Series **157** (1968) 107.

DISCUSSION

W. KLINGLER: Have you made a comparison between your assay and one with extraction procedure?

L. HUMMER: No, I haven't, but Dr. Lesley H. Rees in London has performed a cytochemical assay of ACTH on samples which had also been assayed by this RIA procedure, and has found a good correlation.

G. HEYNEN: Since you immunized with the 1–24 fragment, how do you explain the better sensitivity for the 1–39 ACTH than for the 1–24 fragment?

L. HUMMER: This could be due to a difference in purity between the synthetic 1–39 ACTH and the 1–24 ACTH used in the assay for the determination of cross-reactivity.

F. DIEL: I must say that the sensitivity of your RIA for ACTH is very high. Your mentioning that it is a direct assay for blood plasma reminds me that 10 years ago Berson and Yalow reported a similar good sensitivity in the case of direct immunochemical measurement of ACTH.

As you know, blood sampling is a problem in the case of ACTH. Did you measure the half-life of ACTH in vitro as well as in vivo?

L. HUMMER: We measured the degradation of ACTH in blood at room temperature and found a half-life of 20–30 min. For this reason the blood samples are centrifuged at 4°C within 5–10 min of sampling. I did not perform an in-vitro measurement.

IAEA-SM-220/74

DOSAGE RADIOIMMUNOLOGIQUE DU FRAGMENT BIOLOGIQUEMENT ACTIF DE L'HORMONE PARATHYROIDIENNE HUMAINE

C. DESPLAN, A. JULLIENNE, D. RAULAIS,
P. RIVAILLE, J.P. BARLET,
M.S. MOUKHTAR, G. MILHAUD

Unité 113 INSERM,
Laboratoire associé 163 CNRS,
Hôpital Saint-Antoine,
Paris, France

Abstract–Résumé

RADIOIMMUNOASSAY OF THE BIOLOGICALLY ACTIVE FRAGMENT OF HUMAN PARATHYROID HORMONE.

The paper describes a radioimmunoassay of the biologically active part (N-terminal) of the human parathyroid hormone. This homologous assay uses antibodies obtained from the goat against an N-terminal 1-34 fragment of hPTH synthesized in accordance with the sequence proposed by Niall and co-workers. In this system natural hPTH of different origins (extract of parathyroid adenomas, culture medium of adenomas, hyperparathyroid plasma, extract of normal human plasma obtained by affinity chromatography) behaves identically with the synthetic reference hormone 1-34 hPTHN. The radioimmunoassay detects PTH in 65% of the normal subjects and distinguishes between the normal values and those obtained in hyperparathyroidism patients. In this way the assay can be used for clinical purposes.

DOSAGE RADIOIMMUNOLOGIQUE DU FRAGMENT BIOLOGIQUEMENT ACTIF DE L'HORMONE PARATHYROIDIENNE HUMAINE.

Le mémoire décrit un dosage radioimmunologique de la partie biologiquement active (N-terminale) de l'hormone parathyroïdienne humaine; ce dosage homologue utilise des anticorps obtenus chez la chèvre contre un fragment N-terminal 1-34 de la hPTH synthétisé selon la séquence proposée par Niall et al. Dans ce système la hPTH naturelle provenant de différentes origines (extrait d'adénomes parathyroïdiens, de milieu de culture d'adénomes, plasma hyperparathyroïdien, extrait par chromatographie d'affinité de plasma humain normal) se comporte de manière identique à l'hormone de référence synthétique 1-34 hPTHN. Le dosage radioimmunologique détecte de la PTH chez 65% des sujets normaux et distingue les valeurs normales de celles obtenues chez des malades hyperparathyroïdiens, permettant une utilisation clinique de ce dosage.

Le système hormonal comporte les étapes suivantes : biosynthèse du messager, sécrétion, transport dans le sang, actions au niveau des récepteurs, enfin son inactivation. Ce système est encore plus complexe puisqu'il faut faire intervenir la biosynthèse d'une prohormone, le clivage en hormone active suivi d'une fragmentation. Les molécules hormonales circulantes sont hétérogènes ; on observe une majorité de "grosses" hormones et de fragments, et une minorité d'hormone intacte. Il peut paraître déraisonnable de vouloir étayer un diagnostic sur le résultat d'un dosage radioimmunologique. Toutefois, la situation est favorable dans le cas de l'hormone parathyroïdienne (PTH) qui circule sous plusieurs formes (5, 6, 7, 8) parmi lesquelles on distingue deux fragments, l'un qui possède l'activité biologique (9) et qui est amino-terminal (séquence 1-34) et l'autre qui est dépourvu d'activité biologique et qui est carboxy-terminal (séquence 35-84).

Depuis plus de 13 années (1), le dosage radioimmunologique de la PTH humaine a été mis au point. Il s'agissait de système de dosage hétérologue, comportant la possibilité d'une réaction croisée partielle avec de l'hormone circulante humaine (2, 3, 4). Selon que les anticorps utilisés dans le dosage radioimmunologique sont dirigés vers des sites N- ou C-terminaux de la molécule, le dosage mesurera soit les fragments possédant une activité biologique, soit ceux qui sont dépourvus d'activité biologique.

La plupart des dosages radioimmunologiques utilisés sont à la fois hétérologues et dirigés vers la portion C-terminale de la molécule, ce qui présente quelques inconvénients. Seule, la synthèse permet d'obtenir en quantité suffisante le fragment 1-34 pour immuniser les animaux. La séquence 1-34 hPTH (10) est controversée (11). La divergence porte sur Glu au lieu de Gln^{22}, Leu au lieu de Lys^{28} et Asn au lieu de Leu^{30}. Les études immunochimiques relatives à l'une ou l'autre séquence ont donné des résultats contradictoires (12, 13, 14).

Les résultats des dosages radioimmunologiques N-terminaux homologues ou hétérologues discriminent imparfaitement le sujet normal de l'hyperparathyroïdien (12, 3, 4).

Nous avons mis au point un dosage radioimmunologique homologue de la séquence 1-34 hPTH Niall (1-34 hPTH N), dans lequel le comportement de l'hormone humaine naturelle est identique à celui de la 1-34 hPTH N. De plus, les valeurs relatives aux sujets normaux se distinguent nettement de celles de sujets atteints d'hyperparathyroïdie primaire ou secondaire à une insuffisance rénale. Ce dosage est donc une aide à la décision diagnostique (15).

1. MATERIEL ET METHODES

1.1. Synthèse du fragment 1-34 hPTH N

Cette synthèse a été réalisée par la méthode de Merrifield (16, 17). Le profil de la première élution en milieu acétique à 1 % ("Biogel P6", 100-200 meshs) présente trois pics. Pour le premier, la composition en acides aminés est la plus proche de la théorie ; le produit est le plus homogène sur l'électrophorétogramme et l'activité biologique la plus élevée (88 U MRC/mg) ; elle tombe à 40 U pour le second pic et à 0 U pour le troisième. La courbe dose-effet est parallèle à celle obtenue avec de la PTH bovine MRC. La seconde filtration sur "Biogel P6" (200-400 meshs) dans le même solvant donne trois pics partiellement confondus ; l'activité biologique est de 180 U MRC/mg dans les deux premiers et de 40 U dans le troisième. Les deux premiers pics sont chromatographiés sur carboxyméthyl cellulose (CM 52, pH 4,5, gradient de conductivité de 4 à 20 mmhos). Différents pics sont élués à 7,5, 9, 9,5, 11, 13, 15, 16 et 20 mmhos. Après désalage sur "Biogel P2", l'analyse en acides aminés ne permet pas de différencier les pics entre eux ; mais le dosage biologique montre un maximum d'activité dans la fraction éluée à 9 mmhos. Une certaine activité biologique est présente dans les fractions éluées à 9,5 et 11 mmhos. Le peptide présent dans le pic principal est homogène sur chromatographie en couche mince

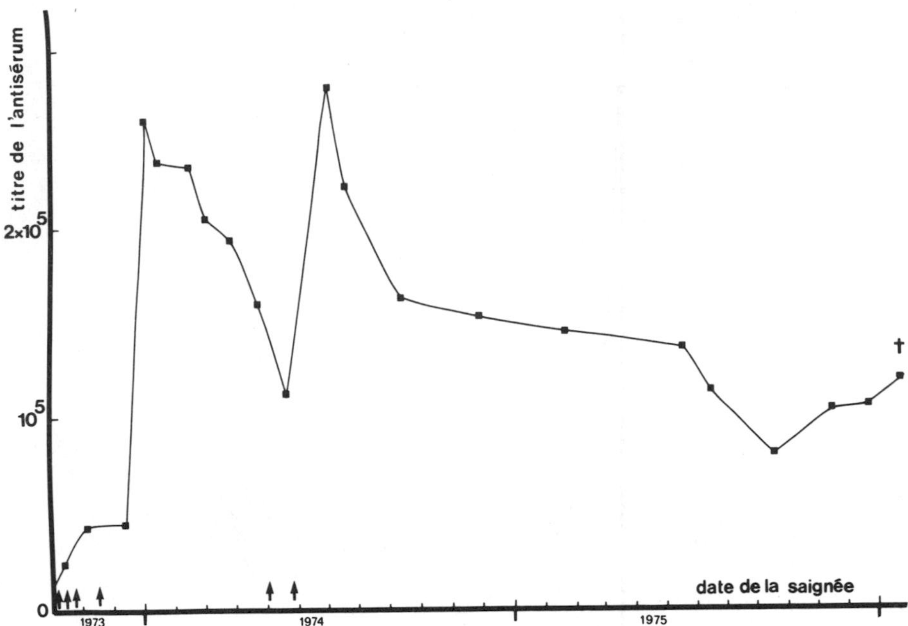

FIG.1. Evolution du titre des antisérums au cours de l'immunisation.
Le titre est la valeur de la dilution de l'antisérum qui capture la moitié d'une faible dose (10 pg) de 1–34 hPTH N^{125}I (B/F = 1). On injecte 150 µg de 1–34 hPTH en présence de charbon végétal et d'adjuvant complet de Freund.

(Silice, ButOH, AcOH, H_2O 4 : 1 : 5) et électrophorèse sur papier et sa composition en acides aminés est conforme à la formule : Arg 2,09 (2), Asp 4,87 (4), Glu 5,08 (5), Gly 0,98 (1), His 2,33 (3), Ile 0,57 (1), Leu 4,98 (5), Lys 3,02 (3), Met 1,70 (2), Phe 1,18 (1), Ser 1,85 (3), Trp 0,65 (1), Val 2,75 (3).

L'analyse séquentielle confirme que l'enchaînement des vingt premières étapes est correcte ; la pureté du produit est de l'ordre de 70 à 75 %. Le rendement est de 85 mg de 1-34 hPTH NH_2/g de résine ; l'activité biologique, déterminée chez le rat (18) en se référant à l'étalon A 67/342 d'hormone parathyroïdienne bovine MRC, varie selon les préparations de 1200 à 351 U/mg.

De la même manière, le peptide correspondant à la séquence proposée par Brewer a été synthétisé (19).

1.2. Obtention d'anticorps

Plusieurs chèvres reçoivent par voie sous-cutanée le mélange de 150 µg de peptide, de charbon végétal et d'adjuvant complet de Freund. Des prises de sang sont effectuées quinze jours après chaque immunisation. Le sang est recueilli sur héparine, centrifugé à froid ; le plasma est réparti dans les tubes et immédiatement congelé. Les antisérums sont dilués progressivement, titrés en fonction de leur capacité à lier une dose traceuse de 1-34 hPTH N marquée à l'Iode-125. Les anticorps de titres les plus élevés sont sélectionnés selon leur sensibilité au déplacement du peptide marqué par le peptide froid.

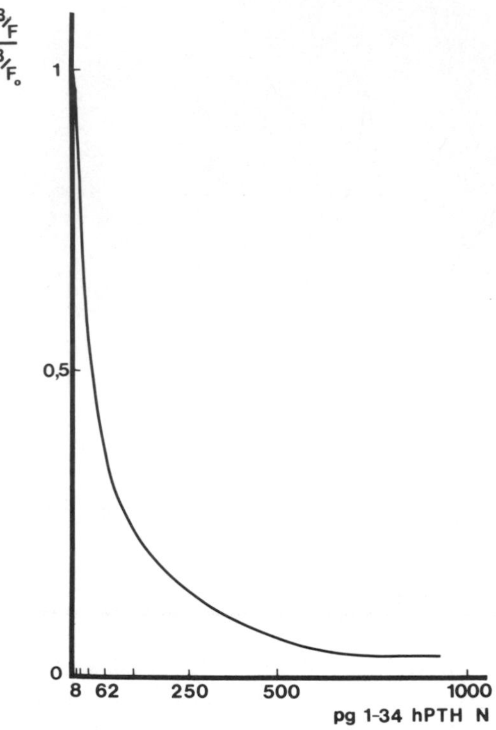

FIG.2. Déplacement de la radioactivité par l'hormone de référence.
L'anticorps est dilué 250 000 fois en présence de 2000 cpm (~10 pg) de 1–34 hPTH N ^{125}I.

1.3. Iodation du peptide

La 1-34 hPTH est marquée à l'Iode 125 sur les résidus histidines et phénylalanine, selon la technique à la chloramine T de Hunter et Greenwood modifiée (20). La séparation des iodures, des fragments et du peptide met en jeu l'adsorption du peptide sur de la silice précipitée (QuSo G 32) (21) suivie d'une élution par le mélange acide acétique-eau-acétone. La pureté de l'indicateur radioactif est vérifiée par la chromatoélectrophorèse dans des conditions standardisées.

L'activité spécifique du peptide est d'environ 50 à 100 µCi/µg.

1.4. Système immunochimique

L'antisérum est préincubé à la dilution normale de 1/250.000, pendant trois jours, dans un milieu contenant du tampon véronal 0,05 M, pH 8,6, 1/6 en volume de plasma humain débarrassé de PTH par chromatographie d'affinité, 0,2 % d'azide de sodium, en présence d'hormone de référence ou du plasma à doser. On rajoute alors 2000 cpm de 1-34 hPTH N, soit environ 10 pg ; le volume final est de 500 µl. L'incubation est prolongée pendant quatre jours ; on adsorbe l'hormone libre (F) sur du charbon dextran (22).

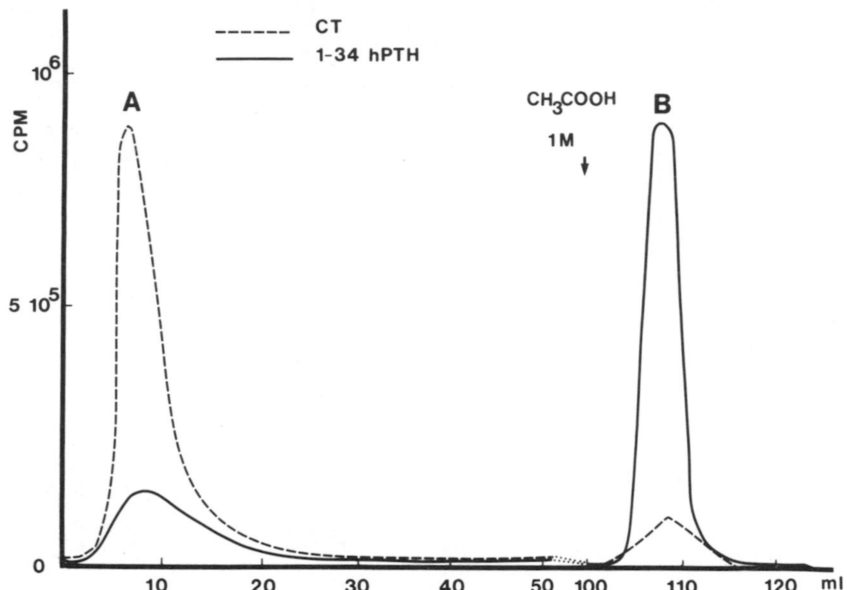

FIG. 3. Profil d'élution de la 1–34 hPTH N ^{125}I sur colonne d'affinité.
Les anticorps couplés sont obtenus contre la 1–34 hPTH N. La fixation de la 1–34 hPTH (–) se fait en tampon véronal 0,05 M, pH = 8,6; l'élution est réalisée par l'acide acétique 1 M. Une autre hormone comme la calcitonine (. . . .) n'est pas fixée.

La gamme de l'hormone étalon est comprise entre 8 et 200 pg par tube. Le plasma à doser est introduit à raison de 100 µl.

Les témoins nécessaires à la détermination de l'adsorption non spécifique sont incubés lors de chaque dosage.

1.5. Chromatographie d'affinité

Deux types d'anticorps sont couplés sur un support solide d'agarose (23) :

- Les anticorps qui sont utilisés pour le dosage et qui ont été obtenus à l'aide de 1-34 hPTH N (As 10/107).
- Les anticorps de cobaye obtenus à l'aide d'un extrait ATC impur de PTH bovine (b PTH). Ces anticorps sont dirigés vers des sites C-terminaux de la molécule (24) ; la réaction croisée avec l'hormone humaine extractive est bonne.

Les globulines des antisérums sont précipitées par du sulfate d'ammonium 33 %, dialysées et concentrées à 4°C sur Amicon PM 30, puis couplées sur du Sépharose 4B (Pharmacia) activé par du bromure de cyanogène une nuit à 4°C (25). Ce gel est chargé dans de petites colonnes, lavé alternativement par de l'acide acétique 1 M et du tampon véronal pH 8,6.

Un litre de plasma humain normal est passé successivement sur l'une et l'autre colonne ; la PTH liée aux anticorps est éluée par l'acide acétique 1M. L'éluat est neutralisé par de la soude puis utilisé à dilutions croissantes dans le dosage radioimmunologique (26).

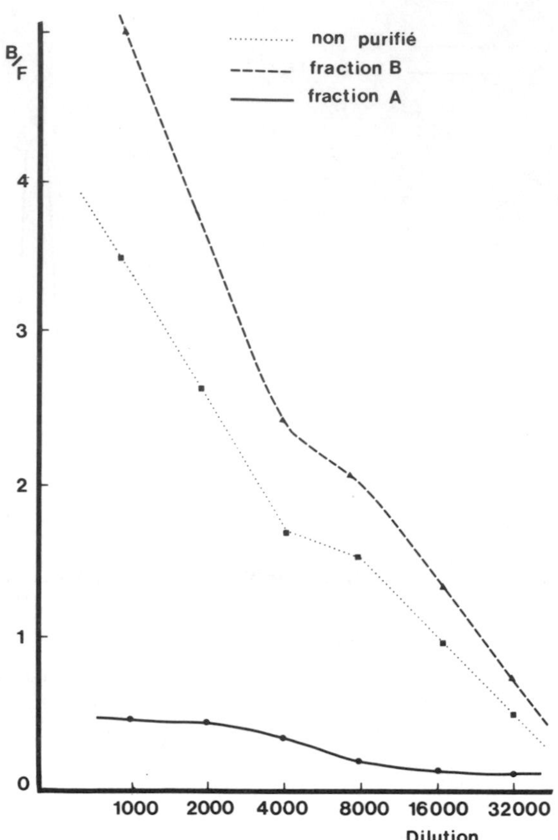

FIG.4. Augmentation d'immunoréactivité de la 1–34 hPTH N ^{125}I par chromatographie d'affinité.
L'hormone iodée non purifiée (. . . .), ainsi que les fractions éluées en milieu pH 8,6 (–) ou acide (- - - -) sont testées d'après leur possibilité de fixation par l'anticorps 10/017.

Les extraits 1 et 2 ont été obtenus respectivement à partir des colonnes I (anti 1-34 hPTH N) et II (anti bPTH).

Le plasma filtré successivement sur les deux colonnes est débarrassé de toute PTH immunoréactive ; il sert à préparer le tampon utilisé lors du dosage.

Une autre colonne type I sert à purifier la 1-34 hPTH N marquée à l'Iode 125.

1.6. Hormones naturelles

1.6.1. *Extraits d'adénomes parathyroïdiens*

Des adénomes parathyroïdiens prélevés au cours d'intervention chirurgicale sont immédiatement congelés dans l'azote liquide puis lyophilisés ; la poudre acétonique est alors extraite par du phénol : l'hormone est purifiée jusqu'au stade de poudre ATC (27).

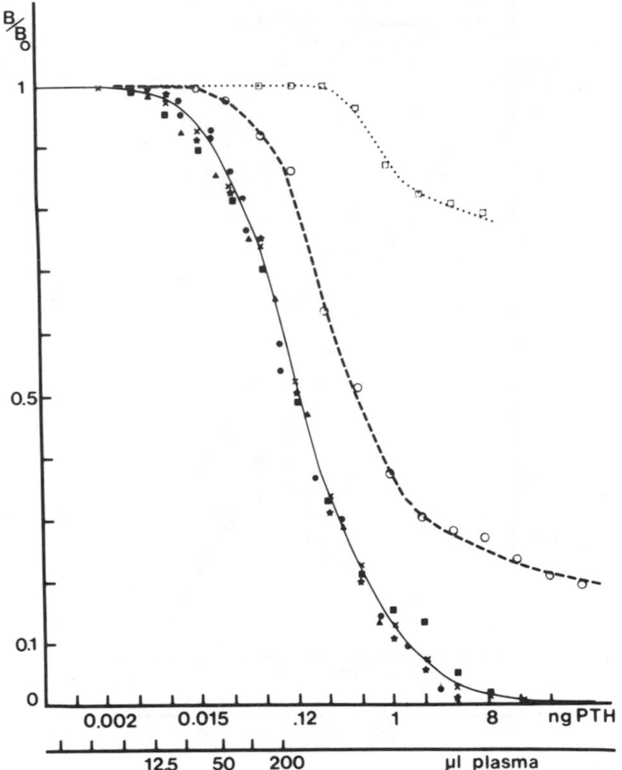

FIG.5. Comportement immunochimique de différentes hormones.
On teste le déplacement de la 1–34 hPTH ^{125}I par des dilutions successives de différentes PTH:

× *1–34 hPTH N*
○ *1–34 hPTH B*
□ *1–84 bPTH*
■ *1–84 hPTH extraite d'adénomes parathyroïdiens*
▲ *milieu de culture d'adénomes parathyroïdiens*
★ *extrait de plasma humain par la colonne d'affinité I*
● *extrait de plasma humain par la colonne d'affinité II*
✸ *plasma hyperparathyroïdien.*

1.6.2. *Extraits du milieu de culture d'adénomes parathyroïdiens*

Ce produit, obtenu par adsorption sur de la silice précipitée (QuSo), a été généreusement offert par le British Medical Research Council à Londres, référence 72/3.

1.6.3. *Plasmas humains*

Cent µl de plasmas provenant de sujets normaux ou de patients atteints d'hyperparathyroïdie primaire, confirmée ultérieurement lors de l'intervention chirurgicale, ou d'hyperparathyroïdie secondaire à une insuffisance rénale, sont dosés. L'hormone radioactive est incubée dans les mêmes conditions avec les plasmas, en l'absence d'anticorps, pour déterminer l'adsorption non spécifique de la radioactivité en cours de dosage.

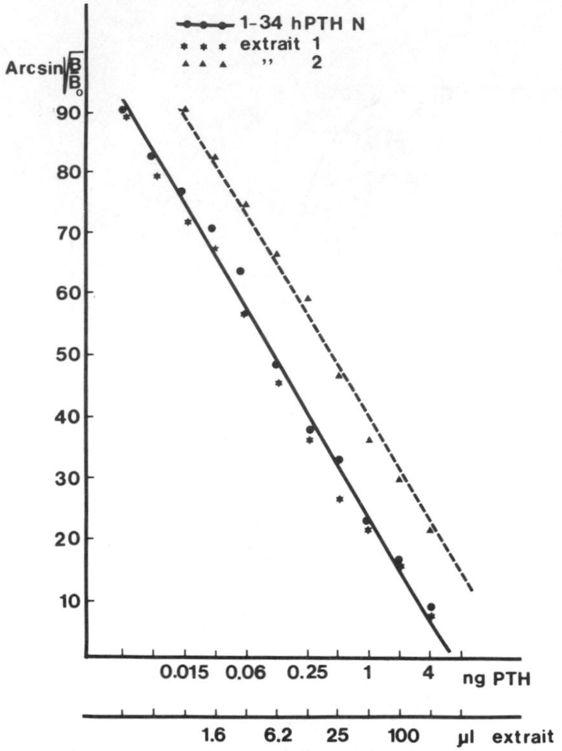

FIG. 6. Concentration des extraits d'affinité N et C terminaux.
Dans les mêmes conditions de la PTH est extraite du plasma par les colonnes anti-bPTH (▲) ou anti 1–34 hPTH (★) et comparée à la 1–34 hPTH N (●).

2. RESULTATS

2.1. Production et choix de l'antisérum

L'évolution du titre des antisérums au cours de l'immunisation est rapportée sur la fig. 1. L'antisérum est choisi pour son affinité pour la 1-34 hPTH iodée et la sensibilité du déplacement par l'hormone froide.

Cet antisérum (10/017) dilué au 1/250.000 capte environ la moitié de la 1-34 hPTH N marquée (B/F = 1). La sensibilité du dosage exprimée par la plus petite dose de 1-34 hPTH de référence susceptible de provoquer une modification significative de la radioactivité liée par l'anticorps est de 7 pg/tube (fig. 2).

2.2. Purification de l'hormone iodée

Préalablement à chaque dosage, l'hormone marquée est purifiée par chromatographie d'affinité : la radioactivité effluente est mesurée au cours de la fixation et de l'élution (fig. 3) et le comportement des différentes fractions vis-à-vis de l'anticorps est étudié (fig. 4).

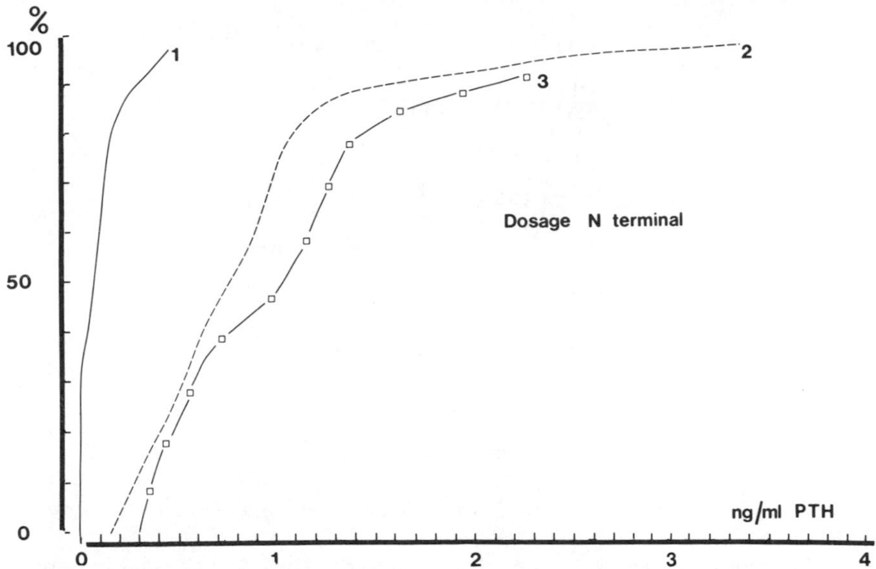

FIG. 7. Distribution en fréquence cumulée de la PTH circulante (N-terminale). Chez des sujets normaux (1 ——), atteints d'hyperparathyroïde primaire (2 - - - -) ou secondaire à une insuffisance rénale (3 □ — □).

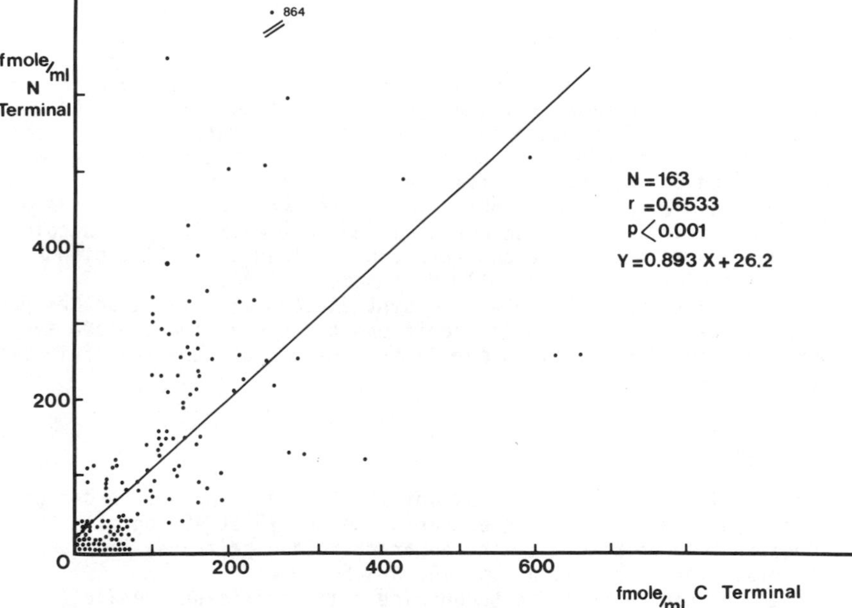

FIG. 8. Corrélation entre les résultats de dosages C ou N terminaux. Des plasmas normaux ou hyperparathyroïdiens sont dosés par deux systèmes C ou N terminaux. Les résultats sont exprimés en femtomoles d'équivalent bPTH (C-terminal) ou 1–34 hPTH N (N-terminal). 1 fmole = 9,4 pg de bPTH ou 3,8 pg de 1–34 hPTH N.

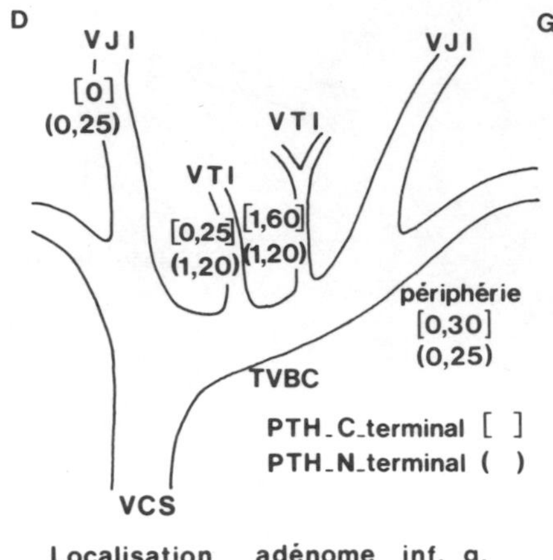

FIG. 9. Localisation d'un adénome par dosage radioimmunologique N et C terminaux de la PTH.
VJI: veine jugulaire interne; VTI: veine thyroïdienne inférieure; TVBC: tronc veineux brachio-céphalique; VCS: veine cave supérieure.

2.3. Comparaisons immunochimiques

La hPTH, extraite d'adénomes parathyroïdiens ou sécrétée dans le milieu de culture d'adénomes, a le même comportement que la 1-34 hPTH N synthétique. Il en est de même pour l'hormone circulante dans le plasma du sujet hyperparathyroïdien et pour les hormones extraites du plasma normal à l'aide des colonnes d'affinité I ou II (fig. 5).

Toutefois, la quantité de hPTH immunoréactive extraite à l'aide de la colonne I est 4 fois plus forte que celle qui est extraite par la colonne II (fig. 6). Dans le sang, la concentration du fragment 1-34 (colonne d'affinité I) est plus élevée que celle du fragment 35-84.

Avec ces anticorps, la 1-34 hPTH synthétisée selon la structure proposée par Brewer (1-34 hPTH B) présente une bonne réaction croisée avec les hormones précédentes, alors que la bPTH ne déplace que très faiblement la 1-34 hPTH (fig. 5).

2.4. Applications cliniques

Quatre-vingt un sujets normaux ont été étudiés ; dans 65 % des cas, le taux circulant était détectable et variait entre 70 et 450 pg/ml.

Chez 61 malades atteints d'hyperparathyroïdie primaire, les taux étaient plus élevés, s'étageant de 150 à 3250 pg/ml.

Dans l'hyperparathyroïdie secondaire à l'insuffisance rénale (17 cas), les valeurs variaient entre 300 et 1750 pg/ml (fig. 7).

Le chevauchement entre les valeurs du sujet normal et celles de l'hyperparathyroïdien est de 14 %. Il est compatible avec l'utilisation du dosage radioimmunologique du fragment amino-terminal de l'hormone parathyroïdienne pour le diagnostic de l'hyperparathyroïdie.

La comparaison de ces résultats avec ceux obtenus à l'aide d'un dosage radioimmunologique C-terminal fait apparaître une forte corrélation positive ($r = 0,65$; $P < 0,001$) (fig. 8).

L'une des autres applications cliniques du dosage radioimmunologique de l'hormone parathyroïdienne consiste à prélever du sang de façon étagée dans différentes veines du cou avec l'intention de localiser un éventuel adénome parathyroïdien. Grâce au gradient de la sécrétion hormonale, les résultats des dosages de PTH immunoréactive obtenus par des dosages C et N terminaux sont rapportés dans la fig. 9 : le chirurgien a enlevé un adénome situé dans la région inférieure gauche de la thyroïde.

3. DISCUSSION

L'incertitude relative à la séquence exacte des 34 premiers aminoacides de l'hormone parathyroïdienne n'est pas un obstacle insurmontable à la mise au point du dosage radioimmunologique de ce fragment. Nous avons montré que l'hormone humaine extractive a le même comportement immunochimique que le fragment synthétique 1-34 hPTH répondant à la formule de Niall. Nous avons ensuite constaté que le comportement immunochimique des formes circulantes de la hPTH est identique à celui de la séquence 1-34 de référence.

Nous confirmons non seulement l'identité de réaction de la hPTH extraite d'adénomes parathyroïdiens avec celle de la séquence 1-34 hPTH de Niall (13, 14), mais nous élargissons cette comparaison aux hormones circulantes du sujet normal ou sécrétées par l'adénome parathyroïdien en culture.

Dans notre système, la réaction croisée avec la 1-34 hPTH répondant à la séquence de Brewer et les hormones humaines extractives est relativement bonne. Ceci s'accorde avec les résultats de Fisher et coll. (12) qui ne peuvent distinguer la 1-34 hPTH B de la hPTH hautement purifiée dans plusieurs systèmes homologues. Le fait que la bPTH ne déplace la 1-34 hPTH-125I que pour des doses très élevées peut impliquer soit que les anticorps du dosage sont dirigés vers des sites dont la structure primaire diffère de l'homme au boeuf, soit que les modifications de la séquence selon l'espèce induisent des changements conformationnels de la molécule, laquelle serait alors mal reconnue par l'anticorps.

La colonne II, dont les anticorps reconnaissent particulièrement des sites ultérieurs à la séquence 1-34, retient certains composés qui sont également reconnus par les anticorps utilisés pour le dosage du fragment 1-34. Une partie des molécules extraites possède donc à la fois des sites antigéniques situés dans la partie médiane ou C-terminale et des sites N-terminaux. Il s'agit soit des molécules intactes (1-84) ou de fragments relativement longs, doués d'activité biologique. Toutefois, l'extrait 2 contient 4 fois moins de substances immunoréactives N-terminales que l'extrait 1 (colonne 1-34). On en conclut que ces fragments ne représentent qu'une petite partie de la population de la PTH immunoréactive circulante dosée par l'anticorps N-terminal.

Ces résultats justifient l'utilisation du fragment 1-34 de Niall pour mettre au point le dosage homologue du fragment N-terminal de la PTH humaine. Le chevauchement des valeurs normales avec celles de l'hyperparathyroïdien n'est pas lié au dosage du fragment biologiquement actif, puisque nous observons une discrimination satisfaisante, contrairement à d'autres auteurs (12, 3, 4).

Le dosage radioimmunologique du fragment amino-terminal reflète directement l'activité de la glande parathyroïde.

REFERENCES

(1) BERSON, S.A., YALOW, R.S., AURBACH, G.D., POTTS, J.T. Jr., Proc. Natl. Acad. Sci. USA 49 (1963) 613.
(2) AURBACH, G.D., POTTS, J.T. Jr., Arch. of Intern. Med. 124 (1969) 413.
(3) ARNAUD, C.D., TSAO, H.S., LITTLEDIKE, T., J. Clin. Invest. 50 (1971) 21.
(4) ARNAUD, C.D., GOLDSMITH, R.S., BORDIER, P.J., SIZEMORE, G.W., Am. J. Med. 56 (1974) 785.
(5) BERSON, S.A., YALOW, R.S., J. Clin. Endocrinol. Metab. 28 (1968) 1037.
(6) ARNAUD, C.D., SIZEMORE, G.W., OLDHAM, S.B., FISHER, J.A., TSAO, H.S., LITTLEDIKE, E.T., Am. J. Med. 50 (1971) 630.
(7) CANTERBURY, J.M., REISS, E., Proc. Soc. Exp. Biol. Med. 140 (1972) 1393.
(8) SILVERMAN, R., YALOW, R.S., J. Clin. Invest. 52 (1973) 1958.
(9) SEGRE, G.V., NIALL, H.D., HABENER, J.F., POTTS, J.T. Jr., Am. J. Med. 56 (1974) 774.
(10) BREWER, H.B., FAIRWELL, T., RONAN, R., SIZEMORE, G.W., ARNAUD, C.D., Proc. Natl. Acad. Sci. USA 69 (1972) 3585.
(11) NIALL, H.D., SAUER, R.T., JACOBS, J.W., KEUTMANN, H.T., SEGRE, G.V., O'RIORDAN, J.L.H., AURBACH, G.D., POTTS, J.T. Jr., Proc. Natl. Acad. Sci. USA 71 (1974) 384.
(12) FISHER, J.A., BINSWANGER, U., DIETRICH, F.M., J. Clin. Invest. 54 (1974) 1382.
(13) HENDY, G.N., BARLING, P.M., O'RIORDAN, J.L.H., Clin. Sci. Mol. Med. 47 (1974) 567.
(14) SEGRE, G.V., POTTS, J.T. Jr., Endocrinology 98 (1976) 1294.
(15) DESPLAN, C., JULLIENNE, A., MOUKHTAR, M.S., MILHAUD, G., Lancet ii (1977) 199.
(16) MILHAUD, G., RIVAILLE, P., STAUB, J.F., JULLIENNE, A., C. R. Acad. Sci. Paris Série D 279 (1974) 1015.
(17) RIVAILLE, P., STAUB, J.F., JULLIENNE, A., RAULAIS, D., MILHAUD, G., Peptides 1974 (Y. Wolman Ed.), J. Wiley, New York (1975).
(18) MUNSON, P.L., The Parathyroids (R.O. Greep, R.V. Talmage, Eds), C. Thomas, Springfield (Ill.) (1961) 94.
(19) RIVAILLE, P., BADER, C.A., MONET, J.D., GAUBERT, C.H., MOUKHTAR, M.S., MILHAUD, G., Peptides 1976 (A. Loffet Ed.), Editions de l'Université de Bruxelles (1977) 555.
(20) HUNTER, W.M., GREENWOOD, F.C., Nature London 194 (1962) 495.
(21) YALOW, R.S., BERSONS, S.A., Nature London 212 (1966) 357.
(22) HERBERT, V., LAU, K.S., GOTTLIEB, C.W., BLEICHER, S.J, J. Clin. Endocrinol. Metab. 25 (1965) 1375.
(23) AXEN, R., PORATH, J., ERNBACK, S., Nature London 214 (1967) 1302.
(24) MILHAUD, G., JULLIENNE, A., CALMETTES, C., MOUKHTAR, M.S., "Rencontres Biologiques 1976", Expansion scientifique Paris Ed. (1976).
(25) MOUKHTAR, M.S., JULLIENNE, A., THARAUD, D., TABOULET, J., MILHAUD, G., C. R. Acad. Sci. Paris 276 (1973) 3445.
(26) RIVAILLE, P., JULLIENNE, A., DESPLAN, C., BARLET, J.P., BADER, C.A., MILHAUD, G., Proc. 5th Int. Symp. Medical Chemistry, Paris, 1976, in press.
(27) KEUTMANN, H.T., BARLING, P.M., HENDY, G.N., SEGRE, G.V., NIALL, H.D., AURBACH, G.D., POTTS, J.T. Jr., O'RIORDAN, J.L.H., Biochemistry 13 (1974) 1646.

DISCUSSION

J.L.E. GUERIS: Theoretically, the use of a homogeneous system is indeed more satisfactory than that of a heterogeneous system, obtained moreover against an ill-defined immunogen. However, C- and N-terminal assays have been described since the very beginning of the development of human parathyroid hormone assays, and the reason why so far the C-terminal systems have been given preference in clinical practice is that they provide better correlations, as has been shown especially by Arnaud and Bordier.

From this point of view, it would be interesting to know the correlation of the system here proposed (a) with calcaemia and the weight of adenoma in primary hyperparathyroidism and (b) with the data on bone histomorphometry in hyperparathyroidism secondary to chronic renal insufficiency.

C. DESPLAN: I would go further, and say that so far PTH assays have been essentially C-terminal because the N-terminal assays did not give clinically usable information.

Since our assay gave a good discrimination between the levels in normal subjects and subjects with hyperparathyroidism, we were not interested in the likely correlation between the assay results and the more precise points of clinical observation.

J.L.E. GUERIS: Even when the results are expressed in terms of molar concentration, it is difficult to correlate the data provided by a homogeneous system, expressed directly, with those provided by a heterogeneous system, expressed as equivalent concentrations of a hormone of another species.

C. DESPLAN: We studied the correlation between the C- and N-terminal results because the important factor is the relative levels of the different subjects. Furthermore, measurement of the PTH present in a human parathyroid adenoma extract by the two systems gave results in terms of 1–34 hPTH and bovine PTH which were very close in molar concentration.

G. HEYNEN: I am astonished to see such low values of immunoreactive PTH measured with your anti-C-terminal antiserum. What antiserum do you use?

C. DESPLAN: The PTH values obtained obviously depend on the antiserum used. For our C-terminal assay, the results are expressed in nanogram equivalents of bovine PTH with an antiserum against extracted bovine PTH obtained from the guinea-pig. Furthermore, there is a good discrimination with this assay (8% overlap) between normal values and values obtained in hyperparathyroid subjects, so its purpose is served, regardlesss of the absolute values.

G. HEYNEN: Your presentation illustrates our ignorance and the imperfection of our scientific language when we speak about N- and C-terminal fragment; there are certainly several antigenic sites on the N-terminal fragment, since your results differ from those published by other authors using an anti-N-terminal serum.

C. DESPLAN: There are not only an N-terminal fragment and a C-terminal fragment resulting from the splitting of the whole molecule, but also metabolites of these fragments; those that we measure by our N-terminal system reflect the activity of the gland, and those measured by other N-terminal antisera can reflect non-specific products unrelated to the activity of the gland.

D. RODBARD: In Fig.8 you show the correlation between results using RIAs for the carboxy-terminal and the amino-terminal segments of parathyroid hormone. This illustrates two statistical problems: non-uniformity of variance, and presence of errors in both the x- and y-variables. The first problem can be partially alleviated by the use of logarithmic transformations of both axes. In this case we would be likely to find a slope significantly greater than unity, corresponding to a curvilinear, rather than a linear, correlation in terms of the original measurements. Thus, I would suggest the use of a power function in preference to a simple linear regression. The problem of errors in both x and y is discussed in Appendix E of paper SM-220/58.

CALCITONIN RADIOIMMUNOASSAY
*Clinical application**

F. RAUE, H. MINNE,
W. STREIBL, R. ZIEGLER
Zentrum für Innere Medizin,
Kinderheilkunde und Dermatologie,
Universität Ulm,
Ulm, Federal Republic of Germany

Abstract

CALCITONIN RADIOIMMUNOASSAY: CLINICAL APPLICATION.

A radioimmunoassay for human calcitonin (hCT) was established. Antisera were produced by immunizing goats with synthetic hCT; 7.5 μg of hCT was labelled with 1 mCi of ^{125}I; hCT served as a standard in the range between 0.1 to 20 ng/ml. Separation of free from antibody-bound tracer was done with a charcoal procedure. The RIA system had a sensitivity of 0.1 ng/ml, the normal range lying below 0.5 ng/ml. The assay was used to study the following clinical problems: (1) In 35 patients with a thyroid tumour, diagnosis of calconin-producing medullary thyroid carcinoma was proven. Serum CT of these patients lay between 1.7 and 120 ng/ml. Clinical signs of this disease are non-specific, so CT determination is important for early diagnosis and control of therapy. In patients with a high tumour risk, pentagastrin stimulation of the C-cells reveals CT secretion above normal if a medullary thyroid carcinoma is present. (2) Two patients with pheochromocytoma showed elevated levels of hCT before operation; after removal of the tumour, the serum CT levels became normal. Extracts of the adrenomedullary tumour revealed immunoreactive CT corresponding to 1 and 4 ng/mg wet weight. (3) hCT is used in the therapy of Paget's disease of the bone, so it is necessary to check the production of antibodies in the patient. In 25 patients with Paget's disease no antibody production against the injected hormone was evident.

I. MATERIAL AND METHODS

A. Radioimmunoassay for human calcitonin (hCT)

Antisera were produced by immunizing goats with multiple intracutaneous injections of 100 μg of synthetic hCT (a gift of Ciba-Geigy, Basel). The hCT was emulsified with complete Freund's adjuvant and charcoal. The antiserum was used in a final dilution of 1:40 000.

---

* Supported by Deutsche Forschungsgemeinschaft, SFB 87.

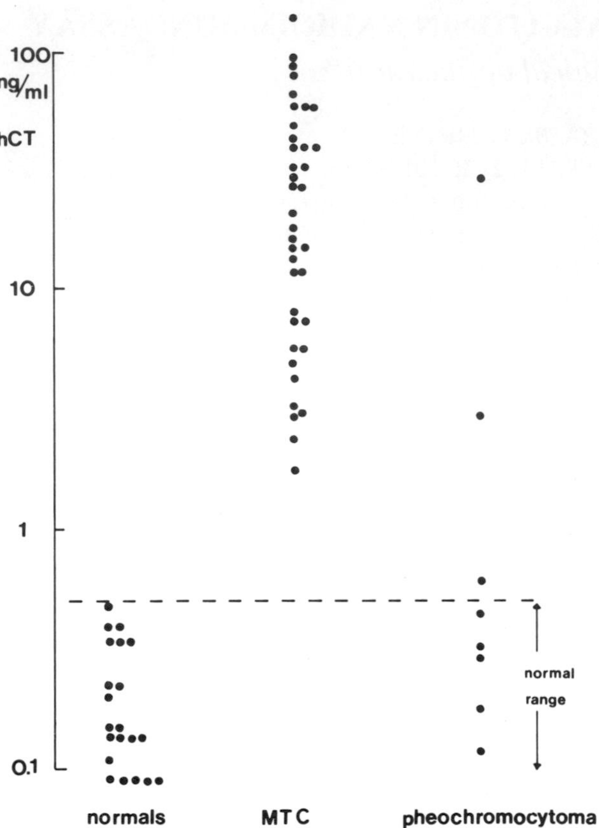

FIG.1. Human calcitonin values of normal persons, patients with medullary thyroid carcinoma and patients with pheochromocytoma.

An amount of 7.5 μg of hCT was labelled with 1 mCi of ^{125}I (Hoechst, Frankfurt) using a modified Chloramine-T method according to Hunter and Greenwood [7].

hCT served as a reference standard in the range of 0.1–20 ng/ml.

The incubation procedure was carried out as follows: after preincubation of the serum samples and standards with antiserum for two days at 4°C, tracer was added for an additional incubation period of 16 h. The total incubation volume was 500 μl.

Control serum with a low hCT concentration was obtained by pooling normal sera that had no measurable hCT and diluting them 1:10 with assay buffer. Separation was performed with a charcoal procedure (1000 μl of a 1% charcoal, 0.1% dextran suspension). Samples to be measured were run in three dilutions (native, 1:1, and 1:4); this procedure allowed one to check whether or not the plotted results diluted parallel to the standard curve [1, 3, 8, 15].

B. Serum sampling and pentagastrin (PG) stimulation test

In 22 normal subjects, 37 patients with medullary thyroid carcinoma (MTC) and 10 with pheochromocytoma, several blood samples were collected in the morning before and after surgery (Fig.1). The blood was allowed to clot, then it was centrifuged and the serum was immediately deep-frozen and stored at −20°C until required for hCT determination.

In serum samples of 25 patients treated with hCT for Paget's disease of the bone, the capacity for binding radioiodinated synthetic hCT was checked (Fig.2).

A PG stimulation test was performed as follows [6, 14]: 0.5 μg PG/kg body weight (Gastrodiagnost., Merck, Darmstadt) was rapidly injected into a cubital vein. Blood samples for hCT determination were taken 15 min and immediately before administration of PG as well as 2, 5, 10 and 15 min after administration (Fig.3).

C. Extraction procedure for tumour tissue

Pheochromocytomata were deep-frozen immediately after removal and stored at −20°C until extraction. Tumour slices of about 1 g were homogenized in 4 ml of cooled 0.1N HCl and then centrifuged for 4 h at 20 000 × g. The hCT immunoreactivity of the supernatant was analysed.

II. RESULTS

A. Radioimmunoassay for hCT

The assay had a sensitivity of 0.1 ng/ml: in 22 normal subjects, 0.283 ng/ml ± 0.160 ng/ml serum were found and in five sera, hCT was not detectable.

Cross-reaction with other proteohormones such as insulin, STH, ACTH, gastrin, pentagastrin, cholecystokinin, bovine PTH, 1-34-hPTH and porcine CT was not detectable; only salmon CT displaced human tracer in a thousandfold higher concentration.

B. Studies in patients with medullary thyroid carcinoma (MTC)

Thirty-five patients with histologically proven MTC showed hCT values between 1.7–120 ng/ml (mean 33.6 ± 5.7 ng/ml) before neck exploration (Fig.1).

After total extirpation of the thyroidal tumour, the hCT levels became normal in three patients. The dilution curves of serum from patients with MTC paralleled the standard curve produced with synthetic hCT.

In patients with borderline basal values, hypercalcitoninaemia may be proven by a pentagastrin stimulation test.

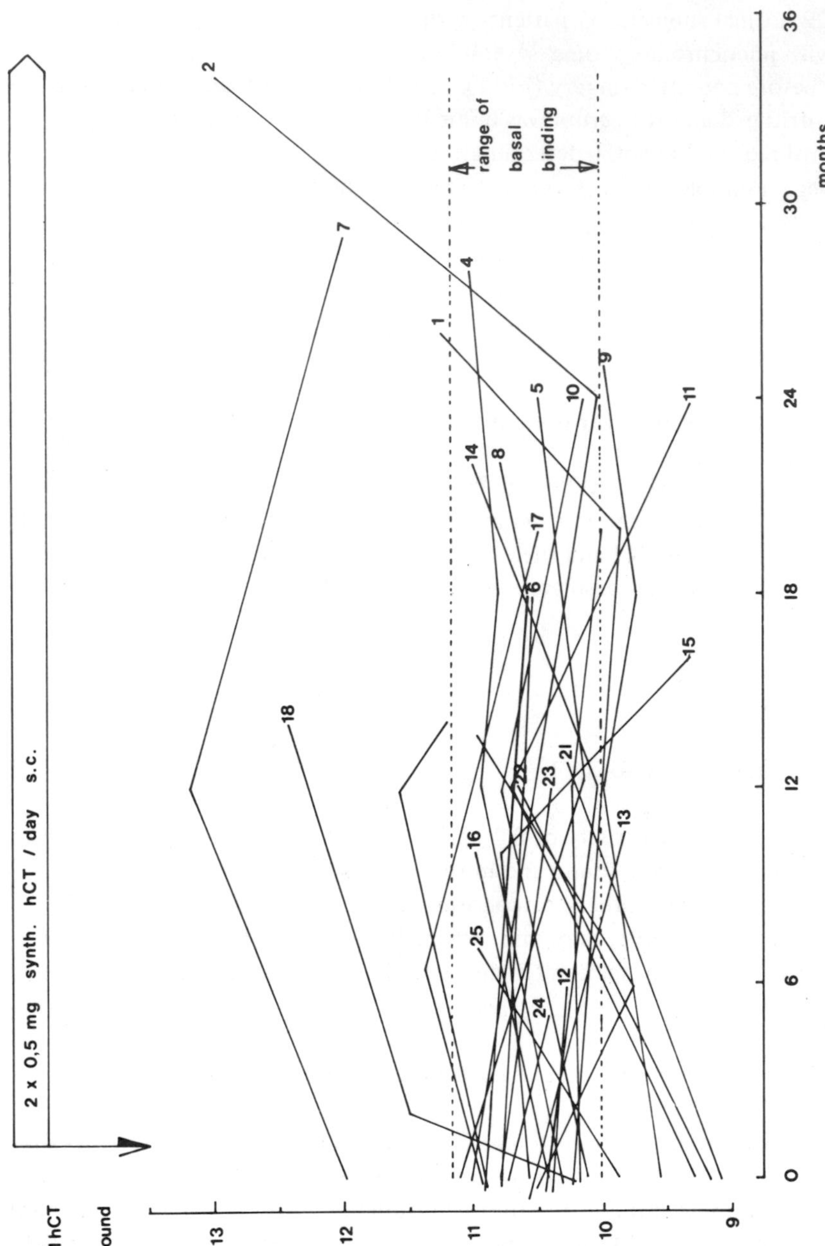

FIG.2. Basal binding of human calcitonin tracer in patients with Paget's disease of the bone.

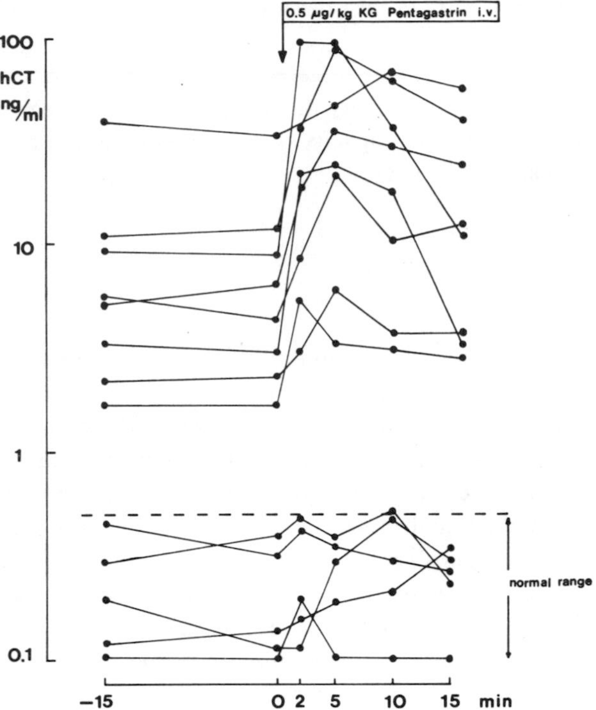

FIG. 3. Pentagastrin stimulation test in normal persons and patients with medullary thyroid carcinoma.

In four normals there was no response to the stimulus, whereas in eight patients with MTC there was a rapid and exaggerated increase in serum CT, the maximum level being found 2 min after injection of PG (Fig.3).

C. Studies in patients with pheochromocytoma

Two of 12 patients with pheochromocytoma revealed elevated levels of hCT before operation (3 ng/ml and 30 ng/ml) (Fig.1). After extirpation of the adrenal medullary tumours, the serum CT was checked and found to be normal in both cases. The extracts of pheochromocytoma tissue from the two patients with the high preoperative values displaced the human tracer from the anti-hCT antibody. The dilution curves of these extracts paralleled the standard curves. They contained 1 ng of hCT/mg and 4 ng of hCT/mg wet weight. In four other tissue extracts, no hCT was detectable.

D. Studies in patients with Paget's disease of bone

Antibody production was investigated in 25 patients who were given subcutaneous injections of hCT every day for periods of between 3 months and 3 1/2 years. In no case did the capacity of the patient's serum to bind the tracer increase during treatment (Fig.2).

III. DISCUSSION

A specific and sensitive radioimmunoassay for hCT has been developed to study states of increased serum CT. Such a system has been proven to be of value for clinical use since its first introduction by Tashjian and coworkers in 1970 [15].

Since patients with MTC suffer only from non-specific clinical signs like tumour growth in the neck region (comparable to a thyroid nodule, goitre or metastatic lymph nodule) and sometimes diarrhoea, hCT measurements are of importance for early diagnosis [2, 3, 12].

After the successful removal of a malignant tumour there is a normalization of the amount of hCT in the serum; the level remains above normal if the surgery has been incomplete. Recurrence of the tumour or the occurrence of metastases is accompanied by increased basal or pentagastrin stimulated serum CT, sometimes before any detectable clinical signs.

Hereditary occurrence of MTC represents about 10% of cases so it is necessary to screen the siblings of patients with MTC. This is easy to perform. Pentagastrin stimulation reveals increased hCT secretion capacity of small tumours in patients with normal basal values [16].

Other substances like glucagon, calcium infusion and ethanol are also able to stimulate hCT secretion, but PG seems to be the most reliable stimulus in a comparative test [6, 14].

To exclude a Sipple syndrome, a hereditary occurrence of pheochromocytoma and MTC [13], serum CT was measured in 12 patients with pheochromocytoma. Before extirpation of the adrenomedullary tumour, serum CT was distinctly elevated in two patients. After removal of the tumour, the basal and the pentagastrin stimulated calcitonin levels remained within the normal range. In extracts from the two corresponding pheochromocytoma tissues, immunoreactive CT was detected. Compared with the hCT concentration in extracts from MTC, pheochromocytoma tissues yielded only one thousandth of the amount [10, 11]. But, as hCT is only found in pheochromocytoma tissue from patients who had preoperative elevated CT levels, it is suggested that hypercalcitoninaemia in patients with pheochromocytoma may be of other than thyroidal origin and does not always indicate a medullary thyroid carcinoma. Similar results are reported by Voelkel and colleages [17], who found two hCT-positive cases among 10 patients with adrenomedullary tumour. The relationship between the two tumours may depend on their common origin from the neural crest [9].

The therapeutic effect of hCT in patients with Paget's disease of the bone is generally acknowledged [18]. As hCT is injected subcutaneously once or twice a day, the antibody level may rise. In our series, no antibody production against the injected hormone was evident, which is in agreement with the observations of Greenberg and colleagues [4]. When salmon or porcine CT was used, the phenomenon of refractoriness to therapy was attributed to neutralizing antibodies against these calcitonins [5].

IV. CONCLUSIONS

The radioimmunoassay for hCT is useful for early diagnosis and therapeutic control of patients with MTC. Hypercalcitoninaemia is not specific for C-cell carcinoma, as it also occurs in patients with pheochromocytoma. In patients with pheochromocytoma, but without Sipple syndrome in which MTC is also present, CT is presumably secreted by the pheochromocytoma tissue itself. Antibodies to synthetic hCT did not appear during treatment with hCT in Paget's disease of the bone.

REFERENCES

[1] DEFTOS, L.J., Radioimmunoassay for calcitonin in medullary thyroid carcinoma, JAMA **227** (1974) 403.

[2] DEFTOS, L.J., BURY, A.E., HABENER, J.F., SINGER, F.R., POTTS, J.T., Immunoassay for human calcitonin, II. Clinical studies, Metabolism **20** (1971) 1129.

[3] FRANCHIMONT, P., HEYEN, G., Parathormone and Calcitonin Radioimmunoassay in Various Medical and Osteoarticular Disorders, Masson, New York (1976).

[4] GREENBERG, P.B., DOYLE, F.H., FISHER, M.T., HILLYARD, C.J., JOPLIN, G.F., PENNOCK, J., MacINTYRE, I., Treatment of Paget's disease of bone with synthetic human calcitonin, Am. J. Med. **56** (1974) 867.

[5] HADDAD, J.G., CALDWELL, J.G., Calcitonin resistance: Clinical and immunologic studies in subjects with Paget's disease of bone treated with porcine and salmon calcitonin, J. Clin. Invest. **51** (1972) 3133.

[6] HENNESSY, J.F., GRAY, T.K., COOPER, C.W., ONTJES, D.A., Stimulation of thyreocalcitonin secretion by pentagastrin and calcium in two patients with medullary carcinoma of the thyroid, J. Clin. Endoctrinol. Metab. **36** (1972) 200.

[7] HUNTER, W.M., GREENWOOD, F.C., Preparation of iodine-131-labelled human growth hormone of high specific activity, Nature (London) **194** (1962) 495.

[8] MINNE, H., RAUE, F., SCHÄFER, A., ZIEGLER, R., Bestimmung von Parathormon, Calcitonin sowie Serumantikörpern gegen Calcitonin beim Menschen, Ärztl. Lab. **21** (1975) 336.

[9] PEARSE, A.G.E., POLAK, K.M., Endocrine tumors of neural crest origin: neurolophomas, apudomas and the APUD concept, Med. Biol. **52** (1974) 3.

[10] RAUE, F., MINNE, H., BAYER, J.M., Studies in endogenous hypercalcitoninaemia in man, Vth Int. Cong. Endocrinol., Hamburg (Abstract) **386** (1976).

[11] RAUE, F., MINNE, H., KLÜBER, S., ZIEGLER, R., Comparison of bioassay and radio-immunoassay of calcitonin in medullary carcinoma of the thyroid, Symp. Dtsch. Ges. Endokrinol. (Abstract) 34 (1975); Acta Endocrinol. Suppl. **193** (1975) 34.

[12] RAUE, F., MINNE, H., SCHÄFER, D., ZIEGLER, R., Die Calcitoninbestimmung in der Klinik, Münchner Med. Wochenschr. **119** (1977) 219.

[13] SIPPLE, J.H., Association of pheochromocytoma with carcinoma of the thyroid gland, Am. J. Med. **31** (1961) 163.

[14] SIZEMORE, G.W., GO, V.L.W., Stimulation test for diagnosis of medullary thyroid carcinoma, Mayo Clinic Proc. **50** (1975) 53.

[15] TASHJIAN, A.H., HOWLAND, B.G., MELVIN, K.E.W., HILL, C.S., Immunoassay for human calcitonin: clinical measurement, relation to serum calcium and studies in patients with medullary carcinoma, New Engl. J. Med. **283** (1970) 890.

[16] WELLS, S.A., ONTJES, D.A., COOPER, C.W., HENNESSY, J.F., ELLIS, G.J., McPHERSON, H.T., SABISTON, D.C., The early diagnosis of medullary carcinoma of the thyroid gland in patients with multiple endocrine neoplasia type II, Ann. Surg. **182** (1975) 362.

[17] VOELKEL, E.F., TASHJIAN, A.H., DAVIDOFF, F.F., COHEN, R.B., PERLIA, C.P., WURTMAN, R.J., Concentration of calcitonin and catecholamines in pheochromocytomas, a mucosal neuroma and medullary thyroid carcinoma, J. Clin. Endocrinol. Metab. **37** (1973) 297.

[18] ZIEGLER, R., HOLZ, G., RAUE, F., MINNE, H., DELLING, G., "Therapeutic studies with human calcitonin", Human Calcitonin and Paget's Disease (Proc. Int. Workshop London, 1976) (MacINTYRE, I., Ed.), Hans Huber Publisher, Bern, Stuttgart, Vienna (1977) 167.

DISCUSSION

C. DESPLAN: Have you observed any increasing levels of calcitonin in the families of medullary carcinoma patients?

F. RAUE: We have tested several families of patients with medullary thyroid carcinoma but haven't so far observed a familial occurrence of C-cell carcinoma.

K.D. BAGSHAWE: It has been reported that patients with various types of lung carcinoma have increased serum concentrations of calcitonin. Have you any data on this point?

F. RAUE: We have tested about 100 patients with different tumours, of whom only two had slightly elevated calcitonin values, 0.8 ng/ml and 1.3 ng/ml, respectively, and after control they were normal. Both patients had tumours of the chest.

ETUDE DE LA SPECIFICITE DU DOSAGE RADIOIMMUNOLOGIQUE DU PROCOLLAGENE DE TYPE I ET DE TYPE III

G. HEYNEN*, M. BROUX**, B. NUSGENS**,
C.M. LAPIERE**, J.A. KANIS*,
S. GASPAR*, P. FRANCHIMONT*
Université de Liège,
Belgique

Abstract–Résumé

STUDY OF THE SPECIFICITY OF RADIOIMMUNOASSAY OF TYPE I AND TYPE III PROCOLLAGEN.

Bovine procollagens of Type I and Type III are highly antigenic molecules. The paper describes the radioimmunoassay of these polypeptides and gives details concerning their specificity. The authors describe the application of this method to biological media and present some examples.

ETUDE DE LA SPECIFICITE DU DOSAGE RADIOIMMUNOLOGIQUE DU PROCOLLAGENE DE TYPE I ET DE TYPE III.

Les procollagènes bovins de type I et de type III sont des molécules fortement antigéniques. Le mémoire décrit la méthode de dosage radioimmunologique de ces deux polypeptides, en précisant leur spécificité. L'application de cette méthode aux milieux biologiques est décrite et on en donne quelques exemples.

La dermato-sparaxie est une maladie héréditaire du tissu conjonctif des bovidés se caractérisant par une fragilité particulière de la peau. Les fibres formant les faisceaux désorganisés du collagène dermique résultent de l'accumulation d'une molécule anormale: le collagène dermato-sparaxique (dPC). Ce dPC représente une des formes précurseur du collagène proprement dit, et se compose de deux chaînes polypeptidiques alpha 1 et une chaîne alpha 2, semblables aux chaînes alpha 1 et alpha 2 du collagène de type I normal avec, en plus, une extension polypeptidique à leur extrémité amino-terminale [1]. Il est admis que le dPC I s'accumule à cause d'un défaut enzymatique: la pro-collagène peptidase [2].

De la même façon qu'il existe plusieurs types de collagène, on connaît actuellement plusieurs types de pro-collagène (PC), c'est-à-dire le collagène avec au moins en plus une extension polypeptidique amino-terminale [3]. Le poids moléculaire de ces différents types de PC est supérieur à 300 000 et leur antigénicité est nettement plus marquée que chez le collagène correspondant [4].

---

* Laboratoire de radioimmunologie.

** Laboratoire de dermatologie expérimentale.

L'objet de notre travail est de décrire la méthode et la spécificité du dosage radioimmunologique des PC de type I et de type III, ainsi que son application à la détermination quantitative de ces substances dans les milieux biologiques.

MATERIEL ET METHODE

Matériel

Les différentes substances utilisées dans notre étude sont les suivantes: le collagène normal, le dPC I, le dPC III, et le d-peptide. Ce dernier représente le peptide amino-terminal additionnel à la chaîne alpha 1 du dPC I. Toutes ces substances ont été obtenues par des méthodes antérieurement décrites [3, 4].

Méthode

Immunisation. L'antisérum a été obtenu en immunisant un lapin par trois injections mensuelles de 0,25 mg de dPC I émulsifié dans l'adjuvant incomplet de Freund.

Marquage. Le marquage des dPC I et III s'effectue selon une modification de la méthode de Greenwood et al. [5]. A une solution de 25 μl de Na ^{125}I (1 mCi) sont ajoutés successivement 50 μl de tampon phosphate 0,25 M pH 7,4, 5 μg de substance à marquer puis 10 μg de chloramine T, chacun dissous dans 25 μl de tampon phosphate 0,5 M. Après une minute de mélange à 4°C, 10 μg de métabisulfite dans 50 μl de tampon phosphate 0,5 M sont ajoutés pour arrêter la réaction d'oxydation. La purification du mélange des produits de la réaction de marquage s'effectue en réalisant une chromatographie sur colonne de Sephadex G 50 M (1 X 25 cm).

Incubations. Les incubations sont réalisées à 4°C pendant 4 jours. Le volume total, de 0,50 ml, se répartit de la façon suivante: 0,1 ml de produit marqué (10^3 à 2×10^3 cpm); 0,1 ml de l'antisérum à la dilution finale de 4×10^{-5} lorsque le traceur est le dPC I et 10^{-4} lorsque le traceur est le dPC III; 0,2 ml de tampon phosphate 0,05 M pH 7,4 contenant 500 UI par ml de Trasylol, 0,09 g/l de EDTA et 0,5% d'albumine bovine; 0,1 ml de l'antigène à tester ou 0,1 ml de sérum dilués dans le même tampon phosphate. Après 4 jours d'incubation à 4°C le complexe antigène-anticorps est précipité par addition d'une quantité optimale de sérum anti-IgG de lapin fixé sur de la cellulose.

Divers. Dans le but de préciser la localisation du site immunoréactif, le dPC a été traité par la collagénase animale [6]. Les produits de la réaction ont été

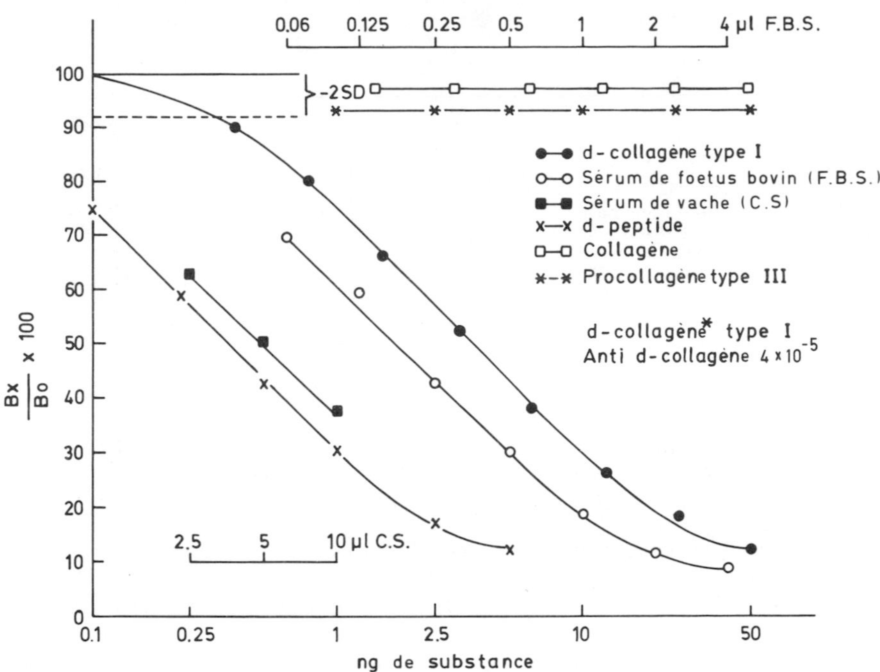

FIG.1. Courbe de dosage radioimmunologique représentative du dPC I. La dilution progressive du sérum de fœtus bovin et du sérum de vache donne des courbes parallèles à celles obtenues avec le dPC I et le d-peptide. Par contre aucune réaction immunologique n'est décelée pour la molécule de collagène ni pour la molécule de procollagène de type III.

soumis à une électrophorèse en gel de polyacrylamide (7,5%) à pH 5,5. Le gel a ensuite été coupé en portions égales de 2 mm et extrait. Les groupements antigéniques réactionnels ont été déterminés sur ces extraits. Par ailleurs des prélèvements sanguins hebdomadaires ont été effectués chez une vache gestante à partir de la quatrième semaine jusqu'au onzième jour après la mise bas. Enfin le d-peptide a été dosé dans les extraits de peau normale et dermato-sparaxique.

RESULTATS

Le rendement du marquage est de 22% ± 4 (écart type; n = 10) et l'activité spécifique du dPC I* se situe entre 40 et 50 μCi par μg. La figure 1 montre que le d-peptide et le dPC I ont un déterminant antigénique commun, puisqu'ils sont capables l'un et l'autre d'entraîner un déplacement complet du dPC I* de son anticorps. De plus, les courbes obtenues sont parallèles. Cette même figure

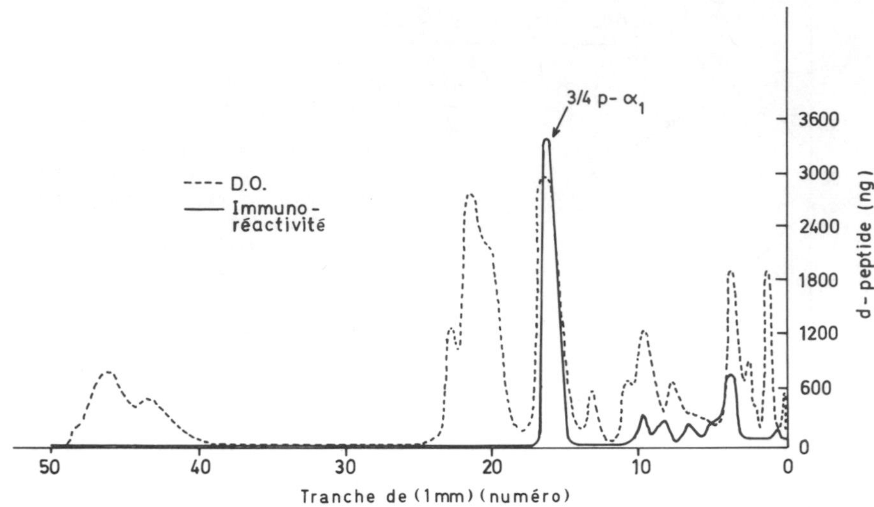

FIG. 2. Profil de l'immunoréactivité et de la densité optique décelée dans les éluats de l'électrophorèse en gel de polyacrylamide du dPC I traité par la collagénase animale. On voit que l'immunoréactivité principale est décelée dans la zone de migration de la partie amino-terminale de la chaîne pro-alpha 1 du dPC I. Par contre, aucune immunoréactivité n'est décelée dans les zones d'élution ultérieures, à savoir au niveau de l'extension amino-terminale de la chaîne pro-alpha 2, et au niveau de l'extension carboxy-terminale. L'immunoréactivité décelée dans les zones antérieures à l'extension amino-terminale de la chaîne pro-alpha 1 est due à la présence de polymères et de dPC I non clivé par la collagénase.

démontre également que ce déterminant antigénique n'est pas présent sur le collagène normal, ni sur le dPC III. Par contre, le sérum de fœtus dermato-sparaxique et le sérum bovin normal contiennent un déterminant antigénique semblable à celui présent sur le dPC I et d-peptide. Il y a 20 à 30 fois plus de déterminant de type d-peptide dans le sérum du fœtus que dans celui de la vache adulte. La détermination de l'immunoréactivité dans les éluats des fractions de l'électrophorèse en gel de polyacrylamide à pH 5,5 de dPC I traité par la collagénase animale est montrée à la figure 2. On y voit que l'immunoréactivité est principalement décelée dans la zone de migration de la partie amino-terminale du pro-alpha 1, et que la partie carboxy-terminale ne présente aucune activité immunologique décelable. De même, nous ne décelons aucune activité immunologique dans la zone d'élution de la chaîne polypeptidique pro-alpha 2. Exprimée en équivalents immunologiques de d-peptide, la concentration normale de d-peptide dans le sérum de la vache après mise bas est de 100,8 ng/ml ± 34 (1 écart type, S.D.). Elle est significativement plus élevée pendant la gestation et cela d'autant plus que la gestation est moins avancée en âge (fig. 3). La peau normale de veau contient 3 μg de d-peptide par mg de collagène alors que la peau de veau dermato-sparaxique en contient 69 μg/mg de collagène, soit 23 fois plus.

Lorsque le dPC III est utilisé comme traceur et l'anti-sérum à la dilution finale de 1/10 000, la figure 4 montre qu'il est également possible d'établir un dosage spécifique pour le dPC de type III. En effet la sensibilité permet la détection de 0,35 ng de dPC III par tube. Le dPC I et le d-peptide induisent un déplacement du dPC III de sa fixation à l'anticorps mais seulement à des concentrations respectivement 12 fois et 350 fois supérieures à celle de ce dernier (fig. 4).

DISCUSSION ET CONCLUSION

Le dPC I est une forme précurseur du collagène fortement antigénique puisqu'il a suffi d'un lapin et de trois injections mensuelles d'une faible quantité de ce matériel pour obtenir un antisérum anti-pro-collagène dont le titre en anticorps est élevé. La sensibilité de la méthode est telle qu'elle permet la détection de 0,35 ng de dPC I et III, et de 0,035 ng de d-peptide. En se basant sur un poids moléculaire de 350 000 pour les dPC et de 17 500 pour le d-peptide, la méthode radioimmunologique permet donc la détection de 1 femtomole de dPC I et III, et de 2 femtomoles de d-peptide.

L'absence d'immunoréactivité du collagène normal (fig. 1), des chaînes pro-alpha 2 et de la partie carboxy-terminale du dPC I (fig. 2), alors que le d-peptide entraîne une réaction croisée complète (fig. 1), indique que le site antigénique du dPC I est situé sur l'extension amino-terminale de la chaîne pro-alpha 1. Cette observation est semblable aux observations antérieures [2] et à celle de Sherr et Goldberg [7] qui ont montré que les immuns-sérums obtenus avec du pro-collagène humain contiennent des anticorps dirigés uniquement contre la partie amino-terminale.

L'utilisation de traceurs de type I et de type III démontre que l'antisérum contient des anticorps dirigés contre ces deux molécules. Ces anticorps sont différents pour deux raisons. D'une part l'absence de réactivité du dPC III dans le système utilisant le dPC I comme traceur et l'antisérum à la dilution de 4×10^{-5} indique que le dPC I réagit avec des anticorps qui ne reconnaissent pas le dPC III. D'autre part, dans le système utilisant le dPC III comme traceur et l'antisérum à la dilution de 10^{-4}, il faut, en mole, 12 fois plus de dPC I et $1,47 \times 10^4$ fois plus de d-peptide pour entraîner le même degré d'inhibition de la réaction que celui provoqué par une mole de dPC III. Le(s) site(s) antigénique(s) du dPC III est donc différent de celui du d-peptide, qui est, pour rappel, immunologiquement semblable au dPC I dans l'autre système. Cette observation est donc compatible avec la présence, dans la préparation de dPC I, de 8,3% de dPC III. Cette contamination de dPC I par le dPC III expliquerait de surcroît la génération d'anticorps anti-dPC III avec la préparation de dPC I comme agent immunogène. Ainsi donc l'utilisation du traceur correspondant et de dilutions appropriées de l'antisérum permet la détection spécifique des déterminants antigéniques propres au type I et au type III.

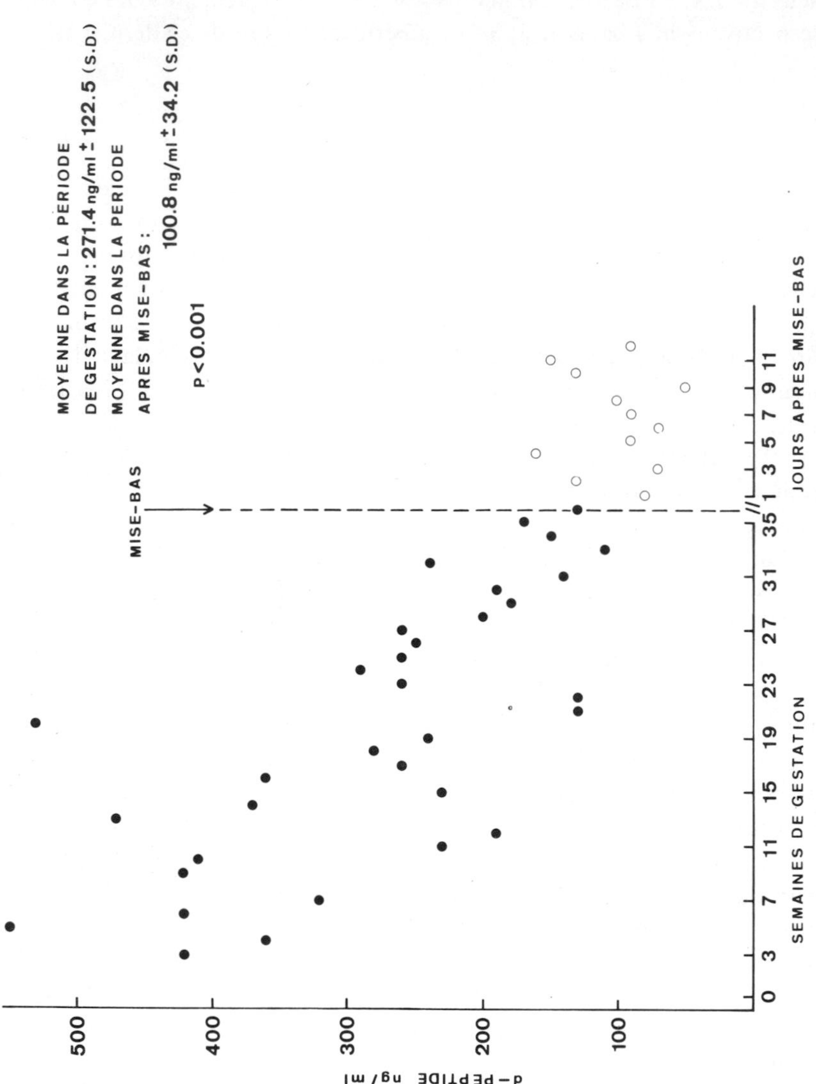

FIG.3. Taux sériques de d-peptide aux différents âges de la gestation avant (●) et après (○) la mise bas chez une vache.

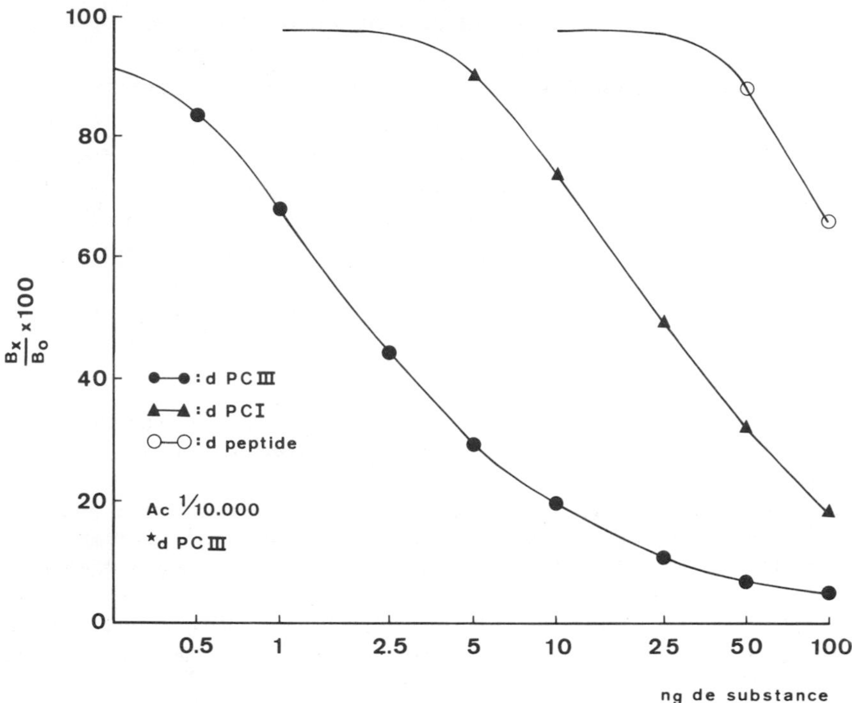

FIG.4. Courbe de dosage représentative du dPC III utilisant comme traceur le dPC III et l'antisérum à la dilution de $1/10^{-4}$. Une réaction croisée complète est notée avec le dPC I, alors que le d-peptide n'est que faiblement immunoréactif.

Le déterminant antigénique semblable au d-peptide est présent en très grande quantité dans les extraits de peau et les sérums de sujets dermato-sparaxiques, mais également, quoique en moindre quantité, de sujets normaux. La concentration sérique de ce déterminant antigénique décroît avec l'âge et varie selon les conditions physiologiques, comme la grossesse. Ces résultats démontrent que le déterminant antigénique du dPC n'est pas exclusif de la dermato-sparaxie et suggèrent qu'il pourrait également être présent sur la molécule de pro-collagène bovin normal de type I. Cette hypothèse est d'autant plus vraisemblable que des molécules immunologiquement semblables au pro-collagène humain ont été décelées dans le sérum humain par une méthode radioimmunologique [8]. Cependant, la nature moléculaire du déterminant sérique n'est pas encore connue: il pourrait s'agir de pro-collagène, de d-peptide, ou encore d'autres formes moléculaires contenant ce déterminant antigénique du d-peptide. La signification précise de sa concentration et son rôle éventuel dans le plasma restent encore à préciser.

En conclusion, la méthode de dosage radioimmunologique peut donc être appliquée au pro-collagène et utilisée pour étudier in vivo dans le sérum et les extraits tissulaires le métabolisme de l'extension polypeptidique amino-terminale du pro-collagène bovin dans les conditions normales et pathologiques. En outre, les déterminants antigéniques du dPC I et du dPC III sont différents et les anticorps correspondants en permettent la détermination spécifique. En particulier, il est possible d'étudier, in vitro, les facteurs qui induisent ou répriment la biosynthèse par les fibroblastes de l'un de ces deux types de pro-collagène.

REFERENCES

[1] LENAERS, A., ANSAY, M., NUSGENS, B.V., LAPIERE, C.M., Collagen made of extended alpha chains, procollagen in genetically-defective dermatosparaxic calves, Eur. J. Biochem. **23** (1971) 533.

[2] LAPIERE, C.M., LENAERS, A., KOHN, L.O., Procollagen peptidase: an enzyme excising the coordination peptides of procollagen, Proc. Natl Acad. Sci. **68** (1971) 3054.

[3] LENAERS, A., LAPIERE, C.M., Type III procollagen and collagen in skin, Biochim. Biophys. Acta **400** (1975) 121.

[4] TIMPL, R., WICK, G., FURTHMAYER, H., LAPIERE, C.M., KÜHN, K., Immunochemical properties of procollagen from dermatosparaxic calves, Eur. J. Biochem. **32** (1973) 584.

[5] GREENWOOD, F.C., HUNTER, W., GLOVER, J., Preparation of ^{131}I labelled human growth hormone of high specific radioactivity, Biochemistry **89** (1963) 114.

[6] McCROSKERY, R.A., WOOD, D.S., Jr., HARRIS, E.D., Jr., Gelatin: a poor substrate for mammalian collagenase, Science **182** (1973) 70.

[7] SHERR, C.T., GOLDBERG, B., Antibodies to a precursor of human collagen, Science **180** (1973) 1190.

[8] TAUBMAN, M.B., GOLDBERG, B., SHERR, C.J., Radioimmunoassay for human procollagen, Science **186** (1974) 1115.

DISCUSSION

D.K. HAZRA: Is this disease in cattle an animal model of human Ehlers-Danlos syndrome, and has this test been applied to patients with this syndrome?

G. HEYNEN: Yes, it is a model of the human disease. The assay has not been applied to such patients.

Invited review paper

TUMOUR-ASSOCIATED ANTIGENS

K.D. BAGSHAWE
Charing Cross Hospital,
London, United Kingdom

Abstract

TUMOUR-ASSOCIATED ANTIGENS.

The identification of tumour markers relates to the diagnosis of malignant disease, to monitoring the course of the disease and its response to therapy and to membrane-located substances which may provide targets for chemotherapeutic attack. Substances characteristic of cancer cells may be defined by (1) the detection of reactive responses by the host to the presence of tumour, (2) the response of host lymphocytes in vitro to previously encountered antigens, and (3) the detection in body fluids of secretions by cancer cells. Radioimmunoassay is applicable to the third of these alternatives. A substantial number of tumour products have been defined as eutopic or ectopic products. None of the substances so far defined has proved to be unique for cancer cells and the value of a particular marker depends upon the regularity of its association with a particular form of cancer, its correlation with staging or total burden of tumour cells and the biological range of concentrations observed in both health and disease states. Two excellent marker substances, alpha-foetoprotein and human chorionic gonadotrophin, relate to uncommon cancers but full use of these markers has not yet been achieved. Carcinoembryonic antigen provides less critical information for a more common group of cancers. The identification of other tumour markers can be anticipated and the place in clinical practice of some substances already defined requires continued evaluation.

One of the anomalies of cancer therapy is that as treatment becomes more effective so it becomes more important to achieve early diagnosis. When treatment is ineffective, micrometastatic disease often carries a similar prognosis to advanced disease, but with effective therapy the prognosis and the duration and hazards of treatment are often profoundly affected by the 'stage' of the disease or extent of tumour burden at the time of diagnosis. Thus, attempts to achieve early diagnosis will become increasingly important and the problem of detecting asymptomatic disease will eventually confront us.

No less important is the process of monitoring the response of a tumour to therapy because one of the outstanding features of the changes in therapy in the last two decades has been the matching of therapeutic methods to specific types of cancer with the use of more than 30 different chemotherapeutic agents, radiotherapy and surgery.

Three broad approaches to the problem of detecting substances characteristic of cancer cells can be defined. (1) One is based on the detection of biochemical responses of host tissues to the presence of a tumour. (2) The second depends on the presence on cancer cells of membrane markers which are not secreted in detectable amounts into body fluids. (3) A third approach is the detection of specific secretions by the cancer cells into body fluids.

These three approaches have already provided a large number of leads and it would not be possible to review all these adequately here. Although I shall be concerned principally with the third of these categories the other two merit some mention.

1. SUBSTANCES APPARENTLY PRODUCED BY HOST CELLS IN RESPONSE TO TUMOURS

These substances are interesting but show relatively low specificity. Changes in concentration may have some value in monitoring the course of malignant disease in the absence of more specific markers. Multiparametric analysis of non-specific markers may add some information to that provided by individual measurements, but convincing evidence for this has not yet been provided [1].

Muramidase (lysozyme)

Muramidase, which has a molecular weight of 14 000, is present in the serum of normal subjects in a concentration of about 5 – 8 mg/litre and is thought to originate from disintegrating neutrophil granulocytes [2]. Macrophages within solid tumours make a contribution to the serum concentration but the most marked elevations are found in monocytic, myelomonocytic and myelocytic leukaemia [3 – 5]. Spinal fluid values have been elevated in the presence of both primary and secondary tumours within the central nervous system, especially with histiocytic lymphoma [6]. High serum values also result from Crohn's disease and chronic renal failure. Values may be increased in spinal fluid by infection.

α_2-H-Ferritin

The ferritins have molecular weights of the order of 450 000 and form a widely distributed family of isomeric proteins associated with iron metabolism. Normal serum values are about 200 μg/litre. The α_2-H-protein was first described in serum of children with cancer [7] and subsequently it was found in the sera of adults with haematological neoplasias, lymphomas, hepatomas and breast cancer [8, 9] in concentrations up to 6000 μg/litre. Elevations also occur in myocardial infarction, cirrhosis and non-malignant gastrointestinal tract disease.

Pregnancy-associated α_2-glycoprotein (pregnancy-associated macroglobulin)

This protein, with a molecular weight of 326 000 – 760 000, is present at concentrations of 20 – 200 ng/litre in normal adult serum but increases 40- to 80-fold in late pregnancy and during estrogen and progestagen therapy. Increased values have been observed in patients with various cancers and particularly in carcinoma of the breast where a correlation between the course of the disease and its serum concentration has been reported [10, 11].

Hydroxyproline

This amino acid is derived from collagen metabolism and is excreted in the urine bound to peptides. Excretion increases in a variety of disease states, in the presence of bone metastases and sometimes with soft-tissue metastases [12, 13]. Hydroxyproline secretion may be increased before bone metastases are demonstrable by other techniques.

Other changes

Other responses to foci of cancer cells include endocrine changes such as abnormal adrenal function [14] and changes in so-called acute phase proteins [15].

The polyamines [16 – 18, 83] and methylated nucleic acid bases [19, 20] have also merited some interest as potential tumour markers, although these might be more properly regarded as products both of malignant and normal cell death rather than as products of biochemical responses.

It would however be unduly optimistic to expect changes in substances within this broad category to revolutionize cancer diagnosis and provide all the information we require.

2. CELL-MEMBRANE-RESTRICTED MARKERS

Markers on the cancer cell membrane which are not released into body fluids in detectable amounts may nevertheless be detectable indirectly. Such markers may, for instance, act as receptors for substances which are present in blood. An example of this is suggested by recent work relating to modified blood-group substances which indicates that whereas normal cells express the MN blood substances, many tumours express instead 'T' antigen, its desialylated derivative. 'T' antigen occurs widely on bacteria and antibodies to 'T'. antigen are universal. The 'T' antigen on cancer cells has been claimed to absorb out the antibody resulting in lowered serum concentrations [21].

Another approach to membrane-bound antigens depends on their recognition by the host's circulating lymphocytes. Although this would have wide application if there were appropriate specific antigens and responding lymphocytes, much of the interest so far has been directed at responses to myelin basic protein and a possibly related substance described as cancer basic protein. This originated with the observations of Field and Caspary [22] that when the lymphocytes of patients with cancer were incubated with myelin basic protein, they apparently released a lymphokine which could be detected by its ability to cause a reduction in the net electrostatic charge of macrophages obtained from guinea-pig ascites, as shown by their slowing in an electrophoretic field. The implication that a similar substance was presumptively present on cancer cells lead to the preparation of cancer basic protein. Although most cancer patients appear to give positive results in this test its specificity is not high and technical difficulties with the test have, so far, excluded it from clinical application.

Another lymphocyte-based method measures rotation of polarized light emitted by fluorescein molecules released within lymphocytes by enzymatic hydrolysis of fluorescein diacetate [23]. It depends on rapid distinctive responses by lymphocytes to previously encountered antigens and it is claimed to be specific if cancer extracts corresponding to the patient's tumour are employed as the stimulogen. It still remains to be seen whether these claims can be fully supported in other laboratories [24].

Experience with these methods in my laboratory has led us to the view that these are phenomena which are interesting but we are cautious about their dependability. It seems probable that changes occur in lymphocytes within an hour, possibly within minutes, of contact with previously encountered antigens and that it may prove possible to exploit these responses for diagnostic purposes, although it is unlikely that they will have much role in monitoring the course of disease. Lymphocytes may however be modified non-specifically in the presence of disease and the exclusion of aberrant responses resulting from such changes is a necessary step towards achieving the necessary reliability.

3. SECRETED TUMOUR PRODUCTS

General considerations

Tumour markers secreted by tumours which display the required specificity are likely to be some form of protein. They can be classified in several ways. They may be eutopic or ectopic, that is appropriate or inappropriate to the tumour according to its tissue of origin. They may be hormones, enzymes, antibodies or may have no known biological function. They may be adult or embryonic in type and the last group can be divided into placental or foetal.

The ectopic production of hormones by tumours is of considerable theoretical interest since it is presumed to indicate genetic derepression in the tumour cells. It includes the well-known examples of Cushing's syndrome with ACTH-producing tumours [25], galactorrhoea with prolactin [26], hypercalcaemia with calcitonin [27], prostaglandins and parathyroid hormone production [28], malabsorption associated with glucagon [29], hyponatraemia with arginine vasopressin [30], gyanecomastia with gonadotrophins and placental lactogen [31] and the gastrointestinal tract hormone syndromes [32, 33].

The incidence of ectopic hormone production probably exceeds 20% of all cancers. Ectopic products are, however, generally found after rather than before the diagnosis is established. Moreover, the incidence is not high enough to be valuable in screening, and recent studies [34, 35] have shown that it would be unrewarding to attempt this with present markers.

We are therefore left with a few tumours for which good markers exist and where measurements are very important to the management of the individual patient. These also throw light on the problems of tumour elimination in a more general context. Whilst we can lament our slow progress in defining and refining suitable markers for the common tumours we seem slow to make proper use of the few good markers already known. Part of the reason for this is that the good tumour markers relate to rather rare tumours and, also, to make good use of them it is necessary to accumulate experience. This can only be done through some form of regional centralization either of the patients, or of the laboratory services, or of both.

Quantitative measurements of one of the important tumour markers, human chorionic gonadotrophin (hCG), have been available for 20 years and semi-quantitative measurements for half a century. Yet most patients with hCG-producing tumours in Europe still do not benefit as they might from frequent, precise measurements in a sensitive assay system coupled with an informed and experienced interpretation of the marker measurements.

The question whether tumour markers are identical with the corresponding normal tissue product has often been examined and it is evident that variations occur. However, 'normal' glycoproteins, for example, may show heterogeneity and the extent to which tumour products differ within this spectrum in a consistent and specific fashion is not fully established for any antigen. 'Big' ACTH has been described as an ectopic product [35] and the 'C' and 'N' terminal fragments and melanocyte-stimulating hormone [36] may be largely, perhaps exclusively, associated with neoplasms. The number of sialic acid moieties in a glycoprotein molecule may vary substantially.

The most useful markers are those that reflect the total body burden of cells. Thus α-foetoprotein (AFP) and hCG can both be present in concentrations up to 10^7 times the normal value and correspond to a substantial part of the range of tumour burden. However, it is necessary to take account of the fact that patients with advanced disease have tumour burdens in the range $10^{11} - 10^{12}$ cells compared with estimated total body cells of the order of 5×10^{13}. Ideally a tumour marker would cover the whole range but even with hCG and AFP the limit of detection is probably of the order of $10^4 - 10^5$ cells. Failure to recognize the critical importance of this limit and its implications for management results in many unnecessary therapeutic failures by discontinuing therapy too early. The question of who should be responsible for interpreting measurements of tumour markers is critical to this issue. Ideally, tumour marker measurements are made within oncology departments so that there is no hindrance to correlation of all the many clinical and laboratory factors that bear on the problems of interpretation.

In essence, we have two good markers for a few uncommon tumours, some second-rate markers for some of the common cancers and a few which still await full evaluation. I shall restrict myself to more detailed discussion of hCG, AFP and carcinoembryonic antigen (CEA), and summarize other potential markers in Tables I–IV at the end of this paper.

Carcinoembryonic antigen

CEA is a glycoprotein with beta mobility (mol. wt 200 000) generally obtained from colonic primary or secondary tumours and defined, directly or indirectly, by a line of continuity in immunoprecipitative tests with the original antigen-antibody pair prepared by Gold and Freedman [84]. Heterogeneity within purified CEA preparations has been demonstrated by various techniques [85] chiefly in the carbohydrate moieties. In addition, two closely related glycoproteins now known as NCA_1 and NCA_2 share antigenic determinants with CEA, and antisera can be directed wholly or partially at these determinants with consequent loss of specificity. Absorption of antisera with extracts of normal colon therefore form an essential part of the preparation of anti-CEA sera, but it is a critical process and it seems clear that CEA is expressed in normal mucus-secreting cells. The variations in carbohydrate moieties of the molecule continue to be studied to see whether they provide a basis for improved specificity in CEA determinations.

Assays for CEA have developed from the Farr technique [86] and zirconyl phosphate gel separation [87], both of which use perchloric-acid-extracted serum and various double-antibody methods [88, 89] on extracted or non-extracted serum or plasma. Direct comparisons between the different assay methods have shown little or no consistent superiority for one method [90]. In our hands a pre-precipitated double-antibody system with a one-stage incubation of unextracted serum has proved the most convenient and readily automated. Differences in numerical values between assays may arise from the use or non-use of serum in the reference standards [91].

The application of CEA measurements for diagnostic purposes is well established in certain clinical situations and there is agreement that it has no place in the screening of asymptomatic subjects for cancer. In most diagnostic situations involving gastrointestinal tract cancer, CEA measurements have ancillary rather than primary importance since in most instances histological confirmation of the diagnosis will be necessary. In geriatric patients, gross elevations of CEA values together with clinical evidence consistent with inoperable malignant disease may spare the patient more distressing and more expensive investigations. Its main application has however been in following up patients who have had apparently successful resections for colo-rectal cancer. Regular, monthly estimations may provide evidence of disease progression several months in advance of clinical evidence in about 70% of patients [92]. The fact that it is far from completely reliable even in this context must be emphasized. At present it is not established whether the early detection of disease progression in these patients is therapeutically advantageous. It may provide a basis for a second-look operation in some instances. Undoubtedly, when more effective chemotherapeutic agents become available, evidence of early relapse will assume new importance.

In following the response of colo-rectal cancer to existing chemotherapy there is a broad correlation between CEA values and therapeutic response, but in our experience dissociation is not uncommon.

Placental and foetal products

Human chorionic gonadotrophin (hCG)

This glycoprotein is synthesized predominantly by syncytiotrophoblast and to a lesser extent by the cytotrophoblast. Recent evidence indicates however that there are small amounts of hCG-like material in the testes [93] and pituitary gland [94]. It is possible that as more sensitive techniques are developed hCG will be detected in normal serum, but in our hands it has only rarely been detected at a sensitivity level of 10 pg/ml (0.2 mIU/ml). hCG is cleared from blood to urine at a rate of approximately 1.0 – 1.5 ml/min; plasma and urine concentrations of hCG are therefore of similar magnitude at average urine flow rates of 1.0 – 1.5 ml/min.

hCG consists of two non-covalently bound subunits. The α-subunit (mol.wt 14 900) has a similar sequence homology to the α-subunit of luteinizing hormone (LH), follicle-stimulating hormone and thyroid-stimulating hormone. The β-subunit (mol.wt 23 000) has similarities with the same pituitary polypeptides but is larger by some 30 amino acid residues at the C-terminal end than luteinizing hormone. This tail protein has a high proportion of proline and serine residues. Both subunits have a high content of sialic acid [95].

Most antisera raised to intact hCG cross-react with luteinizing hormone, but a few antisera raised to β-hCG are highly discriminating and 50 – 100 times more sensitive to hCG than LH. Assays with antisera raised to intact hCG are therefore generally hCG/LH assays whereas with anti-β-hCG sera, assays detecting hCG at concentrations < 1 mIU/ml without interference from LH can be achieved [96]. β-hCG assays measure both intact hCG and free β-hCG, and with normal, non-pregnant subjects, values < 1 mIU/ml are found. With hCG/LH assays the 'normal' values are determined by the subjects' physiological status with respect to LH; thus, values are in the range 100 – 400 IU hCG/24 h in menopausal subjects and 5 – 100 IU hCG/24 h in pre-menopausal women. At ovulation in women and in adult males, values of 60 – 150 IU hCG/24 h are found by hCG/LH assay.

To distinguish between assays sensitive to both hCG and LH and those which detect only hCG, the terms hCG/LH assay and β-hCG assay are used in this paper.

Hydatidiform mole, invasive mole and choriocarcinoma

Since the 1930s, hCG has been detected in the blood and urine of patients with tumours which consist wholly or partially of trophoblast as a eutopic product and also in a wide variety of patients with other tumours as an ectopic product [97].

The measurement of hCG in relation to gestational trophoblastic tumour exemplifies the use of tumour products in screening, diagnosis, monitoring and follow-up care. Following the evacuation of hydatidiform mole, hCG excretion persists for a variable period of time in most patients and reflects surviving trophoblastic cells in the myometrium or elsewhere. In 90 – 95% of patients, these trophoblastic lesions die out spontaneously within 6 months [98]. Of the remaining 5 – 10% of cases about half or less have, or develop, choriocarcinoma and the remainder have invasive moles which can be dealt with successfully by surgery at the cost of sterility, or by cytotoxic chemotherapy with preservation of reproductive function. The indications from hCG measurements which point to the need for treatment include progressively rising values after evacuation of the mole and levels persisting at a high rate (> 20 000 IU/24 h in urine) more than 6 weeks after evacuation. The urinary assay, though less sensitive than the plasma β-hCG assay, has the substantial advantage of convenience and avoidance of venepuncture for this purpose.

About 1% of those requiring treatment (i.e. about 0.1% of all mole patients) develop choriocarcinoma after a period of weeks or months during which hCG/LH values are normal. The number of such 'missed' cases could be reduced by serum β-hCG assay after hCG/LH values have become normal.

For monitoring the response of trophoblastic tumours the β-hCG assay is advantageous at low levels of production, and the limit of sensitivity corresponds to the rate of production of $10^4 - 10^5$ viable choriocarcinoma cells [99].

Metastases in the central nervous system (CNS) may be detected before clinical, radiological or isotope scanning manifestations are apparent by comparing the serum and cerebrospinal fluid (CSF) concentrations. In the absence of brain metastases the serum/CSF ratio is > 60:1 and values below this figure indicate their presence unless sampling is performed during a period of precipitate fall in serum hCG concentration when equilibrium is disturbed. CSF values may exceed serum values in cases where metastatic disease is present predominantly within the CNS. Serial measurements of serum/CSF hCG provide a means of monitoring the response of the CNS lesions to therapy more or less independently of the extra-CNS disease [100].

It is conceptually useful to translate hCG values into the corresponding number of tumour cells, particularly when considering how long to continue chemotherapy in patients whose tumours have responded and where hCG has become undetectable. Failure of hCG levels to fall in response to therapy is an indication for changing the mode of therapy and it is frequently possible to detect drug resistance even with sub-clinical disease. Progressive increase in hCG values or sustained high levels of hCG in body fluids has always been accompanied, or followed by, evidence of disease progression.

Follow-up care of patients successfully treated for gestational choriocarcinoma by hCG monitoring is essential. The risk of relapse is highest in the first few months after stopping treatment but relapses up to 3 years, and in one case 7 years, have been recorded without intervening pregnancies. hCG values should be checked approximately 3 weeks after any pregnancy subsequent to hydatidiform mole or choriocarcinoma.

Malignant teratoma

The proportion of malignant teratoma producing hCG is not known and estimates have varied widely according to the method of assessment and case selection. Histological evidence of trophoblast in primary testicular tumours is as low as 2%, but radioimmunoassay for hCG in one study revealed that 90% of teratoma patients had detectable levels at some stage in the disease.

Malignant mediastinal and ovarian teratomas appear to have a similar high probability of hCG production. hCG production by putatively benign teratoma would be strong evidence of malignancy.

With 'pure' trophoblastic teratomas, hCG values reflect the course of the disease as reliably as for the gestational form, but in general, hCG is a less complete marker for teratomas than for gestational choriocarcinoma since the hormone reflects the activity and mass of only one cell line within a tumour which may be multi-clonal [101, 102].

Brain metastases in malignant teratoma are frequently but not invariably due to choriocarcinoma and serum/CSF values must be interpreted accordingly.

Multiple markers are available for some malignant teratomas, and these include hCG, AFP, HPL, placental alkaline phosphatase, CEA and casein. Dissociation between the responses of hCG-producing and AFP-producing cells within a teratoma have been recognized. Measurements of these two markers at intervals of 3 – 7 days by RIA is now a minimum requirement for proper clinical management.

Investigation of complaints of swelling, pain or confirmed tumour in the testis should include serum hCG and AFP measurements. They are also appropriate in the investigation of anterior mediastinal masses.

Non-trophoblastic tumours

hCG may be produced by dysgerminomas and occasionally by hepatomas and a few other tumours in amounts comparable to choriocarcinoma. In the plasma of patients with a wide variety of other tumours small amounts of hCG are also often detectable [97]. The data available at present are inadequate to define the probability of hCG production for each tumour type, especially since improvements in sensitivity of the assay appear to yield an increased number of hCG-positive tumours. The distribution of values obtained from a variety of cancer patients suggests that we are still at one end of a distribution curve which may embrace most patients with cancer.

In contrast to the situation with gestational choriocarcinoma where a 10^7-fold range of values is observed, it is clear that hCG measurements for these other tumours may have diagnostic value but are limited in value for monitoring the response to therapy unless assay sensitivity and specificity can be still further extended.

hCG subunits

Tumours producing intact hCG have also been found to produce one or other subunit in excess [103]. Some tumours produce only the 'alpha' subunit of the glycoprotein hormones and others produce only 'beta'-hCG [104]. In some cases the amounts of the subunits detected have been adequate for monitoring purposes.

The significance of the production of hCG and its subunits by a wide variety of tumours has yet to be defined, but it has been claimed that a high proportion of human tumours can be demonstrated by immunoperoxidase techniques to express hCG, HPL or other placental polypeptides on their surfaces [104, 105].

$\beta_1 - SP_1$

This glycoprotein, which is also known as β-foetoprotein and PAPP C, has a molecular weight of 90 000 and was found independently by several groups of workers [106, 107] in the serum of pregnant women at concentrations of 5 – 25 mg/100 ml. It has been detected in the serum of patients with trophoblastic tumours before treatment [108] and localized in the syncytiotrophoblast by immunofluorescent methods. In general, it is far less effective than hCG for monitoring trophoblastic tumours but present evidence indicates that it is occasionally detectable after hCG is no longer present. Recently it has been demonstrated in 80% of breast tumours by immunoperoxidase enzyme bridge techniques [105] although confirmation of this observation is awaited.

Placental alkaline phosphatase

The alkaline phosphatase isoenzyme produced by the placenta exists as several phenotypic variants which were found by Fishman and his colleagues [109] to be heat stable and L-phenylalanine sensitive. Placental-type alkaline phosphatase (PAP) was found in the serum and tumour of a patient (Regan) with carcinoma of the lung. Since then it has been identified in association with tumours at various sites sometimes in large amounts but more often at low levels. The early studies with enzymatic or immunoenzymatic methods indicated that it was detectable in the sera of up to 14% of cancer patients, but the specificity of these methods for low concentrations of antigen was questionable and with radioimmunoassay no PAP-positive case was found in 100 patients with various types of cancer [110]. Later studies with a more sensitive immunoenzymatic method demonstrated activity in all normal sera examined whilst a somewhat less sensitive method gave positive results in 2% of normal subjects and 9% of cancer patients [111]. It appears that although PAP and other AP variants have been described in cancer patients, particularly those with ovarian and lung cancer, the amounts identified in most cases are small. At present it seems that measurements of PAP are likely to be useful only for exceptional patients.

Fishman's recent studies [112] have shown that PAP is trophoblastic in origin and that three specific phosphatases exist at different phases of the organ's existence. It has been postulated that the alkaline phosphatase of human tumour tissues reflects the expression of placental genes corresponding to one or more phases of trophoblastic development. Studies on a monophenotypic cell line have shown that DNA synthesis is not required for induction of the enzyme.

α-Foetoprotein

Human α-foetoprotein (AFP) is a glycoprotein which has a molecular weight of 70 000 and contains about 4% sugar with an average sialic acid content of two resudies per molecule [113]. It is present in the yolk sac and in foetal liver and is synthesized by the hepatocyte. Levels of AFP are high in the foetus and fall rapidly after birth. Although values remain variable in the first post-natal year, the adult normal range is established by five years. In the non-pregnant adult, very high levels of AFP in the serum are generally associated with hepatocellular carcinoma or malignant teratoma, although hepatic regeneration associated with any cause may give increased values.

AFP has been isolated from human cord serum, foetal serum, serum from patients with hepatoma and hepatoma tissue.

AFPs derived from hepatoma and foetal sources have been compared electrophoretically [114]. The hepatoma-serum-derived preparations usually had several subcomponents in comparison to a single component from most foetal sera. Neuraminidase treatment reduced the hepatoma-derived AFP to a single detectable component. However, not all the microheterogeneity resides in the sialic acid, whose removal incidentally can lessen the immunological activity of AFP. While amino-acid composition and peptide maps of several purified preparations of AFPs from foetuses and hepatoma patients show no difference, three isoproteins have been identified after neuraminidase treatment of which only two were immunoprecipitable [115]. Other workers obtained two variants of AFP, one of which was bound to concanavalin A, the other was not. Despite the microheterogeneity it is evident from collaborative studies designed to prepare a reference standard for AFP that results between preparations can be correlated successfully [116].

The first assays for AFP were based on immunodiffusion and counter-immuno-electrophoresis. More sensitive radioimmunoassays have been developed by which AFP can be measured at the level present in normal human serum. Double-antibody systems have been devised by Ruoslahti and Seppälä [117] and a convenient one-day double-antibody assay has been automated [118]. The range of concentration of 2-16 μg/litre in normal human serum was defined by Seppälä and Ruoslahti [119].

Some of the differences in the reported numbers of patients with hepatocellular carcinoma who have increased serum values of AFP are attributable to the sensitivity of detection of the method used. In general, about 80% are positive [120]. Values exceeding 500 μg/litre are common in primary liver cancer. The elevated values occasionally found in cirrhosis or chronic hepatitis, or infective hepatitis, tend to be transient.

Primary gastrointestinal tract and other cancers sometimes produce AFP [120]. A case of bronchogenic carcinoma has been described with metastases in the liver and AFP present only in the liver parenchyma adjacent to the secondary tumour [121]. Conversely, in a carcinoid tumour of the stomach with metastases to the liver, immunohistological localization of AFP was evident only in some of the primary stomach tumour cells [122].

Some ovarian and testicular tumours produce large amounts of AFP. About 75% of testicular teratocarcinomas are associated with values greater than 40 μg/litre [120]. A similar incidence probably applies to ovarian teratoma and expression of AFP has been related to histological identification of yolk-sac endoderm in the tumour [123].

AFP levels can be used to monitor the course of the disease. In a Japanese series of patients with hepatomas, those who showed a good clinical response to chemotherapy showed a decline in their serum AFP levels, while ineffective chemotherapy was mirrored by a steady rise in AFP levels [124]. The relationship between AFP concentration and tumour bulk has been questioned [125], but in making such assessments viable tumour mass needs to be distinguished from gross mass.

Malignant teratomas of testis, ovary or other sites producing both AFP and hCG are now regularly monitored. In some cases, both markers decline in parallel in response to therapy, in others one marker may remain elevated, indicating persistence of the corresponding cell line. Where elevation of either persists after treatment, persistence or recurrence of the disease is observed clinically.

Some other tumour markers

Calcitonin

This hormone is produced by the para-follicular or C cells of the thyroid and by medullary carcinoma of the thyroid which arises from these cells. It is a tumour which tends to be familial and associated with parathyroid hyperplasia or adenoma, phaeochromocytoma and Cushing's syndrome. A raised serum calcitonin value in a patient with a familial syndrome with or without mucosal neuromas points to phaeochromocytoma or to medullary carcinoma. In a low percentage of cases the basal calcitonin level is normal [$<$ 100 pg/ml] but a calcium infusion or gastrin or whisky may demonstrate abnormality [126]. These tumours are also associated with raised serum values of carcinoembryonic antigen.

More recently it has been reported that calcitonin is produced in relatively small amounts as an ectopic product by a wide range of tumours, particularly by carcinoma of breast and oat cell carcinoma of bronchus [127].

Casein

Casein is present in the exocrine secretion of the mammary gland and is apparently under the control of prolactin. Immunologically detectable K-casein is present in the serum of lactating women [128]. It is not normally detectable at levels greater than 100 μg/litre in men or in women who are not lactating.

Hendrick and Franchimont [128], exploring the value of K-casein as a tumour index substance, isolated a "first-cycle soluble casein" fraction of casein from human milk following the work of earlier authors and proceeded to a further purification of the K-fraction, a β-globulin which produced a single precipitin line on immunoelectrophoresis against an antiserum raised to whole casein.

A radioimmunoassay for K-casein has been established in which K-casein is labelled by modification of the Chloramine-T method. Serum of 361 samples from subjects who were neither pregnant nor lactating had serum casein values < 60 μg/litre. Although elevated levels were found in 57% patients with metastatic carcinoma of the breast, the correlation with disease stage was poor and high values were found in 9% of patients with benign breast disease [129].

TABLE I. SUMMARY OF PROPOSED TUMOUR MARKERS

Substance	Regular or appropriate association	Ectopic production or non-neoplastic associations	Ref.
Placental products			
Human chorionic gonadotrophin	Hydatidiform and invasive mole, gestational chorio-carcinoma, malignant teratoma of testis, ovary, mediastinum, etc.	Hepatocellular carcinoma Lung and various tumours	T[a]
Alpha-hCG subunit			T
Beta-hCG subunit	As hCG	Lung and various others	T
Human placental lactogen			T
$Beta_1$-SP_1			
(Beta-foetoprotein)	As hCG	Not recorded	T
Placental alkaline phosphatase	No regular association but could be "appropriate" to choriocarcinoma	Various tumours in small amounts, occasionally large amounts	T
Foetal antigens			
Carcinoembryonic antigen	Carcinoma of colon, rectum, pancreas, stomach, gall-bladder, lung, breast, ovary, testes, prostate, cervix, bladder, kidney, medullary ca., thyroid etc.	Inflammatory disease of bowel, peptic ulcer, liver disease, pulmonary infection, tissue necrosis, heavy smoking	T

[a] See text

TABLE I (cont.)

Substance	Regular or appropriate association	Ectopic production or non-neoplastic associations	Ref.
Alpha-foeto-protein	Hepatoma, malignant teratoma, endodermal sinus (yolk sac) tumours	Hepatic regeneration with metastatic cancer or non-cancerous conditions	T
Beta-oncofoetal antigen	Colon, melanoma, endometrial carcinoma	Foetal tissues	[37]
DNA binding protein (C3DP)	Reported in 60% of various cancer sera	Foetus	[38], [39]
Foetal sulphoglycoprotein	Gastric secretions in stomach carcinoma		
Alpha $_2$-H (an isoferritin)	Malignant haemopathies, head and neck, stomach and colonic cancer, breast, lung	Foetus, rheumatoid arthritis, cirrhosis, myocardial infarction	T
Leukaemia associated, Hodgkin's disease associated	Various leukaemias Spleen and nodes	Foetal haemopoietic tissue Foetal haemopoietic tissue	[40] [41]
Pancreatic oncofoetal antigen	Carcinoma body of pancreas colon, gall-bladder	Pancreatitis Pancreatic cysts	[42]
Sarcoma associated S_1, S_2	Sarcomas, carcinomas	Various normal adults	[43]

TABLE I (cont.)

Substance	Regular or appropriate association	Ectopic production or non-neoplastic associations	Ref.
Pituitary polypeptide			
Adrenocortico-trophine (ACTH) CLIP, N-terminal fragments, 'big' ACTH and melanocyte stimulating hormone	Pituitary (chromophobe) adenoma and carcinoma	Carcinoma of lung (adeno-squamous, undiff.)	T
		Colon, pancreas, medullary, thyroid, prostate, cervix, ovary, thymoma, phoceochromocytoma, carcinoid, etc.	T
Anti-diuretic hormone (ADH) (arginine vasopressin)		Lung, Ewing's sarcoma, etc.	T
Corticotrophin releasing factor-like-activity		Carcinoma of pancreas, lung	[44]
Follicle stimulating hormone (FSH)		Carcinoma of lung	[45]
Growth hormone (GH)	Pituitary adenoma	Lung, stomach	[46]
Neurophysin	Pituitary, hypothalamus	Lung carcinoma and carcinoid, lung, kidney	[47]
Prolactin			[48]
Thyrotrophic hormone (TSH)	Pituitary		[49]

TABLE I (cont.)

Substance	Regular or appropriate association	Ectopic production or non-neoplastic associations	Ref.
Gastrointestinal tract associated hormones			
Insulin	Insulinomas (beta cells, pancreatic islets)	Various ectopic sites, lymphosarcomas, other sarcomas	[50]
Glucagon	Glucagonomas (a-z cells, pancreatic islets)	Kidney	[51]
Gastrin	Zollinger-Ellison syndrome, pancreatic islets	Ovary	[52]
Vasoactive inhibitory peptide (VP)	Islet cell tumours		[32]
Gastric inhibitory peptide (GIP)	Islet cell tumours		[32]
Pancreatic polypeptide	Insulinoma, glucagonoma, vipoma, gastrinoma		[33]
Pancreatic somatostatin	Somatostatinoma	(Growth hormone release-inhibiting hormone)	[53]
Other polypeptide hormones			
Calcitonin	Medullary carcinoma of thyroid	Pancreas, lung (oat cell), prostate, body of uterus, bladder, breast, etc.	T
Erythropoietin	Renal carcinoma, nephroblastoma, renal cysts	Phaeochromocytoma, uterine fibromyoma, cerebellar haemangiosarcoma	[54]

TABLE I (cont.)

Substance	Regular or appropriate association	Ectopic production or non-neoplastic associations	Ref.
Parathyroid hormone	Parathyroid adenomas, carcinomas	Kidney, lung, liver, adrenal, parotid, spleen, breast, testis	[55]
Renin	Juxta-glomerular-cell tumours	Cerebellar haemangioblastoma	[56]
Other hormones			
Prostaglandins	Medullary carcinoma of thyroid, etc.	Breast	[57]
Catecholamines	Phaeochromocytoma, haemoblastoma		[58]
Enzymes			
Amylase	Lung		[59]
Lymphocyte adenosine triphosphate	Gastrointestinal cancer		[60]
Acid phosphatase	Prostate		[61]
Alkaline phosphatase bone isoenzyme	Osteosarcoma, bone metastases, especially breast, prostate, thyroid	Paget's disease	[61]
Liver isoenzyme	Liver metastases	Hepatocellular disease	[61]
Placental	See placental products		T
Histaminase	Medullary carcinoma of thyroid, pleural and ascitic fluid in lung, etc., carcinoma ovary		[62]

TABLE I (cont.)

Substance	Regular or appropriate association	Ectopic production or non-neoplastic associations	Ref.
Muramidase	Monocytic, mydomonocytic leukaemia, colorectal carcinoma, central nervous system (CSF)	Inflammatory disease, especially Crohn's disease	T
5-Nuclotide phosphodiesterase	Primary or secondary liver metastases		[63]
Prolyl hydroxylase	Hepatocellular carcinoma breast		[64]
Sialyl transferase	Breast, lung, colon, leukaemia and others	Rheumatoid arthritis and probably others	[65]
Tyrosinase	Melanoma, breast cancer		[66]
Other antigens			
Stomach antigen	Stomach		[67] and T
EDCL	Acute myeloid and monocytic leukaemia, carcinoma of ovary, colon, etc.		[68]
JBB5	Various leukaemias, lymphomas, melanoma, carcinoma of gastro-intestinal tract, ovary, cervix, lung	Cardiovascular disease, muscular dystrophy, hepatic and renal disease	[69]
Milk proteins			
Casein	Carcinoma of breast, bronchus and others	Pregnancy, lactation, benign tumours	T
Lactoferrin	Breast tumours	Circulating monocytes	[70]
Alpha-lactalbumin	Breast tumours		[71]

TABLE I (cont.)

Substance	Regular or appropriate association	Ectopic production or non-neoplastic associations	Ref.
Pregnancy associated			
(Non-foetal non-placental origin)			
Pregnancy associated $alpha_2$-globulin (Pregnancy associated macroglobulin)	Breast, bronchus, gastrointestinal tract, genito-urinary tract, lymphoma, sarcoma	Pregnancy, estrogen therapy, Damber et al. found no difference between cancer patients and normal controls	T
Plasma glycoprotein			
Acute phase proteins ($alpha_1$, see also $alpha_2$-H)	Cancer generally	Injury, surgery, infection, inflammation	[72]
$Alpha_2$	Colorectal metastatic disease	Injury, surgery, infection, inflammation	
$Alpha_1$-antitrypsin	Cancer generally	" "	[73] [74]
Haptoglobin	Cancer generally	" "	
Hemopexin	Cancer generally	" "	
Seromucoid	Cancer generally	" "	[75]
Modified cell surface glycoprotein	Leukaemia	" "	
Immunoglobulins	Myeloma	Various	[76] [77]
Rheumatoid factor	Carcinoma bladder	Rheumatoid diseases	[78]

TABLE I (cont.)

Substance	Regular or appropriate association	Ectopic production or non-neoplastic associations	Ref.
Plasma lipoproteins			
Alpha$_1$-lipoprotein	Decreased except with estrogen excess		[79]
Other proteins			
Myelin and cancer basic protein	Virtually all tumours, cell-mediated responses	Damage to nervous tissue, necrosis, cirrhosis	T
Ferritin (see also placental and foetal antigens and text)	Acute leukaemia, lymphomas	Cirrhosis	T
T antigen		Wide spectrum of tumours	T
Nerve growth factor	Liposarcoma, neuroblastoma, medullary cancer thyroid		[80] [81]
Plasminogen activator	Lung		[82]
Metabolic products			
Hydroxyproline	Bone and soft tissues metastases	Various	T
Methylated nucleosides and pseudouridine	Breast, lung, ovary, testis, melanoma, lymphoma, leukaemia	Inflammatory disease, psoriasis, arthritis	T
Polyamines, spermine, spermidine, putrescine	Cell death and proliferation	Inflammation and tissue regeneration	T and [83]

TABLE II. CEA: % POSITIVE VALUES IN MALIGNANT DISEASES

For assays I, II, IV, V a = 5 – 20 μg/l b > 20 μg/l
III a = 2.5 – 10 μg/l b > 20 μg/l
VI a = 12.5 – 40 μg/l b > 40 μg/l

Reference	I [130]		II [131]		III [87]		IV [132]		V [88]		VI [133]	
Site	a	b	a	b	a	b	a	b	a	b	a	b
Colorectal												
Localized	88	34	28	20	47	35	18	60	15	51	42	47
Disseminated	93	56		67								
No. in series	91		100		544		126		39		68	
Stomach												
Localized	88	34			50	19	15	25	17	29	40	6
Disseminated	93	56										
No. in series	67				79		5		17		15	
Pancreas				100	56	35	10	40	9	36	27	36
No. in series					55				11		11	
Liver											33	66
No. in series											3	
Lung												
Localized	74	17	36	30	50	26			44	16	54	16
Disseminated	88	44										
No. in series	33		30		181				50		37	
Breast												
Localized	74	17	22	22					45	0	29	18
Disseminated	88	44							3	7		
No. in series	32		9						100		79	

TABLE II (cont.)

Reference	I [130]		II [131]		III [87]		IV [132]		V [88]		VI [133]	
Site	a	b	a	b	a	b	a	b	a	b	a	b
Female genital tract												
Pre-invasive	37	0										
Localized	52	11									26	5
Disseminated	74	15										
No. in series	171										19	
Leukaemia					37	5						
Lymphoma					35	0						
Sarcoma					31	0						
No. in series					150							
Other	36	0	12	9	49	1						
No. in series	64		10		78							
Leukaemia					35	5						
Lymphoma					35	0						
Sarcoma					31	0						
Other	36	0	12	9	49	1						

TABLE III. CEA ASSAYS: NON-MALIGNANT DISEASES AND HEALTHY CONTROLS: % POSITIVES

Disease	I [130]		II [131]		III [87]		IV [132]		V [88]		VI [133]	
	a	b	a	b	a	b	a	b	a	b	a	b
G.I. tract			30	10								
No. in series			39									
Ulcerative colitis	25	8					17	8	16	4	29	0
No. in series	75						40		51		31	
Polyps	73	0			3	0	14	4			18	0
No. in series	11				90		76				11	
Diverticulitis	20	0					20	12			52	0
No. in series	14						25				8	
Pancreatitis	64	0										
No. in series	14											
Cirrhosis							15	0				
No. in series							21					
Chronic bronchitis											38	0
No. in series											16	
Hospital controls	47	0							16	0		
No. in series	100								100			
No apparent disease	3	0	5	0	1.5[a]	0	0	0[b]	2	0	8	0
No. in series	130				1425				161		60	

[a] Age dependent

[b] Studies referred to

TABLE IV. SERUM K-CASEIN VALUES IN PATIENTS WITH CARCINOMA OF BREAST

Serum K-casein (μg/litre)	< 100	100 – 200	> 200	Total + ve
Before treatment	3	5	3	8/11
Stage I post-treatment	24	7	10	17/41
Stage II post-treatment	27	8	19	27/54
Recurrent	5	3	18	21/26

REFERENCES

[1] COOPER, E.H., TURNER, R., MILFORD-WARD, A., NEVILLE, A.M., "Multiparametric tests in the monitoring of cancer", Cancer Related Antigens (FRANCHIMONT, P., Ed.), North Holland, Amsterdam (1976).

[2] HANSEN, N.E., KARLE, H., ANDERSEN, V., OLGAARD, K., Lysozyme turnover in man, J. Clin. Invest. **51** (1972) 1146.

[3] CURRIE, G.A., ECCLES, S.A., Serum lysozyme as a marker of host resistance. 1. Production by macrophages resident in rat sarcomata, Br. J. Cancer **33** (1976).

[4] SKARIN, A.T., MATSUO, Y., MOLONEY, W.C., Muramidase activity in leukaemia and myeloproliferative disorders, Oncology **27** (1973) 406.

[5] COOPER, E.H., TURNER, R., STEELE, L., GOLIGER, J.C., Blood muramidase activity in colorectal cancer, Br. Med. J. **iii** (1974) 662.

[6] NEWMAN, J., JOSEPHSON, A.S., CACATIAN, A., TSANG, A., Spinal fluid lysozyme in the diagnosis of central nervous system tumours, Lancet **ii** (1974) 755.

[7] BUFFE, D., RIMBAULT, C., BURTIN, P., Presence d'une proteine d'origine tissulaire, l'alpha$_2$-H-globuline, dans le serum de sujets atteints d'affections malignes, Int. J. Cancer **3** (1968) 850-6.

[8] CRAGG, S.J., JACOBS, A., PARRY, D.H., WAGSTAFF, M., WORWOOD, M., Isoferritins in acute leukaemia, Br. J. Cancer **35** (1977) 635.

[9] MARCUS, D.M., ZIMBERG, N., Measurement of serum ferritin by RIA: Results in normal individuals and breast cancer, J. Natl. Cancer Inst. **55** (1975) 791.

[10] STIMSON, W.H., Pregnancy associated macroglobulin, Lancet **i** (1975) 777.

[11] COOMBES, R.C., GAZET, J.C., SLOANE, J.P., POWLES, T.J., FORD, H.T., LAURENCE, D.J.R., NEVILLE, A.M., Biochemical markers in human breast cancer, Lancet **i** (1977) 132.

[12] CUSHIERI, A., FELGATE, R.A., Urinary hydroxy-proline excretion in carcinoma of breast, Br. J. Exp. Pathol. **53** (1972) 237.

[13] POWLES, T.J., LEESE, C.L., BONDY, P.K., Hydroxy-proline excretion in patients with breast cancer and response to treatment, Br. Med. J. **ii** (1975) 164.

[14] MARMOSTON, J., WEINER, J.M., HOPKINS, C.E., STEM, E., Cancer **19** (1966) 1327.

[15] NEVILLE, A.M., COOPER, E.H., Ann. Clin. Biochem. **13** (1976) 283.

[16] STEVENS, L., The biochemical role of naturally occurring polyamines in nucleic acid synthesis, Biol. Rev. **45** (1970) 1.

[17] RUSSELL, D.H., RUSSELL, S.D., Relative usefulness of measuring polyamines in serum plasma and urine as biochemical markers of cancer, Clin. Chem. **21** (1975) 860.

[18] LIPTON, A., SHEEHAN, L., MORTEL, P., HARVEY, H.A., Urinary polyamine levels in patients with localised malignancy, Cancer **38** (1976) 1344.

[19] WAALKES, T.P., GEHRKE, C.W., BLEYER, W.A., ZUMWAIT, R.W., OLWENY, C.L.M., KUO, K.C., LAKINGS, D.B., JACOBS, S.A., Potential biologic markers in Burkitt's Lymphoma, Cancer Chem. Rep. **59** (1975) 721.

[20] LEVINE, L., WAALKES, T.P., STOLBACH, L., Serum levels of N^2, N^2 dimethylguanosine and pseudouridine as determined by radioimmunoassay, J. Natl. Cancer Inst. **54** (1975) 341.

[21] SPRINGER, G.F., DESAI, P.R., YANG, H.J., MURTHY, M.S., Clin. Immunol. Immunopathol. (in press).

[22] FIELD, E.J., CASPARY, E.S., Lymphocyte sensitization. An in vitro test for cancer? , Lancet **ii** (1970) 1337.

[23] CERCEK, L., CERCEK, B., Application of the phenomenon of changes in the structuredness of cytoplasmic matrix (SCM) in the diagnosis of malignant disorders: a review, Europ. J. Cancer **13** (1977) 903.

[24] BAGSHAWE, K.D., Workshop on macrophage electrophoretic mobility (MEM) and structuredness of cytoplasmic matrix (SCM) tests, Br. J. Cancer **35** (1977) 701.

[25] BAGSHAWE, K.D., Hypokalaemia, carcinoma and Cushing's syndrome, Lancet **ii** (1960) 284.

[26] TURKINGTON, R.W., Ectopic production of prolactin, New Eng. J. Med. **285** (1971) 1455.

[27] ELLISON, M.L., WOODHOUSE, D., HILLYARD, C., DOWSETT, M., COOMBES, R.C., GILBY, E.D., GREENBERG, P.J., NEVILLE, A.M., Immunoreactive calcitonin production by human lung carcinoma cells in culture, Br. J. Cancer **32** (1975) 373.

[28] TASHJIAN, A.H., LEVINE, L., MUNSON, P.L., Immunochemical identification of parathyroid hormone in non-parathyroid neoplasma associated with hypercalcaemia, J. Exp. Med. **119** (1964) 467.

[29] MALLINSON, C.N., BLOOM, S.R., WARIN, A.P., SALMON, P.R., COX, B., A glucagon syndrome, Lancet **ii** (1974) 1.

[30] ZIMBLER, H., ROBERTSON, G.L., BARTTER, F.C., DELEA, C.S., POMEROY, T., Ewing's sarcoma as a cause of the syndrome of inappropriate secretion of antidiuretic hormone, J. Clin. Endocrinol. Metab. **41** (1975) 390.

[31] GREENWOOD, S.M., GOODMAN, J.R., SCHNEIDER, G., FORMAN, B.H., KRESS, S.C., GELB, A.F., Choriocarcinoma in Man. The relationship of gynaecomastia to chorionic somalomammotrophin and estrogens, Am. J. Med. **51** (1971) 416.

[32] PEARSE, A.G.E., The gut as an endocrine organ, Br. J. Hosp. Med. **11** (1974) 697.

[33] WILLIAMS, R.R., McINTIRE, K.R., WALDMANN, T.A., FEINLEIB, M., GO, V.L.W., KANNEL, W.B., DAWBER, T.R., CASTELLI, W.P., McNAMARA, P.M., Tumor-associated antigen levels (carcinoembryonic antigen, human chorionic gonadotrophin, and alpha-fetoprotein) antedating the diagnosis of cancer in the Framingham Study, J. Natl. Cancer Inst. **58** (1977) 1547.

[34] FRANCHIMONT, P., ZANGERLE, P.F., Present and future clinical relevance of tumour markers, Europ. J. Cancer **13** (1977) 637.

[35] YALOW, R.S., BERSON, S.A., Characteristics of 'Big ACTH' in human plasma and pituitary extracts, J. Clin. Endocrinol. Metab. **36** (1973) 415.

[36] BLOOMFIELD, G.A., HOLDAWAY, I.M., CORRIN, B., RATCLIFFE, G.M., REES, M.E., REES, L.H., Lung tumours and ACTH production, Clin. Endocrinol. (Oxf.) **6** (1977) 95.

[37] FRITSCHE, R., MACH, J.P., Identification of new oncofetal antigen associated with several types of human carcinoma, Nature (London) **258** (1975) 734.

[38] HOCH, S.C., LONGMIRE, R.L., HOCH, J.A., Unique DNA binding protein in the serum of patients with various neoplasms, Nature (London) **255** (1975) 560.

[39] PARSONS, R.G., LONGMIRE, R.L., HOCH, S.O., HOCH, J.A., A clinical evaluation of Serum C3DP in individuals with malignant diseases, Cancer Res. **37** (1977) 692.

[40] BROWN, G., CAPELLARO, D., GREAVES, M., Leukaemia-associated antigens in man, J. Natl. Cancer Inst. **55** (1975) 1281.

[41] CHISM, J.E., ORDER, S.E., HELLMAN, S., Tumor-fetal antigens in Hodgkin's disease: an immunoelectrophoretic analysis, Am. J. Roentgenol., Radium Ther. Nucl. Med. **117** (1973) 5.

[42] BANWO, O., VERSEY, J., HOBBS, J.R., New oncofetal antigen for human pancreas, Lancet **i** (1974) 643.

[43] HIRSHAUT, Y., PEI, D.T., MARCOVE, R.C., MULCHERJI, B., SPIELWOGEL, A.R., ESSNER, E., Seroepidemiology of human sarcoma antigen (S_1), New Eng. J. Med. **291** (1974) 1103.

[44] UPTON, V., AMATRUDA, T.T., Evidence for the presence of tumour peptides with corticotrophin-releasing-factor-like activity in the atopic ACTH syndrome, New Eng. J. Med. **285** (1971) 419.

[45] FAIMAN, C., COLWELL, J.A., RYAN, R.J., HERSHMAN, J.M., SHIELDS, T.W., Gonadotrophin secretion from a bronchogenic carcinoma, New Eng. J. Med. **277** (1967) 1395.

[46] NIEWENHJYGEN, K., BOTS, G.T., LINDEMAN, J., SCHABERG, A., Use of immunohistochemical and morphologic methods for the identification of human growth hormone producing pituitary adenomas, Cancer **38** (1976) 1162.

[47] HAMILTON, B.P., Presence of hemophysin proteins in tumours associated with the syndrome of inappropriate ADH secretion, Ann. N.Y. Acad. Sci. **248** (1975) 153.

[48] FRANKS, S., NABARRO, J.D.N., JACOBS, H.S., Prevalence and presentation of hyperprolactinaemia in patients with 'functionless' pituitary tumours, Lancet **i** (1977) 778.

[49] FAGLIA, G., FERRARI, C., NERI, V., BERK-PECCOZ, P., AMBROSI, B., VALENTINI, F., High plasma thyrotropin levels in two patients with pituitary tumour, Acta Endocrinol. **69** (1972) 649.

[50] MARKS, V., Diagnosis of Insuloma, Gut **12** (1971) 835.

[51] MALLINSON, C.N., BLOOM, S.R., WARIN, A.P., SALMON, P.R., COX, B., A Glucagon syndrome, Lancet **ii** (1974) 1.

[52] COCCO, A.E., CONWAY, S.J., Zollinger Ellison syndrome associated with ovarian mucous cystadenocarcinoma, New Eng. J. Med. **293** (1975) 485.

[53] LARSSON, L., HIRSCH, M.A., HOLST, J.J., INGEMANSSON, S., KUHL, C., JENSEN, S.L., LUNDQUIST, G., REHFELD, J.F., SCHWARTZ, T.W., Pancreatic somatostatinoma, Lancet **i** (1977) 666.

[54] DONATI, R.M., McCARTHY, J.M., LANGE, R., GALLAGHER, N.I., Erythropoietin and neoplastin tumors, Ann. Int. Med. 58 (1963) 47.

[55] PALMIERI, G.M.A., NORDQUIST, R.E., OMENN, G.S., Immunochemical localisation of parathyroid hormone in cancer tissue from patients with ectopic hyperparathyroidism, J. Clin. Invest. **53** (1971) 1726.

[56] VOUTE, P.A., VAN DER MEER, J., STANGAARD-KLOOSTERZIEL, W., Plasma renin activity in Wilm's tumour, Acta Endocrinol. **67** (1971) 197.

[57] JAFFE, B.M., Prostaglandins and cancer: an update, Prostaglandins **6** (1974) 453.

[58] KASER, H., Circular thin-layer chromatography for diagnosis and follow-up of neural crest tumours, J. Chromatog. 82 (1973) 127.

[59] AMMANN, R.W., BERK, E., FRIDHANDLER, L., UEDA, M., WEGMANN, N., Hyperamylasaemia with carcinoma of lung, Ann. Intern. Med. 78 (1973) 521.

[60] DIMITROV, N.V., ELLEGAARD, J., Elevated lymphocyte adenosine triphosphate activity in patients with gastrointestinal carcinoma, New Eng. J. Med. 286 (1972) 353.

[61] BODANSKY, O., Biochemistry of Human Cancer, Academic Press (1975).

[62] LIN, C.W., OREUTT, M.L., STOLBACH, L.L., Elevation of histaminase and its concurrence with Regan isoenzyme in ovarian cancer, Cancer Res. 35 (1975) 2762.

[63] TSOU, K.C., McCOY, M.G., LO, K.W., An isoenzyme of 5-nucleotide phosphodiesterase and α-fetoprotein in human hepatic cancer patient sera, Cancer Res. **34** (1974) 2459.

[64] BAILLIE, J., AL ADNANI, M.S., PATRICK, R.S., KIRRANE, J.A., McGEE, J. O'D., The expression of prolyl hydroxylase and collagen by premalignant and malignant hepatocytes, Proc. Path. Soc. Great Brit. and Ireland, July 1975, p.21.

[65] KESSEL, D., ALLEN, J., Elevated plasma sialyltransferase in the cancer patient, Cancer Res. 35 (1975) 670.

[66] CHEN, Y.M., CHAVIN, W., Serum tyrosinase in malignant disease, Oncology **31** (1975) 147.

[67] DEUTSCH, E., APFFEL, C.A., MORI, H., WALKER, J.E., A tumor associated antigen in gastric cancer secretions, Cancer Res. 33 (1973) 112.

[68] RUDMAN, D., CHAWLA, R.K., HEYMSFIELD, S.B., BETHEL, R.A., SHOJI, M., VOGLER, W.R., NIXON, D.W., Urinary excretion of the cancer related glycoprotein EDCL, Ann. Intern. Med. 86 (1977) 174.

[69] CHAWLA, R.K., HEYMSFIELD, S.B., WADSWORTH, A.A., SHOJI, M., RUDMAN, D., Isolation and characterisation of a patient with carcinoma of colon, Cancer Res. **37** (1977) 873.

[70] RUMKE, P.H., VISSER, D., KWA, H.G., HART, A.M., Radio-immunoassay of lactoferrin in blood plasma of breast cancer patients, lactating and normal women, Folia Med. Nederl. **14** (1971) 156.

[71] ROSE, H.N., McGRATH, C.M., α-Lactalbumin production in human mammary carcinoma, Science **190** (1975) 673.

[72] COOPER, E.H., TURNER, R., STEELE, L., NEVILLE, A.M., MACKAY, A., The contribution of serum enzymes and carcinoembryonic antigen to the early diagnosis of metastatic colorectal cancer, Br. J. Cancer **31** (1975) 111.

[73] KEMP, J.H., JOHNSTONE, J.M., Evaluation of serum trypsin inhibitor activity in the detection of malignant disease, Br. J. Cancer **8** (1964) 390.

[74] TALERMAN, A., HAIJE, W.G., BAGGERMAN, L., Alpha-1-antitrypsin and alpha-fetoprotein in sera of patients with germ cell neoplasms, Int. J. Cancer **19** (1977) 741.

[75] HARSHMAN, S., REYNOLDS, V.H., NEWMASTER, T., PATIKAS, T., WORRALL, T., The prognostic significance of serial seromucoid analysis in patients with cancer, Cancer **34** (1974) 291.

[76] HOBBS, J.R., Immunochemical classes of myelomatosis. Including data from a therapeutic trial by a Medical Research Council Working Party, Br. J. Haematol. **16** (1969) 599.

[77] SALMON, S.E., SMITH, B.A., Immunoglobulin synthesis and total body tumor cell number in IgG multiple myeloma, J. Clin. Invest. **49** (1970) 1114.

[78] PYRHONEN, S., TIMONEN, T., HEIKKINEN, A., PENTTINEN, K., OLFTAN, O., SAKSELA, E., WAGER, O., Rheumatoid factor as an indicator of serum blocking activity and tumour recurrences in bladder tumours, Europ. J. Cancer **12** (1976) 87.

[79] NYDEGGER, U.E., BUTLER, R.E., Serum lipoprotein levels in patients with cancer, Cancer Res. **32** (1972) 1756.

[80] HERSHMAN, H.R., LERNER, M.P., Production of a nervous-system-specific protein by human neuroblastoma cells in culture, Nature (London) New Biol. **241** (1973) 242.

[81] BIGAZZI, M., REVOLTELLA, R., CASCIANO, S., VIGNETI, E., High level of a nerve growth factor in the serum of a patient with medullary carcinoma of thyroid, Clin. Endocrinol. (Oxf.) **6** (1977) 105.

[82] DAVIDSON, J.F., McNICOL, G.P., FRANK, G.L., ANDERSON, J.J., DOUGLAS, A.S., Plasminogen-activator-producing tumour, Br. Med. J. **i** (1969) 88.

[83] DURIE, B.G.M., SALMON, S.E., RUSSELL, D.H., Polyamines as markers of response and disease activity in cancer chemotherapy, Cancer Res. **37** (1977) 214.

[84] GOLD, P., FREEDMAN, S.O., Demonstration of tumour-specific antigens in human colonic carcinomata by immunological tolerance and absorption techniques, J. Exp. Med. **121** (1965) 439.

[85] ROGERS, G.T., LEAKE, B.A., SEARLE, F., BAGSHAWE, K.D., Heterogeneity and specificity of circulating carcinoembryonic antigen, Eur. J. Cancer **13** (1977) 293.

[86] THOMSON, D.M.P., KRUPEY, J., FREEDMAN, S.O., GOLD, P., The radioimmunoassay of circulating carcinoembryonic antigens of the human digestive system, Proc. Natl. Acad. Sci. USA **64** (1969) 161.

[87] HANSEN, H.J., SNYDER, J.J., Carcinoembryonic antigen assay. A laboratory adjunct in the diagnosis and management of cancer, Hum. Pathol. **5** (1974) 138.

[88] SEARLE, F., LOVESEY, A.C., ROBERTS, B.A., ROGERS, G.T., BAGSHAWE, K.D., Radioimmunoassay methods for carcinoembryonic antigen, J. Immunol. Methods **4** (1974) 113.

[89] KHOO, S.K., HUNT, P.S., MACKAY, I.R., Studies of carcinoembryonic antigen activity of whole and extracted serum in ulcerative colitis, Gut **14** (1973) 545.

[90] BAGSHAWE, K.D., SEARLE, F., "Tumour markers", *in* Essays in Medical Biochemistry, No.3, The Biochemical Journal (in press).

[91] DAS, S., DAS, B.R., TERRY, W.D., Modifications and evaluation of double antibody radioimmunoassay of human carcinoembryonic antigen, Cancer Res. **36** (1976) 1954.

[92] MACKAY, A.M., PATEL, S., CARTER, S., STEVENS, V., LAURENCE, D.J.R., COOPER, E.H., NEVILLE, A.M., Role of serial plasma carcinoembryonic antigen assays in detection of recurrent and metastatic colorectal carcinoma, Br. Med. J. **iv** (1974) 382.

[93] BRAUNSTEIN, G.D., HCG in testis, New Eng. J. Med. **293** (1975) 1339.

[94] CHEN, H.C., HODGEN, G.D., MATSUURA, S., LIN, L.J., GROSS, E., REICHERT, L.E., BIRKEN, S.V., CANFIELD, R.E., ROSS, G.T., Proc. Natl. Acad. Sci. **73** (1976) 2885.

[95] MITCHELL, H.D., BAGSHAWE, K.D., Human Chorionic Gonadotrophin in Hormone Assays and their Clinical Application (LORAINE, J.A., BELL, E.T., Eds), Churchill Livingstone, Edinburgh (1976).

[96] KARDANA, A., BAGSHAWE, K.D., A rapid, sensitive and specific radioimmunoassay for human chorionic gonadotrophin, J. Immunol. Methods **9** (1976) 297.

[97] MUGGIA, F.M., ROSEN, S.W., WEINTRAUB, B.D., HANSEN, H.H., Ectopic placental proteins in non-trophoblastic tumours. Serial measurements following chemotherapy, Cancer **36** (1975) 1327.

[98] BAGSHAWE, K.D., WILSON, H., DUBLON, P., SMITH, A., BALDWIN, M., KARDANA, A., Follow-up after hydatidiform mole. Studies using radioimmunoassay for urinary human chorionic gonadotrophins, J. Obstet. Gynaecol. Br. Commonw. **80** (1973) 461.

[99] BAGSHAWE, K.D., "Recent observations related to the chemotherapy and immunology of gestational choriocarcinoma", Advances in Cancer Research 18, Academic Press, New York (1973) 231.

[100] BAGSHAWE, K.D., HARLAND, S., Immunodiagnosis and monitoring of gonadotrophin-producing metastases in the central nervous system, Cancer **38** (1976) 112.

[101] PERLIN, E., ENGELER, J.E., EDSON, M., KARP, D., McINTIRE, K.R., WALDMANN, T.A., The value of serial measurement of human chorionic gonadotropin and alpha-fetoprotein for monitoring germinal cell tumors, Cancer **37** (1976) 215.

[102] HOFFKEN, K., SCHMIDT, C.G., Z. Krebsforsch. 87 (1976) 37.

[103] VAITUKAITIS, J., Immunologic and physical characterisation of human chorionic gonadotrophin (hCG) secreted by tumours, J. Clin. Endocrinol. Metab. **37** (1973) 505.

[104] NAUGHTON, M.A., MERRILL, D.A., McMANUS, L.M., FINK, L.M., Localization of the β chain of human chorionic gonadotrophin on human tumour and placental cells, Cancer Res. **35** (1975) 1887.

[105] HORNE, C.H.W., REID, I.N., MILNE, G.D., Prognostic significance of inappropriate production of pregnancy proteins by breast cancers, Lancet ii (1976) 279.

[106] BOHN, H., Studies on the pregnancy-specific β_1-glycoprotein (SP_1), Arch. Gynaekol. 216 (1974) 347.

[107] LIN, T.M., HALBERT, S.P., SPELLACY, W.N., Measurement of pregnancy-associated plasma proteins during human gestation, J. Clin. Invest. **54** (1974) 576.

[108] TATARINOV, Y.S., MESNYANKINA, N.V., NIKOULINA, D.M., NOVIKOVA, L.A., TOLOKNOV, B.O., FALALEEVA, D.M., Immunochemical identification of beta$_1$-globulin of the "pregnancy zone" in serum of patients with trophoblastic tumors, Inst. J. Cancer **14** (1974) 548.

[109] FISHMAN, W.H., Immunologic and biochemical approaches to alkaline phosphatase isoenzyme analysis. The Regan isoenzyme, Ann. N.Y. Acad. Sci. **166** (1969) 745.

[110] JACOBY, B., BAGSHAWE, K.D., A radioimmunoassay for placental-type alkaline phosphatase, Cancer Res. **32** (1972) 2413.

[111] CADEAU, B.J., BLACKSTEIN, M.E., MALKIN, A, Increased incidence of placenta-like alkaline phosphatase activity in breast and genito-urinary cancer, Cancer Res. **34** (1974) 729.

[112] FISHMAN, L., MIYAYAMA, H., DRISCOLL, S.G., FISHMAN, W.H., Developmental phase-specific alkaline phosphatase isoenzymes of human placenta and their occurrence in human cancer, Cancer Res. **36** (1976) 2268.

[113] RUOSLAHTI, E., SEPPALA, M., Studies of carcinofoetal proteins: physical and chemical properties of human α-foetoprotein, Int. J. Cancer **7** (1971) 218.

[114] RUOSLAHTI, E., PIHKO, H., Effect of chemical modification on the immunogenicity of homologous α-foetoprotein, Annals N.Y. Acad. Sci. **259** (1975) 85.

[115] ALPERT,E., PERENCEVICH, R.C., Human α-foetoprotein: immunochemical analysis of isoproteins, Annals N.Y. Acad. Sci. **259** (1975) 131.

[116] SIZARET, P., BRESLOW, N., ANDERSON, S.G.,et al., Collaborative study of a preparation of human cord serum for its use as a reference in the assay of α-foetoprotein, J. Biol. Standardization 3 (1975) 201.

[117] RUOSLAHTI, E., SEPPÄLÄ, M., Studies of carcinofoetal proteins III: Development of a radioimmunoassay for α-foetoprotein in the serum of healthy adults, Int. J. Cancer 8 (1971) 374.

[118] BAGSHAWE, K.D., Computer controlled automated radioimmunoassay, Lab. Pract. **24** (1975) 573.

[119] SEPPÄLÄ, M., RUOSLAIITI, E., α-Foetoprotein in normal and pregnancy sera, Lancet i (1972) 375.

[120] WALDMANN, T.A., McINTIRE, K.R., The use of a radioimmunoassay for α-fetoprotein in the diagnosis of malignancy, Cancer **34** (1974) 1510.
[121] TSUNG, S.H., α-Foetoprotein in lung cancer metastatic to the liver, Arch. Pathol. **99** (1975) 267.
[122] ZISHORSKY, N., KORDAC, V., MASOPUST, J., OBROVSKA, D., STEPAN, J., α-Foetoprotein and carcinoembryonic antigen in a patient with carcinoid of stomach, Gann **65** (1974) 193.
[123] TEILUM, G., ALBREDITSEN, R., NORGAARD-PEDERSEN, B., Histogenetic embryologic basis for reappearance of α-foetoprotein in endodermal sinus tumour and teratoma, Acta. Pathol. Microbiol. Scand., 83A **i** (1975) 80.
[124] MATSUMOTO, Y., SUZUKI, T., ONO, H., NAKASE, A., HONJO, I., Response of alpha-fetoprotein to chemotherapy in patients with hepatomas, Cancer **34** (1974) 1602.
[125] PURVES, L.R., Primary liver cancer in man as a possible short duration seasonal cancer, S. African J. Science **69** (1973) 173.
[126] MELVIN, K.E.W., MILLER, H.H., TASHJIAN, A.H., Early diagnosis of medullary carcinoma of thyroid gland by means of calcitonin assay, New Eng. J. Med. **285** (1971) 1115.
[127] COOMBES, R.C., HILLYARD, C., GREENBERG, P.B., MacINTYRE, I., Plasma immunoreactive calcitonin in patients with non-thyroid tumours, Lancet **i** (1974) 1080.
[128] HENDRICK, J.C., FRANCHIMONT, P., Radioimmunoassay of casein in the serum of normal subjects and patients with various malignancies, Eur. J. Cancer **10** (1974) 725.
[129] WOODS, R.L., SEARLE, F.S., BAGSHAWE, K.D., K-casein concentrations in patients with benign and malignant breast diseases, Br. J. Cancer **35** (1977) 256.
[130] KHOO, S.K., Radioimmunoassay for carcinoembryonic antigen: its application to diagnosis and post-treatment follow-up of human cancer, Med. J. Aust. **1** (1974) 1025.
[131] MACH, J.P., PUSZTASZERI, G., DYSLI, M., KAPP, F., BIERENS de HAAN, B., LOOSLI, R.M., GROB, P., ISLIKER, B., Dosage radio-immunologique de l'antigène carcinoembryonnaire (CEA), Schweiz. Med. Wochenschr. **103** (1973) 365.
[132] JOINT NAT. CANCER INST. CANCER/AM. CANCER SOC. INVESTIGATION, A collaborative study of a test for carcinoembryonic antigen in the sera of patients with carcinoma of colon and rectum, Can. Med. Assoc. J. **107** (1972) 25.
[133] LAURENCE, D.J.R., STEVENS, U., BETTELHEIM, R., DARCY, D., LEESE, C., TURBERVILLE, C., ALEXANDER, P., JOHNS, E.W., NEVILLE, A.M., Role of plasma carcinoembryonic antigen in diagnosis of gastrointestinal, mammary and bronchial carcinoma, Br. Med. J. **iii** (1972) 605.

DISCUSSION

D.W. WILSON: We at the Tenovus Institute, together with the British Prostate Study Group, are involved in the determination of various steroids and polypeptides, as well as tumour markers, in the plasma of patients with cancer of the prostate. The initial objective of the study was to relate concentrations of these substances, before treatment, to the stage of the disease according to the TNM classification of the Union Internationale contre le Cancer.

To accomplish this satisfactorily, we found it necessary: (a) to establish efficient internal quality-control schemes that would ensure reliability of assay performance over a number of years; (b) to lay down definitive mass-spectroscopic methods to evaluate the accuracy of the steroid RIA procedures; and (c) to utilize sophisticated multivariate statistical techniques such as canonical variate and discriminant function analyses to elicit valuable information which may not otherwise be revealed.

We have reviewed facets of curve-fitting for standard hormone concentrations, internal quality controls and statistical analysis (Wilson, D.W. and Tan, S.E., Tenovus Workshop on Tumour Markers, Alpha Omega Publishers, Cardiff (1977)) but I would appreciate your comments on some of these points.

K.D. BAGSHAWE: I agree, of course, that quality control is important in relation to tumour markers as it is in all other areas of assay measurement; the problems are not specific to tumour markers.

P. VASSILAKOS: Have you any information about the stability of CEA when the serum samples are stored at – 20°C?

K.D. BAGSHAWE: Although – 20°C is said by some biochemists to be unsuitable for long-term storage of peptides, we have evidence that the loss of immunoreactivity of CEA in specimens of serum stored at this temperature for periods of three months is not significant.

A. MALKIN: Would you care to comment on the use of markers in helping to "stratify" patients among prognostic groups for analysing the effect of treatment?

K.D. BAGSHAWE: In some situations marker values are of critical importance in staging and "stratification". In choriocarcinoma and in malignant teratoma the markers have important prognostic implications since they reflect total tumour burden. For tumours where marker measurements provide less decisive and less reliable information it is not possible to "stratify" on the basis of marker information but marker data may be incorporated in some form of multivariate analysis. In general, clinicians do not feel they can make decisions affecting the treatment of individual patients with breast cancer, on the basis of group data, unless the probability that a marker value is associated with metastatic disease is very high.

J. HAMMERSTEIN (*Chairman*): In his lecture at the start of the Symposium (SM-220/201) Dr. Odell mentioned that pro-ACTH, β-lipotropin, the α-unit of glycopeptide hormones and some octapeptides were suitable as markers for lung cancer. Would you care to comment on this?

K.D. BAGSHAWE: Dr. Odell's report of his findings was most interesting, and the incidence of pro-ACTH in lung cancer which he mentioned was substantially higher than in previous reports from other workers. The range of concentrations he reported in the tumour tissue was very great although the range of serum concentrations was of a lower order of magnitude. The problem is of course that an association between a substance and the clinical presence of tumour is not, by itself, enough to make it a useful marker. To be useful in the clinic it must provide information not available from other means. This is why I have tried to emphasize the ability to detect sub-clinical disease as the primary attribute of a useful marker. With the markers to which Dr. Odell referred it will be interesting to see whether they provide such information.

IAEA-SM-220/90

A DIFFERENT APPROACH TO THE RADIOIMMUNOASSAY OF THYROTROPHIN-RELEASING HORMONE

T.J. VISSER, W. KLOOTWIJK,
R. DOCTER, G. HENNEMANN
Medical Faculty,
Erasmus University,
Rotterdam, The Netherlands

Abstract

A DIFFERENT APPROACH TO THE RADIOIMMUNOASSAY OF THYROTROPHIN-RELEASING HORMONE.

Thyrotrophin-releasing hormone (TRH) was linked to haemocyanin by means of a dinitrophenylene moiety. TRH (pGlu-His-Pro-NH_2) was reacted with a large excess of 1,5-difluoro-2,4-dinitrobenzene to yield N^{im}-[5-fluoro-2,4-dinitrophenyl]TRH. After removal of excess reagent the derivative was coupled to haemocyanin with a minimum of side-reactions. From two rabbits out of four immunized with this material, valuable antisera were obtained which were used in the radioimmunoassay of the hypothalamic hormone at a final dilution of 1:7 500 and 1:15 000, respectively. The properties, especially with regard to specificity, of these antisera were studied and compared with another antiserum which was obtained using a conjugate having TRH linked to thyroglobulin via a p-azophenylacetyl moiety. Despite the difference between the derivatives, i.e. the nature and the point of attachment of the side chains, the specificities of the assays were very similar. Deamidation of TRH, deletion of either one of the terminal residues, hydrolysis of the lactam of the pyroglutamyl residue, and replacing Pro-NH_2 by Pro-Gly-NH_2 or by an octapeptide chain, yield peptides with strongly diminished cross-reactivities. However, N^{im}-benzyl-TRH and pGlu-Phe-Pro-NH_2 were 5–10 times more active than TRH, probably because of a closer physico-chemical similarity to the arrangement of the haptens in the conjugates. This suggests that the sensitivity of the radioimmunoassay may be increased markedly by converting TRH into the N^{im}-dinitrophenyl derivative and by using a related compound for radioiodination.

INTRODUCTION

For the production of antisera to thyrotrophin-releasing hormone (TRH; pGlu-His-Pro-NH_2; compound *1* [1] in Fig.1), the hormone has to be rendered antigenic by coupling it to immunogenic proteins. Bis-diazotized benzidine (BDB) has been used almost exclusively in the preparation of TRH-protein conjugates [1]. In this procedure, BDB is reacted simultaneously with an equimolar amount of TRH and protein to yield, among others, compound *2*. Obviously this is only one

[1] Numbers in italics refer to the compounds listed in Fig.1.

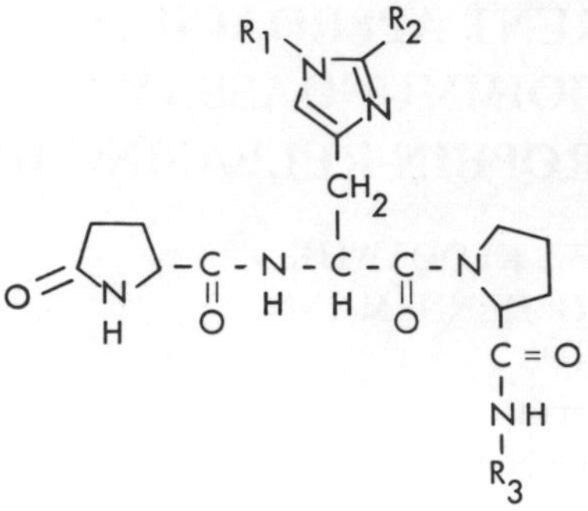

Compound	R_1	R_2	R_3
1	H	H	H
2	H	-N=N-⟨O⟩-⟨O⟩-N=N-Ⓟ	H
3	H	-N=N-⟨O⟩-CH_2-COOH	H
4	H	-N=N-⟨O⟩-CH_2-C(=O)-Ⓟ	H
5	H	H	-Ⓟ
6	-⟨O⟩(F)(NO_2)-NO_2	H	H
7	-⟨O⟩(Ⓟ)(NO_2)-NO_2	H	H
8	H	I	H
9	-CH_2-⟨O⟩	H	H
10	-⟨O⟩(NO_2)-NO_2	H	H

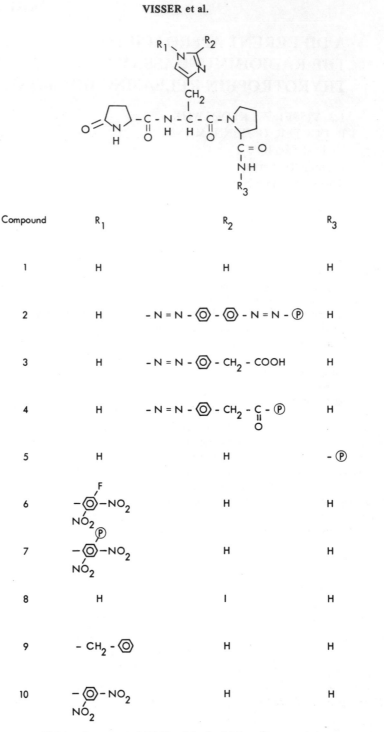

FIG.1. Structure of TRH and its derivatives (Ⓟ, protein).

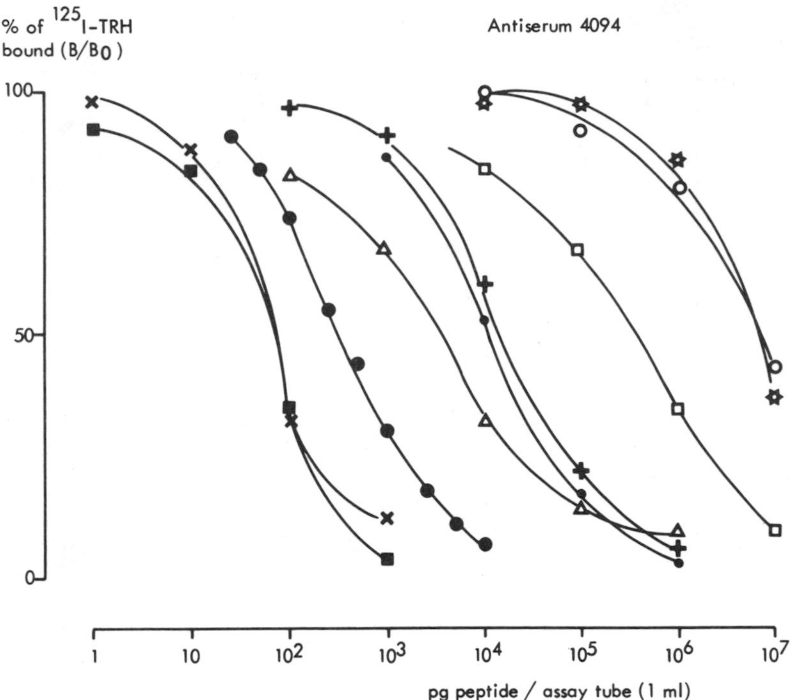

FIG.2. Displacement of [^{125}I]TRH from antiserum 4094 (final dilution 1:15 000) by increasing concentrations of TRH(●), Glu-His-Pro-NH$_2$ (·), His-Pro-NH$_2$ (○), pGlu-N^{im}Bzl-His-Pro-NH$_2$ (■), pGlu-N^{im}Bzl-His-Pro-OCH$_3$ (Δ), pGlu-N^{im}Bzl-His-Pro-OH (□), LH-RH (★), pGlu-Phe-Pro-NH$_2$ (x) and pGlu-His-Pro-Gly-NH$_2$ (+).

of the possible reactions since one mole of reagent can react with two moles of TRH or with reactive groups on the protein, e.g. ϵNH_2-groups, tyrosyl and histidyl residues [2], resulting in the formation of intra- and inter-molecular cross-links. Consequently, much of the reagent is lost and large, insoluble complexes are formed.

To circumvent these problems one can use an asymmetrical bifunctional reagent. For this approach, p-aminophenylacetic acid was chosen [3, 4]. This reagent is diazotized and subsequently reacted with TRH; the derivative *(3)* is then attached via the COOH-group to protein with the aid of a carvodiimide *(4)*. Another TRH-protein conjugate, which does not involve the imidazole of the tripeptide, has been obtained [5] by the formation of an amide bond between pGlu-His-Pro-OH and NH_2-groups of a protein carrier *(5)*.

We have recently reported [6, 7] the coupling of TRH to keyhole limpet haemocyanin (HC) according to the method of Tager [8]. In this method, TRH is reacted with a large excess of 1,5-difluoro-2,4-dinitrobenzene (DFDNB) giving

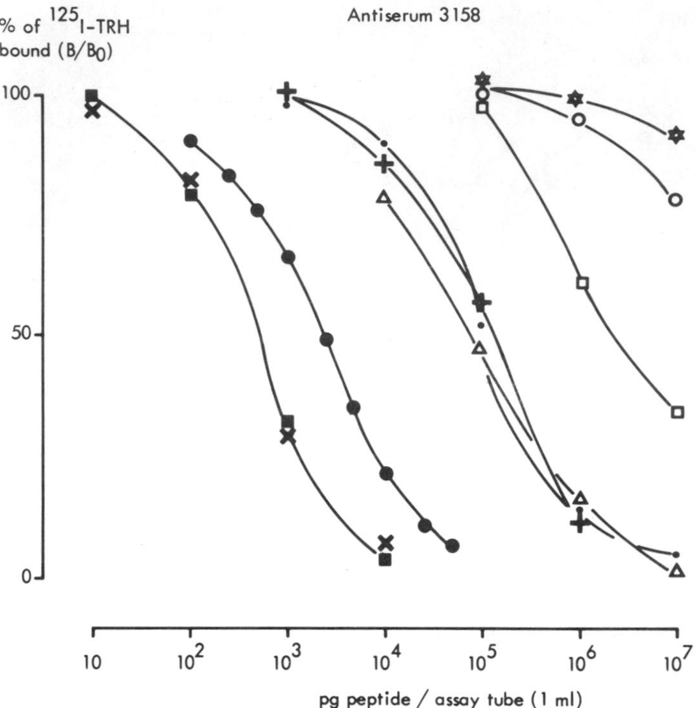

FIG. 3. Displacement of [^{125}I]TRH from antiserum 3158 (final dilution 1:2 000) by TRH and analogous peptides. (For explanation of symbols see legend to Fig. 2.)

compound *6* which, after the removal of excess reagent, is attached to haemocyanin *(7)*.

In the present paper we describe and compare the characteristics of antisera raised against conjugates with TRH anchored either by way of the p-azophenylacetyl (APA) *(4)* or through the dinitrophenylene (DNP) *(7)* moiety.

METHODS

Preparation of TRH-protein conjugates

TRH was coupled to bovine thyroglobulin (Tg) with the APA bridge (TRH-APA-Tg) as previously described [4].

The TRH-DNP-HC conjugate was prepared as follows [6–8]. TRH (2.5 mg in 0.2 ml 0.1M phosphate, pH 7.2) was reacted with DFDNB (30 mg in 1 ml methanol) for 15 min at 22°C. Excess reagent was removed by several washings

TABLE I. CROSS-REACTIVITY OF VARIOUS TRH ANALOGUES WITH ANTI-TRH ANTISERA

Analogue	Cross-reactivity (%)[a]		
	Antiserum 4094[b]	Antiserum 4101[b]	Antiserum 3158[b]
pGlu-His-Pro-NH_2 (TRH)	100	100	100
Glu-His-Pro-NH_2	3.3	4.0	2.4
pGlu-His-Pro-OH	$<$0.005	$<$0.005	$<$0.025
Glu-His-Pro-OH	$<$0.005	$<$0.005	$<$0.025
His-Pro-NH_2	0.006	0.006	0.025
pGlu-His-OH	$<$0.005	$<$0.005	$<$0.025
pGlu-His-OCH_3	$<$0.005	$<$0.005	$<$0.025
pGlu-N^{im}Bzl-His-Pro-NH_2	560	1100	560
pGlu-N^{im}Bzl-His-Pro-OCH_3	11.6	0.8	3.7
pGlu-N^{im}Bzl-His-Pro-OH	0.11	0.03	0.13
pGlu-His-Trp-Ser-Tyr-Gly-Leu-Arg-Pro-Gly-NH_2 (LH-RH)	0.02	0.02	$<$0.05
pGlu-Phe-Pro-NH_2	460	580	460
pGlu-His-Pro-Gly-NH_2	2.6	4.6	2.1

[a] Cross-reactivity is defined as the ratio (X 100) of the concentration of TRH over that of the analogue, both of which displace 50% of [^{125}I]TRH from the antiserum.

[b] 4094, antiserum raised against TRH-DNP-HC; final dilution, 1:15 000.
4101, antiserum raised against TRH-DNP-HC; final dilution, 1:7 500.
3158, antiserum raised against TRH-APA-Tg; final dilution, 1:2 000.

with ether. To the aqueous phase containing N^{im}-[5-fluoro-2,4-dinitrophenyl]TRH (FDNP-TRH) was added HC (25 mg in 0.8 ml 0.1M borate, pH 10.0) and the reaction was allowed to proceed for 24 h at 22°C. The mixture was dialysed exhaustively against water and from the recovery of added [^{3}H]TRH it was calculated that approx. 450 mols TRH were attached to each mol. HC.

Radioimmunoassay (RIA) of TRH

Antisera against the conjugates were raised in rabbits as described elsewhere [4, 7]. A useful antiserum was raised against TRH-APA-Tg in one animal (No.3158) out of four and against TRH-DNP-HC in two (Nos. 4094 and 4101) out of four. [^{125}I]TRH *(8)* was prepared using a modification [4] of the Chloramine-T method [9]. The specific activity of [^{125}I]TRH was always better than 300 μCi/μg. The antiserum dilution chosen bound approx. 30% of the added [^{125}I]TRH (20 000 counts/min). RIA of TRH was performed as set out before (final volume, 1 ml) using the second antibody method [4].

RESULTS

Figure 2 shows a typical standard curve for TRH from the assay using one of the anti-(TRH-DNP-HC) antisera (No.4094). Very similar results were obtained with antiserum 4101. The sensitivity of the RIAs was found to be approx. 10–25 pg/tube. Figure 3 shows the standard curve of the assay utilizing the anti-(TRH-APA-Tg) antiserum 3158. Here, the sensitivity amounted to approx. 50 pg TRH/tube. The dose-response curves for several analogues are also displayed in Figs 2 and 3. Table I gives the relative affinity of the various peptides for the three antisera.

DISCUSSION

The use of a large excess of the symmetrical bifunctional reagent DFDNB to convert TRH into the N^{im}-FDNP derivative *(6)* assures a high degree of reaction and minimizes dimerization (TRH-DNP-TRH formation) of the hormone [8]. Under the conditions used at this stage, hydrolysis of the reagent does not take place [8]. After removal of excess DFDNB, coupling of FDNP-TRH to HC is accomplished conveniently. Because of the lack of serious side-reactions, this method seems to be advantageous over techniques described so far [1, 3–5] for the preparation of TRH-protein conjugates.

An essential difference between the methods used in this paper is that the diazonium reagents add to the C-2 and C-4 positions of the imidazole [2], as does radioactive iodine [10], whereas the reaction with DFDNB takes place at one of the nitrogens [11]. Despite this difference in point of attachment of the side chains connecting the hormone with the protein carrier, the properties of the antisera are strikingly similar (Table I). Deamidation of TRH (yielding pGlu-His-Pro-OH), deletion of one of the terminal residues (pGlu-His-OH and His-Pro-NH_2), hydrolysis of the lactam of the pyroglutamyl residue (Glu-His-Pro-NH_2) and replacement of Pro-NH_2 by Pro-Gly-NH_2 (pGlu-His-Pro-Gly-NH_2) or by an octapeptide chain (luteinizing hormone-releasing hormone, LH-RH) result in an almost complete loss of immunoreactivity. Substitution of a benzyl (Bzl) group for the N^{im}-hydrogen in TRH and pGlu-His-Pro-OH to yield pGlu-N^{im}Bzl-His-Pro-NH_2 *(9)* and pGlu-N^{im}Bzl-His-Pro-OH, respectively, favours the interaction of the peptides with all antisera to a large extent. Replacement of His by Phe (pGlu-Phe-Pro-NH_2) also results in an increased affinity for the antisera.

The high activity of pGlu-N^{im}Bzl-His-Pro-NH_2 compared with that of TRH may be caused by its closer resemblance to the structural arrangement of the haptens in the conjugates. The aromatic moiety attached to the imidazole of TRH may be part of the antigenic determinant in the conjugates.

Recently, similar observations have been made by other investigators involved with the development of RIAs of steroids (e.g. Ref. [12]). In these studies it was noted that radioiodinated derivatives of steroids showed increased affinities for antibodies if the latter were raised against conjugates in which similar derivatives of the hapten were coupled to protein. We have also shown previously [5] that antibodies developed against the condensation product of pGlu-His-Pro-OH and albumin bind TRH approx. 100 times more avidly than the free acid. This – although to a lesser extent – has also been observed in the RIA of prostaglandins [13]. Halsey et al. [14] demonstrated that anti-DNP antibody binds DNP-lysine 10–100 times more strongly than dinitroaniline. These findings indicate that the moiety linking the hapten to the protein carrier is recognized by the antibody even if this side-chain was originally part of the protein.

It may therefore be expected that the N^{im}-DNP derivative of TRH will possess an affinity for antisera 4094 and 4101 which exceeds that of the N^{im}-Bzl derivative. Since N^{im}-DNP-TRH *(10)* is easily obtained [15], studies are now in progress in our laboratory to investigate the possibility to increase the sensitivity of the RIA by prior conversion of TRH into this compound and by using an analogous derivative for labelling with ^{125}I.

The high potency of pGlu-Phe-Pro-NH_2 may be explained by assuming that the basicity of the imidazole of TRH in the conjugates is decreased because of the electron-withdrawing properties of the side-chain bridging the hapten to the carrier. This effect may also contribute to some extent to the increased potency of N^{im}-Bzl-TRH.

ACKNOWLEDGEMENTS

The authors would like to thank Prof. Dr. H.C. Beyerman and Dr. J.L.H. Syrier (Technische Hogeschool, Delft, The Netherlands), Dr. A.O. Geiszler (Abbott, North Chicago, Ill., USA), Drs. D. Gillessen and R.O. Studer (Hoffman-LaRoche, Basel, Switzerland) and Dr. M. von der Ohe (Hoechst, Frankfurt, FRG) for providing them with the various synthetic peptides. Thanks are also due to Mrs. C. Boot for secretarial assistance.

REFERENCES

[1] BASSIRI, R.M., UTIGER, R.D., Endocrinology **90** (1972) 722.
[2] GLAZER, A.N., DeLANGE, R.J., SIGMAN, D.S., "Laboratory techniques in biochemistry and molecular biology, Vol.4, part I, Chemical Modifications of Proteins (WORK, T.S., WORK, E., Eds), Elsevier, Amsterdam (1975) 157.
[3] KOCH, Y., BARAM, T., FRIDKIN, M., FEBS Lett. **63** (1976) 295.
[4] VISSER, T.J., KLOOTWIJK, W., DOCTER, R., HENNEMANN, G., Neuroendocrinol. **21** (1976) 204.
[5] VISSER, T.J., DOCTER, R., HENNEMANN, G., Acta Endocrinol. **77** (1974) 417.
[6] VISSER, T.J., KLOOTWIJK, W., DOCTER, R., HENNEMANN, G., 6th Int. Conf. Endocrinol., 11–15 July 1977, London, Abstr. No.59.
[7] VISSER, T.J., KLOOTWIJK, W., DOCTER, R., HENNEMANN, G., (Submitted for publication).
[8] TAGER, H.S., Anal. Biochem. **71** (1976) 367.
[9] GREENWOOD, F.C., HUNTER, W.L., GLOVER, J.J., Biochem. J. **89** (1963) 114.
[10] LING, N., LEPPÄLUOTO, J., VALE, W., Anal. Biochem. **76** (1976) 125.
[11] GLASS, J.D., SCHWARTZ, I.L., WALTER, R., J. Am. Chem. Soc. **94** (1972) 6209.
[12] GOMEZ-SANCHEZ, C., MILEWICH, L., BRYAN, O., J. Lab. Clin. Med. **89** (1977) 902.
[13] SORS, H., MACLOUF, J., PRADELLES, P., DRAY, F., Biochim. Biophys. Acta **486** (1977) 553.
[14] HALSEY, J.F., CEBRA, J.J., BILTONEN, R.L., Biochemistry **14** (1975) 5221.
[15] McKELVY, J.F., Brain Res. **65** (1974) 489.

DISCUSSION

P. PRADELLES: I think the specific activity of your tracer could be improved considerably by chromatographic separation procedures, up to a factor of 10 perhaps, which would allow you to use one-tenth the mass of tracer in the RIA.

T.J. VISSER: It is of course possible to increase the specific activity of the tracer by certain chromatographic techniques. However, we have found that at the present time the specific activity is not a limiting factor in the sensitivity of the assay.

P. PRADELLES: You obtain strong cross-reactions with APA-type antisera whilst they are very weak with the BDB-type. How do you explain this? Have you performed cross-reactions with N^{im}-1-methyl and N^{im}-2-methyl-TRH for the same antisera? If so, what are the results?

T.J. VISSER: Addition of a benzyl group to the imidazole ring in the case of the DNP- and APA-type antisera results in increased immunoreactivities for the reasons given. In the case of the BDB-type antisera the 'bridge' is larger, and this apparently makes the antibody recognize the difference in the sites of attachment of the benzyl group and the side chain linking the hapten to the carrier.

We have not tested the activities of N^{im}-methyl analogues.

M. TORTEN: Did you find differences in antibody levels in rabbits receiving conjugates with different 'bridges' (PAPA versus DNP)? Do you have any data on the number of rabbits with no or low response to each conjugate?

T.J. VISSER: We found that by far the best method of preparing antibodies is that involving the dinitrophenylene bridge. This is so whether the number of rabbits responding to immunization or the titres of the antisera obtained are considered.

NEW IMMUNOGENIC FORM FOR VASOPRESSIN

Production of high-affinity antiserum and development of an RIA for plasma arginine-vasopressin

G. ROUGON-RAPPUZI[1], B. CONTE-DEVOLX[2],
Y. MILLET[2], M.A. DELAAGE[1]
[1]Centre d'immunologie de Marseille-Luminy,
Marseille
[2]Faculté de médecine,
Marseille, France

Abstract

NEW IMMUNOGENIC FORM FOR VASOPRESSIN: PRODUCTION OF HIGH-AFFINITY ANTISERUM AND DEVELOPMENT OF AN RIA FOR PLASMA ARGININE-VASOPRESSIN.

A highly sensitive and specific radioimmunoassay (RIA) for arginine-vasopressin (AVP) was developed and applied to the measurement of AVP in human plasma. High-affinity anti-vasopressin antobodies with limited association constant heterogeneity were induced by immunizing rabbits with lysine-vasopressin (LVP) coupled to a human immunoglobulin (IgA). The yields of AVP were increased significantly when the acetone-petroleum ether extracts were lyophilized instead of air dried. Equilibrium dialysis was used to separate bound and free antigen, thus reducing the total time required for the assay to 48 h. Only 1 ml of plasma was required for routine determinations because of a sensitivity threshold of better than 0.5 pg/ml. Plasma AVP levels of normal subjects and of patients with inappropriate ADH secretion (SIADH) were determined during different hydratation states and after nicotine or ethanol infusions.

INTRODUCTION

A more general use of radioimmunoassay (RIA) for plasma arginine-vasopressin (AVP) [1–3] has been hampered by several difficulties. The poor immunogenic character of the AVP molecule has prevented most laboratories from obtaining antibodies sensitive enough to detect the very low levels of circulating hormone. Whereas the volume of plasma required can be reduced to 1 ml [4–6], other technical constraints still remain. For example, incubation times of 4 to 7 days are needed and the samples have to be concentrated before being assayed. In this study, we reinvestigated the problems dealing with the development and practical use of the AVP RIA.

Starting with a new immunogenic form of the hormone, we obtained anti-vasopressin antisera with high titres. The extraction procedure of plasma vasopressin was also improved and an RIA based on equilibrium dialysis was developed. Thus, we were able to reduce the incubation time considerably while increasing both the reproducibility and the convenience of the assay.

MATERIALS AND METHODS

Antisera to vasopressin

The immunogenic form of VP was prepared by coupling lysine-vasopressin (LVP) to IgA by a carbodiimide reaction. Two milligrams of LVP (Sigma grade III) and 20 mg of human IgA were incubated with 15 mg of 1-ethyl-3-(3-dimethyl-aminopropyl) carbodiimide, in 1 ml of water at pH5.5 for 24 h at room temperature. The molar ratio of the conjugate was 3 moles LVP/mole IgA.

Solutions of conjugate were prepared in 0.15M NaCl and emulsified with an equal volume of complete Freund's adjuvant: 2 ml of the mixture was administered subcutaneously to each of five rabbits. Four immunizations over a period of four months were needed to obtain a maximum response.

The rise in VP antibody titre was measured by the ability of the antiserum to bind 50% of an added radioactive tracer.

Iodination

AVP (Sigma grade VI) or LVP (Sigma grade IV) were iodinated according to the method of Hunter and Greenwood, except that the reaction was stopped by adding 100 μl of a 25% albumin solution instead of metabisulphite.

Purification was carried out according to Robertson and coworkers [1]: the reaction mixture was immediately applied to a 90 cm × 1 cm column of Sephadex G25, and eluted with 0.2M acetic acid.

Stock solutions

Large batches of labelled ^{125}I-AVP and antibody were diluted in 0.01M dibasic potassium phosphate, 0.15M chloride and 1 mg/ml albumin, pH7.2, and stored frozen in suitable aliquots. By using the same batch of reagents, we obtained virtually superimposable standard curves in different experiments, thus eliminating the need for frequent redrawing of standard curves.

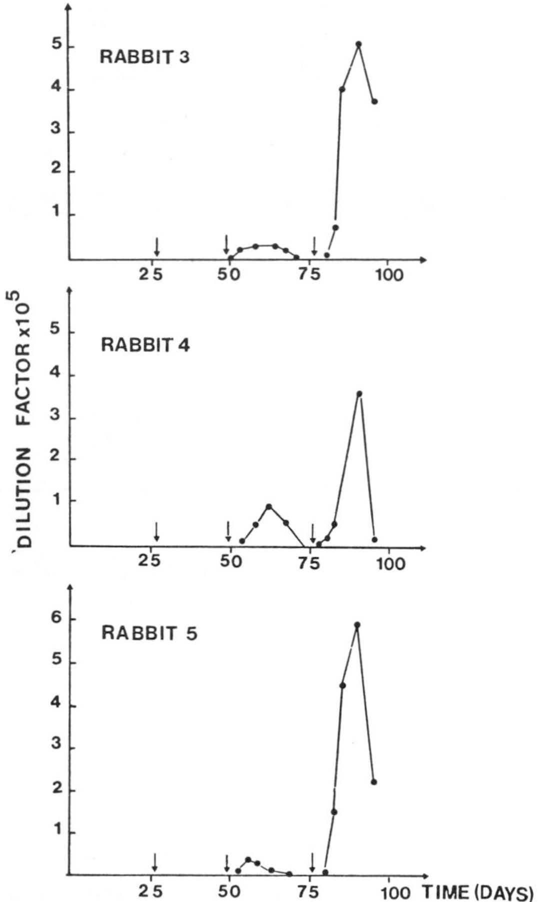

FIG.1. Time course of antibody production of three rabbits. The results are expressed as the reciprocal of the dilution which is able to bind 50% of the iodinated derivative. The days of immunization are indicated by arrows.

Extraction and concentration of plasma AVP

Heparinized venous blood was centrifuged at 4°C. Plasma was frozen immediately at −20°C for subsequent extraction and assay. AVP was extracted according to a modified form of the methods of Robertson and coworkers [5] and Husain and coworkers [4] in which air-drying was replaced by lyophilization in long glass tubes (Corex) to prevent the danger of blowing over part of the powdery sample as it dried.

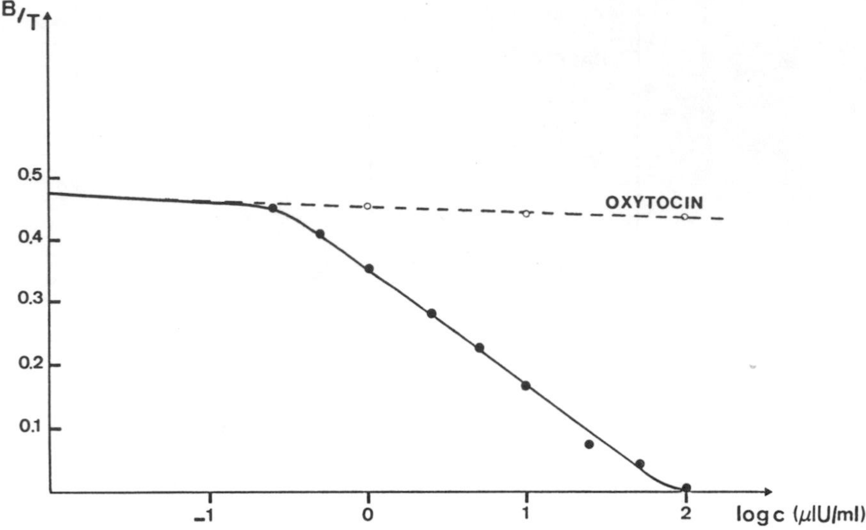

FIG.2. Standard curve for radioimmunoassay using AVP Sigma (360 IU/mg). The concentration is expressed in µIU of AVP/ml of the solution to be tested, i.e. 1 µIU = 2.5 pg.

In an ice bath, 2 ml of acetone were added to 1 ml of plasma. The lipid phase was then removed by washing the solution with 3 ml of petroleum ether. The acetone phase was lyophilized for 2 h and redissolved in a suitable volume of the above-mentioned buffer.

Assay

Incubation was carried out in the dialysis devices previously used by Delaage and colleagues [7, 8]. Equal volumes of the diluted sample and the ^{125}I-AVP solution were mixed and then 150 µl of the mixture was placed on one side of the device. The other side contained 150 µl of the antibody dilution.

Each unknown sample was assayed in duplicate at two different dilutions.

After shaking for 48 h at 4°C, equilibrium was established and 100 µl were taken from each side and counted. The ratio B/T was computed and the concentration of hormone was deduced from the standard curve.

The standard curve was drawn by replacing the diluted sample by 75 µl of unlabelled AVP in varying quantities (0.25, 0.5, 1, 2.5, 5, 10, 25, 50 and 100 µl/ml of solution).

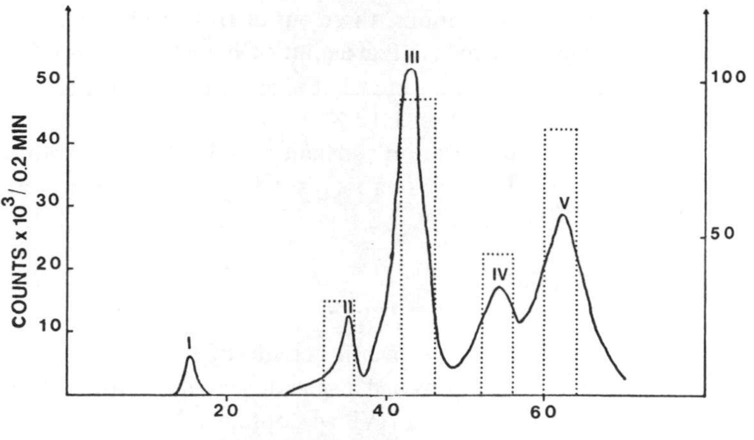

FIG.3. Elution pattern of a representative AVP iodination.
Peak I : ^{125}I-albumin
Peak II : free iodide
Peak III : ^{125}I-AVP
Peak IV : may represent diiodo-AVP
Peak V : is attributed to a by-product formed during iodination.
Left : radioactivity
Right : immunoreactivity of the different peaks expressed as the per cent of radioactivity that could be bound by an excess of antibody.

Human studies

AVP levels were determined under the following conditions:
- after an overnight water restriction
- 30 min after an oral water load
- 15 min after an i.v. infusion of 25 ml of 95% ethanol
- 2, 5, 10, 15, 30 and 60 min after an i.v. infusion of a dose of 2 mg of nicotine diluted in 10 ml of saline.

RESULTS AND DISCUSSION

Antisera

As first observed by Miller and Moses [9] and then by Morton [10], the formation of antibodies in rabbits is indicated by the onset of polyuria of varying severity. The rabbits' responses have been remarkably homogeneous both in titre and affinity. After four immunizations, three out of five rabbits gave antisera which bound 50% of the iodinated AVP at a dilution higher than 1/300 000 (Fig.1).

Antiserum from rabbit 5 had a somewhat higher titre throughout (dilution 1/600 000, binding site concentration 1.12×10^{-5}M). It showed a strong avidity for AVP, as indicated by its dissociation constant of 3.75×10^{-11} M which was determined from a Scatchard plot. No cross-reactions with oxytocin were observed (Fig.2).

Purity of iodinated hormone

For monoiodinated ^{125}I-AVP, a specific activity of 1700 μCi/mg can be calculated. Our purified preparations had a specific activity of over 1450 μCi/mg. Further proof of the purity of the ^{125}I-AVP was obtained by incubating with an excess of antibody to test its immunoreactivity. As shown in Fig.3, more than 95% of the labelled hormone can be bound by the antibody.

There was a detectable decrease in the binding of the labelled peptide with storage up to two months from the date of preparation.

Extraction yield

In one series of five separate experiments, ^{125}I-AVP was added to duplicate human blood samples and submitted to our extraction procedure. The yield was 87.2% ± 1.85 D (range 89.7–85.1%).

In a second series of six separate experiments, AVP was added to human blood samples containing only negligible amounts of hormone. Extraction and RIA were then performed. The mean recovery for all samples was again close to 87% (range 89–83%). This value compares favourably with previously reported yields [2, 4–6]. All results for AVP concentrations in plasma samples are corrected assuming a recovery of 87%.

Performance of the RIA

The precision of any RIA depends essentially on the precision of the binding measurement and on the slope of the standard curve. Using equilibrium dialysis, the standard deviation of the B/T ratio was close to 0.5% for the linear portion of the standard curve, corresponding to a standard deviation for the hormone concentration of about 4.5%. Repeated incubations of the same extract confirm this analysis: in a typical experiment we found 9.477 ∓ 0.52 pg/ml ($\bar{x} \mp$ SD, n = 8).

Other separation methods were tested with the same batches of reagents: compared with double-antibody precipitations, the incubation time was reduced by half. On the other hand, the use of polyethylene glycol leads to a notable decrease in sensitivity.

Normal human subjects

AVP was measured in 23 normal subjects after overnight dehydratation; the mean of the plasma concentrations was 4.24 ± 2.19 pg/ml ($\bar{x} \pm$ SD, n = 23; range 8 – 1).

A significant correlation was found between plasma AVP concentrations and plasma osmolality ($p < 0.001$, n = 23).

Fifteen minutes after i.v. infusion of 25 ml of ethanol, the plasma AVP concentration was reduced to 0.9 ± 0.6 pg/ml ($\bar{x} \mp$ SD, n = 23) without significant changes in plasma osmolality.

An oral water load of 15 ml/kg body weight in ten normal subjects resulted in a fall of the concentration from 5.39 ∓ 2.1 pg/ml ($\bar{x} \mp$ SD, n = 10) to 1.9 ± 0.9 pg/ml (n = 10).

After nicotine infusion, an AVP hypersecretion was observed, showing a maximum between the 5th and 15th min after the infusion. Peak values of more than four times the basal level were obtained.

Pathological cases

In nine patients suffering from different illnesses implicating SIADH, basal values were always higher than 20 pg/ml for a low plasma osmolality. The level did not change after ethanol infusion or a water load.

Six cases of diabetes insipidus were tested. Basal plasma levels were low (0.8 ∓ 0.67 pg/ml, n = 6; range 0 to 1.6); hypersecretion of AVP after injection of nicotine was not observed.

Among four cases of potomania, the plasma levels after water restriction and after overload were comparable to those of diabetes insipidus (range 0.50 ∓ 1.7 pg/ml), but nicotine infusion was followed by increased plasma levels. The low levels of basal AVP and the very weak response to nicotine in the potomania cases can be explained by the classical notion of the secondary and temporary diabetes insipidus induced by potomania.

CONCLUSION

An anti-AVP antiserum with a high titre has been obtained in three out of five rabbits by immunizing with a novel AVP derivative, AVP coupled to human IgA. By combining a new extraction procedure with equilibrium dialysis to separate bound from free antigen, a simple rapid and accurate RIA for AVP has been developed. This method is now used routinely in several laboratories. The levels of circulating hormone measured in normal and pathological states correspond well to the values reported in the literature [3–5, 11]. With our method, the genetics of the AVP response to nicotine administration have been established. As demonstrated by our results, the nicotine test may be useful for differentiating pathological states of AVP production and secretion from potomania.

REFERENCES

[1] ROBERTSON, G.L., KLEIN, L.A., ROTH, J., GORDON, P., Proc. Natl. Acad. Sci., U.S.A. **66** (1970), 1298.

[2] BEARDWELL, C.G., J. Clin. Endocrinol. Metab. **33** (1971) 254.

[3] OYAMA, S.N., KAGAN, A., GLICK, S.M., J. Clin. Endocrinol. Metab. **33** (1971) 739.

[4] HUSAIN, M.L., FERNANDO, N., SHAPIRO, M., KAGAN, A., GLICK, S.M., J. Clin. Endocrinol. Metab. **37** (1973) 616.

[5] ROBERTSON, G.L., MAHR, E.A., ATHAR, S., SINHA, T., J. Clin. Invest. **52** (1973) 2340.

[6] SKOWSKY, W.R., ROSENBLOOM, A.A., FISCHER, D.A., J. Clin. Endocrinol. Metab. **38** (1974) 278.

[7] CAILLA, H.L., RACINE WEISBUCH, M.S., DELAAGE, M.A., Anal. Biochem. **56** (1973) 394.

[8] DE REGGI, M.L., HIRN, M., DELAAGE, M.A., Biochem. Biophys. Res. Commun. **66** (1975) 1307.

[9] MILLER, M., MOSES, A.M., Endocrinology **84** (1969) 557.

[10] MORTON, J.J., WAITE, M.A., J. Endocrinol. **54** (1972) 523.

[11] MORTON, J.J., PADFIELD, P.L., FORSLING, M.L., J. Endocrinol. **65** (1975) 411.

DISCUSSION

V. KRUSE: Have you measured the endogenous vasopressin in the antiserum? Figure 1 shows a late drop in the titre. This could be due to saturation with endogenous vasopressin. It may be possible to remove such endogenous material by a stripping method (Kruse, V., Abstracts, 2nd European Congress on Clinical Chemistry, Prague (1976)). This should enable you to obtain a higher sensitivity of the assay and to utilize the slowly dissociating antibodies in the antiserum after a relatively short incubation period.

What was the purpose of using the dialysis devices – to obtain a lower misclassification error?

G. ROUGON-RAPPUZI: I of course tried to measure endogenous vasopressin in my antisera but I did not succeed in obtaining a quantitative result because of the difficulty of fully eliminating the antibodies which interfere during the assay. I agree with you that there is partial saturation of antibodies by the endogenous hormone because the immunized animals exhibit diabetes insipidus; so there was "trapping" of the circulating vasopressin. However, I do not know any de-saturation technique which does not cause a loss in antibody activity; I shall try your method.

Equilibrium dialysis is a method used both for incubation and for separation of the free hormone complexes since the antibody is not dialysable. It avoids the artefacts due to the addition of a precipitating agent and the need to make blanks. The value of B/T can in fact vary from 0 to 100%.

M.A. DELAAGE: I should point out that it is the rate of the hapten-antibody reaction and not the rate of dialysis which constitutes the limiting factor during the incubation.

RADIOIMMUNOASSAY OF ARGININE-VASOPRESSIN AND CLINICAL APPLICATION*

H. WAGNER, V. MAIER, M. HÄBERLE,
H.E. FRANZ
Zentrum für Innere Medizin und
Kinderheilkunde der Universität Ulm,
Ulm, Federal Republic of Germany

Abstract

RADIOIMMUNOASSAY OF ARGININE-VASOPRESSIN AND CLINICAL APPLICATION.

The low circulatory levels of vasopressin have necessitated an initial extraction procedure before it could be radioimmunoassayed. As this extraction affected the specificity and reproducibility of the extracted hormone, a radioimmunoassay was developed without an extraction step. The AVP was coupled to rabbit-albumin by glutaraldehyde condensation for the immunization of rabbits. Synthetic AVP was iodinated by the method of Greenwood and Hunter and purified by the addition of Dowex. The antibody cannot differentiate between lysine-, arginine-, ornithine- and glycerine-vasopressin and oxytocin. 1–24-ACTH and gastrin did not cross-react. Normal subjects were found to have AVP levels of 5.7 ± 4.4 μU/ml after a dehydration period of 12 h. Subjects suffering from psychogenic polydipsia had normal levels, though different forms of stress yielded higher levels in normal subjects. In patients suffering from liver cirrhosis, the values normalized when ascites was under control.

INTRODUCTION

There are several publications on the development of a radioimmunoassay for arginine-vasopressin (AVP) [1–4]. Although radioimmunoassay has been used successfully to measure vasopressin in buffer solution, problems have arisen in its application to biological fluids like serum and plasma. These problems, together with the low circulatory levels of vasopressin, necessitated an initial extraction procedure, but the extraction itself presented problems with regard to the specificity and reproducibility of the extracted hormone. Therefore, an assay without an extraction procedure was developed.

MATERIALS AND METHODS

Iodination and purification

Synthetic AVP (Ferring AB, Malmö, Sweden) was iodinated with carrier-free Na ^{125}I (Hoechst, Frankfurt, FRG) by a modification of the method of Greenwood

* Supported by Deutsche Forschungsgemeinschaft Bonn – Bad Godesberg, SFB 87 Ulm.

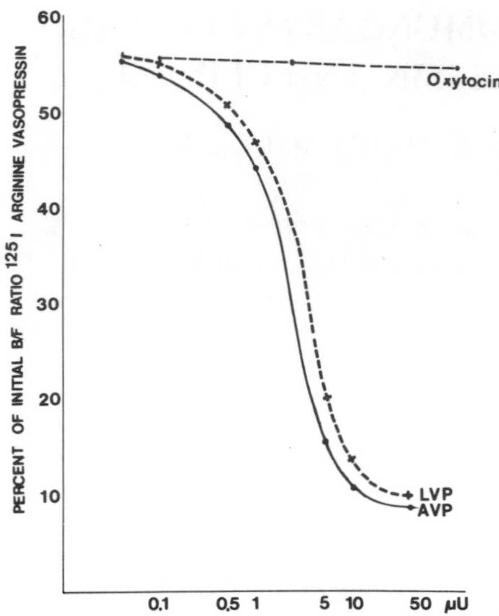

FIG.1. Standard curves for arginine-vasopressin (AVP) and lysine-vasopressin (LVP). Oxytocin shows no displacement of the labelled hormone.

and coworkers [5]. Synthetic AVP (5 μg in 5 μl of 0.15M phosphate buffer, pH 9.0) was added to 1 mCi of Na ^{125}I and oxidized by 20 μl of 0.035% Choramine-T. The reaction was stopped by adding 20 μl of 0.045% metabisulphite after 8 s. Free Na ^{125}I was removed from ^{125}I-AVP by adding to each batch 2 g of Dowex ion-exchange resin (2 × 8, 50–100 mesh, Dow Chemical Co.) in 20 ml of 0.05M Tris-HCl at pH8.0 [1]. The supernatant of ^{125}I-AVP was stable for periods of up to 6 weeks when stored at –20°C. The specific activity of labelled AVP was 180–210 mCi/mg. Gel filtration on a 1.5 cm × 20 cm Sephadex G-25 column (equilibrated with 1M acetic acid) was found to have no well-delineated peak coinciding with the data described by Oyama [6]. This observation can be explained by the adhesiveness of labelled AVP to the Sephadex gel and by the damaged immunoreactive hormone [1, 7]. Therefore we used an ion-exchange resin (Dowex 2 × 8) as described by Edwards and coworkers [1].

Radioimmunoassay

The total reaction volume of the assay was 500 μl. The first incubation period was 24 h, then 10 μl of anti-rabbit γ-globulin was added and incubation was continued for a further 24 h. After subsequent centrifugation, the activity in the supernatant was measured.

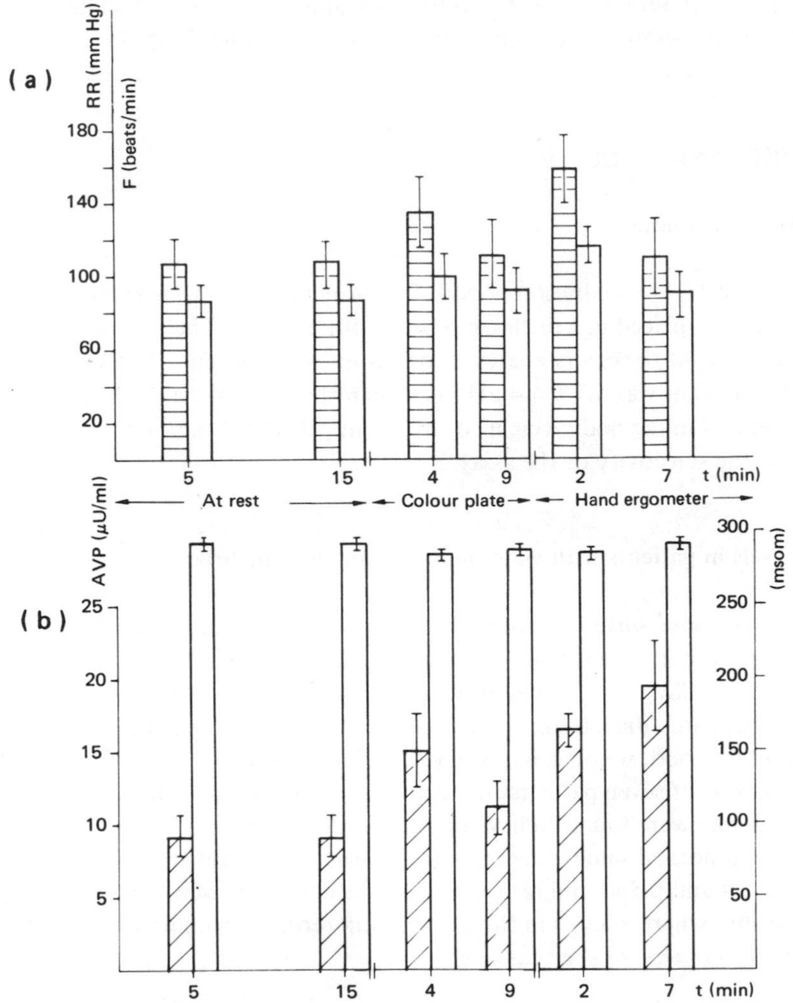

FIG.2. (a) Effect of stress on blood pressure and pulse rate.
(b) Effect of stress on AVP release.

Figure 1 shows typical standard curves. The antibody cannot differentiate between lysine-vasopressin (LVP) and arginine-vasopressin (AVP). The curve for the former shows a slight shift to the right. Heparin (100 U/ml) and EDTA (1 μM) did not interfere with the assay. Oxytocin (Sandoz, Basel, Switzerland), ornithine-vasopressin and glycine-vasopressin (Sandoz, Berlin (West)), synthetic bradykinin (Sandoz, Basel), 1–24 ACTH (Ferring AB, Malmö) and gastrin (ICI, UK) did not cross-react in the assay. All hormones were added in physiological concentrations and in 100 times higher concentrations. To each millilitre of vasopressin-free serum, synthetic arginine-vasopressin was added. The resulting standard curve shows a slight difference in the lower range (Fig. 1).

RESULTS AND DISCUSSION

Physiological studies

After a 12-h dehydration period, 56 normal subjects were given vein punctures and were then placed in a reclining position for 20 min. The blood samples were taken in ice-cold flasks and analysed for vasopressin content. The basic value of the AVP content was 5.7 ± 4.4 μU/ml. When the subjects had drunk a glass of tap water (20 ml/kg body weight) over 15 min, the AVP values decreased to values at the sensitivity of the assay.

AVP levels in patients with water metabolism abnormalities

Five persons suffering from psychogenic polydipsia and with free access to drinking water were found to have normalized AVP levels (i.e. 7.2 μU/ml) in spite of drinking 8–12 litres of water each day. In the serum of three patients with documented diabetes insipidus centralis and without hormone substitution over a 48-h period, we determined levels of 0.6 μU/ml.

Five out of seven patients suffering from liver cirrhosis and ascites with hyponatremia were found to have increased AVP levels (mean 15.5 μU/ml) which approached normal values when the ascites was under control. Two patients had levels of 2.4 and 0.5 μU/ml respectively. These patients were not treated successfully, whereas levels in the other group returned to normal after administration of diuretics for 4 weeks.

Stress experiments

By reading a colour plate (first described by Shapiro) and by performing 'hand-grip' exercises it was possible to show that AVP values are influenced by stress (Fig. 2). In the initial stress, the subjects were exposed to a colour plate of words in which, for example, the word "green" was written in "red" letters and the person had to say "green" quickly. As an index of stress, blood pressure (mmHg) and pulse rate (beats/min) were measured. Although a clear-cut rise in AVP release was shown, no influence on osmolality (mosm) could be detected. To exclude the possibility that the elevated AVP was due specifically to colour-plate stress, the influence of stress caused by a hand ergometer was also measured.

SUMMARY

1. The authors have developed a sensitive and specific RIA without an extraction procedure.

2. The AVP levels in pathophysiological states of water metabolism in man were found to agree with the data reported for bioassay methods.

3. Normal values for AVP were found in subjects suffering from psychogenic polydipsia. However, different forms of stress were found to increase the AVP levels. These findings are in agreement with bioassay measurements of the anti-diuretic substance in the plasma of rats exposed to ether, pain or other noxious stimuli [8]. On the other hand, RIA measurements by Keil and Severs [9] showed a decline in AVP levels in the plasma of rats.

REFERENCES

[1] EDWARDS, C.R.W., CHARD, T., KITAU, M.J., FORSLIN, M.L., LANDON, J., The development of a radioimmunoassay for arginine vasopressin; production of antisera and labeled hormone; separation techniques; specificity and sensitivity of the assay in aqueous solution, J. Endocrinol. **52** (1972) 279.

[2] ROBERTSON, G.L., MAHR, E.A., ATHAR, S., SINHA, T., Development and clinical application of a new method for the radioimmunoassay of arginine vasopressin in human plasma, J. Clin. Invest. **52** (1973) 2340.

[3] BEARDWELL, C.G., GEELEN, G., PALMER, H.M., ROBERTS, D., SALAMONSON, L., Radioimmunoassay of plasma vasopressin in physiological and pathological states in man, J. Endocrinol. **67** (1975) 189.

[4] UHLICH, E., WEBER, P., GRÖSCHEL-STEWART, U., RÖSCHLAU, T.C., Radio-immunoassay of arginine vasopressin in human plasma, Horm. Metab. Res. **7** (1975) 501.

[5] GREENWOOD, F.C., HUNTER, W.M., GLOVER, J.S., The preparation of ^{131}I-labeled human growth hormone of high specific radioactivity, Biochem. J. **89** (1963) 114.

[6] OYAMA, S.M., KAGAN, A., GLICK, S.M., Radioimmunoassay of vasopressin: application to unextracted human urine, J. Clin. Endocrinol. Metab. **33** (1971) 739.

[7] LEGROS, J.J., FRANCHIMONT, P., "The purification and modification of immunological and physicochemical behavior of iodinated posterior pituitary hormones", Radio-immunoassay Methods (KIRKHAM, K.E., HUNTER, W.M., Eds), Churchill and Livingstone, Edinburgh and London (1971) 40.

[8] MARTIN, L., The Pituitary Gland, Vol.3 (HARRIS, G.W., DONOVAN, B.T., Eds), University of California Press (1966) 535.

[9] KEIL, L.C., SEVERS, W.B., Reduction in plasma vasopressin levels of dehydrated rats following acute stress, Endocrinology **100** (1977) 30.

DISCUSSION

G. ROUGON-RAPPUZI: The plasma levels of vasopressin given by you always appear to be much higher than those reported in the literature. Could you please explain why this is so?

M. HÄBERLE: As long as an international standard is not available for AVP, our interest centres on relative changes and not on absolute AVP levels in the serum.

G. ROUGON-RAPPUZI: What is the value of the affinity constant of the immunoserum used in the assays?

M. HÄBERLE: At 1 : 20 000 dilution of our antiserum 57% of the tracer is bound.

A. MALKIN: How do you explain the fall in vasopressin following treatment of patients with hepatic cirrhosis and ascites?

M. HÄBERLE: The immunoreactive AVP was significantly increased in five patients with ascites. We believe that our values are in correlation with the biological activity of the hormone, as in the case of the two patients with normal values but displaying therapeutic resistance to diuretic treatment (furosemide). Successful treatment of ascites and hyponatremia normalized the circulating AVP levels. The metabolic clearance of AVP by the liver and the kidney may be diminshed, and we conclude that the normalization of the AVP level is due to restoration of kidney and liver functions.

A. SCHELLEKENS: Quite a few authors have stressed the addition of blocking agents for proteolytic enzymes to plasma samples as well as to the immunoassay incubates. What did you use?

M. HÄBERLE: We do not use substances for the inhibition of proteolytic enzymes but keep our samples at a temperature of exactly 4°C.

DOSAGE RADIOIMMUNOLOGIQUE DES ENKEPHALINES

P. PRADELLES, C. GROS, C. ROUGEOT,
O. BEPOLDIN, F. DRAY
Unité de radioimmunologie analytique,
Institut Pasteur, Paris

C. LLORENS-CORTES, H. POLLARD, J.C. SCHWARTZ
Unité de neurobiologie de l'INSERM (U.109),
Centre Paul Broca, Paris

M.C. FOURNIE-ZALUSKI, G. CRACEL, B.P. ROQUES
Département de chimie organique, ERA 613,
Université Paul Descartes, Paris,
France

Abstract–Résumé

RADIOIMMUNOASSAY OF ENKEPHALINS.

Using iodine (^{125}I) tracers of high specific radioactivity, the authors have developed the specific radioimmunoassay of methionine-enkephalin (Met-Enk) and leucine-enkephalin (Leu-Enk). The immunosera are obtained by immunizing rabbits with Met-Enk or Leu-Enk combined with ovalbumin by means of carbodiimide. The specificity and the sensitivity of these radioimmunoassays (IC_{50} of 0.57 nM and 0.55 nM for the assay of Met-Enk and Leu-Enk, respectively) afford a means of estimating the enkephalin levels in extracts of various regions of the rat brain. The highest levels are in the striatum and the hypothalamus and the lowest in the cerebellum and the hippocampus.

DOSAGE RADIOIMMUNOLOGIQUE DES ENKEPHALINES.

Les auteurs ont mis au point le radioimmunodosage spécifique de la méthionine-enképhaline (Met-Enk) et de la leucine-enképhaline (Leu-Enk) en utilisant des traceurs iodés (^{125}I) de hautes radioactivités spécifiques. Les immunsérums sont obtenus en immunisant des lapins avec de la Met-Enk ou de la Leu-Enk couplée à l'ovalbumine à l'aide de carbodiimide. La spécificité et la sensibilité de ces radioimmunodosages (IC_{50} de 0,57 nM et 0,55 nM pour le dosage de la Met-Enk et de la Leu-Enk respectivement) permet d'estimer les taux des enképhalines dans des extraits de plusieurs régions du cerveau de rat. Les taux les plus élevés se trouvent dans le striatum et l'hypothalamus et les plus bas dans le cervelet et l'hippocampe.

INTRODUCTION

La découverte récente [1] de substances capables d'entrer en compétition avec les opiacés pour les récepteurs cérébraux spécifiques de la morphine a ouvert une nouvelle voie d'étude du rôle et du mode d'action de ces récepteurs. Ces substances morphino-mimétiques, appelées endorphines, pourraient être les précurseurs de molécules plus petites: les enképhalines, deux pentapeptides (H-Tyr-Gly-Gly-Phe-Met-OH ou Met-Enk et H-Tyr-Gly-Gly-Phe-Leu-OH ou Leu-Enk) [2] qui serviraient de neurotransmetteurs de l'effet analgésique. Afin de mesurer la répartition de ces dernières substances dans le cerveau ou encore de suivre leur évolution dans certains états psychopathologiques, nous avons développé leur radioimmunodosage.

MATERIELS ET METHODES

Préparation des peptides

La synthèse peptidique de la Met-Enk et de la Leu-Enk a déjà été décrite [3,4]. Tyr-Gly, Tyr-Gly-Gly, Phe-Met et l'α-endorphine nous ont été fournis par Serva (Heidelberg) et la β-endorphine par Peninsula Laboratories. Tous les autres peptides ont été synthétisés par phase liquide et leur pureté testée par chromatographie sur couche mince de silice (CCM) dans le système: n-butanol-acide acétique-eau 4 : 1 : 1. Les R_f sont respectivement pour Tyr-Gly-Gly-Phe, Gly-Gly-Phe-Met, Gly-Phe-Met, Gly-Gly-Phe-Leu, Gly-Phe-Leu et Phe-Leu de 0,50; 0,61; 0,55; 0,72; 0,67 et 0,58.

Préparation des immunogènes

Cinq milligrammes (8,7 μmol) de Met-Enk, 1 μCi de ^{3}H-Met-Enk (CEA) et 15 mg d'ovalbumine (Sigma) sont dissous dans 1 ml d'eau. On ajoute 20 mg de 1-éthyl-3-(3-diméthyl-aminopropyl) carbodiimide HCl (Sigma) et on maintient le pH à 5. La réaction est faite à température ambiante pendant une nuit. On dialyse ensuite le produit de la réaction contre NaCl 0,9% pendant 48 h à + 4°C. Tenant compte de la dilution isotopique nous avons estimé à 23 le nombre des résidus Met-Enk liés par molécule d'ovalbumine.

Pour l'obtention d'immunsérums anti-Leu-Enk, nous avons utilisé les mêmes conditions de couplage que précédemment et nous avons estimé à 5 le nombre de Leu-Enk liés par molécule d'ovalbumine.

Immunisation

Cinq lapins femelles (race Bouscat) adultes ont été immunisés par voie intradermique avec 1 mg de chaque immunogène émulsifié dans de l'adjuvant complet de Freund (Difco). Les injections de rappel, effectuées par la même voie, sont faites 5 semaines après l'injection primaire. On a détecté la présence d'anticorps anti-Met-Enk 15 jours après la première injection de rappel, alors que les anticorps anti-Leu-Enk sont apparus deux semaines après le troisième rappel. Par la suite les animaux sont immunisés tous les mois et les saignées effectuées deux semaines après chaque rappel.

Marquage des enképhalines à l'iode-125

L'introduction d'iode radioactif (^{125}I) sur le noyau tyrosyl des enképhalines est obtenu par la méthode d'iodation enzymatique de Marchalonis [5] pour la Met-Enk et celle à la chloramine T de Hunter et Greenwood [6] pour la Leu-Enk.

Dix microlitres (9 nmol) de Met-Enk en solution dans un mélange méthanol-eau (v/v) sont évaporés. On ajoute successivement 10 μl de tampon phosphate 0,5 M pH 7,4, 4 μl de Na ^{125}I ($\cong$ 400 μCi, Amersham), 10 μl de lactoperoxydase (10 μg) (Calbiochem) dans du tampon phosphate 0,05 M pH 7,4 et 10 μl d'H_2O_2 (110 volumes) dilués au 1/90 000. Le mélange est agité pendant 10 minutes et 10 μl d'H_2O_2 diluée sont de nouveau ajoutés. La réaction est arrêtée par addition de 10 μl (25 μg) de métabisulfite de sodium.

Dix microlitres (2 nmol) d'une solution méthanolique de Leu-Enk sont évaporés. On ajoute ensuite 10 μl de tampon phosphate 0,5 M, 2 μl de Na ^{125}I ($\cong$ 200 μCi) et 4 μl (12 μg) de chloramine T dans le tampon dilué. Après une minute, la réaction est arrêtée par addition de 4 μl (60 μg) de métabisulfite.

Les produits de chaque réaction d'halogénation sont purifiés par CCM sur plaque de silice dans le système de solvant décrit précédemment. Une autoradiographie et une distribution de la radioactivité (Berthold Scanner I) nous permet de les localiser et de déterminer le rendement d'halogénation. Les enképhalines marquées sont extraites de la silice par une solution méthanol-eau (v/v) et conservées à –20°C.

Identification des dérivés iodés mono et disubstitués des enképhalines

On réalise l'iodation des enképhalines à l'iode stable (^{127}I) par la méthode au monochlorure d'iode (ICl) [7]. A 20 μl (0,2 μmol) de chaque enképhaline dans du tampon phosphate 0,5 M pH 7,4 sont ajoutés 20 μl (0,2 μmol) d'ICl (Merck) en solution méthanolique. Après une minute le mélange réactionnel est déposé sur une plaque de silice fluorescente. On développe la CCM dans les conditions précédemment décrites. Les produits chromatographiés, absorbant dans l'ultraviolet à 254 nm, sont extraits de la silice par une solution méthanol-eau (v/v) et analysés dans un spectrophotomètre UV (Unicam). L'identification des dérivés mono et diiodés sur le résidu tyrosyle des enképhalines est faite sur la base des spectres d'absorption UV comparés à ceux de la mono et diiodotyrosine [8].

TABLEAU I. PARAMETRES CHROMATOGRAPHIQUES ET RADIOIMMUNOLOGIQUES DES TRACEURS IODES

Produits	R_f [a]	Capacité de liaison[b] (%)	IC_{50} (nM)[c]
Monoiodo Met-Enk	0,38	80	0,57
diiodo Met-Enk	0,42	30	
Met-Enk	0,61	-	
Monoiodo Met-Enk (modifié)[d]	0,70	0	
diiodo Met-Enk (modifié)	0,75	0	
Leu-Enk	0,85	-	
Monoiodo Leu-Enk	0,72	87	0,55
diiodo Leu-Enk	0,78	62	

[a] CCM sur plaques de silice dans le système n-butanol-acide acétique-eau (4 : 1 : 1).

[b] Calculée pour une dilution finale d'immunsérum au 1/600 en présence de 17 000 dpm de traceur.

[c] Concentration d'inhibiteur nécessaire pour déplacer 50% de la radioactivité liée aux anticorps.

[d] Produits d'une réaction secondaire dans l'étape d'halogénation (voir le paragraphe *Résultats et discussion).*

Technique du radioimmunodosage

Du tampon Tris 0,05 M pH 8,6 est utilisé pour diluer les réactifs dans le radioimmunodosage de la Met-Enk et la Leu-Enk. On introduit successivement dans des tubes en polypropylène 0,1 ml des solutions standard des enképhalines ou des échantillons biologiques à doser, 0,1 ml (17 000 dpm) de traceur iodé et 0,1 ml d'immunsérum dilué. On incube pendant une nuit à +4°C. La séparation du complexe antigène-anticorps de l'antigène libre se fait par addition à +4°C successivement de 0,1 ml d'une solution de gamma-globuline à 0,5% dans le tampon Tris et de 0,5 ml d'une solution de polyéthylène-glycol à 40%. Les tubes sont immédiatement centrifugés pendant 20 minutes à +4°C à 2200 × g. Le surnageant est aspiré et la radioactivité du culot comptée dans un spectromètre gamma. B_0 représente la fraction de radioactivité liée aux anticorps en absence de compétiteur et B celle en présence de compétiteur. Les courbes standard sont représentées en portant en abscisse le nombre de moles de compétiteur présent dans chaque tube d'incubation et en ordonnée la valeur en pourcentage du rapport B/B_0.

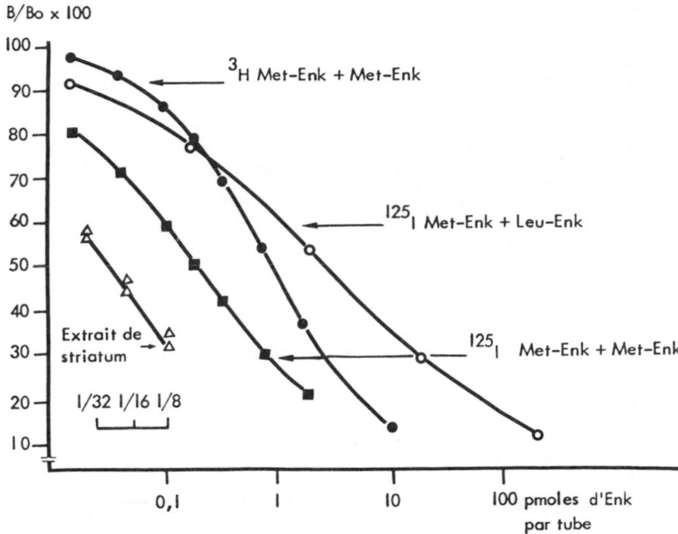

FIG.1. Inhibition de la liaison de ^{125}I-Met-Enk à l'antisérum Met-Enk par Met-Enk, Leu-Enk et un extrait striatal de rat; inhibition de la liaison de ^{3}H-Met-Enk par Met-Enk au même antisérum.

Préparation des extraits biologiques

Immédiatement après le sacrifice, les cerveaux de rats sont disséqués à 0°C et les tissus des différentes régions du cerveau homogénéisés dans de l'HCl 0,1 N à 0°C. On précipite les protéines de l'homogénat (0,3 à 0,5 ml) en portant chaque tube immédiatement à 95°C pendant 15 minutes et en les centrifugeant pendant 5 minutes à 9800 × g. Le surnageant contenant les enképhalines est tamponné à pH 7,4 par une solution de tampon Tris 0,1 M et d'eau distillée.

RESULTATS ET DISCUSSION

Les spectres UV des enképhalines iodées par l'ICl présentent des caractéristiques en milieu alcalin identiques à celles de la monoiodo tyrosine (λ_{max} = 305 nm) et de la diiodotyrosine (λ_{max} = 311 nm). Dans le cas de l'iodation de la Met-Enk nous avons formé deux produits monosubstitués et deux produits disubstitués (tableau I, colonne 1). Nous pensons que l'un de chacun d'entre eux pourrait résulter d'une réaction secondaire d'oxydation du

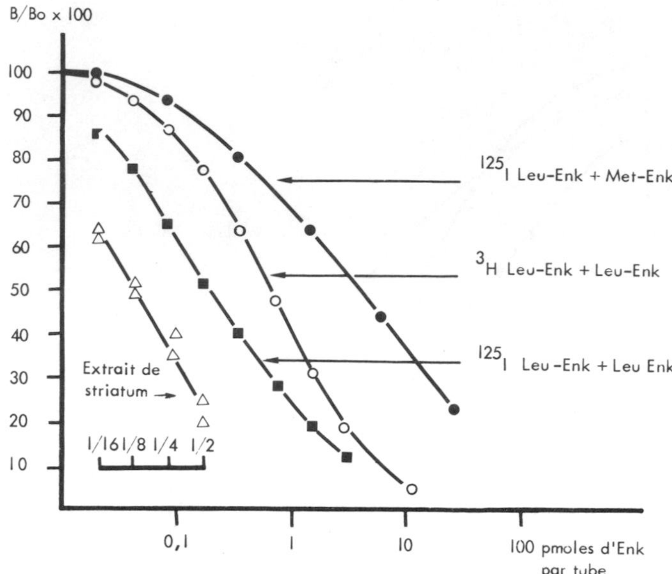

FIG.2. Inhibition de la liaison de ^{125}I-Leu-Enk à l'antisérum Leu-Enk par Leu-Enk, Met-Enk et un extrait striatal de rat; inhibition de la liaison de ^{3}H-Leu-Enk par Leu-Enk au même antisérum.

résidu méthionyle. Les dérivés radioactifs iodés présentent un profil chromatographique identique à celui des dérivés iodés par ICl et nous remarquons qu'un des dérivés mono et diiodés radioactifs de la Met-Enk ne possède pas d'immunoréactivité en présence d'une concentration élevée d'immunsérum (dilution finale 1/600). Ils pourraient correspondre vraisemblablement à une modification chimique de la Met-Enk iodée (tableau I, colonne 2). D'autre part, puisque les dérivés iodés des enképhalines sont entièrement séparés des enképhalines non iodées après CCM (tableau I, colonne 1) nous pouvons leur attribuer une radioactivité spécifique maximale, au moins égale à celle de Na^{125}I (~ 2000 Ci/mmol). Du fait de l'instabilité reconnue des composés diiodés, nous avons choisi d'utiliser comme traceur dans le radioimmunodosage les espèces monoiodées. Dans ce cas pour obtenir un B_0 de 40% nous avons utilisé, pour les meilleures saignées, une dilution finale au 1/6000 pour les antisérums Met-Enk et au 1/18 000 pour ceux de la Leu-Enk.

Nous avons comparé sur les figures 1 et 2 les courbes standard obtenues en utilisant les traceurs iodés et les traceurs tritiés à 30 Ci/nmol (Amersham); l'augmentation de sensibilité observée dans les deux systèmes radioimmunologiques utilisant le traceur iodé par rapport au traceur tritié est le résultat de

TABLEAU II. REACTIONS CROISEES DES ANTISERUMS AVEC DIFFERENTS COMPOSES

Composés	Pourcentage de réactions croisées[a]	
	Met-Enk	Leu-Enk
Tyr-Gly-Gly-Phe-Leu	7	100
Tyr-Gly-Gly-Phe-Met	100	5
Tyr-Gly-Gly-Phe	< 0,1	< 0,1
Tyr-Gly-Gly	"	"
Tyr-Gly	"	"
Tyr	"	"
Leu	"	"
Met	"	"
Phe-Leu	"	"
Phe-Met	"	"
Gly-Phe-Leu	"	"
Gly-Phe-Met	"	"
Gly-Gly-Phe-Leu	"	"
Gly-Gly-Phe-Met	"	"
Tyr-Gly-Gly-(D)Phe-Met	"	0,3
α et β-endorphines	"	< 0,1
Morphine	"	"

[a] Calculé à partir des rapports de IC_{50}.
Les antisérums dilués (dilution finale 1/6000 et 1/18 000 respectivement pour Met-Enk et Leu-Enk) ont été incubés en présence de 10 pM d'enképhalines iodées et de concentrations croissantes des composés indiqués.

deux facteurs: 1 – une augmentation de la radioactivité spécifique, donc une introduction de masse de traceur plus faible dans le dosage; 2 – une modification du traceur iodé entraînant une diminution de son immunoréactivité par rapport à celle du traceur tritié et facilitant par conséquent la compétition vis-à-vis de sa liaison aux anticorps par la molécule standard ou endogène. Dans le cas des systèmes utilisant les traceurs iodés, 0,17 pmol et 0,15 pmol d'enképhaline standard Met-Enk et Leu-Enk respectivement sont nécessaires pour obtenir une valeur de B/B_0 de 50% respectivement pour chaque antisérum. On observe une réaction croisée non négligeable (7% et 5%) avec la Leu-Enk et la Met-Enk respectivement pour les antisérums Met-Enk et Leu-Enk (fig.1 et 2, tableau II)

TABLEAU III. DISTRIBUTION DES TAUX D'ENKEPHALINES DANS DIFFERENTES REGIONS DU CERVEAU DE RAT

Région du cerveau	Met-Enk (nmol/g de tissu)	Leu-Enk (nmol/g de tissu)	Met-Enk/Leu-Enk
Cervelet	0,049 ± 0,006	0,006 ± 0,001	9,4 ± 1,7
Mésencéphale	0,200 ± 0,050	0,011 ± 0,002	29,0 ± 7,1
Hypothalamus	0,468 ± 0,036	0,114 ± 0,005	4,1 ± 0,3
Hippocampe	0,049 ± 0,004	0,005 ± 0,001	10,4 ± 1,9
Striatum	1,230 ± 0,070	0,174 ± 0,005	7,2 ± 0,6
Cortex frontal	0,274 ± 0,043	0,043 ± 0,016	10,1 ± 1,3

Chaque valeur représente la moyenne ± déviation standard de 5 résultats expérimentaux obtenus à partir d'un pool de régions de 2 animaux.

alors qu'elle est minime pour plusieurs fragments peptidiques des enképhalines, analogue α et β-endorphine et morphine (tableau II). Ce résultat peut être expliqué en tenant compte du fait que le couplage avec les protéines antigéniques pour la synthèse des immunogènes a lieu à des endroits de la molécule qui ne sont pas impliqués dans la conformation tertiaire stable de la molécule [4, 9].

Les résultats des radioimmunodosages des enképhalines dans les broyats cérébraux sont groupés dans le tableau III. Nous voyons que: 1 – la majeure partie des enképhalines se trouve dans le striatum et l'hypothalamus alors que les taux les plus bas sont dans l'hippocampe et le cervelet; 2 – la parallélisme de la courbe standard avec celle obtenue avec plusieurs dilutions de ces extraits (fig.1 et 2) est un bon argument en faveur de la spécificité du dosage des enképhalines endogènes; 3 – la grande sensibilité du radioimmunodosage des enképhalines à l'aide des traceurs iodés permet de réduire le poids des échantillons à doser. Par exemple, les extraits de striatum (50 mg de tissu/ml) sont dilués au 1/32 pour le dosage de la Met-Enk et au 1/16 pour celui de la Leu-Enk.

CONCLUSION

La mise au point d'un radioimmunodosage sensible et spécifique des enképhalines utilisant des traceurs iodés nous a permis d'apprécier les taux de ces substances dans différentes régions du cerveau de rat. Des travaux récents [10] utilisant la technique du radiorécepteur pour le dosage des endorphines ont montré une distribution analogue des enképhalines mais avec des taux plus élevés. Il est vraisemblable qu'avec cette technique on dose d'autres produits ayant de l'affinité pour les récepteurs des enképhalines, telles les α et β-endorphines, comme cela a déjà été montré [11]. Aussi, la mise au point d'un dosage radio-immunologique de ces dernières substances devrait nous permettre de confirmer cette hypothèse et d'approfondir nos connaissances sur le mécanisme d'action des endorphines.

REMERCIEMENTS

L'estimation des résidus enképhalines liés par molécule de protéine antigénique a été faite en utilisant des enképhalines tritiées, fournies généreusement par le Dr. J.L. Morgat, du Service de biochimie (CEA, Saclay, France).

REFERENCES

[1] HUGUES, J., Brain Res. **88** (1975) 295.
[2] HUGUES, J., SMITH, T.W., KOSTERLITZ, H.W., FOTHERGIL, L.A., MORGAN, B.A., MORRIS, H.P., Nature (London) **258** (1975) 577.
[3] GARBAY-JAUREGUIBERRY, C., ROQUES, B.P., OBERLIN, R., ANTEUNIS, M., LALA, A.K., Biochem. Biophys. Res. Commun. **71** (1976) 558.
[4] GARBAY-JAUREGUIBERRY, C., ROQUES, B.P., OBERLIN, R., ANTEUNIS, M., COMBRISSON, S., LALLEMAND, J.Y., FEBS Lett. **76** (1977) 99.
[5] MARCHALONIS, J.J., Biochem. J. **113** (1969) 299.
[6] HUNTER, W., GREENWOOD, F., Biochem. J. **91** (1964) 43.
[7] MORGAT, J.L., LAM THANH, H., CARDINAUD, B., FROMAGEOT, P., BOCKAERT, J., IMBERT, M., MOREL, F., J. Labelled Compd **6** (1970) 276.
[8] EDELHOCH, H., J. Biol. Chem. **237** (1962) 2778.
[9] ROQUES, B.P., GARBAY-JAUREGUIBERRY, C., OBERLIN, R., ANTEUNIS, M., LALA, A.K., Nature (London) **261** (1976) 778.
[10] GROS, C., PRADELLES, P., ROUGEOT, C., BEPOLDIN, O., DRAY, F., FOURNIE-ZALUSKI, M.C., ROQUES, B.P., POLLARD, H., LLORENS-CORTES, C., SCHWARTZ, J.C., J. Neurochem. (1977) (soumis pour publication).
[11] LORD, J.A.H., WATERFIELD, A.A., HUGUES, J., KOSTERLITZ, H.W., Nature (London) **267** (1977) 495.

DISCUSSION

M.A. DELAAGE: Is there a cross-reaction with endorphines?

P. PRADELLES: We have examined the cross-reactions with β-endorphine, morphine and all peptide fragments of encephalins. They are below 0.1%.

DOSAGE RADIOIMMUNOLOGIQUE DU FACTEUR THYMIQUE SERIQUE (FTS)

J.M. PLEAU, D. PASQUES, J.F. BACH
INSERM U 25, Hôpital Necker, Paris

C. GROS, F. DRAY
Unité de radioimmunologie analytique,
Institut Pasteur, Paris,
France

Abstract–Résumé

RADIOIMMUNOASSAY OF THE SERUM THYMUS FACTOR (STF).

The serum thymus factor (STF) is a polypeptide involved in the differentiation of T lymphocytes, the primary structure of which has been determined. Preliminary studies based on a semi-quantitative biological assay showed that the serum level of STF is modified in certain immune pathological situations. The authors have developed a radioimmunoassay of this factor. The STF was made immunogenic by combination with bovine albumin; the STF was labelled with iodine-125 previously alkylated with the Bolton Hunter reagent. The dosage sensitivity is such as to permit the detection of 2 pg of STF. However, the presence in the serum of molecules which interfere with the assay make it necessary to develop a method of extraction for the serum assay of STF.

DOSAGE RADIOIMMUNOLOGIQUE DU FACTEUR THYMIQUE SERIQUE (FTS).

Le facteur thymique sérique (FTS) est un polypeptide impliqué dans la différenciation des lymphocytes T, dont la structure primaire a été déterminée. Des études préliminaires, utilisant un essai biologique semi-quantitatif, ont montré que le taux sérique du FTS est modifié dans certaines situations pathologiques immunitaires. Les auteurs ont mis au point un dosage radioimmunologique de ce facteur. Le FTS a été rendu immunogène par couplage à l'albumine bovine; le FTS a été marqué à l'iode-125 préalablement alkylé par le réactif de Bolton Hunter. La sensibilité du dosage permet de détecter 2 pg de FTS. Cependant, la présence dans le sérum de molécules qui interfèrent dans le dosage nécessite la mise au point d'une méthode d'extraction pour réaliser le dosage sérique du FTS.

INTRODUCTION

La sécrétion hormonale du thymus a été suspectée après la découverte de son rôle dans l'immunité par Miller [1]. La restauration de l'immunocompétence par l'injection d'extraits thymiques a permis de mettre en évidence de manière plus directe l'existence d'hormones thymiques [2].

Depuis, plusieurs polypeptides actifs dans de nombreux modèles immunologiques ont été isolés à partir d'extraits thymiques par Goldstein et al. [3, 4] et

Trainin et Small [5]. Bach et al. ont démontré que les extraits thymiques induisent l'apparition de marqueurs T (antigène θ, sensibilité à l'azathioprine) sur des cellules de moelle osseuse initialement dépourvues de ces marqueurs [6]. La démonstration du fait que le sérum contient un facteur ayant la même activité et sa disparition après thymectomie ont établi la preuve de l'origine thymique de ce principe actif, caractérisé par sa capacité d'induire l'antigène θ [7]. Ce facteur, appelé facteur thymique sérique (FTS), a été isolé à partir du sérum de porc par ultrafiltration, chromatographie sur tamis moléculaire et sur échangeur d'ions. Sa séquence a été déterminée (<Gln – Ala – Lys – Ser – Gln – Gly – Gly – Ser – Asn – OH) et l'analogue synthétique possède les mêmes propriétés chimiques et biologiques que le produit naturel [8].

Au cours de la purification le FTS a été caractérisé par un test biologique basé sur l'induction de la sensibilité à l'azathioprine de cellules formant des rosettes de la rate de souris thymectomisée. Cet essai biologique a permis de démontrer que le taux sérique de FTS est modifié dans certaines situations pathologiques immunitaires (lupus, myasthénies, psoriasis) [9]. Cependant, cet essai est semi-quantitatif et il nous a semblé intéressant d'étudier une méthode de dosage radioimmunologique, spécifique du FTS, utilisant une hormone marquée à l'iode-125 et suffisamment sensible pour permettre un dosage direct dans le sang.

PARTIE EXPERIMENTALE

Obtention d'anticorps anti-FTS

Préparation des immunogènes

Le FTS a été rendu immunogène en le couplant à une protéine (la sérum-albumine bovine (BSA)). Nous avons effectué ce couplage de deux manières différentes: soit en présence de glutaraldéhyde, qui se lie aux groupements ϵ aminés du FTS et de la BSA, soit en présence de carbodiimide et de N-hydroxysuccinimide, qui active le groupement COOH terminal du FTS et permet la formation d'une liaison peptidique avec les groupements ϵ aminés de la BSA.

a) Couplage en présence de glutaraldéhyde – Nous avons dissous 2,5 mg de FTS (synthétisé par le groupe des peptides de Merck) et 5 mg de BSA (Behring, A.G.) dans 1 ml de tampon borate 0,1 M, pH 8,4, contenant 1% de glutaraldéhyde, et laissé incuber pendant 16 h à 4°C.

b) Couplage avec formation intermédiaire d'un N-hydroxysuccinimide ester – Nous avons dissous 2,5 mg de FTS dans 0,250 ml de diméthyl-formamide contenant 25 mg de H-hydroxysuccinimide et 50 mg de dicyclohexylcarbodiimide et laissé 16 h à 4°C. Le milieu de réaction est ensuite évaporé sous vide. Le résidu sec est repris avec 0,2 ml d'une solution de BSA (40 mg/ml) dans du tampon borate 0,1 M, pH 8,4. La réaction de couplage se fait pendant 24 h à la température ambiante.

Les deux immunogènes ainsi préparés sont dialysés pendant 48 h à 4°C contre une solution de NaCl à 9‰, puis conservés à −20°C.

Immunisation des animaux

Deux groupes de 4 lapins de race New-Zealand ont été immunisés avec chacun des conjugués.

Nous avons émulsifié des parties égales d'adjuvant de Freund complet et de solution d'immunogène, et injecté l'émulsion selon la méthode de Vaitukaitis [10] intradermiquement en plusieurs points, à raison de 1 mg d'immunogène par lapin. Trois mois après les animaux ont reçu une injection de rappel dans les mêmes conditions d'émulsion, mais à raison de 0,5 mg d'immunogène par lapin. Un mois après la première injection nous avons saigné les lapins chaque semaine et les sérums obtenus ont été testés et conservés dans du glycérol (v/v) à −20°C.

Iodation par $Na^{125}I$ du FTS

Le FTS ne comporte pas dans sa structure d'acide aminé iodable et le marquage direct à l'iode-125 n'a pu être envisagé. Nous avons utilisé la méthode de Bolton et Hunter [11] en alkylant préalablement le FTS par le p-hydroxyphényl-propionate N-hydroxysuccinimide ester et en iodant avec $Na^{125}I$ le produit de l'alkylation.

a) Préparation du dérivé alkylé – Nous avons dissous 0,1 mg de FTS dans 50 μl de tampon borate 0,1 M, pH 8,4, puis incubé avec 0,1 mg de p-hydroxy-phénylpropionate N-hydroxysuccinimide ester pendant 16 h à 4°C. Le produit obtenu est purifié sur une colonne de Sephadex G10 (0,9 × 50 cm) éluée par une solution de NaCl à 9‰. La fraction correspondant au V_0 de la colonne (FTS alkylé) est recueillie et répartie en aliquotes de 2,5 μg puis conservée à −20°C.

b) Iodation par $Na^{125}I$ du FTS alkylé – 2,5 μg de FTS alkylé sont iodés par 1–2 mCi de $Na^{125}I$ en présence de chloramine T suivant la méthode de Hunter et Greenwood [12]. Le mélange est déposé sur une colonne de Sephadex G25 (1,5 × 90 cm) et élué par de l'acide acétique 1M. Cette méthode permet de séparer le dérivé iodé du dérivé non iodé et de l'iode libre. Le pic correspondant à l'hormone marquée est récupéré, réparti en aliquotes et conservé à −20°C. La pureté du ^{125}I FTS est démontrée par la présence d'une seule tache radioactive par chromatographie sur couche mince dans le système de solvants chloroforme, méthanol, ammoniaque 25% 2:2:1 (R_f 0,6).

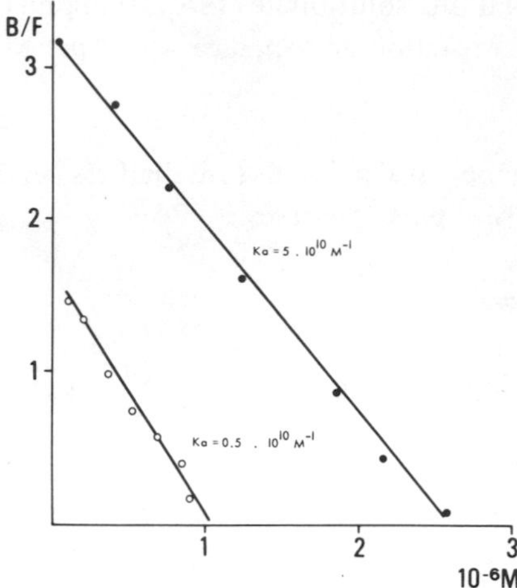

FIG.1. Diagrammes de Scatchard avec différents antisérums d'un même lapin obtenus au cours de l'immunisation.
○ *sérum du 1. 3. 77 (dilution finale 1/15 000),*
● *sérum du 1. 6. 77 (dilution finale 1/300 000).*

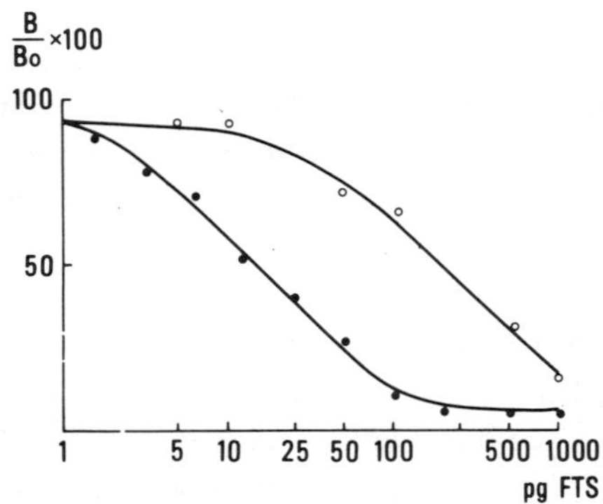

FIG.2. Courbes standard du FTS avec différents antisérums obtenus au cours de l'immunisation.
○ *sérum du 1. 3. 77 (dilution finale 1/15 000),*
● *sérum du 1. 6. 77 (dilution finale 1/300 000).*

Dosage radioimmunologique

Toutes les dilutions sont faites en tampon phosphate pH 7,3 contenant 0,9% de NaCl, 0,01% d'azide de sodium et 0,1% de gélatine (PBSG).

Nous avons incubé pendant 16 h à 4°C, 0,1 ml de ^{125}I FTS (20 000 désint/min), 0,1 ml de solution standard de FTS (contenant 0 à 1000 pg de FTS) ou d'échantillon à doser et 0,1 ml d'antisérum dilué. La séparation des fractions libre et liée du FTS se fait par addition au milieu d'incubation à 4°C de 1 ml d'une suspension de charbon-Dextran (charbon 0,25%, Dextran T 70 0,025% dans PBSG). Au bout de 20 min nous avons centrifugé les tubes à 2000 × g pendant 20 min à 4°C, éliminé le surnageant et mesuré la radioactivité du culot (charbon ayant retenu l'hormone libre).

La dilution d'emploi de l'antisérum a été testée de façon à obtenir une liaison de 40% de l'hormone marquée en l'absence d'hormone standard.

RESULTATS ET DISCUSSION

Obtention des anticorps

Les meilleurs titres d'anticorps ont été obtenus à partir de l'immunogène préparé par couplage en présence de glutaraldéhyde. Les titres d'utilisation de ces antisérums varient de 1/10 000 un mois après l'immunisation primaire à 1/300 000 un mois après le premier rappel. La figure 1 montre les diagrammes de Scatchard obtenus avec les sérums d'un même lapin à partir de deux saignées faites un mois après les injections primaire et secondaire (L_2 1. 3. 77 et L_2 1. 6. 77). Le nombre de sites a fortement augmenté et la constante d'association K_a des anticorps pour l'antigène est passée de $0{,}5 \times 10^{10}\ M^{-1}$ à $5 \times 10^{10}\ M^{-1}$.

Nous retrouvons ces résultats dans les courbes standard, présentées dans la figure 2. En effet, en utilisant les mêmes antisérums, la sensibilité du dosage exprimée comme étant la dose d'hormone capable d'inhiber 50% de la liaison de l'hormone marquée à l'anticorps (IC_{50}) est de l'ordre de 200 pg pour l'antisérum L_2 1. 3. 77 et de 20 pg pour l'antisérum L_2 1. 6. 77. Dans ce dernier cas, la limite de détection ($B_0 \pm 3$ SEM) est de 1 pg, limite que nous espérons abaisser avec les prochaines injections de rappel.

Dosage du FTS dans le sérum

La présence dans le sérum de nombreuses molécules qui interfèrent au niveau du dosage radioimmunologique, que ce soient des molécules liantes ou des peptidases qui dégradent le facteur, nécessite une étude approfondie des conditions d'extraction du FTS et la possibilité de diluer suffisamment le milieu (jusqu'à 1/100) pour éliminer ces interférences. Ce problème ne semble pas exister avec le test biologique.

Différents essais ont été entrepris sur du sérum de porc dans lequel nous avons pu déterminer des taux de FTS de l'ordre de 100 à 500 pg/ml après ultra-filtration et concentration sur membrane Amicon.

D'autres études sont en cours pour étudier des conditions plus simples d'extraction du FTS et la possibilité de sensibiliser le dosage.

REFERENCES

[1] MILLER, J.F., Nature (London) **195** (1962) 1318.

[2] SMALL, M., TRAININ, N., Nature (London) **216** (1967) 377.

[3] GOLDSTEIN, A.L., GUHA, A., ZATZ, M.M., HARDY, H.A., WHITE, A., Proc. Natl. Acad. Sci. USA **69** (1972) 1800.

[4] GOLDSTEIN, G., Nature (London) **247** (1974) 11.

[5] TRAININ, N., SMALL, M., J. Exp. Med. **132** (1970) 885.

[6] BACH, J.F., DARDENNE, M., GOLDSTEIN, A.L., GUHA, A., WHITE, A., Proc. Natl. Acad. Sci. USA **68** (1971) 2734.

[7] BACH, J.F., DARDENNE, M., Transplant. Proc. **4** (1972) 345.

[8] BACH, J.F., DARDENNE, M., PLEAU, J.M., ROSA, J., Nature (London) **266** (1977) 55.

[9] BACH, J.F., DARDENNE, M., SALOMON, J.C., Clin. Exp. Immunol. **14** (1973) 247.

[10] VAITUKAITIS, J., ROBBINS, J.B., NIESCHLAG, E., ROSS, G.T., J. Clin. Endocrinol. Metab. **33** (1971) 988.

[11] BOLTON, A.E., HUNTER, W.M., Biochem. J. **193** (1973) 529.

[12] HUNTER, W.M., GREENWOOD, F., Nature (London) **194** (1962) 495.

DISCUSSION

C. DESPLAN: Have you measured the STF in the thymus by your bioassay or radioimmunoassay? Did you localize this peptide by immunofluorescence?

J.M. PLEAU: We have determined the STF in thymus extract by our bioassay. The work on localization by immunofluorescence in the thymus is now in progress.

C. DESPLAN: Are the interferences observed in RIA due to an identical sequence present in any hormone or serum protein?

J.M. PLEAU: Not as far as we know.

CHAIRMEN OF SESSIONS

Session I	K. OEFF	Federal Republic of Germany
Session II	M. ISTIN	France
Session III	C. BECKERS	Belgium
Session IV	S.L. JEFFCOATE	United Kingdom
Session V	P.E. HALL	World Health Organization
Session VI	R.P. EKINS	United Kingdom
Session VII	R.D. PIYASENA	Sri Lanka/IAEA
Session VIII	C.A. TAFURT	Colombia
Session IX	J. HAMMERSTEIN	Federal Republic of Germany

SECRETARIAT OF THE SYMPOSIUM

Scientific Secretary:	E.H. BELCHER	Division of Life Sciences, IAEA
Administrative Secretary:	C. de MOL van OTTERLOO	Division of External Relations, IAEA
Editor:	A. ERICSON	Division of Publications, IAEA
Records Officer:	S.K. DATTA	Division of Languages, IAEA
Liaison Officer:	G. HERRMANN	Federal Republic of Germany

LIST OF PARTICIPANTS

ARGENTINA

Barmasch, M.	Comisión Nacional de Energía Atómica, Avda. del Libertador 8250, Buenos Aires 1429
Rivarola, M.A.	Centro de Investigaciones Endocrinológicas, Hospital de Niños, Gallo 1330, Buenes Aires

AUSTRALIA

Cairns, B.J.	Pathology Dept., Latrobe Valley Hospital, Moe, Victoria 3838
Smeaton, T.C.	Institute of Medical and Veterinary Science, Box 14, Rundle St., P.O., Adelaide, SA 5000

AUSTRIA

Leb, G.	Medizinische Universitätsklinik, Isotopenstation, Auenbruggerplatz 15, A-8036 Graz
Nowotny, P.J.	I. Medizinische Universitätsklinik, Lazarettgasse 14, A-1090 Vienna
Riedl, P.	Byk-Mallinckrodt, Cottagegasse 94, A-1191 Vienna
Schwarz, S.	Universität Innsbruck, Inst. Exptl. Pathologie, Fritz-Preglstr. 3, A-6020 Innsbruck
Spona, J.	I. Universitäts-Frauenklinik für Geburtshilfe und Gynäkologie, Spitalgasse 23, A-1090 Vienna

BELGIUM

Beckers, C.	Service de médecine nucléaire, UCL 10/17.80, Cliniques universitaires St. Luc, 10 av. Hippocrate, B-1200 Brussels

BELGIUM (cont.)

Bodarwé, L.J.	Laboratoire de radioimmunologie, CHBS, 75 rue Chère-Voie, B-5700 Auvelais
Bossuyt, A.	Labor. voor Farmacologie, Vrije Universiteit Brussel, Eversstraat 2, B-1000 Brussels
Bossuyt Piron, C.	Labor. voor Farmacologie, Vrije Universiteit Brussel, Eversstraat 2, B-1000 Brussels
Bourdoux, P.	Service des radioisotopes, Hôpital universitaire Saint-Pierre, 322 rue Haute, B-1000 Brussels
David, B.	Service de médecine nucléaire, UCL 10/17.80, Cliniques universitaires St. Luc, 10 av. Hippocrate, B-1200 Brussels
De Nayer, Ph.	Service de médecine nucléaire, Cliniques universitaires St. Luc, 10 av. Hippocrate, B-1200 Brussels
Fabry, J.H.	Centre de recherches agronomiques de Gembloux, Station de Zootechnie, Chemin de Liroux, B-5800 Gembloux
Fuld, D.	Centre de diagnostic hormonal, 196 Chaussée d'Alsemberg, B-1180 Brussels
Haustraete, F.R.	Katholieke Universiteit, Dept. Humane Biologie, Afd. Biochemie, Campus Gasthuisberg, Herestraat 49, B-3000 Leuven
Heynen, G.	Laboratoire de radioimmunologie, Université de Liège, Tour de Pathologie, C.H.U., Bâtiment B 23, B-4000 Sart Tilman par Liège 1
Kozyreff, V.	Clinique St. Etienne, 100 rue du Méridien, B-1030 Brussels
Léonard, J. P.	Centre de médecine nucléaire, UCL 54.30, 54 av. Hippocrate, B-1200 Brussels
Reuter, A.M.	Institut national des radioéléments, rue du Wainage, B-6220 Fleurus

Saussez, C.	Institut national des radioéléments, rue du Wainage, B-6220 Fleurus
Vranckx, R.	Institut d'hygiène et d'épidémiologie, 14 rue Juliette Wijtsman, B-1050 Brussels

BRAZIL

Bartolini, P.	Instituto de Energia Atomica – CABRR, CP 11049-Pinheiros, São Paulo -SP
Kuhlmann Russo, E.M.	Escola Paulista de Medicina, Rua Botucatú 720, Vila Clementino, São Paulo
Marques de Assis, L.	Instituto de Energia Atomica – CABRR, CP 11049-Pinheiros, São Paulo-SP

CANADA

Malkin, A.	Dept of Clinical Biochemistry, Sunnybrook Medical Centre, 2075 Bayview Ave, Toronto, Ontario M4N 4M5

CHILE

Pineda, G.	Departamento Endocrinologia y Metabolismo, Hospital Salvador, Rancagua 878, Santiago 9

COLOMBIA

Tafurt, C.A.	Hospital Militar Central, Servicio de Endocrinología, Transv. 5aNo.49-00, Bogotá

DENMARK

Buus, O.	Medi-Lab, Adelgade 7, DK-1304 Copenhagen K
Damkjaer Nielsen, M.	Department of Clinical Physiology, Glostrup Hospital, Nordre Ringvej, DK-2600 Glostrup
Hummer, L.	Dept. of Nuclear Medicine NU 2033, Rigshospitalet, Blegdamsvej 9, DK-2100 Copenhagen ϕ
Kappelgaard, A.-M.	Department of Clinical Physiology, Glostrup Hospital, Nordre Ringvej, DK-2600 Glostrup

DENMARK (cont.)

Kruse, V.
Institut für Physiologie,
Technische Universität München,
D-8050 Freising-Weihenstephan,
Federal Republic of Germany

Kvistgaard, H.J.
Centrallaboratoriet, Centralsygehuset,
DK-7500 Holstebro

Lembøl, H.L.
The Danish National Health Service,
Pharmaceutical Laboratories,
Frederikssundsvej 378, DK-2700 Brønshøj

Lindgreen, P.
Medi-Lab., Adelgade 7, DK-1304 Copenhagen K

Mollerup, C.L.
Rigshospitalet, Blegdamsvej 9,
DK-2100 Copenhagen Ø

EGYPT

El-Dakhakhuy, M.
Faculty of Medicine, Dept. of Pharmacology,
Alexandria University, Alexandria
(see also under Federal Republic of Germany)

FINLAND

Eskola, J.U.
Farmos Group Ltd., Farmos Diagnostica,
P.O. Box 425, SF-20101 Turku 10

Jänne, O.A.
Department of Biochemistry,
University of Oulu, SF-90100 Oulu 10

Juntunen, K.O.
Medica Pharmaceutical Co. Ltd.,
Teollisuuskatu 23-25, SF-00510 Helsinki 51

Mäentausta, O.K.
Clinical Chemistry, University of Oulu,
SF-90220 Oulu 22

Rosenquist, H.
Oy Star AB, Pinninkatu 57,
SF-33100 Tampere 10

Vihko, R.
Dept. of Clinical Chemistry,
University of Oulu, SF-90220 Oulu 22

Viljanen, M.K.
Turku University,
Mäkivaarantie 17, SF-20960 Turku 96

FRANCE

Belleville, F.-L.	Hôpital de Brabois, Route de Maron, F-54500 Vandœuvre-Nancy
Besnard, J.-C.	Faculté de médecine de Tours, 2 bis bld Tonnellé, F-37032 Tours Cedex
Bizollon, Ch.-A.	Service de radiopharmacie et de radioanalyse, Centre de médecine nucléaire, 59 bld Pinel, F-69394 Lyon Cedex 3
Cohen, R.M.	Service de radiopharmacie et de radioanalyse, Centre de médecine nucléaire, 59 bld Pinel, F-69394 Lyon Cedex 3
Courte, C.A.	Bio Merieux, Chemin de l'Orme, Marcy-l'Etoile, F-69260 Charbonnières-lez-Bains
Dechaud, H.	Hospices civils de Lyon, Centre de médecine nucléaire, Hôpital neuro-cardiologique, 59 bld Pinel, F-69394 Lyon Cedex 3
Delaage, M.A.	INSERM-CNRS, Centre d'immunologie de Marseille-Luminy, 70 route Léon-Lachamp, F-13288 Marseille Cedex 2
Desplan, C.	Unité 113 INSERM, Hôpital Saint-Antoine, 184 rue du Faubourg Saint-Antoine, F-75571 Paris Cedex 12
Faivre-Bauman, A.	Groupe de neuroendocrinologie cellulaire, Laboratoire de physiologie cellulaire, Collège de France, 11 place Marcellin Berthelot, F-75005 Paris Cedex 05
Grenier, J.	Fondation de recherche en hormonologie, 67 bld Pasteur, F-94269 Fresnes
Gros, C.	Unité de radioimmunologie analytique, Institut Pasteur, 28 rue du Docteur Roux, F-75724 Paris Cédex 15
Grouselle, D.	Groupe de neuroendrocrinologie cellulaire, Laboratoire de physiologie cellulaire, Collège de France, 11 place Marcellin Berthelot, F-75005 Paris Cedex 05
Guéris, J.L.E.	Laboratoire de radioimmunologie, Hôpital Lariboisière, 2 rue Ambroise Paré, F-75010 Paris

FRANCE (cont.)

Ingrand, J.	Laboratoire de radioimmunologie, CHU-Cochin, 24 rue du Faubourg Saint-Jacques, F-75674 Paris Cedex 14
Istin, M.	Service Hospitalier F-Joliot, Hôpital d'Orsay, F-91400 Orsay
Kadouche, J.	Service des isotopes, Paris Hôpital St. Louis, 40 rue Bichat, F-75010 Paris
Marchand, J.	Dept. des rayonnements ionisant, CEN de Saclay, B.P. no.2, F-91190 Gif-sur-Yvette
Meriadel de Byans, B.M.	Union Carbide France, 4 place des Etats Unis, F-94533 Rungis
Moulin, G.J.	Centre René Huguenin, 5 rue Gaston Latouche, F-92211 Saint-Cloud
Nabet, P.	Hôpital central, Laboratoire de biochimie, 21 av. de Lattre de Tassigny, F-54000 Nancy
Pleau, J.M.	INSERM U 25, Hôpital Necker, Clinique néphrologique, 161 rue de Sèvres, F-75015 Paris Cedex 15
Pradelles, P.	Institut Pasteur, Unité de radioimmunologie analytique, 28 rue du Docteur Roux, F-75724 Paris Cedex 15
Prédine, J.R.	Laboratoire de biochimie hormonale, Hôpital de Bicêtre, 78 rue du Général Leclerc, F-94270 Kremlin-Bicêtre
Prospert, J.	Dept. des rayonnements ionisants, CEN de Saclay, B.P. no. 2, F-91190 Gif-sur-Yvette
Reiffsteck, A.	Fondation de recherche en hormonologie, 67 bld Pasteur, F-94260 Fresnes
Rougon-Rappuzi, G.	INSERM-CNRS, Centre d'immunologie de Marseille-Luminy, 70 route Léon-Lachamp, F-13288 Marseille Cedex 2

GERMANY, FEDERAL REPUBLIC OF

Aderjan, R.E.	Institut für Rechtsmedizin, Universität Heidelberg, D-6900 Heidelberg

Allgeier, V.	Travenol GmbH, Clinical Assays Division, Nymphenburgerstrasse 1, D-8000 Munich 2
Arndts, D.	Biochemische Forschung der Fa. Boehringer, Abt. Biochemie, D-6507 Ingelheim
Arnold, A.	Byk-Mallinckrodt, Chem. Produkte GmbH, Postfach 2060, D-6057 Dietzenbach 2
Arnstadt, K.-I.	Südd. Versuchs- und Forschungsanstalt für Milchwirtschaft, Institut für Physiologie, Weihenstephan, D-8050 Freising
Berthold, F.	Laboratorium Prof. Berthold, Postfach 160, D-7547 Wildbad 1
Beth, H.	Isotopen Dienst West, Einsteinstrasse 9–11, D-6072 Dreieich 1
Biro, G.	Medizinische Universitätsklinik und Poliklinik, Innere Medizin II, D-6650 Homburg/Saar
Bor, D.	Fa. Siemens, UB-Med., Henkestrasse 127, D-8520 Erlangen
Bourvé, H.F.	Boehringer Mannheim, Sandhofer Strasse, D-6800 Mannheim 31
Bozler, G.	Abt. für Biochemie, Dr. Karl Thomae GmbH, D-7950 Biberach
Breuer, H.	Institut für klinische Biochemie, Universitätskliniken, D-5300 Bonn-Venusberg
Buch, K.-U.	Medizinische Klinik, Klinikum Steglitz der Freien Universität Berlin, Hindenburgdamm 30, D-1000 Berlin 45
Büber, V.	Wilhelm-Hauff-Strasse 21, D-1000 Berlin 41
Dauner, H.-O.	Bio-Rad. Laboratories GmbH, Dachauerstrasse 364, D-8000 Munich 50
Diel, F.	Medizinische Klinik, Klinikum Steglitz der Freien Universität Berlin, Hindenburgdamm 30, D-1000 Berlin 45
Distler, W.	Medizinische Einrichungen der Universität Düsseldorf, Frauenklinik, Moorenstrasse 5, D-4000 Düsseldorf

GERMANY, FED. REP. OF (cont.)

Döhler, K.-D.	Abt. für klinische Endokrinologie, Medizinische Hochschule Hannover, Karl-Wiechert Allee 9, D-3000 Hanover 61
Drahovsky, M.	Byk-Mallinckrodt, Chem. Produkte GmbH, Postfach 2060, D-6057 Dietzenbach 2
Düsterberg, B.	Schering AG, Müllerstrasse 170–178, D-1000 Berlin 65
Dwenger, A.	Klinische Biochemie, Medizinische Hochschule Hannover, Karl-Wiechert-Allee 9, D-3000 Hanover 61
Eiletz, J.	Universitäts-Frauenklinik Charlottenburg, Abt. für gynäkologische Endokrinologie, Pulsstrasse 4–14, D-1000 Berlin 19
El-Dakhakhuy, M.	Faculty of Medicine, Dept. of Pharmacology, Alexandria University, Alexandria, Egypt (see also under Egypt)
Endler, J.	Klinikum der medizinischen Hochschule Lübeck, Abt. für Gynäkologie und Geburtshilfe II, Ratzeburger Allee 164, D-2400 Lübeck 1
Eul, A.H.	Boehringer Mannheim, Sandhofer Strasse, D-6800 Mannheim 31
Fehse, P.	Abbott GmbH, Diagnostics Division, Ampèrestrasse 3–5, D-6070 Langen
Fischer, M.	Boehringer Mannheim, Sandhofer Strasse, D-6800 Mannheim 31
Freischmidt, P.	Isotopen Dienst West, Einsteinstrasse 9–11, D-6072 Dreieich 1
Freytag, W.G.	Unilever Forschungsges. mbH, Behringerstrasse 154, D-2000 Hamburg 50
Friedrich, G.	Institut für Rechtsmedizin, Albertstrasse 9, D-7800 Freiburg
Gethmann, U.	Klinikum der medizinischen Hochschule Lübeck, Abt. für Gynäkologie und Geburtshilfe II, Ratzeburger Allee 160, D-2400 Lübeck 1

Hagemann, J.	Abt. für Nuklearmedizin, Universitätskrankenhaus, HH-Eppendorf, D-2000 Hamburg
Hammerstein, J.	Abt. für gynäkologische Endokrinologie, Klinikum Steglitz der Freien Universität Berlin, Hindenburgdamm 30, D-1000 Berlin 45
Hanneck, E.G.	Deutsche Forschungs- und Versuchsanstalt für Luft- und Raumfahrt, D-5000 Cologne 90
Harzer, G.V.	Isotopenlabor Dr. Karl Dirr, Paul-Hösch-Strasse 25a, D-8000 Munich 60
Hasan, S.H.	Schering AG, Müllerstrasse 170–178, D-1000 Berlin 65
Häberle, M.	Zentrum für innere Medizin und Kinderheilkunde der Universität Ulm, D-7900 Ulm
Heicke, B.	Bioscientia, P.O. Box 1628, D-6500 Mainz
Hengels, K.-J.	I. Medizinische Klinik A der Universität Düsseldorf, Moorenstrasse 5, D-4000 Düsseldorf
Henkel, M.	Strahlenklinik und nuklearmedizinische Abt., Stadtkrankenhaus, D-6050 Offenbach
Hesch, R.-D.	Abt. für klinische Endokrinologie, Medizinische Hochschule Hannover, Karl-Wiechert-Allee 9, D-3000 Hanover 61
Himmler, V.	Physiologisches Institut, Tierärztliche Hochschule, Bischofsholer Damm 15, D-3000 Hanover
Hintz, H.	LKB Instrument GmbH, Lochhamer Schlag 5, D-8032 Gräfelfing
Hop, E.	Hewlett-Packard, Herrenbergerstrasse 110, D-7030 Böblingen
Hümpel, M.	Schering AG, Müllerstrasse 170–178, D-1000 Berlin 65
Jacobs, A.	Zentralstelle für Atomenergie Dokumentation, D-7514 Eggenstein-Leopoldshafen 2
Joustra, M.	Deutsche Pharmacia GmbH, Abt. Diagnostika, Munzingerstrasse 9, D-7800 Freiburg 1

GERMANY, FED. REP. OF (cont.)

Kaltwasser, J.P.	Zentrum der inneren Medizin, Abt. für Hämatologie, J.W. Goethe-Universität, Theodor-Stern-Kai 7, D-6000 Frankfurt 70
Keogh, H.J.	Bioscientia, P.O. Box 1628, D-6500 Mainz
Keppel, H.	Federal Research Centre of Agriculture, Project Group Isotope Laboratory, D-3300 Brunswick
Kimpel, G.	Facharzt für innere Krankheiten, Max-Beckmann-Strasse 85, D-7920 Heidenheim/Brenz
Kley, R.	Deutsche Gesellschaft für Laboratoriumsmedizin e.V., Manforter Strasse 225, D-5090 Leverkusen 1
Klingler, W.	Amersham Buchler GmbH, Gieselweg 1, D-3300 Brunswick
Knöchel, A.	Institut für anorganische und angewandte Chemie, Universität Hamburg, Martin-Luther-King-Pl. 6, D-2000 Hamburg 13
Koszik, F.K.	Deutsche KABI Diagnostika, Levelingstr. 18, D-8000 Munich
Kuss, E.	I. Frauenklinik der Universität, Maistrasse 11, D-8000 Munich 2
Lambrecht, W.P.	LKB Instrument GmbH, Lochhamer Schlag 5, D-8032 Gräfelfing
Leising, K.	Amersham Buchler GmbH, Gieselweg 1, D-3300 Brunswick
Lohr, R. von	Paul-Ehrlich-Institut des Bundesamtes für Sera und Impfstoffe, Paul-Ehrlich-Strasse, D-6000 Frankfurt 70
Lommer, D.	Institut für Laboratoriumsdiagnostik, Kreiskrankenhaus, D-8360 Deggendorf
Lüben, G.	Behringwerke AG, Postfach 1140, D-3550 Marburg
Marschner, I.	Medizinische Klinik Innenstadt der Universität München, Ziemssenstrasse 1, D-8000 München 2
Matern, S.	Medizinische Universitätsklinik, Hugstetter Strasse 55, D-7800 Freiburg

Meinhold, H.	Nuklearmedizinische Abt., Klinikum Steglitz der Freien Universität Berlin, Hindenburgdamm 30, D-1000 Berlin 45
Meyer, B.	Amersham Buchler GmbH, Gieselweg 1, D-3300 Brunswick
Müller, J.E.	I. Medizinische Klinik A der Universität Düsseldorf, Moorenstrasse 5, D-4000 Düsseldorf
Naegele, W.	Byk–Mallinckrodt, Chem. Produkte GmbH, Postfach 2060, D-6057 Dietzenbach 2
Nennstiel, H.-J.	Med. Diagnost. Institut, Westliche 51, D-7530 Pforzheim
Nevinny-Stickel, J.	Universitäts-Frauenklinik Charlottenburg, Abt. für gynäkologische Endokrinologie, Pulsstrasse 4–14, D-1000 Berlin 19
Niemann, E.	Hoechst AG, D-6230 Frankfurt 80
Nienweboer, B.	Schering AG, Müllerstrasse 170–178, D-1000 Berlin 65
Noah, E.	Universitätsklinik Mainz, Langenbeckstrasse 1, D-6500 Mainz
Nocke-Finck, L.	Institut für klinische Biochemie der Universität Bonn, D-5300 Bonn-Venusberg
Oeff, K.	Institut für Nuklearmedizin, Klinikum Steglitz der Freien Universität Berlin, Hindenburgdamm 30, D-1000 Berlin 45
Parvizi, N.	Institut für Tierzucht und Tierverhalten FAL, Mariensee, D-3057 Neustadt 1
Pfau, A.	Institut für Tierzucht und Tierverhalten FAL, Mariensee, D-3057 Neustadt 1
Phelps, G.	Travenol Clinical Assays Division, Nymphenburger Strasse 1, D-8000 Munich 1,
Pietilä, U.J.	Wallac Oy, P.O. Box 10, SF-20101 Turku 10, Finland
Pollow, K.	Freie Universität Berlin, Institut für Molekularbiologie und Biochemie, Arnimallee 22, D-1000 Berlin 33

GERMANY, FED. REP. OF (cont.)

Quabbe, D.-J.	Klinikum Steglitz der Freien Universität Berlin, Hindenburgdamm 30, D-1000 Berlin 45
Ranke, B.M.	Abt. für diagnostische Endokrinologie, Universitäts-Kinderklinik, Rümelinstrasse 23, D-7400 Tübingen
Raue, F.	Abt. für innere Medizin, Endokrinologie und Stoffwechsel, Universität Ulm, Steinhövelstrasse 9, D-7900 Ulm
Röhle, G.	Institut für klinische Biochemie, Universitäts-Kliniken, D-5300 Bonn-Venusberg
Sackmann, U.	Universitäts-Frauenklinik Charlottenburg, Abt. für gynäkologische Endokrinologie, Pulsstr. 4–14, D-1000 Berlin 19
Sandel, P.	Institut für klinische Chemie am Klinikum, Grosshadern, Ludwig-Maximilians-Universität, D-8000 Munich
Scheuerlein, H.	C.H.F. Müller, Unternehmensbereich der Philips GmbH, Abt. Med. Datenverarbeitung, Röntgenstrasse 22, D-2000 Hamburg 63
Schmid, A.	Amersham Buchler GmbH & Co KG, Gieselweg 1, D-3300 Brunswick
Schmidt-Gollwitzer, K.	Universitäts-Frauenklinik Charlottenburg, Abt. für gynäkologische Endokrinologie, Pulsstrasse 4–14, D-1000 Berlin 19
Schmidt-Gollwitzer, M.	Universitäts-Fraunenklinik Charlottenburg, Abt. für gynäkologische Endokrinologie, Pulsstrasse 4–14, D-1000 Berlin 19
Schneider, P.	Radiologisches Institut, Städtische Kliniken, Pacelliallee 4, D-6400 Fulda
Scholten, T.	I. Medizinische Klinik A der Universität Düsseldorf, Moorenstrasse 5, D-4000 Düsseldorf
Schöneshöfer, M.	Institut für klinische Chemie, Klinikum Steglitz der Freien Universität Berlin, Hindenburgdamm 30, D-1000 Berlin 41

Schroeter, I.	I. Medizinische Klinik der Universität, Schittenhelmstrasse 12, D-2300 Kiel
Schroeter, R.F.	I. Medizinische Klinik der Universität, Schittenhelmstrasse 12, D-2300 Kiel
Schweer, H.-H.	Medizinische Hochschule, Institut für klinische Biochemie, Karl-Wiechert-Allee 9, D-3000 Hanover 61
Siegers, M.P.	Institut für Medizin, Kernforschungsanlage Jülich, Postfach 1913, D-5170 Jülich
Simane, Z.	E. Merck Medical Research, Frankfurter Strasse 250, D-6100 Darmstadt 1
Sippell, W.G.	Dr. v. Haunersches Kinderspital, Lindwurmstrasse 4, D-8000 Munich 2
Sokolowski, G.	Byk-Mallinckrodt, Chem. Produkte GmbH, Postfach 2060, D-6057 Dietzenbach 2
Sourgens, H.	Institut für Pharmakologie und Toxikologie der Universität, Westring 12, D-4400 Münster
Steinmaus, H.	Henning Berlin GmbH, Komturstrasse 19–20, D-1000 Berlin 42
Stengele, E.	Frauenklinik der Universität, Endokrinologische Abt., Hugstetterstrasse 55, D-7800 Freiburg
Stetten, O. von	Byk-Mallinckrodt, Chem. Produkte GmbH, Postfach 2060, D-6057 Dietzenbach 2
Strecker, H.J.	Hoechst AG, Radiochemisches Laboratorium, Postfach 800 320, D-6230 Frankfurt 80
Streibl, W.	Abt. für innere Medizin der Universität, Steinhövelstrasse 9, D-7900 Ulm
Unz, F.C.	Linder Höhe, D-5000 Cologne 90
Uthemann, H.E.	Biotest-Serum-Institut GmbH, Flughafenstrasse 4, D-6000 Frankfurt
Watzek, K.	Wichernstrasse 11, D-8120 Weilheim
Werder, K. von	Medizinische Klinik Innenstadt der Universität München, Ziemssenstrasse 1, D-8000 Munich 2

GERMANY, FED. REP. OF (cont.)

Wernze, H.	Medizinische Klinik der Universität Würzburg, Josef-Schneiderstrasse 2, D-8700 Würzburg
Winterhoff, H.	Institut für Pharmakologie und Toxikologie der Universität, Westring 12, D-4400 Münster
Wirth, H.E.	Berliner Kies Centrale, Uhlandstrasse 6, D-1000 Berlin 19
Wood, W.G.	Medizinische Klinik Innenstadt der Universität München, Ziemssenstrasse 1, D-8000 Munich 2
Zimmermann, H.H.	Hewlett-Packard, Herrenbergerstrasse 110, D-7030 Böblingen

GHANA

Dakubu, S.	Nuclear Medicine Unit, Dept. of Medicine and Therapeutics, University of Ghana Medical School, P.O.Box 4236, Accra

GREECE

Alevizou-Terzaki, V.	Dept. of Clinical Therapeutics, The University of Athens Medical School, Div. of Radioisotopes, "Alexandra" Hospital, Vas. Sofias Ave and K. Lourou St., Athens 611
Gyftaki, E.	Dept. of Clinical Applications of Radioisotopes, The University of Athens Medical School, Alexandra Maternity Hospital, Vas. Sofias Ave and K. Lourou St., Athens 611
Hadzilouka, A.M.	Radioisotope Dept., Vassilefs Paulas Hospital, The University of Athens, Athens
Panaidou, H.	Alexandra Maternity Hospital, Vas. Sofias Ave and K. Lourou St., Athens 611
Solanoglou, M.	Alexandra Maternity Hospital, Vas. Sofias Ave and K. Lourou St., Athens 611

Vassilakos, P.J.	Nuclear Medicine Dept., Saint Savas Hospital, 171 Alexandras Ave., Athens
Vassilakou, O.I.	Saint Savas Hospital, 171 Alexandras Ave., Athens
Vyzantiadis, A.	State Maternity Hospital of Thessaloniki, Alex. Papanastasiou, Thessaloniki

GUATEMALA

Gutierrez Sole, G.R.	Instituto Nacional de Energía Nuclear, 3 Av. "A" 2–68 Zona 1, Guatemala

INDIA

Hazra, D.K.	Sarojini Naidu Medical College, Agra, UP 282005 (see also under UK)
Shah, K.B.	Bhabha Atomic Research Centre, Trombay, Bombay 400 085

ISRAEL

Buchman, O.	Radiochemistry Dept., Nuclear Research Centre – Negev, P.O. Box 9001, Beer-Sheva
Shani, J.	Radiopharmacy Unit, School of Pharmacy, The Hebrew University, P.O. Box 12065, Jerusalem
Teitelbaum, Z.	Radiochemistry Dept., Nuclear Research Centre – Negev, P.O. Box 9001, Beer-Sheva
Torten, M.	Israel Institute for Biological Research, P.O. Box 19, Ness-Ziona

ITALY

Maussier, M.L.	Nuclear Medicine Institute, Università Cattòlica S.C., Policlinico Gemelli, Largo A. Gemelli 8, I-00168 Rome
Troncone, L.	Nuclear Medicine Institute, Università Cattòlica S.C., Policlinico Gemelli, Largo A. Gemelli 8, I-00168 Rome

LUXEMBOURG

Hoffmann, J.P.	Institut d'hygiène et de santé publique, 42 rue du Laboratoire, Luxembourg

NETHERLANDS

Bosch, A.	Organon Int. B.V., Kloosterstraat 6, Oss
Geuskens, L.M.	St. Joseph Hospital, Aalsterweg 259, Eindhoven
Hünteler, J.L.	Psychiatrisch Ziekenhuis "Sancta Maria", Langevelderlaan 1, Noordwijkerhout
Lequin, R.M.	Dept. of Obstetrics and Gynecology, St. Radboudziekenhuis, Geert Grooteplein Zuid 16, Nijmegen
Lombarts, A.J.	Leyenburg Hospital, Leyweg 275, The Hague
Mulder, J.	Laboratorium voor de Volksgezondheit in Friesland, Jelsumerstraat 6, Leeuwarden
Prins, H.	Medisch Chemisch Laboratorium ABL, Nijlandstraat 11, Postbus 232, NL-9400 AE Assen
Raaijmakers, F.J.	Nenimij B.V., Laan Copes van Cattenburch 76–78, Postbus 85502, The Hague
Schellekens, A.P.	Wilhelmina Gasthuis, Afd. Endocrinologie, 1ste Helmersstr. 104, Amsterdam
Segers, M.F.	St. Radboudziekenhuis, Geert Grooteplein Zuid 16, Nijmegen
Tertoolen, J.F.	Laboratory for Nuclear Medicine "Voorburg", Boxtelseweg 48, Vught
Thomas, C.M.	Dept. of Obstetrics and Gynecology, St. Radboudziekenhuis, Geert Grooteplein Zuid 16, Nijmegen
Vader, H.L.	St. Joseph Hospital, Aalsterweg 259, Eindhoven
Visser, J.W.	Laboratory of Nuclear Medicine of the North East Netherlands Hospital Cooperative Foundation (Sazinon), Dr. G.H. Amshoffweg 1, Postbus 174, Hoogeveen

Visser, T.J. — Department of Internal Medicine III and Clinical Endocrinology,
Erasmus Universiteit, Postbus 1738, Rotterdam

Woldring, M.G. — Dept. of Nuclear Medicine,
University Hospital, Oostersingel 59, Groningen

Zanten, A.K. van — Dept. of Nuclear Medicine,
University Hospital, Oostersingel 59, Groningen

NIGERIA

Afolabi, S.K. — Endocrine Unit, Dept. of Clinical Pathology,
Lagos University Teaching Hospital,
PMB 12003, Lagos

NORWAY

Iversen, M.S. — Dr. Fürst Medical Laboratory,
Kr. August Gt. 15 A, Oslo 1

Rødseth, J.S. — Dr. V. Fürst Medical Laboratory,
Kr. August Gt. 15 A, Oslo 1

Silsand, T. — St. Josephs Hospital, Olavsgt. 26,
N-3900 Porsgrunn

PARAGUAY

Diaz-Gill, G.A. — Instituto para el Estudio de la Reproducción Humana (IERH),
Dr. Montero 658 (FCM),
Asunción

ROMANIA

Simionescu, L. — Institute of Endocrinology,
71279 Bd. Aviatorilor 34, Bucharest

SOUTH AFRICA

Pitout, M.J. — Life Sciences Div., Atomic Energy Board,
Private Bag X256, Pretoria 0001

Watt, J.J. van der — Life Sciences Div., Atomic Energy Board,
Private Bag X256, Pretoria 0001

Wyk, A.J. van — Chemistry Division, Atomic Energy Board,
Private Bag X256, Pretoria 0001

SPAIN

Izquierdo, J.M.	Dept. of Clinical Biochemistry, Hospital General de Asturias, Oviedo, Asturias
Ortin, N.	Junta de Energía Nuclear, Avda. Complutense, Madrid 3

SRI LANKA

Piyasena, R.D.	Nuclear Medicine Unit, Faculty of Medicine, University of Sri Lanka, Peradeniya Campus (see also under IAEA)

SWEDEN

Aurell, N.M.	Dept. of Medicine I, University of Göteborg, Sahlgren's Hospital, S-413 45 Göteborg
Delin, B.K.	Dept. of Medicine I, University of Göteborg, Sahlgren's Hospital, S-413 45 Göteborg
Eriksson, O.	AB Kabi, Research Dept., Analytical Chemistry, Fack, S-112 87 Stockholm
Jonsson, S.	Kärnsjukhuset, S-54101 Skövde
Landin, G.E.F.	Stockholms Immunlaboratorium AB, Vanadisvägen 21, S-113 46 Stockholm
Lundahl, P.N.	Dept. of Clinical Chemistry, Centrallasarettet, Västra Klinikerna, S-551 85 Jönköping
Lundberg, P.-A.	Dept. of Clinical Chemistry, Sahlgrens' Hospital, S-413 45 Göteborg
Thorell, J.I.	Dept. of Nuclear Medicine, University of Lund, Malmö General Hospital, S-214 01 Malmö
Wästhed, A.B.	Stockholms Immunlaboratorium AB, Vanadisvägen 21, S-113 46 Stockholm
Wide, L.	Kliniskt-Kemiska Centrallaboratoriet, Akademiska Sjukhuset, S-750 14 Uppsala 14

SWITZERLAND

Abisch, E.	Sandoz AG, Geb. 507/902, Abt. Biopharmazeutik, CH-4002 Basel
Götz, U.	Sandoz AG, Biological and Medical Research Div., CH-4002 Basel
Knobel, H.R.	F. Hoffmann-LaRoche AG, Dept. Diagnostica, CH-4002 Basel
Kompis, A.	F. Hoffmann-La Roche AG, Kontroll Abteilung, CH-4002 Basel
Kopp, H.G.	Medizinische Poliklinik HL 14, Kantonsspital, Rämistrasse 100, CH-8091 Zurich
Kretschmer, R.E.	Chemisches Zentrallabor, Inselspital, CH-3010 Bern
Le Dain, M.Y.	F. Hoffmann-La Roche AG, Grenzacherstrasse 124, CH-4002 Basel
Marbach, P.	Sandoz AG, Biological and Medical Research Div., CH-4002 Basel
Mittelholzer, E.	F. Hoffmann-La Roche AG, Grenzacherstrasse 124, CH-4002 Basel
Petermann, H.-P.	Ciba-Geigy AG, Experiment. Toxikologie, R 1058/632, CH-4002 Basel
Rettenmaier, R.A.	F. Hoffmann-La Roche AG, Dept. of Vitamin and Nutritional Research, CH-4002 Basel
Vitins, P.	Eidgenössisches Institut für Reaktorforschung, CH-5303 Würenligen

SYRIA

Sakka Amini, M.	Centre de médecine nucléaire, Mezze

TURKEY

Akit, A.	Ankara University Medical School, Nuclear Medicine Center, Cebeci-Anakara
Laleli, Y.R.	Hacettepe Medical Center, Ankara

UNITED KINGDOM

Bagshawe, K.D.	Department of Medical Oncology, Charing Cross Hospital, Fulham Palace Road, London W6 8RF
Bayly, R.J.	The Radiochemical Centre, White Lion Road, Amersham, Bucks HP7 9LL
Broughton Pipkin, F.	University of Nottingham, Professional Unit, City Hospital, Hucknall Road, Nottingham NG5 IPB
Cooper, W.	Dept. of Obstetrics and Gynaecology, Medical School, Ninewells Hospital, Dundee
Corker, C.S.	Wellcome Reagents Ltd., Langley Court, Beckenham, Kent BR3 3BS
Cowan S.I.	Hoechst UK Ltd., Walton Manor, Walton, Milton Keynes, Bucks MK7 7AJ
Ekins, R.P.	Dept. of Nuclear Medicine, The Middlesex Hospital Medical School, Mortimer Street, London W1N 8AA
Hazra, D.K.	Sarojini Naidu Medical College, Agra, U.P. 282005, India (see also under India)
Hordle, D.A.	Beecham Pharmaceuticals, Research Division, Chemotherapeutic Research Centre, Brockham Park, Betchworth, Surrey RH3 7AJ
Hurn, B.A.L.	Wellcome Research Laboratories, Langley Court, Beckenham, Kent BR3 3BS
Jeffcoate, S.L.	Chelsea Hospital for Women, Dovehouse Street, London SW3
Joyce, B.G.	Tenovus Institute for Cancer Research, Welsh National School of Medicine, Heath Park, Cardiff CF4 4XX
Lader, S.R.	Wellcome Research Laboratories, Langley Court, Beckenham, Kent BR3 3BS
Lidgard, G.P.	Corning Medical, Braintree, Essex
Lynch, E.P.J.	The Radiochemical Centre, White Lion Road, Amersham, Bucks HP7 9LL

Malan, P.G.	Dept. of Nuclear Medicine, The Middlesex Hospital Medical School, Mortimer Street, London W1N 8AA
McLean, H.A.	Wellcome Reagents Ltd., Langley Court, Beckenham, Kent BR3 3BS
Moody, G.W.	Searle Diagnostic, Division of G.D. Searle & Co.Ltd., Lane End Road, High Wycombe, Bucks HP12 4HL
Read, G.F.	Tenovus Institute for Cancer Research, Welsh National School of Medicine, Heath Park, Cardiff CF4 4XX
Riad-Fahmy, D.	Tenovus Institute for Cancer Research, Welsh National School of Medicine, Heath Park, Cardiff CF4 4XX
Shelton, J.	Beecham Pharmaceuticals Research Division, Clarendon Road, Worthing, West Sussex
Siddiqui, S.A.	Searle Diagnostic, Division of G.D. Searle & Co.Ltd., Lane End Road, High Wycombe, Bucks HP12 4HL
Stafford, J.E.	Dept. of Metabolic Studies, G.D. Searle & Co. Ltd., Lane End Road, High Wycombe, Bucks HP12 4HL
Sufi, S.B.	Chelsea Hospital for Women, Dovehouse Street, London SW3
Walker, R.F.	Tenovus Institute for Cancer Research, Welsh National School of Medicine, Heath Park, Cardiff CF4 4XX
Webb, B.A.	Dept. of Obstetrics and Gynaecology, Medical School, Ninewells Hospital, Dundee
Weston, S.M.	Searle Diagnostic, Division of G.D.Searle & Co.Ltd., Lane End Road, High Wycombe, Bucks HP12 4HL
White, N.	Dept. of Physiology, St. George's Hospital Medical School, Cranmer Terrace, Tooting, London SW 17
Whitworth, A.	The Radiochemical Centre, White Lion Road, Amersham, Bucks HP7 9LL
Wilkins, T.A.	The Radiochemical Centre, White Lion Road, Amersham, Bucks HP7 9LL

UNITED KINGDOM (cont.)

Wilson, D.W.	Tenovus Institute for Cancer Research, Welsh National School of Medicine, Heath Park, Cardiff CF4 4XX
Young, J.L.	Dept. of Obstetrics and Gynaecology, Ninewells Hospital, Dundee University, Dundee

UNITED STATES OF AMERICA

Block, E.	Schwarz/Mann, Division of Becton Dickinson & Co., Mountain View Avenue, Orangeburg, NY 10962
Cathou, P.Y.	Clinical Assays, Division of Travenol Laboratories Inc., 620 Memorial Drive, Cambridge, MA 02139
Decker, R.H.	Abbott Laboratories, Dept. 90D, Abbott Diagnostics Division, North Chicago, IL 60064
Fitzgerald, J.J.	Cambridge Nuclear Corp., 575 Middlesex Turnpike, Billerica, MA 01865
Fox, A.E.	Carter-Wallace Inc., Wampole Laboratories Division, Half Acre Rd, Cranbury NJ 08512
Gasperoni, P.J.	Cambridge Nuclear Corp., 575 Middlesex Turnpike, Billerica, MA 01865
Goldman, S.C.	Picker Corporation, 12 Clintonville Rd, Northford, CT 06472
Litt, G.J.	New England Nuclear Corp., Biochemical Division, 601 Treble Cove Road, N. Billerica, MA 01862
Malya, G.P.A.	Biomedical Research Dept. ICI US Inc., Wilmington, DE 19897
Nisula, B.C.	National Institute of Child Health and Human Development, National Institutes of Health, Room 10-B-09, Building 10, Bethseda, MD 20014
Odell, W.D.	Harbor General Hospital Campus, UCLA School of Medicine, Torrance, CA 90509
Odstrchel, G.	Corning Glass Works, Sullivan Science Park, Corning, NY 14830

Painter, K. — Dept. of Radiology and Radiation Biology,
Colorado State University,
Fort Collins, CO 80523

Parsons, G.H., Jr. — Clinical Assays,
Division of Travenol Laboratories Inc.,
620 Memorial Drive, Cambridge, MA 02139

Rodbard, D. — Endocrinology and Reproduction Research Branch,
National Institutes of Health,
Room 13-N-236, Building 10, Bethesda, MD 20014

Rothchild, S. — Clinical Assays,
Division of Travenol Laboratories Inc.,
620 Memorial Drive, Cambridge, MA 02139

Schiffman, M.B. — Ortho Diagnostics Research Institute,
Raritan, NJ 08869

YUGOSLAVIA

Gall, D. — Odjel Za Nuklearnu Medicinu, Osijek,
Park Lenjina 3, Opca Bolnica

Odavić, M. — Dept. of Nuclear Medicine,
Internal Clinic, Pasterova str. 2,
YU-11000 Belgrade

ORGANIZATIONS

INTERNATIONAL ATOMIC ENERGY AGENCY

Dudley, R.A. — Medical Applications Section,
Division of Life Sciences,
International Atomic Energy Agency,
Kärntner Ring 11, P.O. Box 590,
1011 Vienna,
Austria

Piyasena, R.D.
(IAEA fellow) — Nuclear Medicine Unit, Faculty of Medicine,
University of Sri Lanka, Peradeniya Campus,
Sri Lanka
(see also under Sri Lanka)

UNITED NATIONS

Szendrei, K.

Division of Narcotic Drugs,
New York, NY 10017,
United States of America

WORLD HEALTH ORGANIZATION

Hall, P.E.

Human Reproduction Unit,
World Health Organization,
CH-1211 Geneva 27,
Switzerland

AUTHOR INDEX

Roman numerals are volume numbers.
Italic numerals refer to the first page of a paper by the author concerned.
Upright numerals denote the page numbers of comments and questions in discussions.

Abisch, E.: I 183
Ahene, I.S.: I *155*
Alevizou-Terzaki, V.: II *193*
Assis, L.M.: I *109*
Ayala, A.R.: I *133*
Bach, J.F.: II *505*
Bagshawe, K.D.: II 426, *435,* 466, 467
Barlet, J.P.: II *405*
Bartolini, P.: I *109,* 121
Baumann, H.: I *123*
Bayly, R.J.: I 511; II 76, 125
Beckers, C.: II *199, 341, 379*
Bepoldin, O.: II *495*
Bidlingmaier, F.: I *229*
Bieglmayer, Ch.: II *245*
Bierich, J.R.: I *309*
Bizollon, Ch.-A.: II *91,* 102, 103, 158, 164, 208
Bosch, A.: I 269, 294; II 222
Bouckaert, A.: II *341*
Bourdoux, P.: II *349,* 361, 368
Bozler, G.: II 298, *299,* 308, 315
Breuer, H.: II *81,* 90, 161, 236, 256
Broux, M.: II *427*
Bryant, J.: I *399*
Campo, S.: II *225*
Cathou, P.Y.: II 103
Chadney, D.C.: I *399*
Cohen, R.: II *91*
Cole, J.: I *277*
Conte-Devolx, B.: II *479*
Cornette, C.: II *341*
Cowan, S.I.: I *347,* 358, 359
Cox, M.G.: I *425*
Cracel, G.: II *495*
Cresswell, M.A.: II *149*
Dakubu, S.: I *155,* 160
Decker, R.H.: I 275
De Estrada, R.: II *237*
Delaage, M.A.: II *479,* 487, 503
Delange, F.: II *349*
De Lean, A.: I *469*
De Nayer, Ph.: I 67, 306; II *199,* 208, 209
Desplan, C.: II *405,* 417, 426, 510
Diel, F.: I *123,* 237; II 403
Dirr, W.: I *69*
Docter, R.: II *469*
Döhler, K.-D.: I *297,* 306, 307; II 90
Dray, F.: II *495, 505*
Dudley, R.A.: I *457,* 467, *517*
Dugue, M.A.: II *349*
Dwenger, A.: II *141,* 148
Edwards, R.: I *329*
Eiletz, J.: II *257*
Ekins, R.P.: I 41, 153, *241,* 269, 270, 274, 275, 305, *329,* 346, *425, 437,* 454, 455, 512, 513; II *6, 39,* 54, 55, 56, 73, 74, 75, 76, 78

Faivre-Bauman, A.: I *319,* 328
Felixberger, F.: I *43*
Figdor, H.C.: I *457*
Foli, A.K.: I *155*
Fournie-Zaluski, M.C.: II *495*
Franchimont, P.: II *427*
François, B.: II *341*
Franz, H.E.: II *489*
Friedel, R.: II *141*
Froget, D.: II *91*
Fuld, D.: I 228, 237, 238, 275, 511; II 36, 54, 73, 77, 90, 102, 137, 223, 243
Gaspar, S.: II *427*
Gerok, W.: II *273*
Gloning, K.: I *69*
Glöckner, B.: I *43*
Goebel, R.: I *69*
Goldman, S.C.: I 217, 395
Gottsmann, M.: I *43*
Götz, U.: I *383*
Grenier, J.: I *91,* 107, 210; II 56, 78, 208, 209
Grouselle, D.: I *319*
Gros, C.: II *495, 505*
Guéris, J.L.E.: II 416, 417
Guilford, H.: II *171*
Gupta, D.: I *309*
Gyftaki, E.: II *193,* 197
Häberle, M.: II *489,* 494
Hadzilouka-Mantaka, A.: II 361
Hagemann, J.: II *363,* 368
Hall, P.E.: II 3, 36, 38, 54, 56, 74, 76, 79, *149,* 158, 160, 163, 165, 166, 167
Hammerstein, J.: II 467
Hammond, G.L.: I *221*
Hashimoto, T.: I *297*
Hazra, D.K.: I 139, 140, 153, *329,* 345, 346; II 72, 78, 208, 339, 387, 434
Heicke, B.: I 368
Hennemann, G.: II *469*
Hertl, W.: II *369*
Hesch, R.-D.: I 274, 422, 512; II *319,* 339, 340, 360
Hettiaratchi, N.: II *177*
Heynen, G.: II 402, 417, *427,* 434
Hötzinger, H.: I *69*
Hummer, L.: II *391,* 402, 403
Hurn, B.A.L.: II *149,* 158, 166
Ingrand, J.: I *185,* 210, 217; II 167, *349,* 360, 361
Jänne, O.A.: II 256, 271, *285,* 293
Jeffcoate, S.L.: I 514; II *57,* 72, 77, 165, 166, *213,* 223, 224
Jonsson, S.: I *161,* 175
Joustra, M.: I 358; II 224, 308
Joyce, B.G.: I *289,* 294, 295
Jullienne, A.: II *405*
Jungbluth, D.: II *81*
Kaltwasser, J.P.: I 358, *361,* 368, 369, 370
Kanis, J.A.: II *427*
Kerner, W.: I *43*
Keroe, E.A.: I *457*
Kesse-Elias, M.: II *193*
Klingler, W.: II 402
Klootwijk, W.: II *469*
Knorr, D.: I *229*
Kolm, H.P.: I 107, 328
Kopp, H.G.: I *57,* 66, 67
Kruse, V.: II 55, 486
Kuss, E.: I 40, *69,* 89, 107, 154, 295; II 223
Lader, S.R.: I *177,* 183
Lapière, C.M.: II *427*
Lechat, M.: II *341*
Léonard, J.P.: II *379,* 387, 388
Lequin, R.M.: I 39, 139, 274, 346; II 55, 72, 164
Lindner, R.E.: II *369*
Link, M.: I *69*
Llorens-Cortes, C.: II *495*

Long, E.M.R.: I *425*
Lynch, E.P.J.: II *171*, 176
Machione, M.: I *109*
Mäentausta, O.K.: II *285*
Maier, V.: II *489*
Malan, P.G.: I 120, 183, 395, *425*, 434, 435, *437*, 467, 504, 510, 512, 514; II 36, 79, 124, 160, 167
Malkin, A.: I 55, 328, 358, 512; II 74, 165, 197, 368, 378, 388, 467, 494
Mamarbachi, A.M.: II *349*
Mantzos, J.: II *193*
Marbach, P.: I *383*, 395, 396
Marchand, J.: I 358
Marschner, I.: I 175, 210, 380; II *81* 90, *127*
Mason, R.D.: II *369*
Matern, S.: II *273*, 283, 293
Meinhold, H.: I 294; II 223
Milhaud, G.: II *405*
Millet, Y.: II *479*
Minne, H.: II *419*
Morris, Jr., A.C.: I *457*, *517*
Moukhtar, M.S.: II *405*
Moulopoulos, S.: II *193*
Mühlen, A. von zur: I *297*
Munson, P.J.: I *469*; II *105*
Mutz, O.J.: I *457*
Nicolau, G.: II *225*
Niemann, E.: I *347*, 368
Nisula, B.C.: I *133*, 139, 140, 307, 455, 504
Nusgens, B.: II *427*
Odell, W.D.: I *3*, 40, 41, 54, 66, 139, 306, 317, 453
Odstrchel, G.: II 192, *369*, 377, 378
Pachaly, J.: II *257*
Painter, K.: I *211*, 217, 218, 359; II 77, 138, 167
Pakarinen, A.: I *221*
Palmstrøm, S.H.: I *399*
Pasques, D.: II *505*
Peetermans, M.: I *277*
Pellizari, E.: II *225*
Pfau, A.: I 369, 370
Pieroni, R.R.: I *109*
Pineda, G.: I 55; II 339
Piyasena, R.D.: II 176, *177*, 192, 197
Pleau, J.M.: II *505*, 510
Pöckl, E.: II *245*
Pollard, H.: II *495*
Pollow, K.: II *257*
Pradelles, P.: II 476, *495*, 503
Quabbe, H.-J.: I 317
Ranke, B.M.: I *309*, 317, 318
Raue, F.: II *419*, 426
Raulais, D.: II *405*
Read, G.F.: I 66, 218, *289*; II 235, *295*, 298, *309*
Riad-Fahmy, D.: I *289*; II 158, 166, *295*, *309*
Rivaille, P.: II *405*
Rivarola, M.A.: II *225*, 235, 236
Rodbard, D.: I 88, 160, 269, 287, 317, 345, 346, 379, 380, 396, 420, 433, 454, 467, *469*, 504, 505, 510, 511, 513; II *21*, 36, 37, 72, 73, 75, 77, 78, *105*, 124, 125, 138, 163, 166, 340, 376, 377, 378, 387, 418
Röhle, G.: II *81*
Roques, B.P.: II *495*
Rougeot, C.: II *495*
Rougon-Rappuzi, G.: II *479*, 486, 493
Sandel, P.: I *373*, 379, 380
Schellekens, A.: II 494
Schneider, C.: II *363*
Schneider, E.: I *123*
Schmidt-Gollwitzer, M.: II *257*, 271
Scholler, R.: I *91*

Schroeder, R.: II *245*
Schwartz, J.C.: II *495*
Schwarz, I.: I *109*
Schwarz, S.: I 514; II 243
Scriba, P.C.: II *81, 127*
Siddiqui, S.A.: II 72, 340, 361
Siegenthaler, W.: I *57*
Sippell, W.G.: I 228, *229,* 237, 238
Smeaton, T.C.: I 513, II 148, 377
Souli-Tsimili, E.: II 193
Spona, J.: II *245,* 256
Stagg, B.H.: I *347*
Stetten, O. von: I 55, 294
Stolk, J.M.: I *133*
Stolk, M.D.: I *133*
Stonecypher, T.E.: I *211*
Strauss, N.: I *91*
Streibl, W.: II *419*
Sufi, S.: I *437*
Tafurt, C.A.: II *237,* 243
Taliadouros, G.S.: I *133*
Taymans, F.: II *379*
Thalasso, M.: II *199*
Thoma, H.: I *69*
Tixier-Vidal, A.: I *319*
Torten, M.: I 41; II 298, 308, 477
Tovey, K.C.: II *171*
Trautschold, I.: II *141*
Travis, K.: II *369*
Vassilakos, P.: II 467
Veteau, J.P.: I *383*
Vetter, W.: I *57*
Vihko, R.: I *221,* 228, 238; II 235, 283
Viinikka, L.: I *221*
Visser, T.J.: II *469,* 477
Vitins, P.: I *57,* 121, 139; II 223
Vogt, W.: I *373*
Vranckx, R.: I *277,* 287
Wagner, H.: I *383*
Wagner, H.: II *489*
Walker, R.F.: II *309*
Ward, F.B.: II *369*
Weerasekera, D.A.: II *177*
Werder, K. von: I 40, *43,* 55, 121
Werner, E.: I *361*
Wide, L.: I *143,* 153, 273, 306, 358
Wikramanayake, T.W.: II *177*
Wilkins, T.A.: I *379,* 380, *399,* 420, 422, 435, 511; II 197
Williams, E.S.: I *329*
Wilson, D.W.: I 380, 511; II 466
Winder, R.L.: I *399*
Wood, W.G.: I 218; II 75, *81, 127,* 138, 139, 163
Ziegler, R.: II *419*

CORRIGENDA TO VOLUME I

Paper IAEA-SM-220/8 by E. Kuss et al.
Page 69, bottom line

For estradiol-C6-carboxymethoxime *read* estriol-C6-carboxymethoxime

Page 80, line 4 of the figure caption

For $(0.1\ \mathrm{nmol \cdot litre^{-1}})$ *read* $(0.1\ \mu\mathrm{mol \cdot litre^{-1}})$

Page 80 and page 81

The bottom line of page 80 should read as follows:

flow fluorometry) [16] and for binding of ^{3}H-ouabain by anti-ouabain antiserum [14].

The top line of page 81 should read as follows:

A modification of the latter method was used in this paper. It was suggested that

Page 83, beginning of last sentence

For To further study *read* Because of

Paper IAEA-SM-220/36
Page 401

Eq.(4) should read:

$$X = \frac{P}{Z} - \frac{K_2/2}{(1-Z)} - A + \frac{P}{Z}\sqrt{1 - \frac{K_2}{P^2}\left(K_1 - \frac{K_2}{4}\right)\left(\frac{Z}{1-Z}\right)^2}$$

General discussion on data analysis
Page 511, line 9

For $T^2 y = aY$ *read* $\sigma^2 Y = aY$

The following conversion table is provided for the convenience of readers and to encourage the use of SI units.

FACTORS FOR CONVERTING UNITS TO SI SYSTEM EQUIVALENTS *

SI base units are the metre (m), kilogram (kg), second (s), ampere (A), kelvin (K), candela (cd) and mole (mol).
[For further information, see International Standards ISO 1000 (1973), and ISO 31/0 (1974) and its several parts]

Multiply		*by*	*to obtain*
Mass			
pound mass (avoirdupois)	1 lbm	= 4.536×10^{-1}	kg
ounce mass (avoirdupois)	1 ozm	= 2.835×10^{1}	g
ton (long) (= 2240 lbm)	1 ton	= 1.016×10^{3}	kg
ton (short) (= 2000 lbm)	1 short ton	= 9.072×10^{2}	kg
tonne (= metric ton)	1 t	= 1.00×10^{3}	kg
Length			
statute mile	1 mile	= 1.609×10^{0}	km
yard	1 yd	= 9.144×10^{-1}	m
foot	1 ft	= 3.048×10^{-1}	m
inch	1 in	= 2.54×10^{-2}	m
mil (= 10^{-3} in)	1 mil	= 2.54×10^{-2}	mm
Area			
hectare	1 ha	= 1.00×10^{4}	m^2
(statute mile)^2	1 mile^2	= 2.590×10^{0}	km^2
acre	1 acre	= 4.047×10^{3}	m^2
yard^2	1 yd^2	= 8.361×10^{-1}	m^2
foot^2	1 ft^2	= 9.290×10^{-2}	m^2
inch^2	1 in^2	= 6.452×10^{2}	mm^2
Volume			
yard^3	1 yd^3	= 7.646×10^{-1}	m^3
foot^3	1 ft^3	= 2.832×10^{-2}	m^3
inch^3	1 in^3	= 1.639×10^{4}	mm^3
gallon (Brit. or Imp.)	1 gal (Brit)	= 4.546×10^{-3}	m^3
gallon (US liquid)	1 gal (US)	= 3.785×10^{-3}	m^3
litre	1 l	= 1.00×10^{-3}	m^3
Force			
dyne	1 dyn	= 1.00×10^{-5}	N
kilogram force	1 kgf	= 9.807×10^{0}	N
poundal	1 pdl	= 1.383×10^{-1}	N
pound force (avoirdupois)	1 lbf	= 4.448×10^{0}	N
ounce force (avoirdupois)	1 ozf	= 2.780×10^{-1}	N
Power			
British thermal unit/second	1 Btu/s	= 1.054×10^{3}	W
calorie/second	1 cal/s	= 4.184×10^{0}	W
foot-pound force/second	1 ft·lbf/s	= 1.356×10^{0}	W
horsepower (electric)	1 hp	= 7.46×10^{2}	W
horsepower (metric) (= ps)	1 ps	= 7.355×10^{2}	W
horsepower (550 ft·lbf/s)	1 hp	= 7.457×10^{2}	W

* Factors are given exactly or to a maximum of 4 significant figures

Multiply		*by*	*to obtain*
Density			
pound mass/inch^3	1 lbm/in^3	= 2.768 × 10^4	kg/m^3
pound mass/foot^3	1 lbm/ft^3	= 1.602 × 10^1	kg/m^3
Energy			
British thermal unit	1 Btu	= 1.054 × 10^3	J
calorie	1 cal	= 4.184 × 10^0	J
electron-volt	1 eV	≃ 1.602 × 10^{-19}	J
erg	1 erg	= 1.00 × 10^{-7}	J
foot-pound force	1 ft·lbf	= 1.356 × 10^0	J
kilowatt-hour	1 kW·h	= 3.60 × 10^6	J
Pressure			
newtons/metre^2	1 N/m^2	= 1.00	Pa
atmosphere[a]	1 atm	= 1.013 × 10^5	Pa
bar	1 bar	= 1.00 × 10^5	Pa
centimetres of mercury (0°C)	1 cmHg	= 1.333 × 10^3	Pa
dyne/centimetre^2	1 dyn/cm^2	= 1.00 × 10^{-1}	Pa
feet of water (4°C)	1 ftH$_2$O	= 2.989 × 10^3	Pa
inches of mercury (0°C)	1 inHg	= 3.386 × 10^3	Pa
inches of water (4°C)	1 inH$_2$O	= 2.491 × 10^2	Pa
kilogram force/centimetre^2	1 kgf/cm^2	= 9.807 × 10^4	Pa
pound force/foot^2	1 lbf/ft^2	= 4.788 × 10^1	Pa
pound force/inch^2 (= psi)[b]	1 lbf/in^2	= 6.895 × 10^3	Pa
torr (0°C) (= mmHg)	1 torr	= 1.333 × 10^2	Pa
Velocity, acceleration			
inch/second	1 in/s	= 2.54 × 10^1	mm/s
foot/second (= fps)	1 ft/s	= 3.048 × 10^{-1}	m/s
foot/minute	1 ft/min	= 5.08 × 10^{-3}	m/s
mile/hour (= mph)	1 mile/h	= { 4.470 × 10^{-1}	m/s
		1.609 × 10^0	km/h
knot	1 knot	= 1.852 × 10^0	km/h
free fall, standard (= g)		= 9.807 × 10^0	m/s^2
foot/second^2	1 ft/s^2	= 3.048 × 10^{-1}	m/s^2
Temperature, thermal conductivity, energy/area·time			
Fahrenheit, degrees −32	°F − 32	$\frac{5}{9}$	°C
Rankine	°R		K
1 Btu·in/ft^2·s·°F		= 5.189 × 10^2	W/m·K
1 Btu/ft·s·°F		= 6.226 × 10^1	W/m·K
1 cal/cm·s·°C		= 4.184 × 10^2	W/m·K
1 Btu/ft^2·s		= 1.135 × 10^4	W/m^2
1 cal/cm^2·min		= 6.973 × 10^2	W/m^2
Miscellaneous			
foot^3/second	1 ft^3/s	= 2.832 × 10^{-2}	m^3/s
foot^3/minute	1 ft^3/min	= 4.719 × 10^{-4}	m^3/s
rad	rad	= 1.00 × 10^{-2}	J/kg
roentgen	R	= 2.580 × 10^{-4}	C/kg
curie	Ci	= 3.70 × 10^{10}	disintegration/s

[a] atm abs: atmospheres absolute;
atm (g): atmospheres gauge.

[b] lbf/in^2 (g) (= psig): gauge pressure;
lbf/in^2 abs (= psia): absolute pressure.

HOW TO ORDER IAEA PUBLICATIONS

An exclusive sales agent for IAEA publications, to whom all orders and inquiries should be addressed, has been appointed in the following country:

UNITED STATES OF AMERICA	UNIPUB, P.O. Box 433, Murray Hill Station, New York, N.Y. 10016

In the following countries IAEA publications may be purchased from the sales agents or booksellers listed or through your major local booksellers. Payment can be made in local currency or with UNESCO coupons.

ARGENTINA	Comisión Nacional de Energía Atómica, Avenida del Libertador 8250, Buenos Aires
AUSTRALIA	Hunter Publications, 58 A Gipps Street, Collingwood, Victoria 3066
BELGIUM	Service du Courrier de l'UNESCO, 112, Rue du Trône, B-1050 Brussels
C.S.S.R.	S.N.T.L., Spálená 51, CS-113 02 Prague 1
	Alfa, Publishers, Hurbanovo námestie 6, CS-893 31 Bratislava
FRANCE	Office International de Documentation et Librairie, 48, rue Gay-Lussac, F-75240 Paris Cedex 05
HUNGARY	Kultura, Bookimport, P.O. Box 149, H-1389 Budapest
INDIA	Oxford Book and Stationery Co., 17, Park Street, Calcutta, 700016
	Oxford Book and Stationery Co., Scindia House, New Delhi-110001
ISRAEL	Heiliger and Co., 3, Nathan Strauss Str., Jerusalem
ITALY	Libreria Scientifica, Dott. Lucio de Biasio "aeiou", Via Meravigli 16, I-20123 Milan
JAPAN	Maruzen Company, Ltd., P.O. Box 5050, 100-31 Tokyo International
NETHERLANDS	Martinus Nijhoff B.V., Lange Voorhout 9-11, P.O. Box 269, The Hague
PAKISTAN	Mirza Book Agency, 65, Shahrah Quaid-e-Azam, P.O. Box 729, Lahore-3
POLAND	Ars Polona-Ruch, Centrala Handlu Zagranicznego, Krakowskie Przedmiescie 7, PL-00-068 Warsaw
ROMANIA	Ilexim, P.O. Box 136-137, Bucarest
SOUTH AFRICA	Van Schaik's Bookstore (Pty) Ltd., P.O. Box 724, Pretoria 0001
	Universitas Books (Pty) Ltd., P.O. Box 1557, Pretoria 0001
SPAIN	Diaz de Santos, Lagasca 95, Madrid-6
	Diaz de Santos, Balmes 417, Barcelona-6
SWEDEN	AB C.E. Fritzes Kungl. Hovbokhandel, Fredsgatan 2, P.O. Box 16358 S-103 27 Stockholm
UNITED KINGDOM	Her Majesty's Stationery Office, P.O. Box 569, London SE1 9NH
U.S.S.R.	Mezhdunarodnaya Kniga, Smolenskaya-Sennaya 32-34, Moscow G-200
YUGOSLAVIA	Jugoslovenska Knjiga, Terazije 27, POB 36, YU-11001 Belgrade

Orders from countries where sales agents have not yet been appointed and requests for information should be addressed directly to:

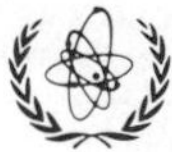

Division of Publications
International Atomic Energy Agency
Kärntner Ring 11, P.O.Box 590, A-1011 Vienna, Austria

78-05965